D1225177

Stacey Tate, M.D.

Cytopathology Review Guide
3rd edition

To my fellow Cytopathology Professors and colleagues in diagnostic cancer and research. Your inspiration has inspired me to strive for what sometimes seems the unimaginable—a solution to this crisis. To my former students, your excitement and thirst for this area of medicine kept me motivated. To my Mother and Father (Carolyn and Ted) thanks for keeping faith in your son throughout the years. And to my wife Liesl and children Caleb, Noah, and Frances, I do this for you and your children.

EBH

E. Blair Holladay, PhD, SCT(ASCP)^CM

Cytopathology Review Guide
3rd edition

Tae W Moon (design/production)
Martin Tyminski (cover)
Joshua Weikersheimer (publishing direction)

Notice

Trade names for equipment and supplies described are included as suggestions only. In no way does their inclusion constitute an endorsement of preference by the Author or the ASCP. The Author and ASCP urge all readers to read and follow all manufacturers' instructions and package insert warnings concerning the proper and safe use of products. The American Society of Clinical Pathology, having exercised appropriate and reasonable effort to research material current as of publication date, does not assume any liability for any loss or damage caused by errors and omissions in this publication. Readers must assume responsibility for complete and thorough research of any hazardous conditions they encounter, as this publication is not intended to be all-inclusive, and recommendations and regulations change over time.

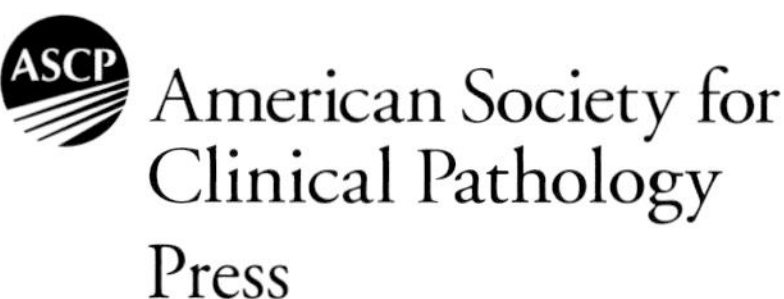

Copyright © 2009 by the American Society for Clinical Pathology. All rights reserved. No part of this publication may be reproduced, stored in a retrieval system, or transmitted in any form or by any means electronic, mechanical, photocopying, recording, or otherwise, without the prior written permission of the publisher.

Printed in Hong Kong

13 12 11 10 09

Contents

Acknowledgments

I'd like to acknowledge several key individuals whose roles in the original development of this text and the third edition have been instrumental in its success. First is Karen Allen, SCT(ASCP), an expert and visionary for the profession, and an individual who served as an author-editor, and also as coauthor for the Liquid-Based Cytology chapter. Secondly, Mac Demay, a former colleague whose myriad textbooks in cytopathology keep this vital field of pathology infused with the most reliable data and techniques for contemporary practice. In the second edition, I also had the privilege of collaborating with a fellow Medical University of South Carolina colleague, Laurine Charles, MHS, MT(ASCP)SBB, in the Laboratory Management and Administration chapter. Lastly, the staff of the ASCP, whose focus on excellence helped keep me focused and aligned throughout the vicissitudes of this important endeavor. God bless you all.

Preface

Since the first edition of Cytopathology Review Guide, I have been pleased that so many have used this textbook as a litmus test for their board examinations, cytotechnology generalist and specialist exams, as well as cytopathology residents and fellows. New innovative technologies in liquid-based preparation, computer-assisted diagnostics, and molecular markers for diagnostic cytopathology have made significant strides since the original publication of this textbook. It is imperative that we serve the needs of our patients by exploring each of these diagnostic venues to their fullest capacity, but as scientists, also keeping in mind that we must carefully scrutinize each of these advancements in technology by scientifically validating their utility for our profession and the field of cytopathology. In addition, quality assurance must be constantly monitored in the cytopathology laboratory in order for it to remain effective and for its continued evolution. For these and many other reasons, the third edition includes one additional chapter (Bethesda System of Classification and 2006 Consensus Guidelines for the Management of Women with Abnormal Cervical Cancer Screening Tests), two enhanced chapters (Liquid-based Cytology and Molecular Diagnostics and Special Stains) and frequent updates throughout the individual chapters. Each of these areas has had significant impact and altered the profession over the past 6 years since the previous edition. As the threads of innovation are woven into the fabric of our profession, rest assured they will continue to be found on current and future qualifying examinations that measure competence for the practice of cytopathology. I hope this text assists you with your board preparations. Best of luck.

E. Blair Holladay, PhD, SCT(ASCP)^CM^

Chicago, IL   September 2008

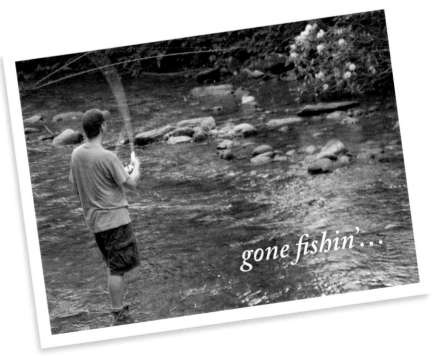

Chapter 1

Basic Science

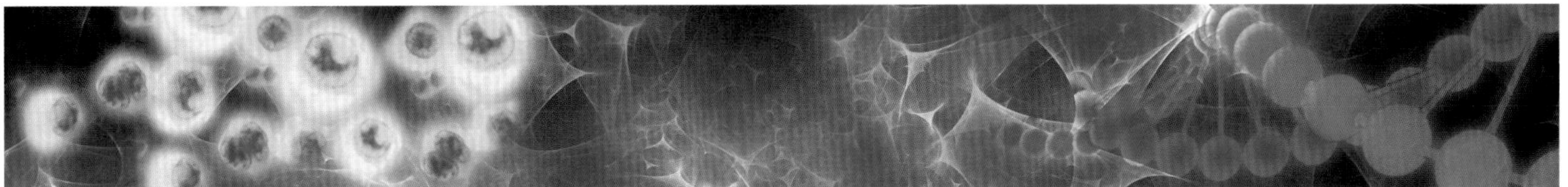

1. **A type of junctional complex focally distributed along the plasma membrane of epithelial cells (aka "spot welds") are:**

   A. gap junctions
   B. zonula occludens
   C. microfilaments
   D. macula adherens

2. **Which cell marker is useful in identifying Reed-Sternberg cells?**

   A. Leu-7
   B. B-72.3
   C. Leu-M1
   D. HMB-45

3. **Intranuclear cytoplasmic invaginations:**

   A. lie free in the nucleoplasm
   B. are pseudoinclusions
   C. stain magenta with the Pap stain
   D. are poorly delineated nonmembranous structures

4. **Granulomatous inflammation is histologically composed of:**

   A. lymphocytes, epithelioid histiocytes, multinucleated histiocytes
   B. neutrophils, eosinophils, fibroblasts
   C. neutrophils, red blood cells, diathesis
   D. basophils

5. **What type of cell contains abundant lysosomes?**

   A. Kupffer
   B. squamous
   C. pneumocyte type I
   D. columnar

6. **Which of the following represents a malignancy in which karyotyping might be useful?**

   A. chronic granulocytic leukemia
   B. esophageal carcinoma
   C. squamous carcinoma
   D. cervical carcinoma

7. **What tumor marker is expressed in germ cell tumors of the testes?**

   A. carcinoembryonic antigen
   B. human chorionic gonadotropin
   C. calcitonin
   D. acid phosphatase

8. **What is the most useful criterion for differentiating normal and malignant cells?**

   A. nuclear sizes are enlarged in malignancies but not in benignities
   B. coarsely granular irregularly distributed chromatin is associated with malignancies but not with benignities
   C. multinucleation is common in malignancies but not with benignities
   D. malignancies generally possess bipolar mitoses whereas benignities possess tetrapolar mitoses

9. **Which of the following lesions has documented cytogenetic abnormalities involving chromosomal changes?**

A. squamous cell carcinoma of the cervix
B. Hürthle cell carcinoma of the thyroid
C. meningioma
D. fibroadenoma of the breast

10. **Which of the following is not considered a true fungus?**

A. *Blastomyces dermatitidis*
B. *Nocardia asteroides*
C. *Cryptococcus neoformans*
D. *Histoplasma capsulatum*

11. **What tumor marker is expressed in hepatocellular carcinoma?**

A. acid phosphatase
B. alpha-fetoprotein
C. estrogen receptor
D. carcinoembryonic antigen

12. **What tumor marker is expressed within medullary carcinoma of the thyroid?**

A. acid phosphatase
B. carcinoembryonic antigen
C. alpha-fetoprotein
D. calcitonin

13. **An indication of good cellular activity prior to specimen collection is:**

A. cellular membrane integrity
B. cytolysis
C. cellular eosinophilia
D. hydrolysis

14. **What phase of the cell cycle has tetraploid DNA?**

A. G/1
B. G/2
C. G/0
D. G/3

15. **What tumor marker is expressed in colonic adenocarcinoma?**

A. alpha-fetoprotein
B. carcinoembryonic antigen
C. calcitonin
D. acid phosphatase

16. **Which of the following cells possess abundant rough endoplasmic reticulum?**

A. plasma cells
B. poorly differentiated squamous cell carcinoma
C. stem cells
D. lymphoblasts

17. **Sarcomas most frequently metastasize via the:**

A. lymphatic channels
B. vascular channels
C. follicular centers
D. nervous tissues

18. **The cellular organelle involved in selective absorption and surface area capacity is the:**

A. endoplasmic reticulum
B. desmosome
C. microtubule
D. microvilli

19. **What structures aid in anchoring cilia?**

A. microvilli
B. flagella
C. basal bodies
D. tonofilaments

20. **Dense core secretory granules containing polypeptide hormones as demonstrated by electron microscopy and special stains indicate:**

A. keratin differentiation
B. mucin production
C. neuroendocrine differentiation
D. hemosiderin pigment

21. **One of the major functions/roles of the plasma membrane is:**

A. to facilitate active transport across a semipermeable membrane
B. to synthesize ribosomal RNA
C. to provide antibody carrying capacity
D. to synthesize DNA

22. **In light microscopy, the breaking up of light waves as they pass by an obstruction is known as:**

A. aperture
B. diffraction
C. resolution
D. magnification

23. **The composition of chromatin includes:**

A. DNA, histones, and nonhistone proteins
B. tonofibrils
C. intermediate filaments
D. lipids, proteins, and carbohydrates

24. **Aneuploid DNA is never found in:**

A. malignant cells
B. normal cells
C. anaplastic cells
D. premalignant cells

25. **An explanation for transformation of a malignant tumor into a benign neoplasm may be:**

A. chemotherapy
B. radiation therapy
C. maturation of an immature tumor
D. small doses of promoting agents

26. **In what syndrome does chromosomal nondisjunction occur?**

A. Klinefelter
B. Chiari-Frommel
C. Stein-Leventhal
D. Forbes-Albright

27. **Neoplastic cells are most sensitive to radiation as they approach which stage of the cell cycle?**

A. G/1
B. S
C. G/2
D. G/0

28. **A malignancy derived from an ectodermal germ tissue is a (an):**

A. osteosarcoma
B. carcinoma
C. lymphoma
D. leukemia

29. **Examples of intermediate filaments found within cells include:**

A. hemosiderin: mesenchymal cells
B. cytokeratin: squamous cells
C. actin: skeletal muscle cells
D. myosin: smooth muscle cells

30. **Which stage of oncogenesis is considered permanent and irreversible?**

A. initiation
B. development
C. promotion
D. retrogression

Basic Science *Answer Key*

1. **D macula adherens**

The three junctional complexes include the occludens (tight junctions which fuse the cell membranes), adherens (nonfusing, allowing materials to pass between the cells, eg, desmosome), and the gap junction (membranes that are very close but separated by small plates, allowing for intercellular communication).

DeMay RM, The Art & Science of Cytopathology.
The cell membrane, p. 51.

2. **C Leu-M1**

Leu-M1 (CD15) may also be used as a marker for epithelial tumors and dermatofibroma.

DeMay RM, The Art & Science of Cytopathology.
Other cell markers, p. 18.

3. **B are pseudoinclusions**

This intranuclear cytoplasmic inclusion type is the most common, a result of a portion of the cytoplasm pushing into the nucleus, thus appearing as "intranuclear." These inclusions, however, actually remain outside of the nucleus and do not represent true intranuclear inclusions.

DeMay RM, The Art & Science of Cytopathology.
The nucleus, p. 43.

4. **A lymphocytes, epithelioid histiocytes, multinucleated histiocytes**

Granulomatous inflammation may be secondary to fungal diseases, tuberculosis, sarcoidosis, as well as carcinomas (lymphomas, seminomas).

DeMay RM, The Art & Science of Cytopathology.
Other manifestations of inflammation, p. 114.

5. **A Kupffer**

Kupffer cells are liver macrophages or phagocytes that contain abundant lysosomes, cellular organelles consisting of hydrolytic enzymes used to digest antigenic substances or to autolyse cellular organelles during necrobiosis.

DeMay RM, The Art & Science of Cytopathology.
The cytoplasm, p. 47.

6. **A chronic granulocytic leukemia**

Chronic granulocytic (myelogenous) leukemia will reveal a translocation between chromosome numbers 22 and 9. Other malignancies with proven genetic abnormalities include meningioma (loss of number 22 chromosome) and retinoblastoma (deletion of the long arm of chromosome 13).

DeMay RM, The Art & Science of Cytopathology.
The nucleus, p. 42.

7. **B human chorionic gonadotropin**

Placental lesions and germ cell tumors of the ovary and testes express human chorionic gonadotropin.

DeMay RM, The Art & Science of Cytopathology.
Hormones, p. 18.

8. **B coarsely granular irregularly distributed chromatin is associated with malignancies but not with benignities**

The chromatin pattern found within nuclei of benign cells is usually finely granular and regularly distributed, whereas that associated with malignancies is often fine to coarse and irregularly distributed.

DeMay RM, The Art & Science of Cytopathology.
Summary of diagnostic features of malignancy, p. 52.

9. **C meningioma**

See 6 for explanation. In addition to malignant lesions, benign tumors including pleomorphic adenoma may present with translocations involving chromosomal numbers 8, 12, or 3. Other benign lesions that involve chromosomal changes include lipoma, leiomyoma, villous adenomas involving the colon, and meningioma.

DeMay RM, The Art & Science of Cytopathology.
Meningioma, p. 1190.

10. **B *Nocardia asteroides***

Nocardia asteroides is a gram-positive, acid-fast bacterium that may cytologically mimic a fungal disease due to its branching hyphae.

DeMay RM, The Art & Science of Cytopathology.
Bacteria, p. 55.

11. **B alpha-fetoprotein**

Hepatocellular carcinomas and testicular and ovarian germ cell tumors express alpha-fetoprotein.

DeMay RM, The Art & Science of Cytopathology.
Oncofetal antigens, p. 18.

12. **D calcitonin**

Calcitonin is expressed within medullary carcinomas of the thyroid, but can be positive in neoplasms from the lung, colon, and pancreas.

DeMay RM, The Art & Science of Cytopathology.
Hormones, p. 18.

13. **A cellular membrane integrity**

Well-preserved nuclear and cytoplasmic structures are helpful in establishing cell life before fixation. The presence of cilia indicates a viable and metabolically active cell before its forcible removal by instrumentation.

DeMay RM, The Art & Science of Cytopathology.
The cell membrane, p. 49.

14. **B G/2**

DNA synthesis is the doubling of 46 chromosomes to 92. Mitosis is then required to restore the cell to its original diploid state. The end of the DNA synthesis phase and the post-synthesis gap (G/2) are the only phases of the cell cycle in which tetraploid DNA exists.

DeMay RM, The Art & Science of Cytopathology.
The nucleus, p. 43.

15. **B carcinoembryonic antigen**

Carcinoembryonic antigen (CEA) is expressed in tumors arising from the gastrointestinal tract and lung.

DeMay RM, The Art & Science of Cytopathology.
Oncofetal antigens, p. 18.

16. **A plasma cells**

Rough endoplasmic reticulum (RER) is abundant in many cells that synthesize proteins, such as plasma cells, pancreatic acinar cells, fibroblasts, and hepatocytes. The endoplasmic membrane appears rough due to the presence of abundant ribosomes (protein-producing organelles) attached or "studded" to its surface. Ribosomes form proteins by capturing amino acids from the cytoplasm that are labeled with transfer RNA and ultimately binding the amino acids together in a sequence that is specified by messenger RNA.

DeMay RM, The Art & Science of Cytopathology.
The cytoplasm, pp. 45–46.

17. **B vascular channels**

Sarcomas most often metastasize via the blood vessels, while carcinomas usually metastasize by way of the lymphatic channels.

18. **D microvilli**

These finger-like projections from the cell membrane serve to increase the surface area of the cells and transport amino acids.

DeMay RM, The Art & Science of Cytopathology.
The cytoplasm, p. 50.

19. **C basal bodies**

Cilia, which function to move material in a synchronous motion, are anchored within the portion of the plasma membrane ultrastructurally composed of dense granules, referred to as the basal body or terminal plate.

DeMay RM, The Art & Science of Cytopathology.
The cytoplasm, p. 50.

20. **C neuroendocrine differentiation**

These secretory granules as demonstrated by electron microscopy are helpful in the identification of neuroendocrine processes, such as small cell squamous carcinoma. Overall, demonstration of secretory granules may prove useful in determining the histogenesis of the cell.

DeMay RM, The Art & Science of Cytopathology.
The cytoplasm, p. 46.

21. **A to facilitate active transport across a semipermeable membrane**

The plasma membrane serves as a selective barrier between the cell's interior and the environment. It is a lipid bilayer with associated intrinsically and extrinsically located hydrophilic and hydrophobic globular proteins.

DeMay RM, The Art & Science of Cytopathology.
The cell membrane, pp. 49–51.

22. **B diffraction**

DeMay eloquently defines diffraction as, "the breaking up of (light) waves as they pass by an obstruction, ie, a hole or aperture, or around objects…diffraction makes an exact point-to-point correspondence between the object and the image possible."

DeMay RM, The Art & Science of Cytopathology.
Lenses, p. 4.

23. **A DNA, histones, and nonhistone proteins**

Chromatin is composed of nucleic acids (DNA), basic nucleoproteins (histones), and acidic nonhistone proteins. In its active state it is referred to as euchromatin while in its inactive state it is called heterchromatin; basic nucleoproteins (histones), and acidic nonhistone proteins.

DeMay RM, The Art & Science of Cytopathology.
The nucleus, p. 41.

24. **B normal cells**

An aberration from the normal number of genes or chromosomes (n = 46, 2N) which compose the DNA of a particular cell is considered aneuploid if the DNA is greater than 2N and results in karyotypic instability (3N, 5N, 7N etc.). Aneuploid DNA is commonly found within anaplastic tumor cells and can be seen in some premalignant processes. Normal cells must be diploid (2N) or have even multiples of the diploid state.

DeMay RM, The Art & Science of Cytopathology.
The nucleus, pp. 42–43.

25. **C maturation of an immature tumor**

Maturation of an immature tumor such as neuroblastoma into a benign ganglioneuroma is an example of malignant reversion. Other malignancies which have been reported to spontaneously regress include kidney carcinoma, melanoma, and choriocarcinoma.

26. **A Klinefelter**

Klinefelter syndrome is a sex chromosome abnormality found in males in which the chromatids fail to separate during meiosis, resulting in a 47XXY karyotype. Turner syndrome, another example of sex chromosome nondisjunction, is found in females where the sperm donates an X chromosome to an ovum void of a donor sex chromosome, resulting in 45XO. Male breast cancer is common in men with Klinefelter syndrome.

DeMay RM, The Art & Science of Cytopathology.
Cancer of the male breast, pp. 890–891.

27. **B S**

As cells approach DNA synthesis (S), they are most sensitive to radiation. However, after cells enter the synthesis phase, they are resistant to radiation.

DeMay RM, The Art & Science of Cytopathology.
Radiation cytology, p. 118.

28. **B carcinoma**

In contrast, mesodermal and endodermal tumors are referred to as sarcomas.

29. **B cytokeratin: squamous cells**

Keratin (both acidic and neutral or basic) intermediate filaments are contained within epithelial cells, vimentin is found within mesenchymal, glial, and rare epithelial cells, and desmin is found within muscle tissue. Neurofilaments and glial fibrillary proteins are contained within neurons and their supportive glial cells, respectively.

DeMay RM, The Art & Science of Cytopathology.
The cytoplasm, p. 48.

30. **A initiation**

Initiation is the primary step in the natural history of neoplasia. This phase of carcinogenesis fixes the DNA, resulting in a permanent, irreversible alteration. Promotion, the second phase, is dependent upon the number of initiated cells; therefore, it is dose-dependent. Progression to malignancy is the result of initiation and promotion and signifies the move of this cell towards aneuploidy.

Chapter 2

Female Reproductive Tract

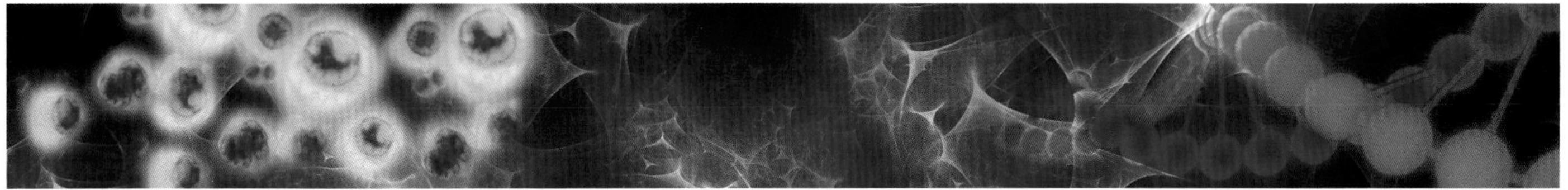

1. **The portion of the menstrual cycle that is constant is:**

   A. follicular phase
   B. secretory
   C. ovulation
   D. proliferative

2. **Which of the following is considered a pituitary gonadotropin?**

   A. luteinizing hormone
   B. estrogen
   C. androgen
   D. glucocorticoid

3. **Cells normally found in the endocervical canal that resemble histiocytes, possess uniform nuclei with fine, regular chromatin distribution, and have discretely vacuolated but poorly defined cytoplasm are:**

   A. reserve cells
   B. cells from microglandular hyperplasia
   C. metaplastic cells
   D. oxyphilic cells

4. **LH peaks at which day of the menstrual cycle?**

   A. 28
   B. 5
   C. 14
   D. 1

5. **The presence of mitotic figures indicates:**

   A. the possibility of neoplasia
   B. reparative/regenerative processes
   C. a current HPV infection
   D. no pathologic information

6. **An example of a protective reaction of the uterine cervix is:**

   A. hyperkeratosis
   B. pemphigus
   C. folic acid deficiency
   D. chronic lymphocytic cervicitis

7. **Which of the following may be associated with a threatened abortion?**

   A. increase in desquamation and cytolysis
   B. boat-shaped intermediate cells
   C. large cells with multiple, tightly clustered nuclei
   D. intermediate cell maturation

8. **A vaginal smear from a 23-year-old woman contains ciliated glandular cells, metaplastic epithelial cells, and mixed mature squamous cells in the presence of a moderate inflammatory exudate. The appropriate diagnosis is:**

   A. negative for squamous intraepithelial lesion
   B. negative for squamous intraepithelial lesion, limited by inflammation
   C. vaginal adenosis
   D. a diagnosis cannot be rendered based on the above cytologic findings

9. **Estrogen reaches its greatest concentration in the bloodstream at which day of the menstrual cycle?**

A. 1
B. 14
C. 21
D. 28

10. **A masculinizing tumor of the ovary is:**

A. Sertoli-Leydig cell tumors
B. Brenner tumor
C. gynandroblastoma
D. endodermal sinus

11. **In order for menses to occur, which structure in the ovary must degenerate?**

A. corpus luteum
B. tunica albuginea
C. Call-Exner bodies
D. medulla

12. **The ratio of estrogen to follicle stimulating hormone in the bloodstream is:**

A. proportional
B. inverse
C. unrelated
D. these two hormones are never found together

13. **Microglandular hyperplasia is most often associated with:**

A. squamous dysplasia
B. broad spectrum antibiotics
C. oral contraceptives
D. chronic lymphocytic cervicitis

14. **Which phase of the menstrual cycle directly follows a degenerated corpus albicans?**

A. menses
B. follicular
C. secretory
D. ovulation

15. **Which pituitary hormone stimulates the primordial follicles of the ovary to grow?**

A. LH
B. FSH
C. estrogen
D. progesterone

16. **A 22-year-old woman presents with primary amenorrhea. Upon clinical investigation, she was found to have a low hairline, large numbers of pigmented nevi, polydactyly, and a short webbing of the neck. A smear from the lateral vaginal wall was collected for hormonal analysis. What maturation index is compatible?**

A. 0/0/100
B. 0/50/50
C. 0/100/0
D. 100/0/0

17. **What may explain why some postmenopausal women have an intermediate cell maturation while others will have deep atrophy?**

A. increased vascularization near the basal lamina in women with intermediate cell atrophy
B. women with deep atrophy are most likely to have undergone castration early in their reproductive years
C. weak adrenal hormonal production in those patients with intermediate cell maturation
D. weak ovarian stromal hormonal production in those patients with intermediate cell maturation

18. **A 64-year-old asymptomatic woman presents for a routine Papanicolaou smear. A vaginal smear is performed for hormonal analysis. Which of the following maturation indices are feasible given this patient's age?**

A. 0/0/100
B. 75/25/0
C. 0/25/75
D. 0/10/90

19. **Which of the following are contraindications for performing hormonal analyses?**

A. mature cycling female
B. correlation of follicular persistency
C. *Trichomonas vaginalis* infection
D. correlation of Turner syndrome

20. A 52-year-old woman with advanced cirrhosis of the liver is likely to show:

A. increased estrogenic effect
B. decreased estrogenic effect
C. increased progesterone effect
D. decreased progesterone effect

21. A patient with secondary amenorrhea would have a maturation index of:

A. 100/0/0
B. 0/100/0
C. 0/0/100
D. cannot be determined based on the above clinical information

22. The significance of hyperkeratosis and/or parakeratosis is that they:

A. may overlie and/or be associated with a possible lesion
B. are usually associated with a high-grade squamous intraepithelial lesion
C. are predictive of reparative/regenerative processes
D. are of no significance

23. Severe hypothyroidism may be represented by which of the following maturation indices?

A. 0/100/0
B. 0/0/100
C. 0/50/50
D. 75/25/0

24. The administration of tamoxifen citrate in postmenopausal breast cancer patients:

A. increases cellular maturation
B. has no effect on cellular maturation
C. promotes formation of navicular-like cells
D. decreases cellular maturation

25. Cells with spine-like processes protruding from the cytoplasmic membrane (spider cells), occurring singularly and rarely in sheets, with smooth nuclear margins found proximal to the endocervical canal are diagnostic of:

A. adenocarcinoma in situ, endocervix
B. endocervical columnar cells
C. immature metaplastic cells
D. mature metaplastic cells

26. *Torulopsis glabrata* is similar in morphologic appearance to *Candida albicans* with the exception that:

A. *Torulopsis glabrata* lacks hyphae
B. *Candida albicans* has true mycelium
C. *Torulopsis glabrata* contains sulfur granules
D. *Torulopsis glabrata* reproduces by binary fission

27. An abortive attempt at keratinization is termed:

A. hyperkeratosis
B. reserve cell hyperplasia
C. parakeratosis
D. Arias-Stella reaction

28. What is the effect of progesterone therapy upon an estrogen-primed epithelium?

A. no change
B. decreased maturation to the intermediate cell level
C. decreased maturation to the deep parabasal cell level
D. increased maturation to a thick superficial cell level

29. A 42-year-old woman suffers from menometrorrhagia of 3 months' duration following an automobile accident involving head injury.What might explain her condition?

A. pituitary hypogonadism
B. glioblastoma multiforme
C. pseudocyesis
D. Sertoli-Leydig cell tumors

30. Useful criteria to employ in the differential diagnosis between "atypical" reparative processes and nonkeratinizing squamous cell carcinoma include:

A. presence of single cells in repair
B. presence of nucleoli in carcinoma
C. coarse, irregular chromatin in carcinoma
D. nuclear polarity in carcinoma

31. A Papanicolaou smear reveals pools of mature and immature lymphocytes found in the company of tingible body macrophages. The diagnosis is consistent with:

A. lymphocytic leukemia
B. lymphoblastic lymphoma
C. follicular cervicitis
D. subacute inflammation

32. The smear pattern for a patient with Stein-Leventhal syndrome would reveal:

A. superficial predominance, intermediate cells without folding or clustering
B. parabasal cells
C. mixed parabasal and intermediate cells
D. intermediate cell predominance with excessive Döderlein cytolysis

33. A 32-year-old patient presents with severe bullous dermatitis and vulvar itching. A vulval smear revealed numerous parabasal squamous cells in sheets with large oval nuclei, perinuclear halos, regular-to-coarse chromatin, and prominent nucleoli. The most likely diagnosis is:

A. well-differentiated squamous cell carcinoma
B. poorly differentiated squamous cell carcinoma
C. *Haemophilus ducreyi*
D. pemphigus vulgaris

34. Which pregnancy-related deficiency produces multinucleated giant cells with relatively normal nuclear-to-cytoplasmic ratios?

A. folic acid
B. benzopyrene
C. birth control pills
D. podophyllin

35. Cells resembling metaplastic cells arranged in sheets, exhibiting cytoplasmic streaming, moderate anisocytosis, fine to coarse chromatin, and prominent macronucleoli are haphazardly scattered throughout a cervical/endocervical smear. The diagnosis is consistent with:

A. poorly differentiated squamous cell carcinoma
B. high-grade squamous intraepithelial neoplasia
C. koilocytic changes associated with HPV infection
D. reparative/regenerative process

36. The cellular effects of radiation include:

A. hyperchromasia, high N/C ratio
B. macrocytic changes, polychromasia
C. intranuclear cytoplasmic inclusions
D. eosinophilic intranuclear inclusions and polymorphonuclear neutrophils

37. Which of the ovarian tumors frequently present with bilateral involvement?

A. serous
B. mucinous
C. endometrioid
D. Sertoli-Leydig cell

38. The Schiller test is performed to identify:

A. glycogenated areas that stain with iodine
B. nonglycogenated areas that stain with methylene blue
C. glycogenated areas that do not stain with methylene blue
D. nonglycogenated areas that do not stain with iodine

39. What microorganism maintains the vaginal pH?

A. *Lactobacillus acidophilus*
B. *Leptothrix*
C. *Bacterionema* sp.
D. staphylococci

40. It has been determined that squamous cell carcinoma of the uterine cervix is associated with:

A. expression of HPV 6, 11 viral DNA
B. expression of HPV 6, 16 viral DNA
C. expression of HPV 16, 18 viral DNA
D. antibody titer against episomal viral DNA

41. **The most common clinical term that describes a benign ovarian tumor is:**

A. embryonal teratoma
B. mature cystic teratoma
C. Krukenberg tumor
D. gynandroblastoma

42. **The Clinical Laboratory Improvement Amendments of 1988 (CLIA '88) implement all of the following conditions except:**

A. all cases of atypical squamous cells of undetermined significance (ASC-US) are considered part of the 5-year retrospective review process
B. a diagnosis of a low-grade squamous intraepithelial lesion mandates follow-up of the patient
C. daily records of the number of slides reviewed as well as the amount of time spent reviewing the slides must be kept on each cytotechnologist
D. board-certified pathologists may not perform primary review of more than 100 slides in any 24-hour period

43. **Which of these diagnostic entities is associated with hyperestrinism and endometrial adenocarcinoma?**

A. endometrial polyps
B. HPV
C. endometrial hyperplasia
D. atypical squamous metaplasia

44. **Abnormal cells originating from endocervical adenocarcinoma may be distinguished from cells originating from endometrial adenocarcinoma by:**

A. presence of granular cytoplasm and columnar cellular shape
B. frothy, delicate cytoplasm and round cellular shapes
C. nucleoli and polymorphonuclear neutrophilic cannibalism
D. diathesis background with 3-D hyperchromatic cell groupings

45. **If a uterine cancer were described as a heterologous mixed müllerian tumor it could be:**

A. endometrial carcinoma only
B. endometrial carcinoma + osteosarcoma
C. endometrial sarcoma only
D. endometrial carcinoma + leiomyosarcoma

46. **The clinical utility of performing molecular HPV testing and the use of cervicography are considered:**

A. specific for determining the likelihood of progression of any one lesion
B. adjunctive methods that currently lack the specificity needed to determine the progression rate of any one lesion
C. important in determining the progression rate for patients with HPV
D. basically equal in comparison

47. **The vagina, uterus, and ovaries are formed embryologically from which germ cell layer(s)?**

A. ectoderm
B. mesoderm
C. endoderm
D. ectoderm and mesoderm

48. **Large numbers of small-to-medium, round, single cells exhibiting hyperchromasia and finely granular, evenly distributed nucleus comprising most of the cellular area is most suggestive of:**

A. spider cells
B. nonkeratinizing dysplasia, severe (high-grade squamous intraepithelial lesion)
C. atypical squamous cells of undetermined significance
D. nonkeratinizing dysplasia, mild (low-grade squamous intraepithelial lesion)

49. **Which of the following variants of endometrial adenocarcinoma are aggressive, arise in atrophic endometrium of older postmenopausal women, and are unrelated to hyperplastic precursor lesions?**

A. well-differentiated type
B. poorly differentiated type
C. secretory type
D. mucinous type

50. **Which characteristic serves as the most important hallmark of ectocervical squamous lesions?**

A. opaque nuclei
B. pleomorphism
C. orangeophilic/amphophilic staining
D. sheets of cells

51. An in situ carcinoma of the vulva is termed:

A. Nabothian cyst
B. Paget disease
C. Gartner disease
D. Bowen disease

52. A benign proliferation of undifferentiated cells under endocervical-type glandular epithelium is termed:

A. reserve cell hyperplasia
B. cervical hypertrophy
C. atrophy
D. neoplasia

53. The histologic presentation of condyloma of the cervix includes:

A. abnormal cells comprising 90% of the epithelial thickness
B. submucosal dyskeratosis
C. smudged nuclear features and cave-like perinuclear vacuoles
D. mononuclear hypochromatic cells

54. Remnants of the mesonephric system found in the lateral vaginal wall are termed:

A. Gartner cysts
B. cloacal fold
C. Bartholin ducts
D. Skene glands

55. The correct order for chromatin degeneration associated with cell death is:

A. karyolysis, pyknosis, karyorrhexis
B. karyorrhexis, cytolysis, pyknosis
C. pyknosis, karyorrhexis, karyolysis
D. karyorrhexis, pyknosis, karyolysis

56. Which of the human papilloma virus (HPV) types have episomal replication and are considered "low risk"?

A. HPV 6, HPV 16
B. HPV 6, HPV 11
C. HPV 11, HPV 16
D. HPV 16, HPV 18

57. Which cytomorphologic criteria are essential when establishing a diagnosis of a reparative process over a malignant one?

A. anisonucleosis, hyperchromasia
B. hyperchromasia, single cells
C. anisonucleosis, syncytial fragments
D. normochromasia, cytoplasmic streaming

58. Which clinical finding would place the patient at risk for infection by *Candida* species?

A. follicular phase of the menstrual cycle
B. diabetes mellitus
C. intrauterine devices
D. antibodies against cytomegalovirus

59. During the embryological development of a female, if the müllerian ducts fail to fuse, the end result may be a (an):

A. pseudohermaphroditic female
B. bicornate uterus
C. improper ovarian ligament support
D. Wolffian duct continuation

60. A 24-year-old woman presented to the clinician with hyperemic, petechial hemorrhages of the vaginal walls and fornices. Which of the following may be responsible for the clinical findings?

A. a yeast infection
B. *Trichomonas vaginalis* infection
C. Bowen disease
D. condyloma acuminata

61. Puerperal endometritis may present cytologically as:

A. reactive trophoblasts
B. psammoma bodies
C. Curshmann spirals
D. folate changes

62. **Cervical smears containing irregular spherical structures that take on a radiated appearance and are associated with hemorrhagic infarcts are:**

A. cockleburs
B. brown artifact ("cornflaking")
C. impossible to identify without special stains
D. hematoidin crystals

63. **Which of the following occurs due to the estrogenic effect upon normal squamous epithelium during the follicular phase of the menstrual cycle?**

A. increased deposition of glycogen in the cytoplasm
B. folding and clustering of intermediate cells
C. desquamation of squamous cells
D. increased Döderlein cytolysis

64. **A morphologic change seen in late secretory phase and pregnancy is:**

A. an increase in the nuclear to cytoplasmic ratio
B. glycogenated navicular cells
C. an increase in cellular eosinophilia
D. the presence of syncytiotrophoblasts

65. **A 42-year-old nulliparous woman complaining of irregular menses frequently sheds fragments of normal endometrium in the mid-luteal phase of her menstrual cycle. Further clinical evaluation might suggest:**

A. dilatation and curettage to rule out hyperplasia of the endometrium
B. conization for endometriosis
C. hysterectomy
D. further evaluation not necessary, endometrial cells are normally found in mid-luteal phase

66. **Radiated crystalline arrays lacking central filaments, found in late pregnancy, formed from stagnating products of degenerated cells and composed of nonimmune glycoprotein, lipid, and calcium are diagnostic of:**

A *Actinomyces* sp.
B. hematoidin crystals
C. cockleburs
D. corpora amylacea

67. **Which clinical feature is associated with an increased risk for well-differentiated endometrial cancer?**

A. a history of opposed estrogen
B. nulliparous
C. early menopause
D. increased number of sexual partners

68. **What has been hypothesized to promote squamous cell carcinoma of the uterine cervix?**

A. oncogene activation secondary to HPV
B. increased progesterone stimulation
C. episomal viral types
D. HPV-induced exophytic lesions

69. **Human chorionic gonadotropin is:**

A. produced by the corpus luteum in early pregnancy
B. found during the third trimester of pregnancy only
C. considered important in menstruation
D. produced by the graafian follicle in early pregnancy

70. **Which embryological duct system develops internal genitalia in the female?**

A. Wolffian
B. mesonephric
C. paramesonephric
D. mesentery

71. **Multinucleated cells with cytoplasmic tails and tightly packed centrally located small hyperchromatic nuclei found in pregnancy are diagnostic of:**

A. cytotrophoblasts
B. endometrial adenocarcinoma
C. syncytiotrophoblasts
D. choriocarcinoma

72. **Of the following tissues, which is considered the most radiosensitive?**

A. muscle
B. brain
C. uterus
D. gastrointestinal epithelium

73. **Which finding is associated with the diagnosis of well-differentiated endometrial adenocarcinoma?**

A. basophilic watery diathesis
B. coarsely granular necrotic diathesis
C. sheets of neoplastic cells
D. papillary groups with associated psammoma bodies

74. **Which condition is associated with the development of endometrial adenocarcinoma?**

A. multiparity
B. exposure to the human papillomavirus
C. granulosa-theca cell tumor
D. exposure to cytomegalovirus

75. **The most common metastatic tumor found in Papanicolaou smears is:**

A. ovarian
B. fallopian tube
C. breast
D. colon

76. **A 51-year-old patient with a history of normal Papanicolaou smears has a large population of malignant cells with hyperchromatic fine, irregular chromatin patterns, seen in sheets and single cells. Cytoplasmic configurations resemble a columnar formation. Endocervical curettings revealed no pathologic abnormality. In determining the origin of these cells, you might consider:**

A. colon for malignancy
B. vagina for malignancy
C. breast for malignancy
D. lung for malignancy

77. **A cervical/endocervical sample from a 38-year-old patient reveals large groups of cells in columnar formation with hyperchromatic nuclei and irregular chromatin. The cells have anisocytosis with intact cilia. These cells represent:**

A. adenocarcinoma in situ, endocervix
B. well-differentiated adenocarcinoma, endocervix
C. well-differentiated adenocarcinoma, colon
D. tubal metaplasia

78. **Which malignancy is often associated with psammoma bodies?**

A. mucinous cystadenocarcinoma, ovarian primary
B. serous adenocarcinoma, ovarian
C. adenocarcinoma, colon
D. endocervical adenocarcinoma

79. **Cells exhibiting multiple frond-like projections arranged in a papillary group with hyperchromatic, fine, irregular chromatin patterns and "bird's eye" macronucleoli were observed in a cervical/endocervical smear from a 40-year-old patient. The background was clean with a mild inflammatory component. Endocervical curetting was negative. The origin of the cells suggests:**

A. vagina
B. fallopian tube
C. ovary
D. colon

80. **The cytoplasm of cells from vulvar intraepithelial neoplasia grade 3 (VIN III) is:**

A. pleomorphic
B. polygonal
C. round-to-oval
D. frothy, lacy, delicate

81. **Which of the following statements is true regarding discrimination of endocervical adenocarcinoma from endometrial adenocarcinoma?**

A. morula configuration and frothy cytoplasm are observed in endocervical adenocarcinoma
B. columnar configuration and granular cytoplasm are observed in endometrial adenocarcinoma
C. columnar configuration and granular cytoplasm are observed in endocervical adenocarcinoma
D. micronucleoli are observed in endocervical adenocarcinoma, while macronucleoli are observed in endometrial adenocarcinoma

82. **Which vulvar infection clinically presents as a vesiculopustule and requires the identification of gram-negative bacilli arranged in pairs or clusters?**

A. *Neisseria gonorrhoeae*
B. *Torulopsis glabrata*
C. molluscum contagiosum
D. *Haemophilus ducreyi*

83. **The most common sarcomatous element associated with a homologous mixed müllerian tumor of the uterus is:**

A. rhabdomyosarcoma
B. endometrial stromal sarcoma
C. leiomyosarcoma
D. osteosarcoma

84. **A differential diagnosis for keratinizing dysplasia is:**

A. dyskeratosis
B. koilocytosis
C. reactive/reparative cells
D. superficial stromal cells

85. **A differential diagnosis for the bare nuclei of normal endocervical cells found in post-menopausal patients is:**

A. atypia of atrophy and maturity
B. parakeratosis
C. pemphigus vulgaris
D. chronic follicular cervicitis

86. **A 41-year-old woman with a history of diabetes presents for an annual Papanicolaou smear. Her last menstrual period, regularly 28 days in length, was three weeks prior to the current date. Cytology reveals large numbers of three-dimensional glandular cells in tight clusters with indistinct cellular outlines, surrounded by a clean background. What clinical follow-up may help determine the origin of these cells?**

A. cervical biopsy to rule out endocervical adenocarcinoma
B. cervical biopsy to rule out infiltrating squamous cell carcinoma
C. endometrial biopsy to rule out cystic hyperplasia
D. ovarian biopsy to rule out endometriosis

87. **A 72-year-old woman presents with pruritus and vaginal dryness. Cytologic examination reveals large numbers of deep parabasal cells masked by severe acute inflammation. A small population of round cells displaying an eosinophilic-to-orangeophilic appearance with India ink nuclei are diagnostic of:**

A. low-grade squamous intraepithelial lesion, mild keratinizing dysplasia
B. high-grade squamous intraepithelial lesion, severe keratinizing dysplasia
C. degenerated parabasal cells of atrophy
D. keratinizing pearls

88. **Which of the following may mimic follicular cervicitis?**

A. metaplastic cells
B. well-preserved neutrophils
C. nonkeratinizing dysplasia
D. malignant lymphoma

89. **When differentiating a reparative process from a malignant one, which of the following criteria is important?**

A. single cells in repair
B. sheets of cells without single cells in repair
C. nucleoli in repair
D. nucleoli in malignancy

90. **Cells from a 62-year-old woman that possess scalloping borders, finely vacuolated cytoplasm often containing polymorphonuclear neutrophils, anisonucleosis, and nuclei with irregular chromatin distribution and slight hyperchromasia are found in concert with mucicarmine-positive signet ring cells among a dense, wispy background demonstrated with the Diff-Quik stain. The diagnosis is consistent with:**

A. adenoacanthoma
B. clear cell endometrial adenocarcinoma
C. papillary serous endometrial adenocarcinoma
D. mucinous endometrial adenocarcinoma

91. Adenoacanthoma is identified cytologically by the presence of:

A. lipophages
B. superficial stromal cells
C. a squamous metaplastic component
D. deep stromal cells

92. A cervical/endocervical smear from a 41-year-old patient reveals cells possessing hyperchromatic nuclei with smooth chromatin patterns. A slight degree of anisonucleosis with a loss of polarity is also found in cells exhibiting a "feathering" effect. In addition, a hyperchromatic population of well-preserved, round-to-oval, bare nuclei are seen. The diagnosis is:

A. endocervical adenocarcinoma
B. endometrial adenocarcinoma
C. AGUS/endocervical dysplasia
D. adenoid basal carcinoma

93. A cervical/endocervical smear reveals cells in sheets, and microbiopsies reveal columnar formation, pseudostratification, granular cytoplasm, fine irregular chromatin, and micronucleoli. Red blood cells and fibrin are also identified. The cytology is diagnostic of:

A. endometrial adenocarcinoma
B. endocervical adenocarcinoma
C. endometrial reparative/regenerative processes
D. endocervical reparative/regenerative processes

94. What cytologic feature found in endometrial cells is associated with patients who have an intrauterine device?

A. macronucleoli
B. coarse, irregular chromatin
C. large, distended vacuoles
D. diathesis

95. Which of the following is not considered a precursor lesion for adenocarcinoma of the endometrium?

A. cystic hyperplasia
B. atypical hyperplasia
C. endometrial CIS
D. endometrial polyps

96. Cells exhibiting coarse, irregular chromatin, irregularly defined cytoplasmic borders, and large distended vacuoles were identified in a cervical/endocervical smear from a 41-year-old patient. Endocervical and endometrial curettings revealed no pathologic abnormality. The diagnosis/origin of these cells is:

A. medullary carcinoma/breast
B. papillary carcinoma/thyroid
C. serous cystadenocarcinoma/ovary
D. mucinous cystadenocarcinoma/ovary

97. The cytologic diagnosis of lichen sclerosus is based on the presence of:

A. hyperkeratosis, plasma cells
B. koilocytosis, polymorphonuclear neutrophils
C. squamous cell carcinoma
D. pseudoepitheliomatous hyperplasia

98. An example of solid primary tumor of the vulva is:

A. granular cell tumor (myoblastoma)
B. minimal deviation adenocarcinoma
C. clear cell adenocarcinoma
D. adenocarcinoma, Skene duct origin

99. In which of the following patients is gonorrheal vulvitis most commonly diagnosed?

A. children
B. mature cycling women
C. postmenopausal women with intermediate cell atrophy
D. lichen sclerosus et atrophicus

100. The best method for diagnosing Bartholin gland infections is a (an):

A. vaginal scraping
B. vulvar scraping
C. fine needle aspiration
D. endocervical curetting

101. Poorly differentiated endometrial adenocarcinomas possess which of the following cytologic features?

A. an increase in sheets over gland formation
B. an increase in gland over sheet formation
C. an increase in the number of oxyphilic cells present
D. a decrease in nucleoli

102. A 42-year-old patient presents with pelvic ascites for a pelvic examination. A Papanicolaou smear was performed and the cytologic evaluation revealed a large population of three-dimensional cells exhibiting anisocytosis, polymorphic nuclear features, and hyperchromatic nuclei with fine irregular chromatin patterns. Macronucleoli and psammoma bodies are seen. The background is clean or free of diathesis. The diagnosis is:

A. cervical polyp
B. well-differentiated endometrial adenocarcinoma
C. serous adenocarcinoma of the ovary
D. endocervical adenocarcinoma

103. As the differentiation of an endometrial adenocarcinoma decreases, the size and number of nucleoli:

A. increase
B. decrease
C. stay the same
D. are not predictable

104. Multinucleation is commonly associated with:

A. folic acid deficiency
B. squamous cell carcinoma
C. cytotrophoblasts
D. lymphocytes

105. Bean-shaped gram-negative bacilli with a "safety pin" appearance found within the cytoplasm of histiocytes are diagnostic of:

A. Donovan bodies, *Calymmatobacterium granulomatis*
B. *Haemophilus ducreyi*
C. *Neisseria gonorrhoeae*
D. *Gardnerella vaginalis*

106. A 22-year-old patient with a history of birth control pill usage (6 years) recently terminated usage. The patient currently suffers from galactorrhea (3 weeks). What condition is associated with the clinical findings?

A. Sheehan syndrome
B. del Castillo syndrome
C. Forbes-Albright syndrome
D. Stein-Leventhal syndrome

107. On colposcopic examination, HPV-related cervical abnormalities may be represented by:

A. mosaic patterns
B. decrease in vascularity
C. uterine prolapse
D. atrophic uterine cervix

108. The pathognomonic indication for HPV infection in cytology is:

A. the presence of chromatin smudging
B. koilocytosis
C. nuclear wrinkling
D. parakeratosis

109. What significant post irradiation finding might raise suspicion of a possible recurrent squamous cell carcinoma?

A. macrocytosis
B. amphophilic staining
C. an abrupt increase in squamous cell maturation
D. intermediate cells with concentric cytoplasmic fibrils

110. Which of the following is (are) a possible treatment regimen for high-grade intraepithelial lesions?

A. LEEP/LLETZ
B. DNA ploidy analysis
C. vitamin D therapy
D. methotrexate

111. What diagnosis might be confused with an HPV infection?

A. changes associated with *Trichomonas* infections
B. repair
C. microglandular hyperplasia
D. squamous cell carcinoma

112. The smear pattern taken from a patient suffering from extreme anorexia nervosa will show:

A. parabasal cell predominance
B. intermediate and superficial cells
C. superficial cell predominance
D. normal cyclic pattern dependent upon the last menstrual period

113. All of the following are possible carcinogenic mechanisms for the initiation and promotion of squamous cell carcinoma except:

A. uncontrolled transcription of E6 and E7
B. HPV integration disrupting the E1-E2 region
C. double point mutations of oncogene p53
D. high-risk HPV types inducing exophytic lesions

114. The presence of malignant cells post irradiation may be considered persistent or recurrent after what length of time?

A. 1 week post irradiation
B. 2 weeks post irradiation
C. 4 weeks post irradiation
D. 8 weeks post irradiation

115. The stem cell from which large cell nonkeratinizing carcinoma arises is:

A. endocervical reserve cell
B. immature squamous metaplasia
C. mature nonkeratinizing squamous epithelium
D. mature keratinizing squamous epithelium

116. Minor (nonspecific) criteria suggestive of condyloma infection include:

A. macrocytes, kite, polka dot, and balloon cells
B. abundant reparative epithelial cells
C. immature squamous metaplastic cells
D. cytoplasmic vacuolization

117. Which of the following is (are) not considered a morphologic variant of carcinoma in situ?

A. immature round dysplastic cell
B. syncytial-like arrangement
C. hyperchromatic crowded groups
D. intermediate-like cells in cobblestone pattern

118. An indication of recurrent post-irradiation adenocarcinoma is:

A. large, round-to-oval stripped nuclei
B. cytoplasmic vacuolization
C. polymorphic cells with orangeophilic cytoplasm
D. opaque nuclear features

119. The most common histologic appearance associated with the "high-risk" HPV viral types is:

A. flat
B. spiked
C. exophytic
D. inverted

120. A 65-year-old woman on long-term, low-dose estrogen therapy will most likely show:

A. parabasal cell predominance
B. intermediate cell predominance
C. superficial cell predominance
D. cannot be predicted

121. Which process mimics a dyskeratotic process but is not considered part of the cytologic spectrum of HPV infection?

A. dyskeratocyte
B. koilocyte
C. parabasal-like cells
D. pseudokeratosis

122. Recurrent carcinoma cells found in patients who have previously received radiation therapy are:

A. smaller than the original tumor cells
B. larger than the original tumor cells
C. the same size as the original tumor cells
D. size cannot be predicted

123. Which of the following histologic criteria are helpful in diagnosing carcinoma in situ instead of dysplasia?

A. abnormal cells throughout the full thickness, differentiated at the surface
B. abnormal cells replacing the full thickness of the squamous mucosa, no differentiation at the surface
C. abnormal cells are present in only 1/3 of the epithelial thickness, normal mature differentiation is present in the upper 2/3
D. abnormal cells are present in only 1/2 of the epithelial thickness, normal mature differentiation is present in the upper 1/2

124. Orangeophilic small parakeratotic cells with enlarged, smudged, and opaque nuclei, exhibiting slight pleomorphism, are:

A. severe keratinizing dysplasia
B. reserve cell hyperplasia
C. dyskeratocytes
D. microglandular hyperplasia

125. What is a useful criterion in distinguishing low-grade squamous intraepithelial lesions from high-grade lesions?

A. cytoplasmic inclusions in low-grade lesions
B. co-infection with HPV in high-grade lesions
C. increased nuclear to cytoplasmic area in high-grade lesions
D. larger nuclear size in high-grade lesions

126. Cells found in three-dimensional syncytial-like arrangements with chaotic architecture, coarse regular chromatin, and hyperchromatic crowded groups are found in a clean background. The diagnosis is:

A. low-grade squamous intraepithelial neoplasia, mild dysplasia
B. high-grade squamous intraepithelial neoplasia, moderate dysplasia
C. high-grade squamous intraepithelial neoplasia, severe dysplasia
D. high-grade squamous intraepithelial neoplasia, carcinoma in situ

127. Which of the following is (are) considered a synonym for carcinoma in situ?

A. Paget disease
B. CIN III
C. infiltrating epithelioma
D. low-grade squamous intraepithelial carcinoma

128. A mechanism that might prove useful to differentiate severe keratinizing dysplasia from invasive keratinizing carcinoma is:

A. diathesis, increased cellular pleomorphism in carcinoma
B. nucleoli in dysplasia
C. increased mitotic activity in dysplasia
D. presence of pearl formation in carcinoma

129. What sexually transmitted condition, related to pelvic inflammatory disease, is the most prevalent in the United States?

A. *Chlamydia trachomatis*
B. gonorrhea
C. human papillomavirus
D. herpes

130. Benign cellular changes related to irradiation include:

A. karyomegaly and macrocytosis
B. viable cells with increased mitosis
C. aneuploidy
D. coarse, irregular chromatin with macronucleoli

131. What benign cellular change mimics dysplasia?

A. irradiation
B. severe inflammation
C. nuclear vacuolation
D. decreased nuclear-to-cytoplasmic ratios

132. **Cytology reveals single cells and syncytial-like aggregates, extreme pleomorphic cytoplasmic features, opaque nuclei, and occasional cells with irregular chromatin distribution. Background material is granular with eosinophilic fibrinous material. The diagnosis is:**

A. high-grade intraepithelial neoplasia, moderate dysplasia
B. squamous cell carcinoma, keratinizing type
C. atypical reparative/regenerative process
D. pleomorphic parakeratosis

133. **The morphogenesis of small cell squamous carcinoma of the uterine cervix is related to the development of:**

A. atypical squamous metaplasia
B. mature squamous metaplasia
C. native squamous epithelium
D. atypical reserve cell hyperplasia

134. **In a subclinical HPV infection, the virus is most likely harbored in:**

A. dysplastic epithelium
B. reserve cells
C. ectocervical cells
D. the underlying stroma

135. **The most common malignancy that involves the uterine cervix is:**

A. keratinizing squamous cell carcinoma
B. nonkeratinizing squamous cell carcinoma
C. small cell squamous carcinoma
D. adenocarcinoma, endocervical type

136. **Which viral genomic segment is responsible for host cellular transformation in vivo?**

A. late region 1,2
B. early region 1,2
C. upstream regulatory region
D. early region 6,7

137. **What is a pitfall in the diagnosis of benign radiation changes?**

A. vitamin C deficiency
B. folic acid deficiency
C. chronic follicular cervicitis
D. vitamin A deficiency

138. **The presence of keratin pearls in a cervical smear is associated with:**

A. keratinizing squamous cell carcinoma
B. keratinizing dysplasia, not otherwise specified
C. keratinizing processes, nonspecific
D. no relation to any process

139. **Small cells exhibiting cell-to-cell compression, high nuclear-to-cytoplasmic ratios, and coarse, irregular chromatin distribution in a "dirty" necrotic background represent:**

A. small cell neuroendocrine carcinoma, cervix
B. squamous cell carcinoma, cervix
C. high-grade intraepithelial neoplasia, carcinoma in situ
D. serous cystadenocarcinoma, metastatic from ovary

140. **The most sensitive technique to identify a specific HPV virotype is:**

A. immunohistochemistry
B. cytologic morphology
C. histomorphology
D. nucleic acid analysis

141. **Which of the following special stains will help verify the neuroendocrine differentiation (ND) found in small cell neuroendocrine carcinoma of the cervix from non-neuroendocrine in poorly differentiated small cell squamous carcinoma?**

A. synaptophysin
B. HMB-45
C. PAS
D. alcian blue

142. **Which technique might be useful in determining the primary site of a carcinoma metastatic to the vaginal/cervical area?**

A. ploidy analysis
B. DNA analysis for human papillomavirus
C. immunohistochemistry
D. flow cytometry

143. The progression rate of immature metaplastic dysplasia compared with the most common dysplasia variant is:

A. greater
B. less
C. the same
D. dependant upon coexisting infections

144. The cytologic features of mucinous/intestinal endometrial adenocarcinoma are which grade?

A. 1
B. 3
C. 4
D. cannot be determined with available information

145. Extrauterine tumors that spread to the vagina via direct extension may be cytologically distinguished from those metastasizing from distant locations (non-implanting) by:

A. diathesis-related changes with malignancies involving direct extension
B. signet ring cells in malignancies involving distant metastasis
C. nuclear chromatin patterns providing delineation
D. pools of mucin, which are more common in malignancies involving direct extension

146. The most helpful cytologic criteria for verifying the "atypical" features associated with cone biopsy artifact as merely benign degenerative changes are:

A. increased crowding resembling neoplasia, large nucleoli
B. increased crowding resembling neoplasia, abundant mitotic figures
C. few "atypical" cells, associated benign epithelial elements
D. increased numbers of hyperchromatic crowded groups, increased crowding resembling neoplasia

147. Hyperchromatic crowded groups and syncytial-like formation as identified by low-power analysis are helpful features for the cytologic identification of:

A. LSIL
B. endometrial adenocarcinoma
C. Arias-Stella reaction
D. carcinoma in situ

148. The risk for development of vaginal adenosis is greatest if exposure to DES is during the:

A. second week of embryonic development
B. eighth week of gestation
C. twelfth week following conception
D. third trimester

149. Which is considered an uncommon protozoan found in the female genital tract?

A. *Vorticella* sp.
B. *Hormodendrum* sp.
C. *Gaffkya* sp.
D. *Aspergillus* sp.

150. Which organism is associated with toxic shock syndrome?

A. *Gardnerella vaginalis*
B. *Staphylococcus aureus*
C. *Chlamydia* sp.
D. *Entamoeba histolytica*

151. Single basophilic cells with variable sizes with scarce, wispy, trailing cytoplasm resembling "rootlets," oval nuclei, and finely granular, evenly distributed chromatin with prominent nucleoli, found in patients with a history of radiotherapy for squamous cell carcinoma, are representative of:

A. recurrent squamous cell carcinoma
B. myofibroblasts
C. leiomyosarcoma
D. post-irradiation dysplasia

152. The vinegar eel found in cervical/vaginal specimens is:

A. *Balantidium coli*
B. *Vorticella* sp.
C. *Enterobius vermicularis*
D. *Turbatrix aceti*

153. The most frequent heterologous constituent of a mixed müllerian uterine tumor is:

A. leiomyosarcoma
B. rhabdomyosarcoma
C. osteosarcoma
D. chondrosarcoma

154. Clear cell adenocarcinomas of the endometrium cytologically present as:

A. well-differentiated cells
B. poorly differentiated, delicate cytoplasm, prominent nucleoli
C. well-differentiated, mucin-positive with signet ring cells
D. poorly differentiated, papillary, psammoma bodies

155. A neuroendocrine malignancy arising in the cervix is:

A. clear cell adenocarcinoma
B. small cell carcinoma
C. nonkeratinizing (large) cell carcinoma
D. adenosquamous carcinoma

156. Difficulties in distinguishing squamous carcinoma in situ (CIS) from endocervical adenocarcinoma in situ (AIS) may arise when:

A. CIS involves the underlying gland-like spaces
B. AIS involves the transformation zone
C. CIS is derived from ectocervical mucosa
D. AIS stains eosinophilic

157. An endometrial adenocarcinoma that cytologically possesses uniform nuclear features and stains positive with periodic acid–Schiff is diagnostic of:

A. secretory adenocarcinoma
B. adenoacanthoma
C. papillary serous adenocarcinoma
D. clear cell adenocarcinoma

158. The possibility of microinvasive squamous carcinoma is suggested when what feature is present?

A. syncytial formation, pronounced chromocenters
B. fine regular chromatin patterns
C. micronucleoli, diathesis
D. macronucleoli

159. Granulomatous cervicitis may be associated with:

A. radiation
B. Arias-Stella reaction
C. psammoma bodies
D. *Candida* sp. infections

160. A normal cell type commonly found in smears from postmenopausal patients is the:

A. superficial squamous cell
B. multinucleated giant histiocyte
C. dyskeratocyte
D. anucleate squame

161. In addition to the human papillomavirus, possible cofactors associated with cervical carcinogenesis may include:

A. the use of progesterone-based birth control pills
B. vitamins A, B, and C deficiency
C. the use of an intrauterine device (IUD)
D. a history of endometritis

162. The most common primary carcinoma of the vulva is:

A. basal cell carcinoma
B. malignant melanoma
C. verrucous carcinoma
D. squamous cell carcinoma, keratinizing type

163. A vulvar smear from a 43-year-old patient shows a large group of columnar cells with anisocytosis, large hyperchromatic nuclei, fine irregular chromatin, macronucleoli, and signet ring formation. A mucinous background was identified. Subsequent endocervical and endometrial biopsies were normal. Which of the following may represent the possible origin of these cells?

A. transitional cell carcinoma, bladder
B. vulvar adenosis
C. Bartholin gland adenocarcinoma
D. ductal carcinoma, breast

164. Which ovarian tumor presents bilaterally and has cells that are positive with the CA-125 monoclonal antibody?

A. serous cystadenocarcinoma
B. mucinous cystadenocarcinoma
C. endometrioid tumor
D. malignant teratoma

165. A pure uterine sarcoma presenting with small, round, and uniform cells with high nuclear-to-cytoplasm ratios, coarse chromatin, and frequent micronucleoli is considered:

A. leiomyosarcoma
B. endometrial stromal sarcoma
C. rhabdomyosarcoma
D. osteosarcoma

166. Psammoma bodies may be seen with all of the following except:

A. endometrial adenocarcinoma
B. fallopian tube adenocarcinoma
C. patients with an IUD
D. Sertoli-Leydig cell tumor

167. The nuclei of adenocarcinoma in situ of the endocervix present with:

A. great pleomorphism
B. little pleomorphism
C. macronucleoli
D. spindle shapes

168. When should one analyze smears taken from patients who have received radiation therapy?

A. within 3–6 days post administration
B. not before 6–8 weeks post administration
C. in patients receiving external beam instead of radium application
D. in patients receiving polonium-induced radiation

169. Which statement is true?

A. atypical glandular cells (AGUS) often accompany squamous dysplasia
B. atypical endocervical repair is associated with Döderlein bacillus metaplasia
C. endometrial adenocarcinoma presents in strips or a "feathering" cellular pattern
D. cells associated with Arias-Stella reaction may be distinguished from squamous carcinoma in situ because of their small cell size

170. Mucicarmine-positive cells presenting in loose aggregates with macronucleoli and cellular cannibalism were found in a vulvar scraping from a 62-year-old woman. The cells are diagnostic of:

A. Paget disease
B. Minimal deviation adenocarcinoma
C. malignant melanoma
D. basal cell carcinoma

171. Stratified strips, rosettes, and columnar shaped cells presenting with palisading, enlarged, (crowded and overlapping), hyperchromatic nuclei possessing coarse chromatin and micronucleoli are diagnostic of:

A. high-grade intraepithelial neoplasia, carcinoma in situ
B. squamous cell carcinoma
C. atypical glandular cells of undetermined significance, favor neoplastic
D. adenocarcinoma, endometrial

172. The cytoplasm of endocervical adenocarcinoma is:

A. diffusely vacuolated
B. generally cyanophilic
C. granular
D. amphophilic

173. Cervical smears containing pleomorphic cells with enlarged, eccentrically located, fine-to-granular hyperchromatic nuclei, prominent nucleoli, PAS-positive vacuolated cytoplasm, and occasional giant cells with low nuclear-to-cytoplasmic ratios resembling chemotherapeutic changes found in a late stage pregnancy are diagnostic of:

A. choriocarcinoma
B. endometrial adenocarcinoma
C. endocervical repair/regeneration
D. Arias-Stella reaction

174. Which cytologic criteria are helpful in distinguishing endocervical adenocarcinoma from endometrial adenocarcinoma?

A. cells with columnar morphology arranged into rosettes and crowded sheets with holes for endocervical adenocarcinoma compared with round, plump cells arranged into balls and molded groups for endometrial adenocarcinoma
B. granular cytoplasm, coarse chromatin in endometrial adenocarcinoma
C. diffusely vacuolated cytoplasm, limited hyperchromasia in endocervical adenocarcinoma
D. cells in sheets, larger cell size, and cyanophilia in endometrial adenocarcinoma

175. Arias-Stella reaction may be normally seen with which of the following?

A. prolonged progesterone stimulation
B. vaginal cuff smears from hysterectomy patients
C. scraping the lower 1/3 of the vaginal wall
D. vulval scrapes

176. A 70-year-old woman complains of vulvar pruritus and bleeding. Cytology reveals a large population of loosely arranged pleomorphic cells with oval nuclei, often binucleated. Nucleoli, often representing 1/3 of the nuclear diameter, are found, as well as intranuclear vacuolization. Intracytoplasmic deposits are seen in many of the cells. The diagnosis is most consistent with:

A. pseudoepitheliomatous hyperplasia
B. basal cell carcinoma
C. bowenoid papulosis
D. malignant melanoma

177. Endocervical adenocarcinoma in situ (AIS) may be distinguished from invasive adenocarcinoma of the endocervix using which criteria?

A. increase in single cells, loosely arranged cell groups, macronucleoli, diathesis present in endocervical adenocarcinoma
B. increase in single cells, loosely arranged cell groups, macronucleoli, diathesis present in endocervical adenocarcinoma in situ
C. three-dimensionality (morula or cell ball formation) of endocervical AIS versus feathering in endocervical adenocarcinoma
D. eosinophilic cytoplasm is found in endocervical AIS, whereas cyanophilia is associated with endocervical adenocarcinoma

178. When discriminating minor endocervical atypia from that of endocervical adenocarcinoma in situ (AIS), which of the following is helpful?

A. chromatin is fine-to-moderately granular and cells present with minimal anisocytosis and lack pseudostratification in endocervical glandular dysplasia
B. chromatin is fine-to-moderately granular and cells present without pseudostratification in endocervical adenocarcinoma in situ
C. apoptosis is present in endocervical glandular dysplasia while absent in adenocarcinoma in situ
D. chromatin is moderate to coarse with prominent pseudostratification in endocervical glandular dysplasia while less pronounced chromatin and pseudostratification are associated with endocervical adenocarcinoma in situ

179. The cytologic criteria most helpful in establishing a diagnosis of large-cell squamous carcinoma from poorly differentiated endometrial adenocarcinoma are:

A. vacuolated cytoplasm, finely granular chromatin with macronucleoli in large cells in squamous carcinoma
B. vacuolated cytoplasm, finely granular chromatin with macronucleoli in endometrial adenocarcinoma
C. syncytial aggregates, micronucleoli in endometrial adenocarcinoma
D. eosinophilic staining cytoplasmic features in endometrial adenocarcinoma versus cyanophilic staining in large cell squamous carcinoma

180. A 3-year-old girl presents with polypoid lesion protruding from the left vaginal wall. Upon cytologic examination, a group of pleomorphic spindle cells is found. They are representative of:

A. vaginal adenosis
B. clear cell adenocarcinoma
C. embryonal rhabdomyosarcoma
D. leiomyosarcoma

181. The mean age of detection of clear cell adenocarcinoma of the vagina is:

A. 10
B. 20
C. 30
D. 50

182. A poorly differentiated uterine glandular tumor presenting as papillary structures lined with stratified cuboidal to columnar cells and accompanying psammoma bodies is a (an):

A. adenoacanthoma
B. clear cell adenocarcinoma, endometrium
C. "hobnail" serous adenocarcinoma, endometrium
D. leiomyosarcoma

183. A differential diagnosis for an endometrial adenocarcinoma that extends into the endocervical canal is:

A. endocervical glandular repair/regeneration
B. grade 1 endocervical adenocarcinoma
C. endocervical glandular dysplasia
D. primary endometrioid endocervical adenocarcinoma

184. A 22-year-old woman presents with multiple papules on the vulva, resembling dysplastic nevi. Polymerase chain reaction revealed HPV positively. The cells have anisocytosis, syncytial formation, and large nuclei with coarse, regular chromatin features. The diagnosis is consistent with:

A. squamous cell carcinoma
B. vulvar intraepithelial neoplasia, grade 1 (VIN I)
C. verrucous carcinoma
D. bowenoid papulosis

185. The cytologic identification of this organism is described best by which of these statements?

A. a spore form predominates in this species
B. this is a true mycelial form lacking the pseudohyphae form of other *Candida* sp.
C. sulfur granules are present in its mature form
D. the mature form is usually peripherally aggregated on an intermediate cell membrane

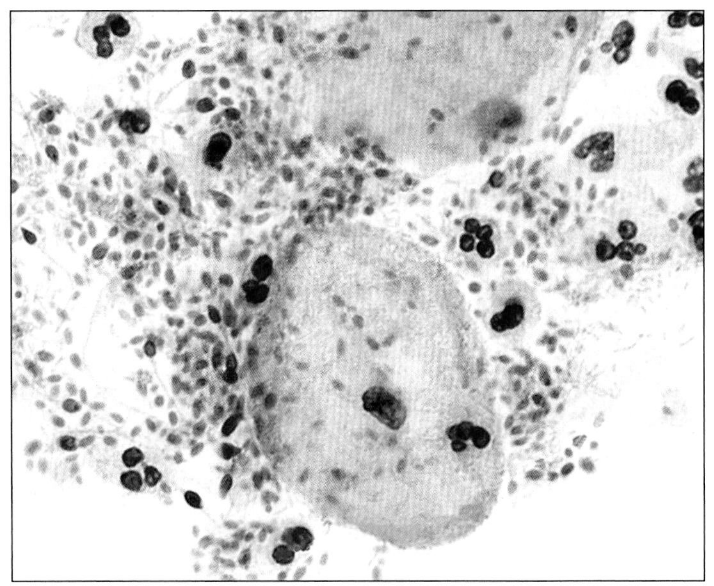

186. The identifiable components within the cytoplasm of these cells are:

A. elementary bodies
B. molluscum bodies
C. Type A inclusions of Cowdry
D. nucleoli

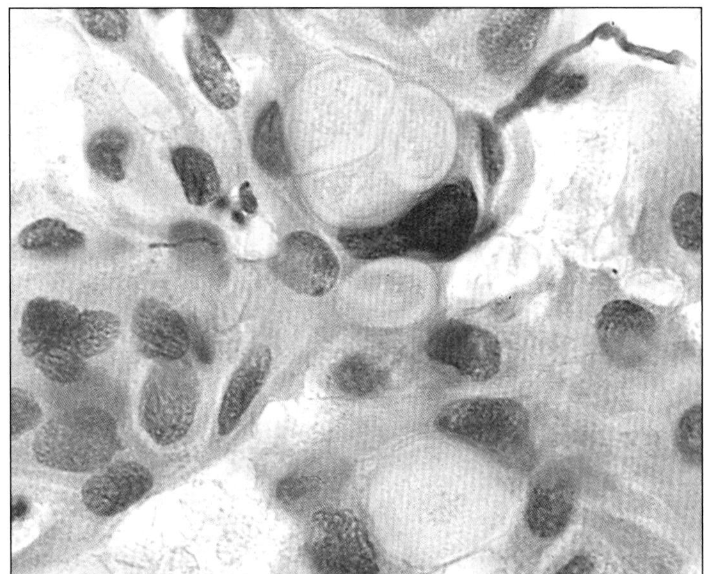

187. The broad alterations in the background (milieu) seen in this specimen are consistent with:

A. coccoid bacteria
B. a mild inflammatory exudate
C. changes secondary to *Trichomonas vaginalis* infection
D. diathesis changes associated with an invasive primary malignancy

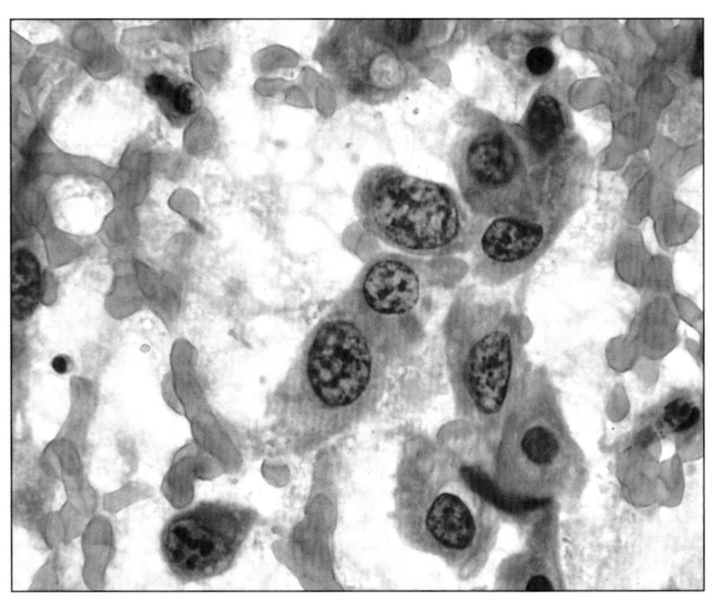

188. What clinical finding is associated with these cytologic findings?

A. increased risk of fetal infection, possibly resulting in death in utero
B. vesicles, erythematous papules
C. *Trichomonas vaginalis* infection
D. *Candida* sp. infections

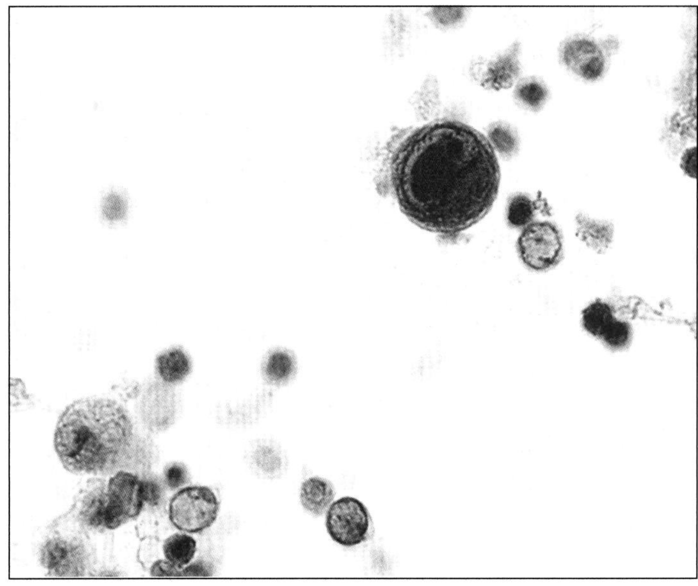

189. These organisms are commonly accompanied by:

A. herpes virus
B. Döderlein bacillus
C. human papillomavirus
D. *Trichomonas vaginalis*

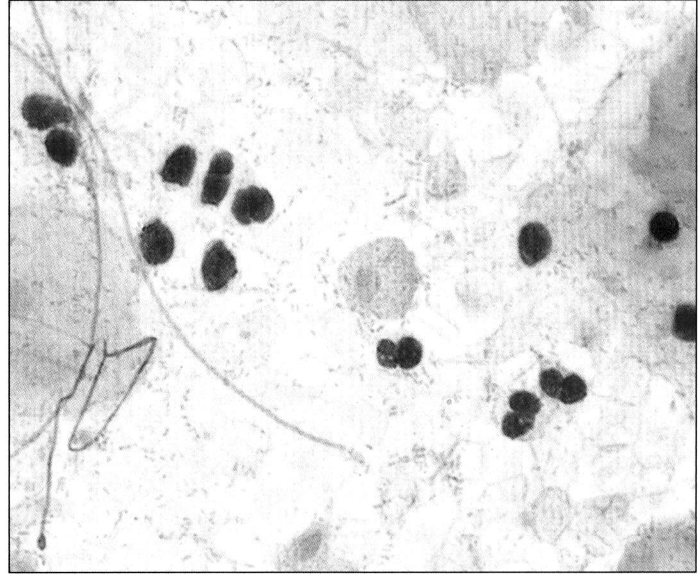

190. These cells are from a vaginal scrape from a 22-year-old woman. The diagnosis is most consistent with:

A. normal endocervical cells
B. normal endometrial glandular cells
C. normal endometrial stromal cells
D. adenosis

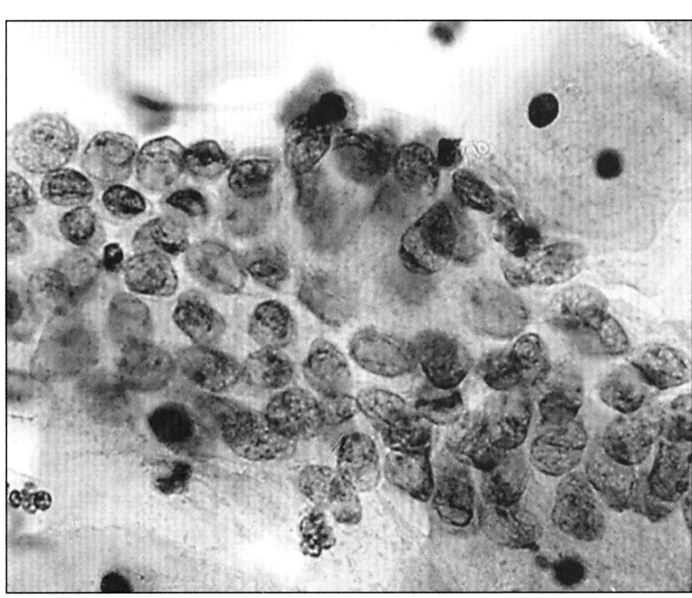

191. Which of the following statements does not correlate with the cytologic findings?

A. these cells are indicative of infection by human papillomavirus
B. the presence of these cells is often associated with keratinizing lesions
C. the cells may be associated with an underlying dysplasia
D. hyperkeratosis may accompany these cells

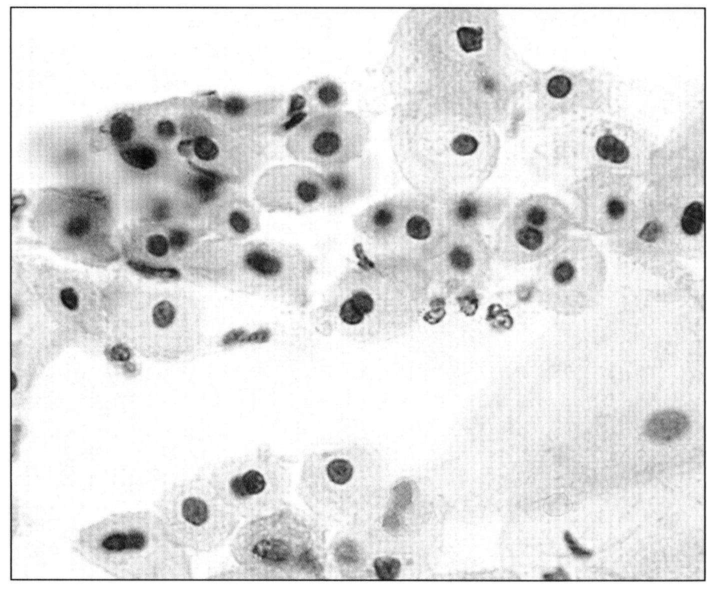

192. These cells are from a cervical scrape and an endocervical brushing from a 23-year-old woman, 4 months pregnant. The diagnosis is consistent with:

A. human papillomavirus
B. cytomegalovirus
C. herpes virus
D. vaccinia virus

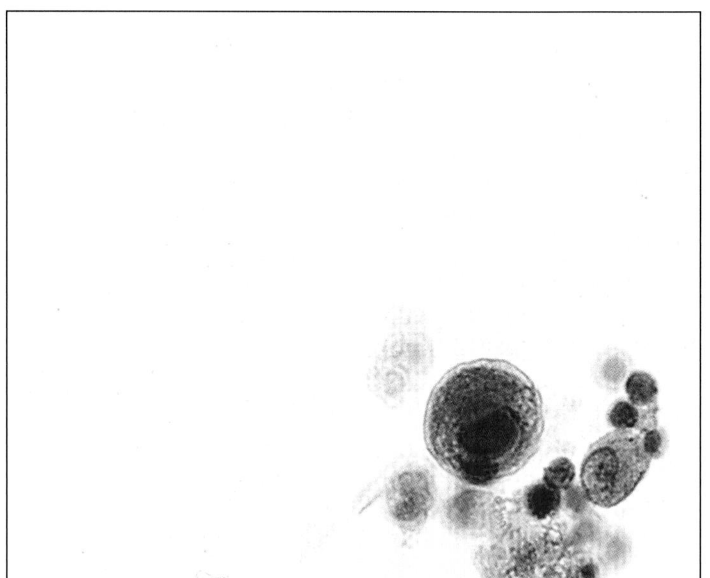

193. What clinical description is associated with these cytologic findings?

A. mature cycling woman
B. use of birth control pills
C. creates a green-yellowish discharge
D. use of an intrauterine device

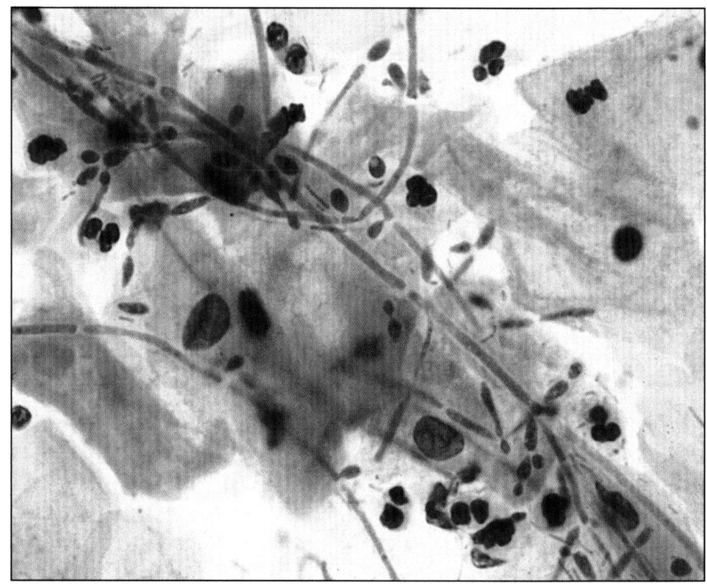

194. **Which of the following applies to these cells observed in a cervical smear?**

A. hyperkeratosis
B. hypodifferentiation
C. an abortive attempt at keratinization
D. histologic differentiation to the stratum spinosum

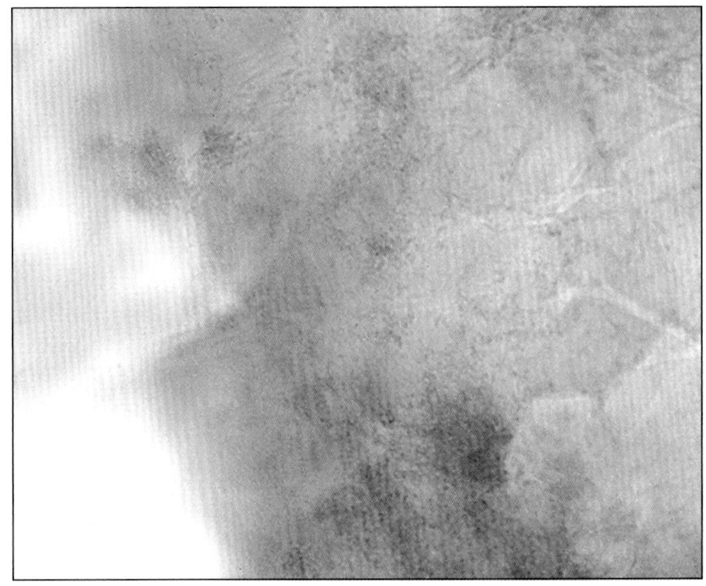

195. **The entities depicted are diagnostic of:**

A. *Candida albicans*
B. *Candida glabrata*
C. *Geotrichum candidum*
D. *Mucor* sp.

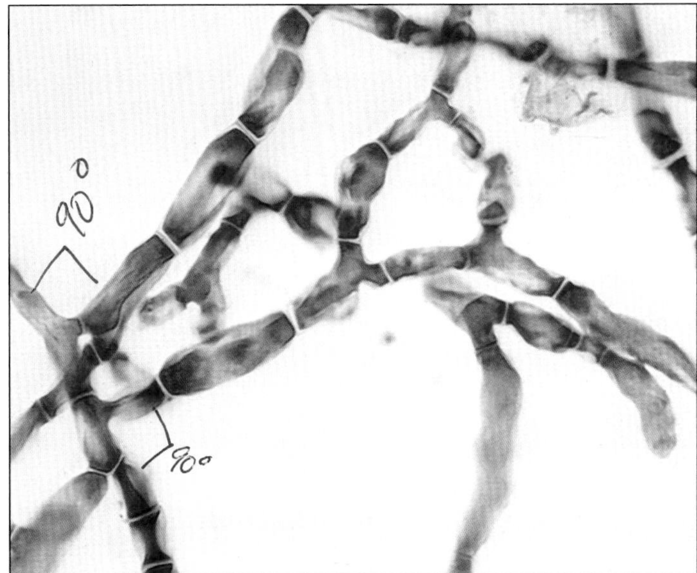

196. **Which of the following clinical histories is compatible with the cytologic findings?**

A. postmenopausal patient on high-dose, short-term estrogen therapy
B. postmenopausal patient with adrenal hyperplasia
C. postmenopausal patient with senile atrophy
D. postmenopausal patient with deep atrophy

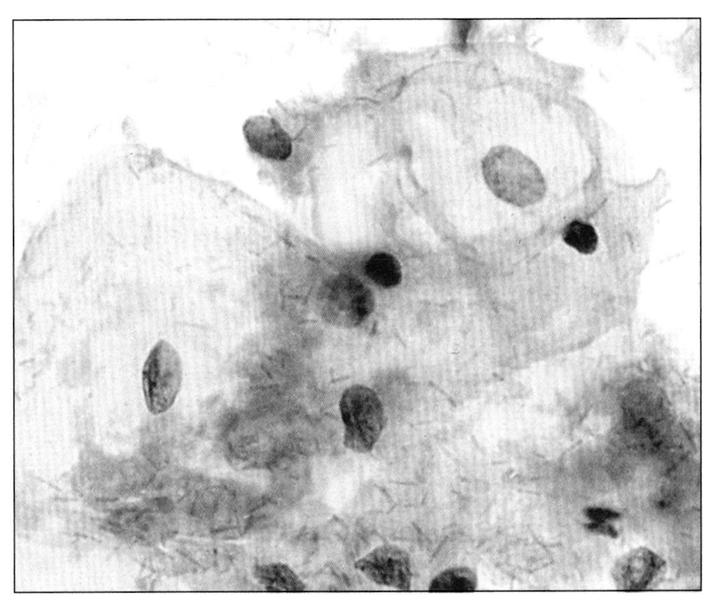

197. These structures found in Papanicolaou smears are:

A. of pathologic significance
B. suggestive of systemic *Cryptococcus* sp. infection
C. suggestive of mites
D. suggestive of pollen

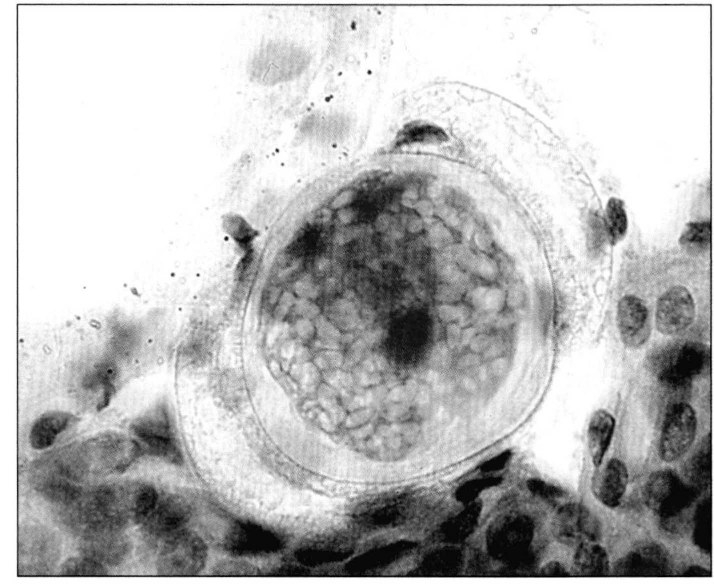

198. What is the significance of these cellular findings?

A. may mask an underlying pathologic condition
B. diagnostic of severe dysplasia and must be treated aggressively
C. suggestive of an invasive lesion
D. associated with progesterone-based birth-control pill usage

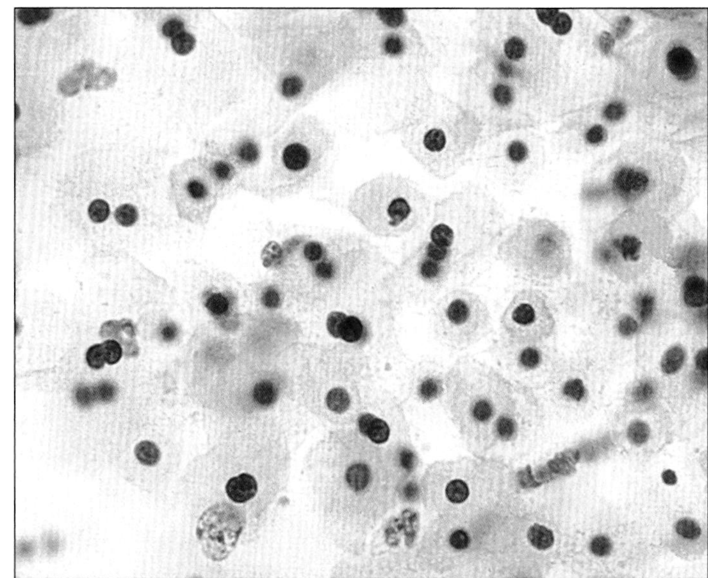

199. These cells are consistent with a:

A. benign protective reaction
B. destructive reaction
C. reparative reaction
D. dysplastic reaction

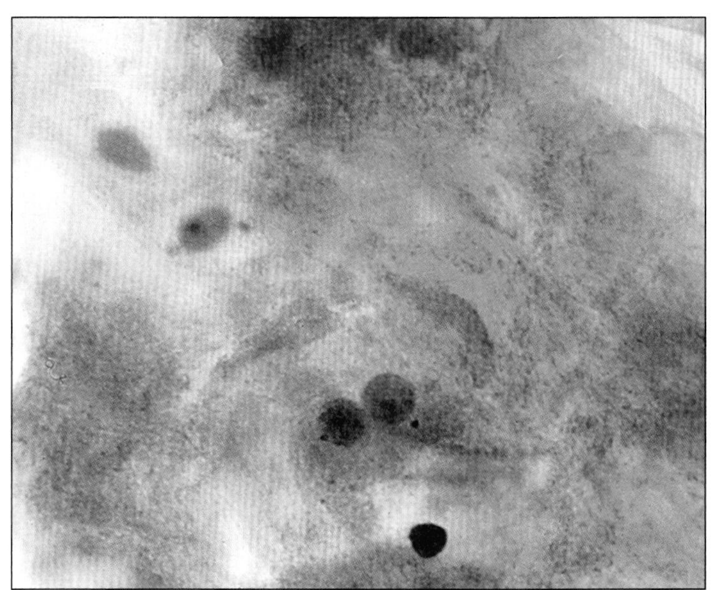

200. **These organisms may be associated with which clinical condition?**

A. endometrial hyperplasia
B. endocervical stenosis
C. vaginal acidity
D. vaginal alkalinity

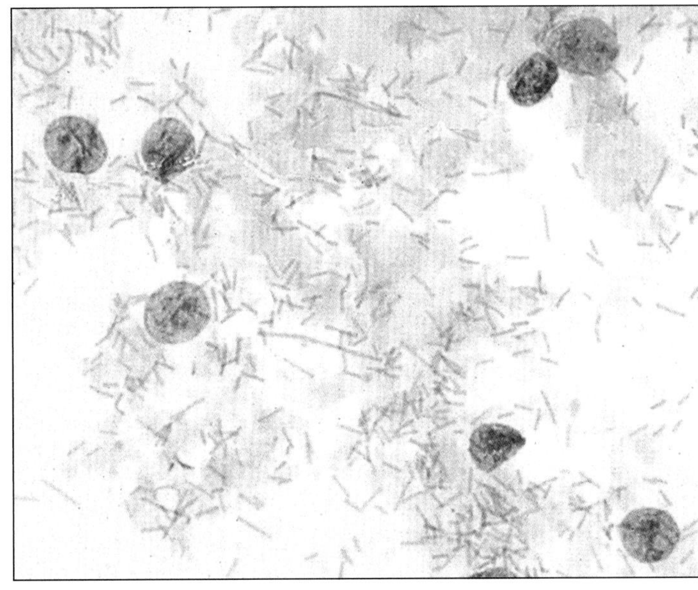

201. **What clinical finding is associated with this organism?**

A. curd-like yeast discharge
B. use of intrauterine devices
C. ulceration of vaginal mucosa
D. vesicles, erythematous papules

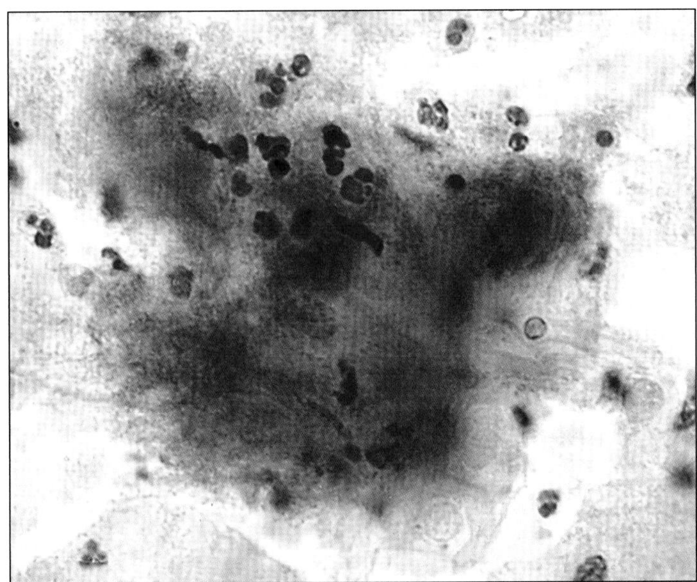

202. **This cytologic sample was taken from a patient with:**

A. atrophy
B. endocervical adenocarcinoma in situ
C. severe parakeratosis
D. small cell carcinoma

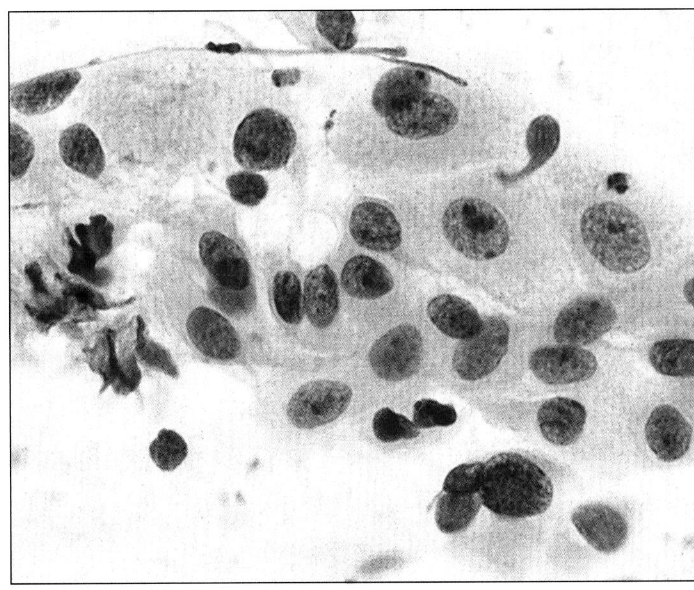

203. The material covering these cells is:

A. hematoxylin sheen
B. endocervical mucus
C. lubricant jelly
D. drying artifact

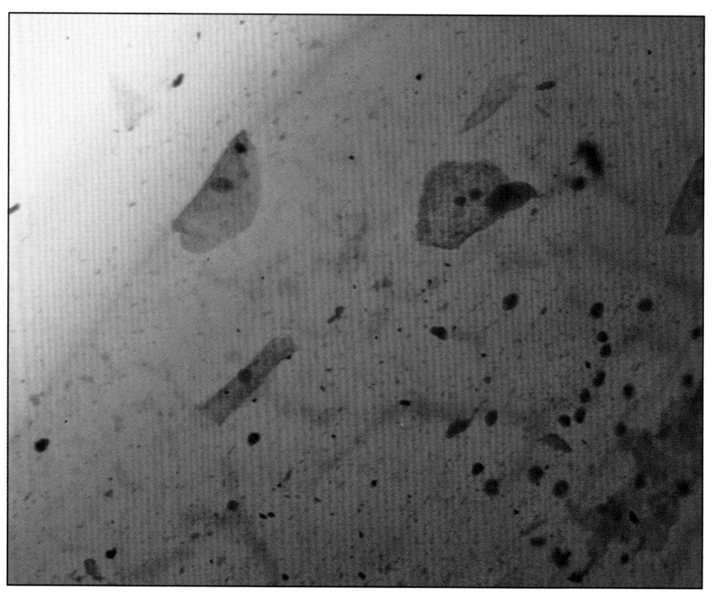

204. What hormonal state is consistent with these cytologic findings?

A. early proliferative
B. ovulation
C. late secretory
D. postpartum with galactorrhea

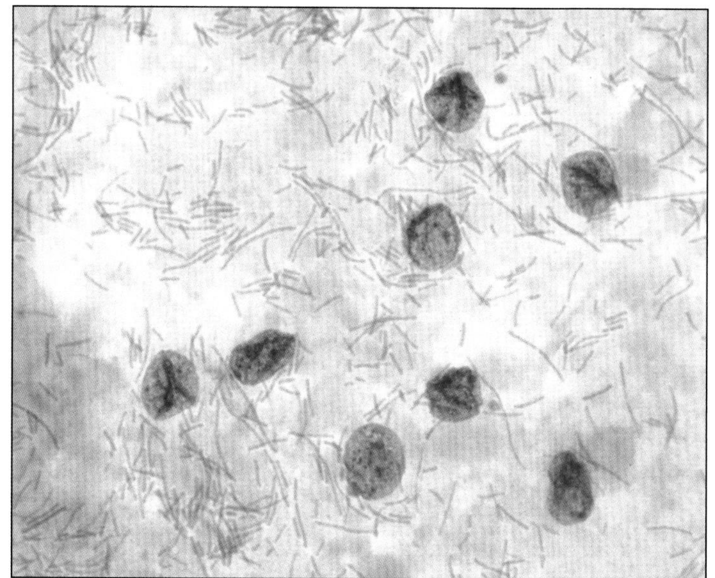

205. These cells are from a cervical scrape and an endocervical brushing from a 18-year-old woman, last menstrual period 3 weeks prior. The findings are consistent with:

A. human papillomavirus
B. multinucleated histiocyte
C. syncytiotrophoblast
D. herpesvirus

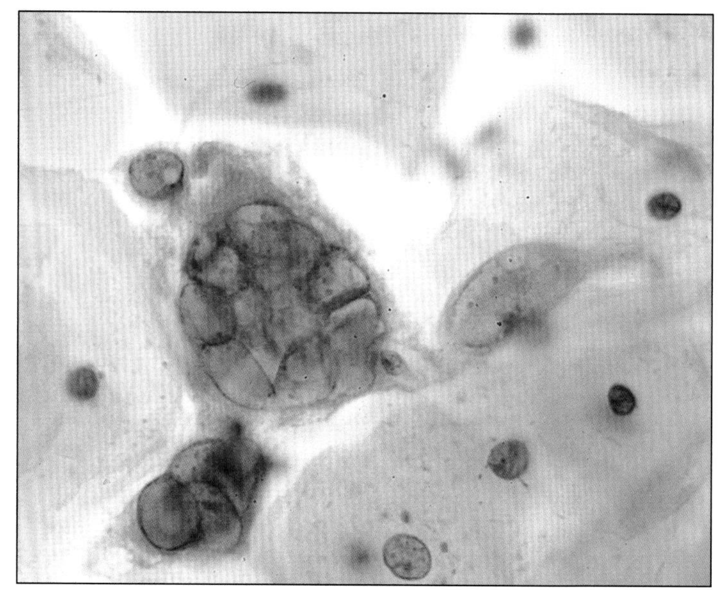

206. **Based on these cytologic findings, which clinical statement applies?**

A. prediction of disease progression is possible
B. it is impossible to predict the progression rate of the lesion
C. increased risk for the development of endometrial cancer
D. high risk of transplacental infection

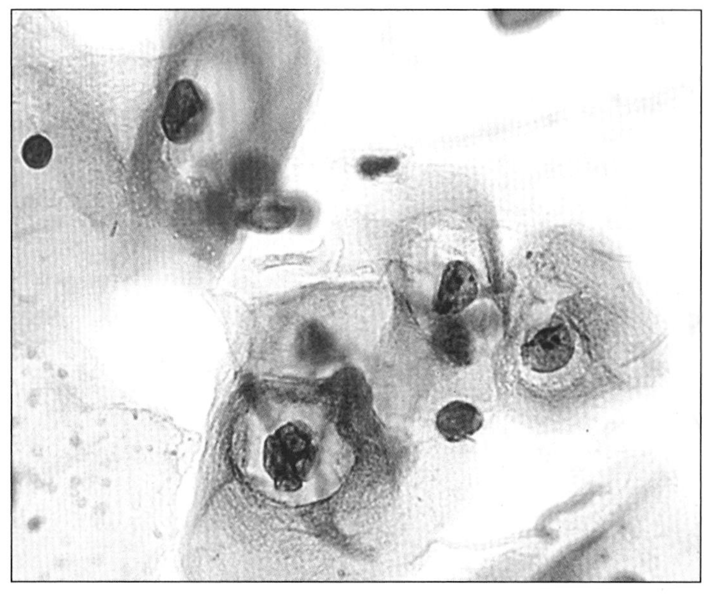

207. **Which of the following is a compatible clinical condition for these cytologic findings?**

A. diabetes mellitus
B. Stein-Leventhal syndrome
C. vaginal adenosis
D. marked estrogen effect

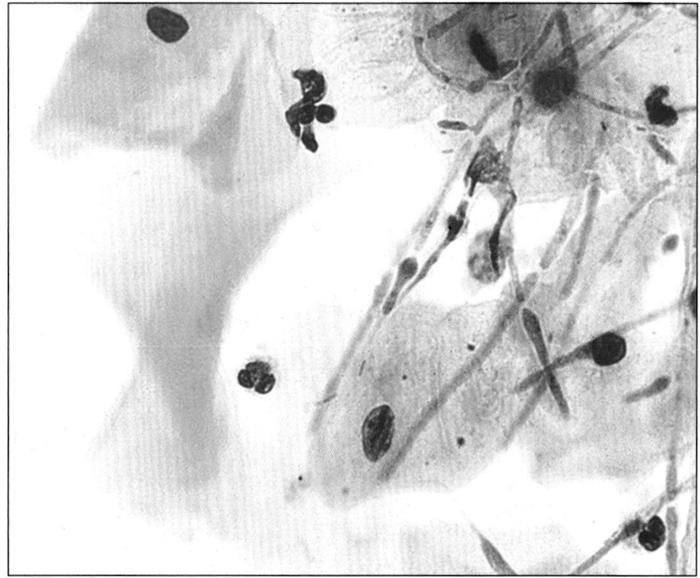

208. **Which of the following is responsible for the nature of this smear taken from the vaginal/cervical area?**

A. improper fixation
B. water in the xylene
C. hardening of the mounting medium
D. too long between application of mounting medium and coverslipping

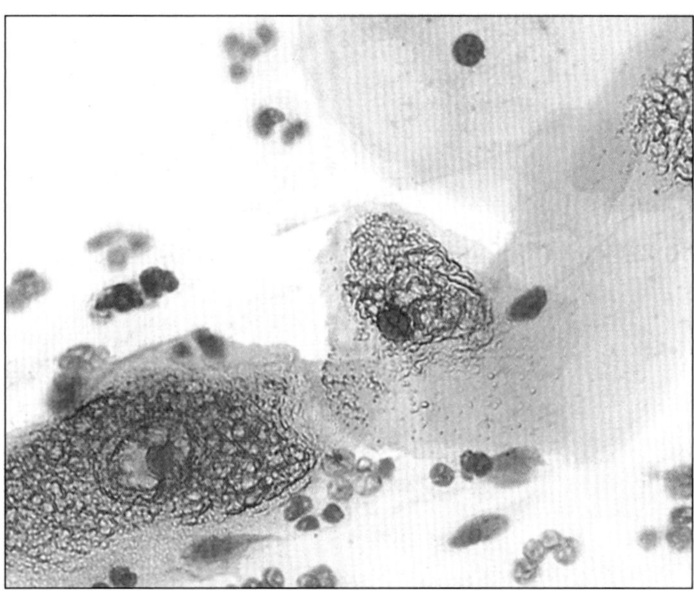

209. **Which of the following is a compatible clinical setting for these cytologic findings?**

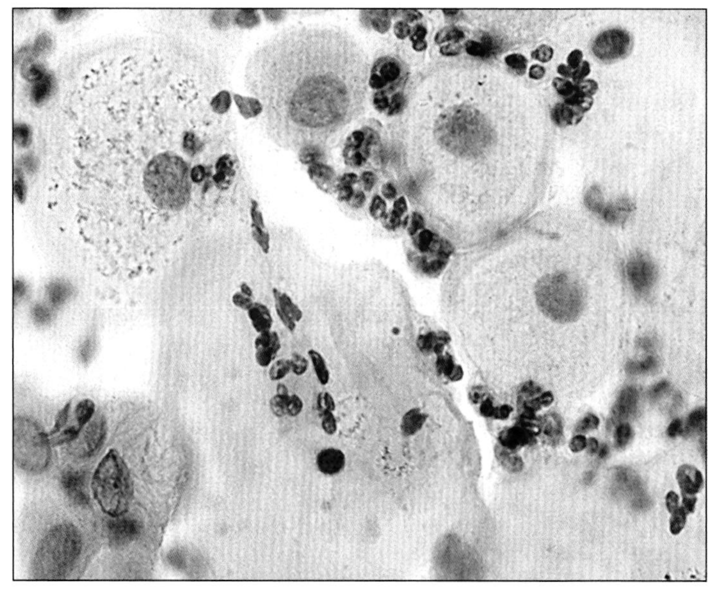

A. perimenarche
B. proliferative phase of the menstrual cycle
C. secretory phase of the menstrual cycle
D. postmenopausal, postcastration (20 years)

210. **The maturation index in the cytologic presentation is:**

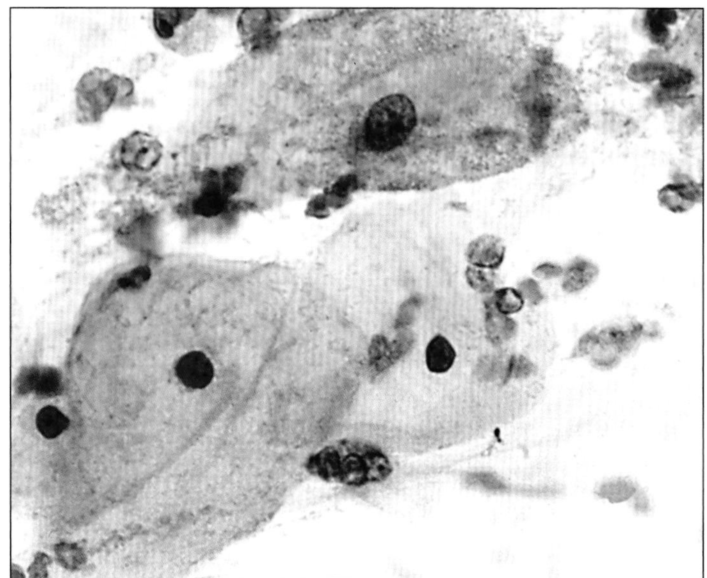

A. 0/50/50
B. 50/50/0
C. 50/0/50
D. cannot be determined

211. **These cells may be associated with which hormonal condition?**

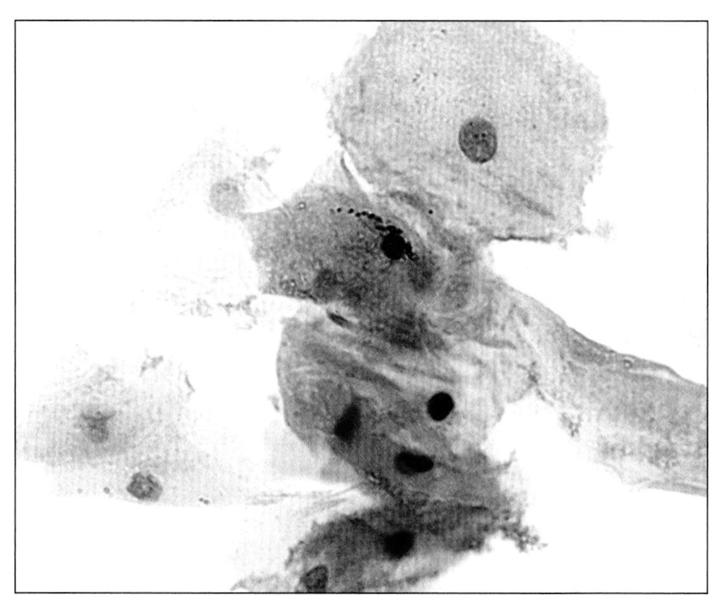

A. menopausal patient on androgenic therapy
B. menopausal patient on high-dose, short-term estrogen therapy
C. menopausal patient on low-dose, long-term estrogen therapy
D. menopausal patient on corticosteroid therapy

212. **These cells are from a vaginal smear of an 18-year-old woman who is currently requesting birth control pills. Which of the following applies?**

A. findings consistent with normal metaplastic epithelium found within the transformational zone
B. vaginal adenosis
C. atypical squamous cells of undetermined significance
D. metaplastic dysplasia

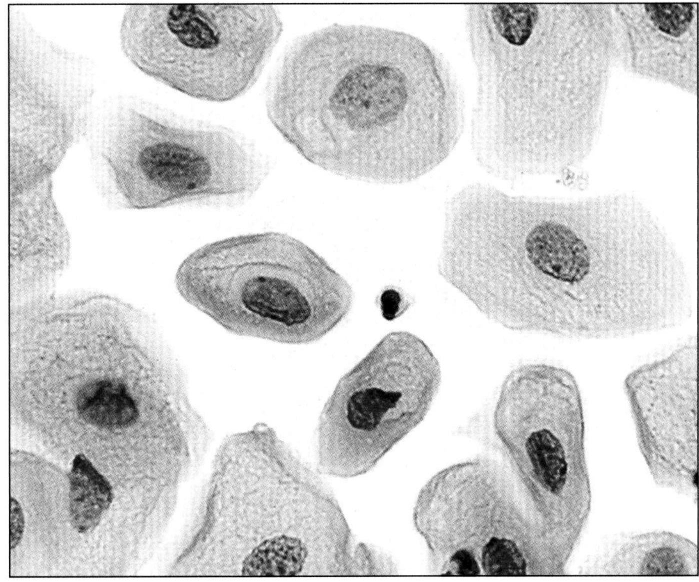

213. **What clinical setting could be associated with these cytologic findings?**

A. 18-year-old woman with primary amenorrhea
B. 28-year-old woman in the early secretory phase
C. 22-year-old woman in late pregnancy
D. 35-year-old woman, last menstrual period 3 days ago

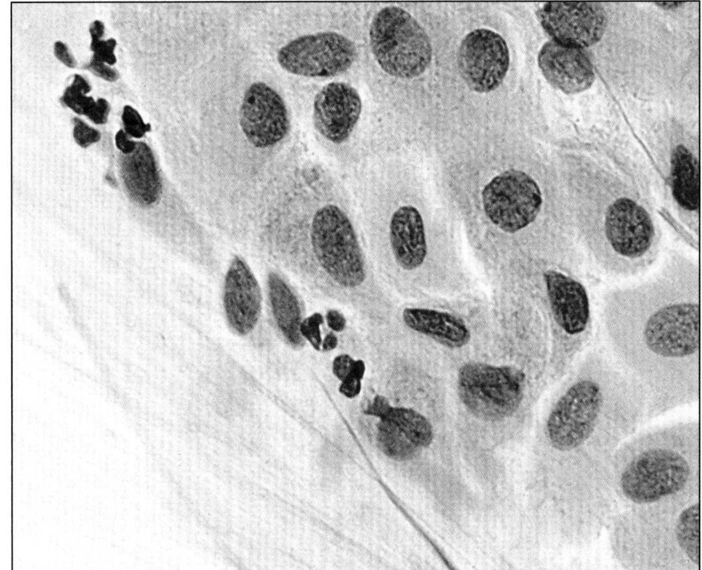

214. **Represented is a vaginal smear from a 32-year-old woman in her 3rd trimester. The presence of this entity is associated with preexisting vaginal:**

A. acidity
B. lesion
C. alkalinity
D. infection

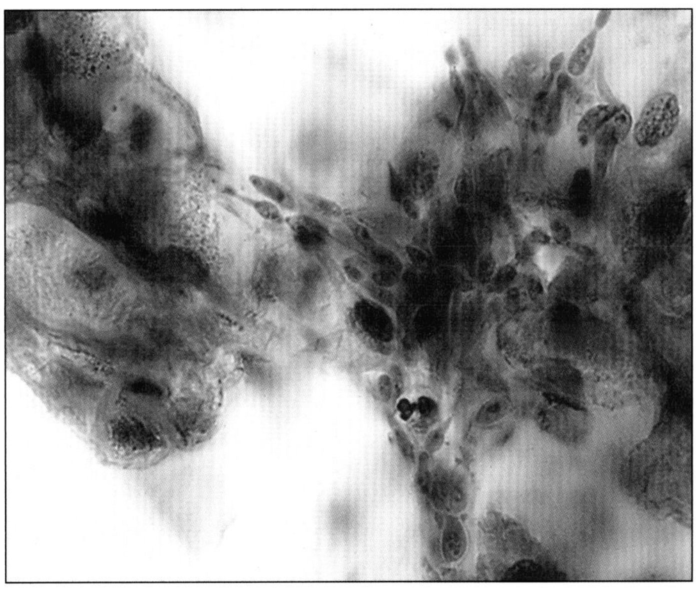

215. These cellular findings represent a sample from a 40-year-old woman with small papillomatous vulval lesions. The most likely diagnosis is:

A. human papillomavirus
B. molluscum contagiosum
C. herpes simplex virus
D. pemphigus vulgaris

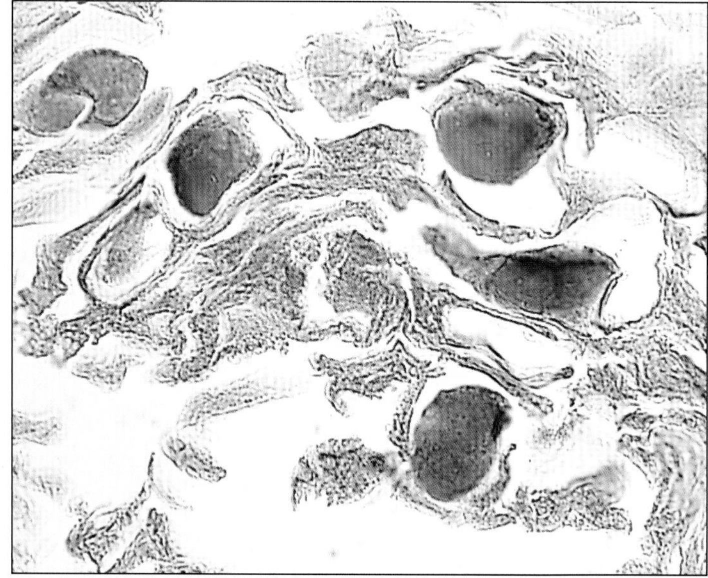

216. These cells are from a 32-year-old woman, 3 months pregnant. Because the patient had previously suffered several spontaneous abortions, the clinician administered estrogen therapy. The cytologic studies are performed 6 weeks post therapy. Based on the cytologic findings, which of the following applies?

A. poor prognostic information
B. good prognostic information
C. A progesterone test should be performed to confirm a threatened pregnancy
D. prognostic information cannot be determined

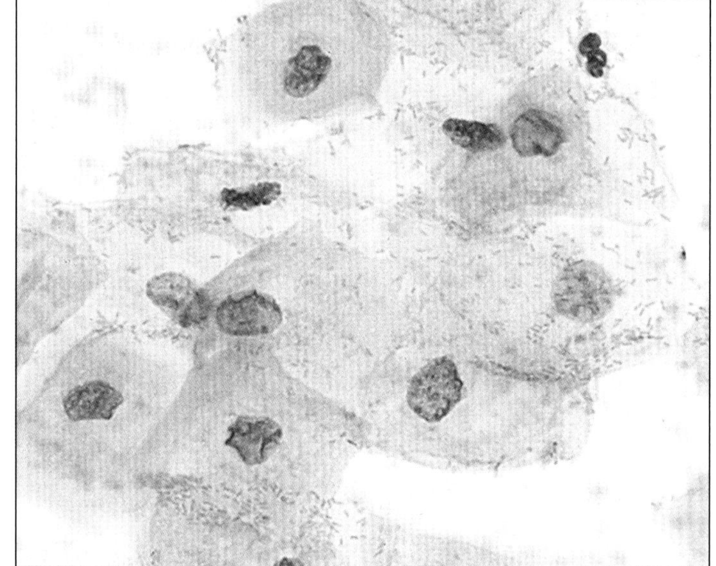

217. These cells represent a vaginal smear from a 50-year-old perimenopausal woman. A hormonal analysis was requested. Which of the following applies?

A. progesterone effect
B. decreased estrogenic effect
C. treat and repeat due to presence of microbiologic agent
D. atrophy

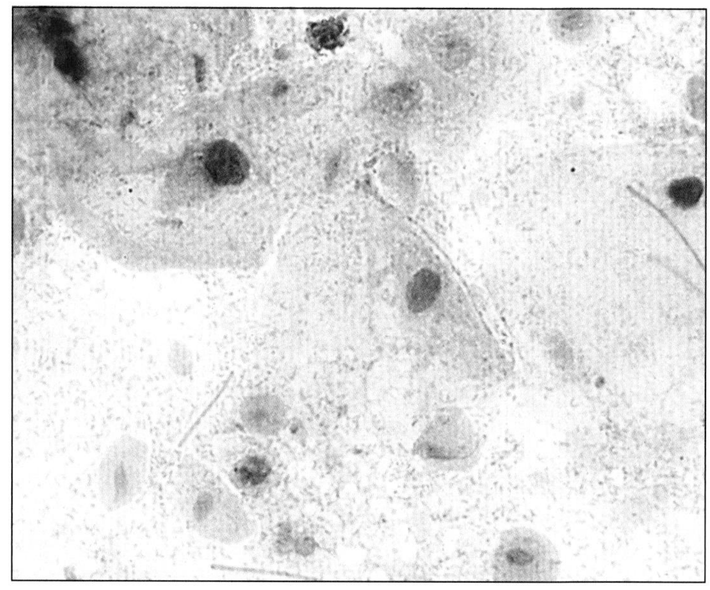

218. **Which of the following clinical settings would not typically support these cytologic findings?**

A. long-term estrogen therapy
B. late secretory phase of the menstrual cycle
C. pregnancy
D. late proliferative phase of the menstrual cycle

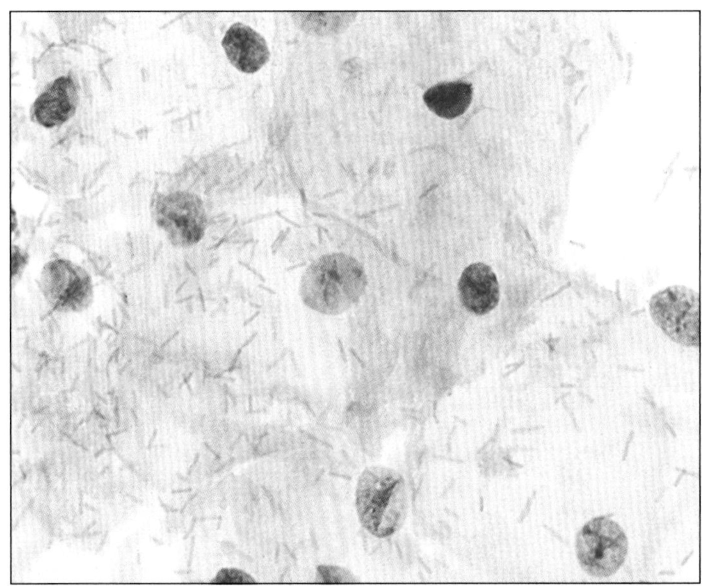

219. **Based on this histologic section, which cytomorphologic features would be seen?**

A. pleomorphism/caudate shape/opaque, irregular chromatin distribution
B. back-to-back glands/increased nuclear size/irregular chromatin distribution
C. spider-like/attenuated processes/regular chromatin distribution
D. cytoplasmic streaming/polygonal shape/regular chromatin distribution

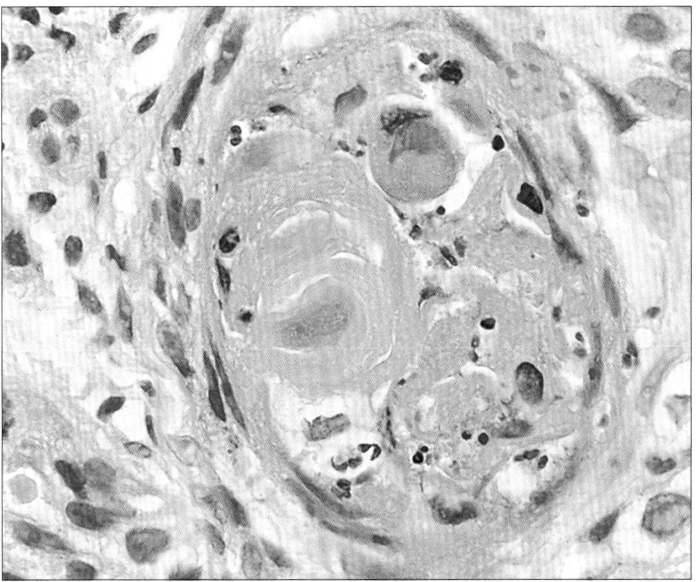

220. **Based on these cells, the differential diagnosis is:**

A. repair/squamous cell carcinoma
B. metaplastic dysplasia/immature metaplastic cells
C. adenocarcinoma in situ/carcinoma in situ
D. deep stromal cells/superficial stromal cells

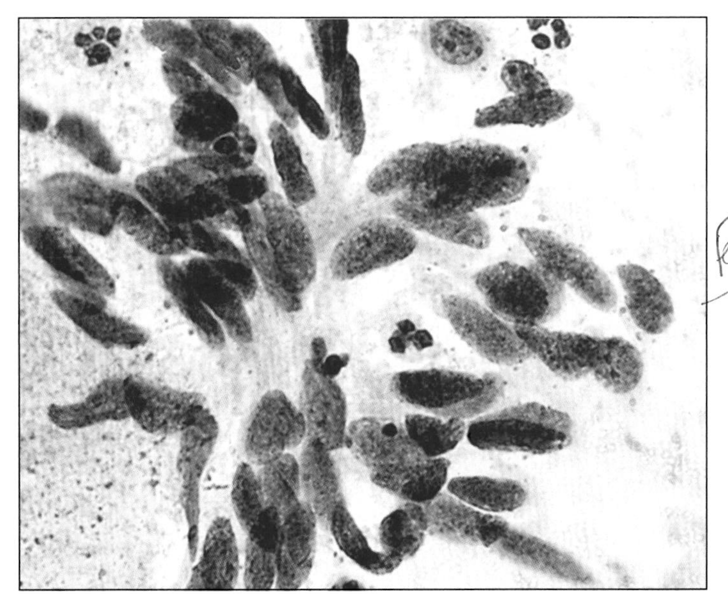

221. **These cells are from a 42-year-old woman who has a lesion on the anterior lip of the cervix. The cytologic pattern is most consistent with a diagnosis of:**

A. atypical repair
B. low-grade squamous intraepithelial lesion (LSIL)
C. endocervical adenocarcinoma
D. squamous cell carcinoma, keratinizing type

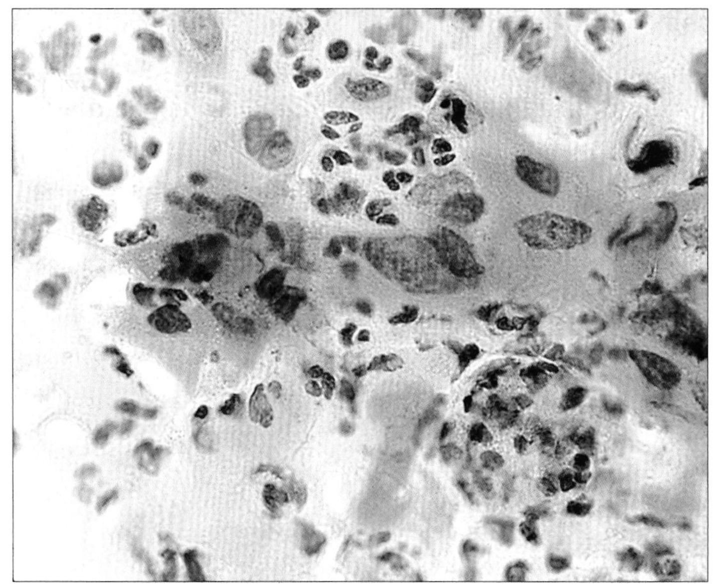

222. **These cells, found in a vaginal pool sample from a 58-year-old woman with a history of Stein-Leventhal syndrome of 20 years' duration, are diagnostic of:**

A. polycystic ovaries
B. endocervical repair
C. endometrial adenocarcinoma
D. deep atrophy

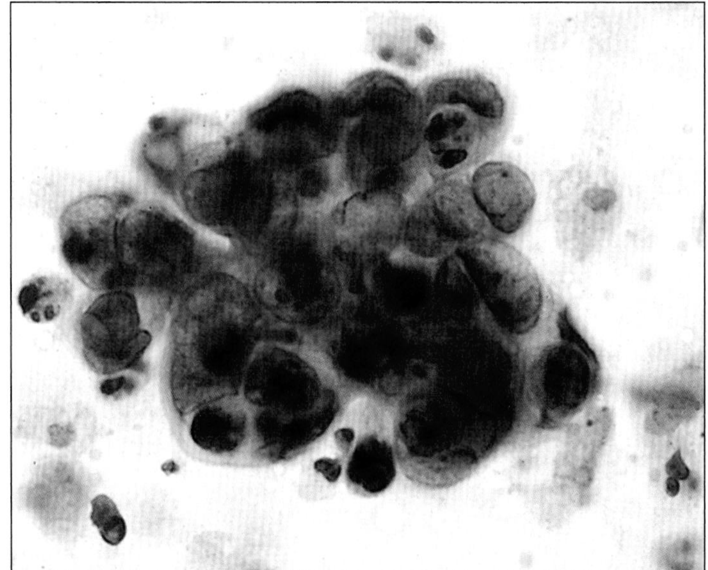

223. **These cells are identified in a cervical smear from a 39-year-old woman on day 9 of her menstrual cycle. They are most consistent with a diagnosis of:**

A. carcinoma in situ, intermediate cell type
B. carcinoma in situ, small cell type
C. small cell carcinoma
D. chronic lymphocytic cervicitis

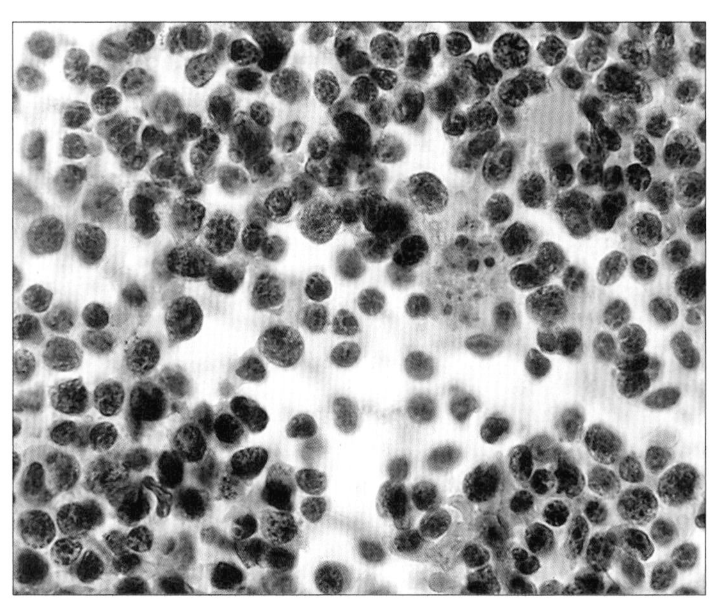

Boards

224. **Using the Bethesda System, this specimen would be classified as:**

A. satisfactory for evaluation but limited by contaminant
B. unsatisfactory for evaluation because of obscuring inflammation
C. unsatisfactory for evaluation because of poor fixation
D. unsatisfactory for evaluation because of drying artifact

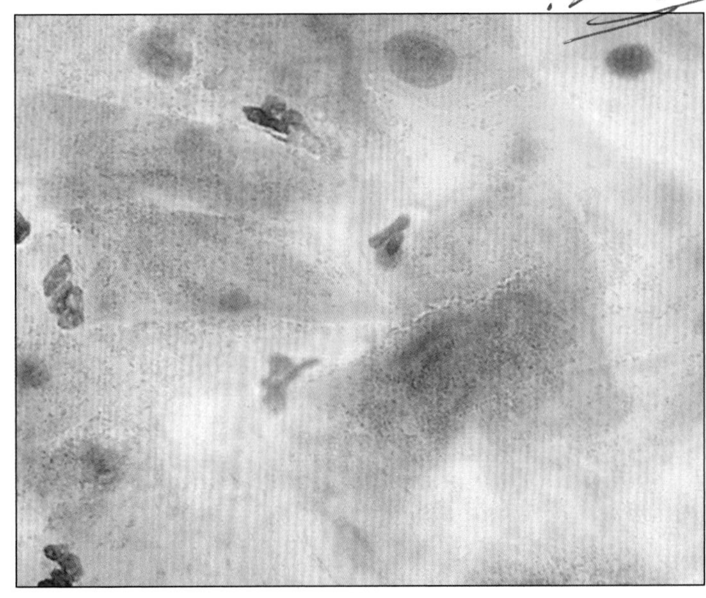

225. **These cells may represent an aspirate from the:**

A. Bartholin glands
B. pouch of Douglas
C. vulval apocrine glands
D. endometrial stroma

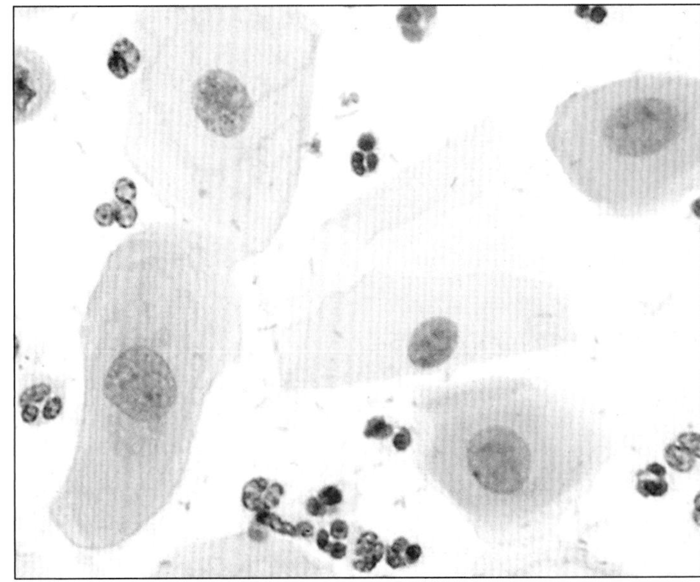

226. **These cells are from a 57-year-old woman with a history of irradiation for squamous cell carcinoma of the uterine cervix. The diagnosis is most consistent with:**

A. radiation changes
B. recurrent carcinoma
C. changes secondary to infection with human papillomavirus
D. carcinoma in situ

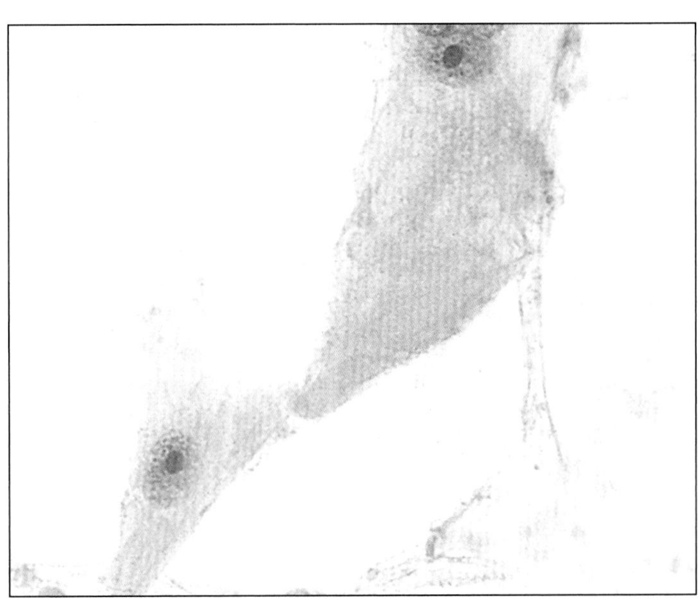

227. These cells represent a process that generally originates from the:

A. native squamous epithelium
B. transformation zone
C. endocervical area
D. endometrial area

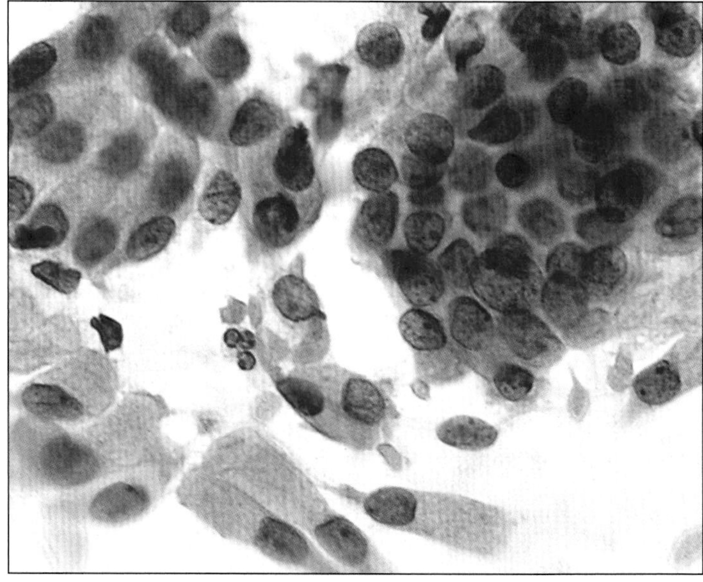

228. These cells represent normal cellular findings from the:

A. endocervix
B. cervical os
C. endometrium
D. fallopian tube

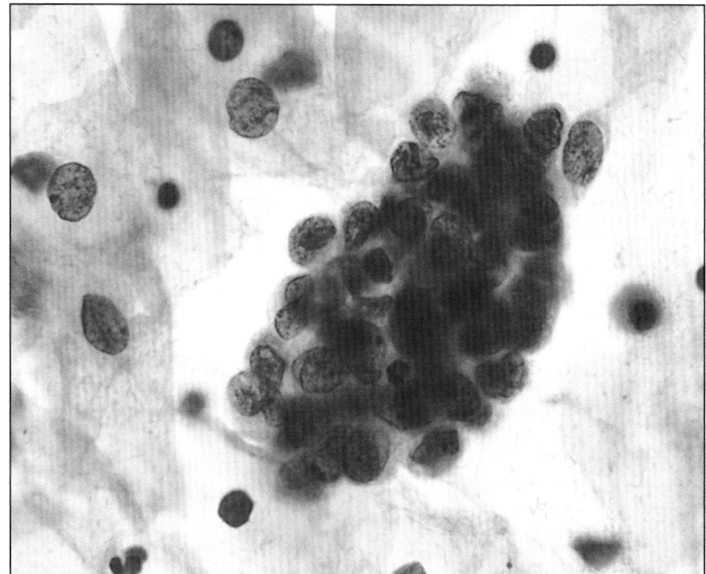

229. A 44-year-old woman presents with an enlarged abdominal girth. A complete work-up, including paracentesis, is performed. These cells, obtained from a cervical scrape and an endocervical brushing, suggest:

A. hepatocellular carcinoma
B. papillary serous cystadenocarcinoma, ovarian primary
C. mucinous cystadenocarcinoma, ovarian primary
D. renal cell carcinoma

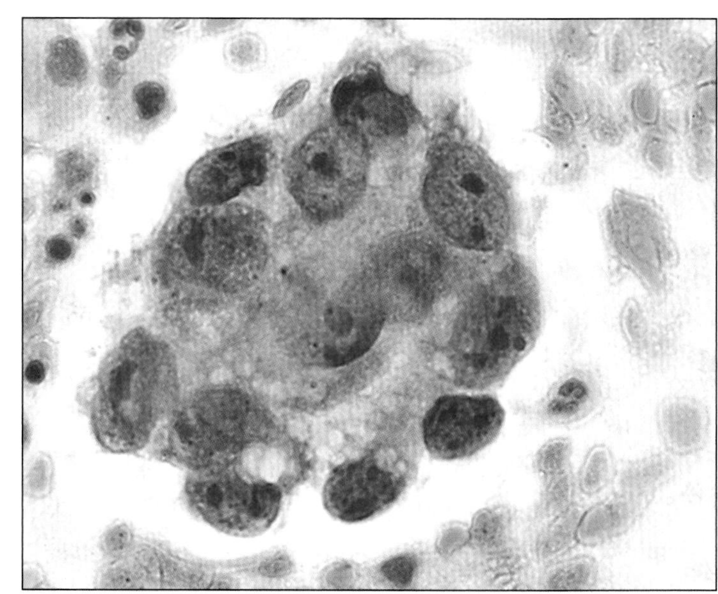

230. The clinical condition depicted in this ectocervical scraping from a 12-year-old girl is:

A. erosion
B. endometritis
C. retroflexion
D. cervicitis

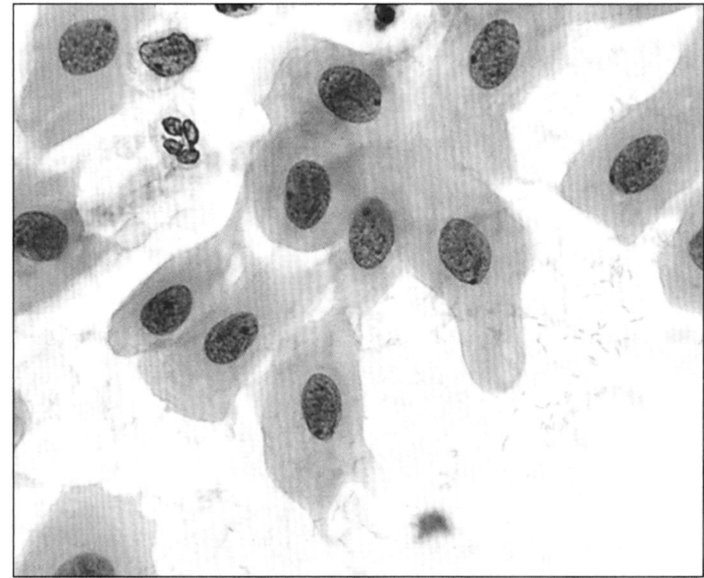

231. A 61-year-old post-menopausal woman presents with a profuse, watery discharge of 4 weeks' duration and lower abdominal cramps. Colposcopic evaluation, endocervical biopsy, and dilatation and curettage of the endometrium are non-confirmatory. The patient has no history of malignant disease. Based on these clinical and cytologic findings, the diagnosis suggests:

A. endometrial adenocarcinoma
B. adenocarcinoma, fallopian tube
C. dysgerminoma
D. endocervical adenocarcinoma

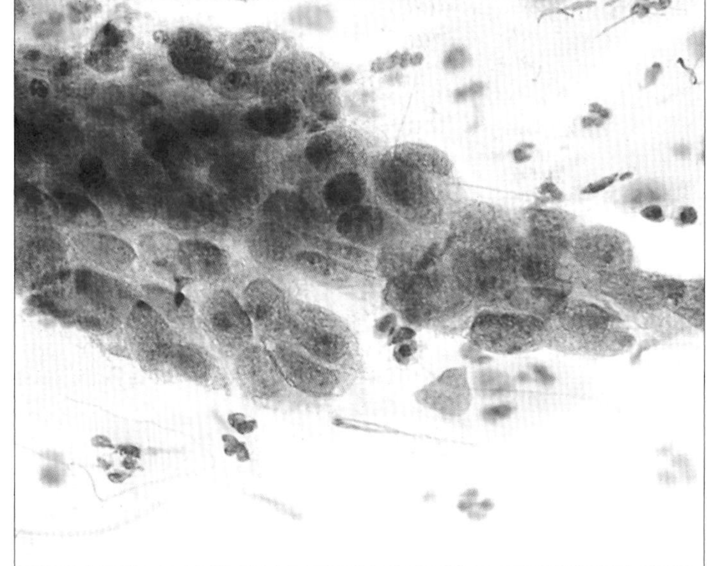

232. These cells are taken from a 43-year-old woman with a history of abnormal cytologic findings. What diagnosis and patient management guidelines apply?

A. HSIL; women with this diagnosis should undergo colposcopy and directed biopsy
B. ASC-US; ablation without histologic confirmation is considered unacceptable
C. LSIL; ablation without histologic confirmation is considered unacceptable
D. negative for squamous intraepithelial lesion; no management is necessary

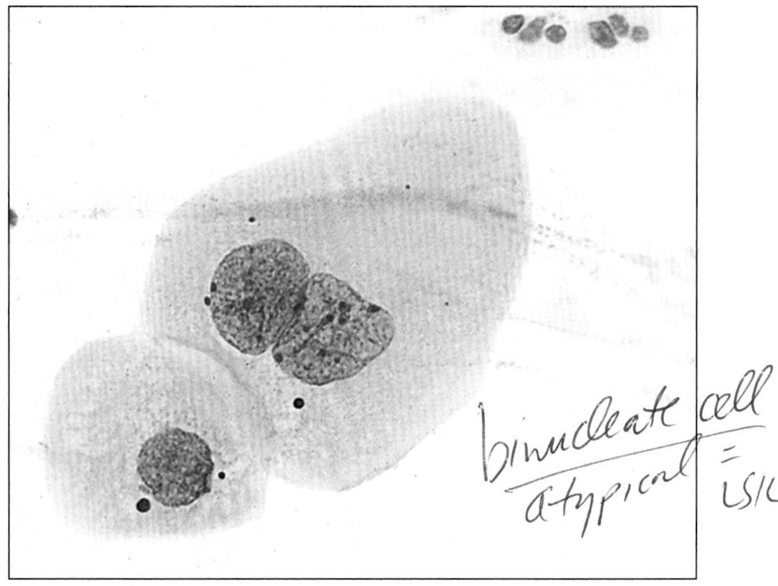

233. These cells are identified in a cellular sample obtained by an ectocervical scrape and an endocervical brushing from a 49-year-old patient complaining of a watery discharge outside of menses. The findings are most consistent with:

A. endocervical adenocarcinoma, grade III
B. metastatic colonic adenocarcinoma
C. endometrial adenocarcinoma, grade I
D. metastatic serous cystadenocarcinoma of the ovary

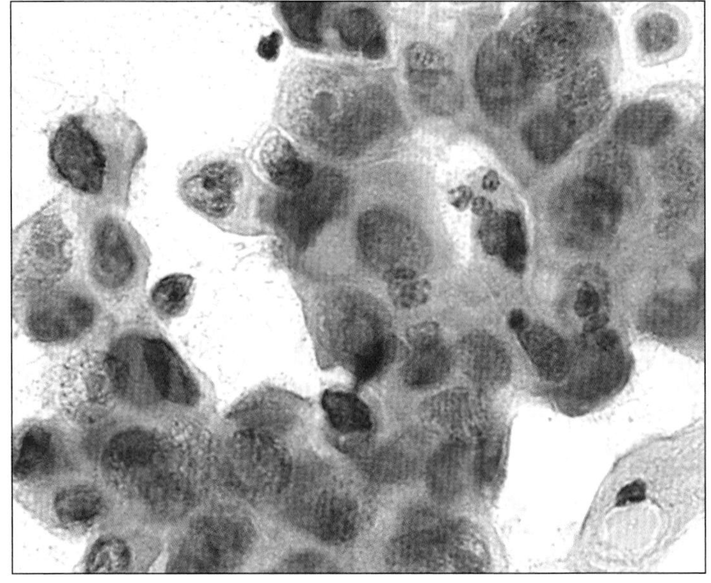

234. These cells are taken from a 22-year-old woman on day 18 of her menstrual cycle. The cytologic picture represents:

A. koilocytosis
B. degenerated squamous cells
C. navicular cells
D. changes secondary to Trichomonas infection

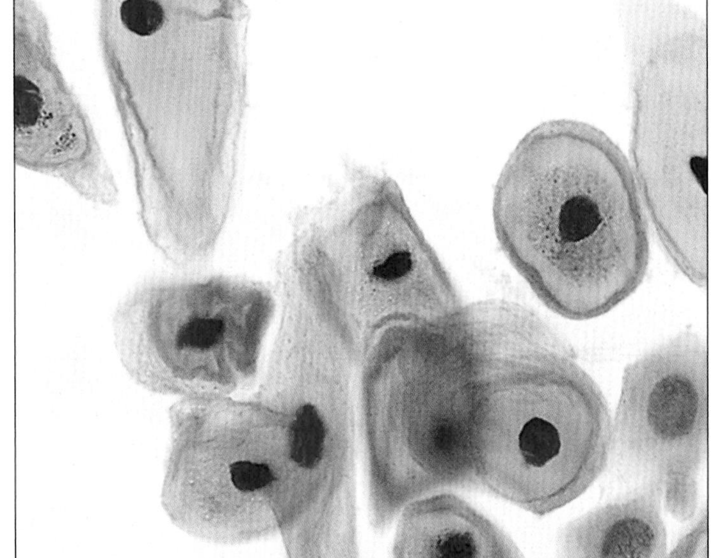

235. The cellular findings represent a vaginal/cervical/endocervical (VCE) sample taken from a 65-year-old woman with a recent onset of vaginal bleeding. The findings are most consistent with:

A. normal endometrial cells
B. endometrial hyperplasia
C. atypical endometrial hyperplasia
D. endometrial adenocarcinoma

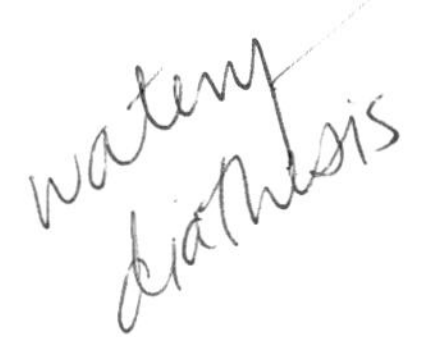

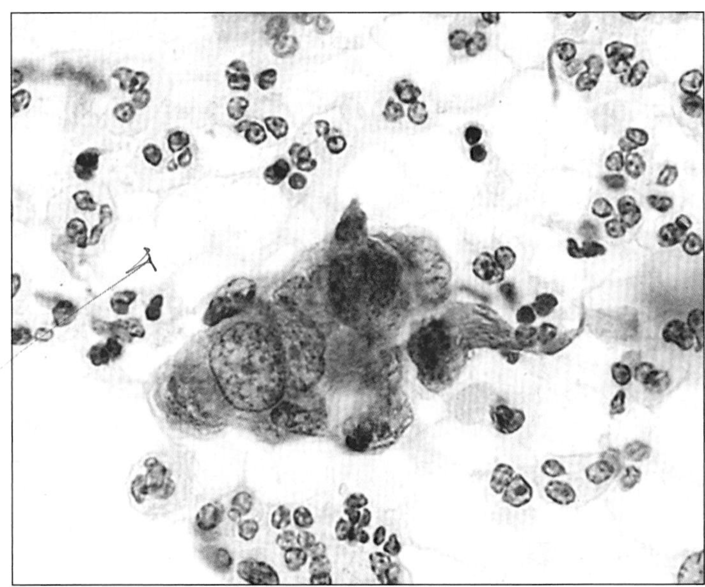

236. The cells depicted are derived from what type of squamous epithelium?

A. native squamous
B. mature metaplastic
C. endocervical glandular
D. immature metaplastic

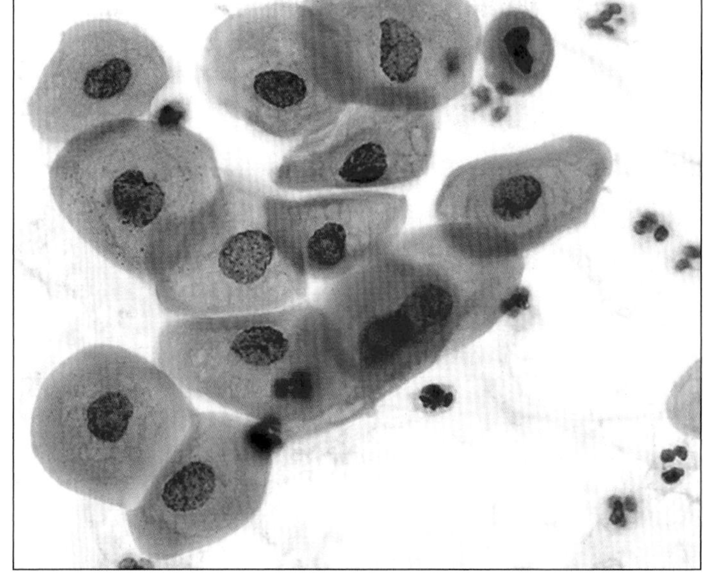

237. The presence of these cells in a vaginal smear suggests:

A. congenital abnormality; maldescension of the paramesonephric ducts
B. congenital abnormality; maldescension of the mesonephric ducts
C. possible exposure to diethylstilbestrol (DES) in utero
D. normal findings

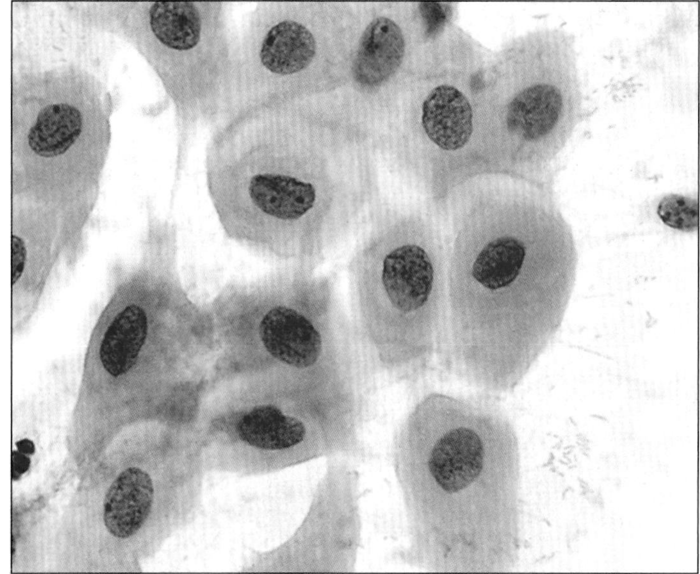

238. These cells were taken from a 40-year-old patient on day 6 of her menstrual cycle. They represent:

A. endometrial stromal cells, in cycle
B. endometrial stromal cells, out of cycle
C. endometrial glandular cells, in cycle
D. endometrial leiomyosarcoma

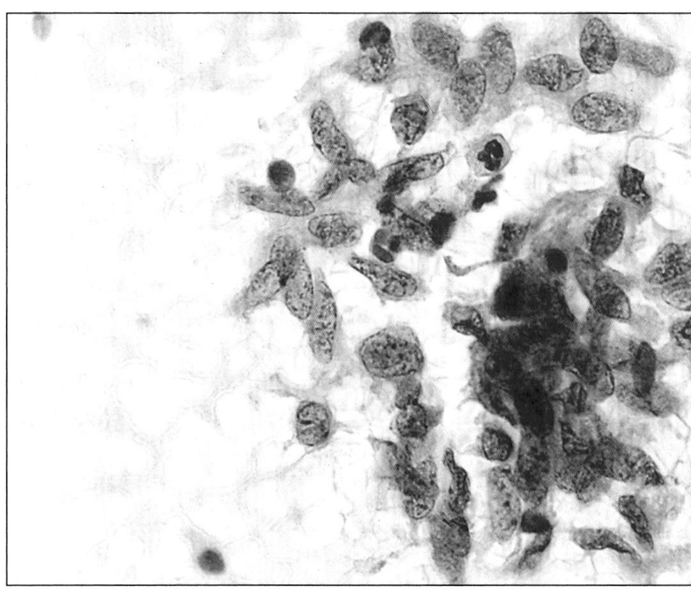

239. Using the 2002 Bethesda System, these cells would be classified as:

A. within normal limits, negative for squamous intraepithelial lesion
B. negative for squamous intraepithelial lesion, reactive cell changes seen
C. epithelial cell abnormality, atypical squamous cells of undetermined significance (ASC-US)
D. epithelial cell abnormality, LSIL

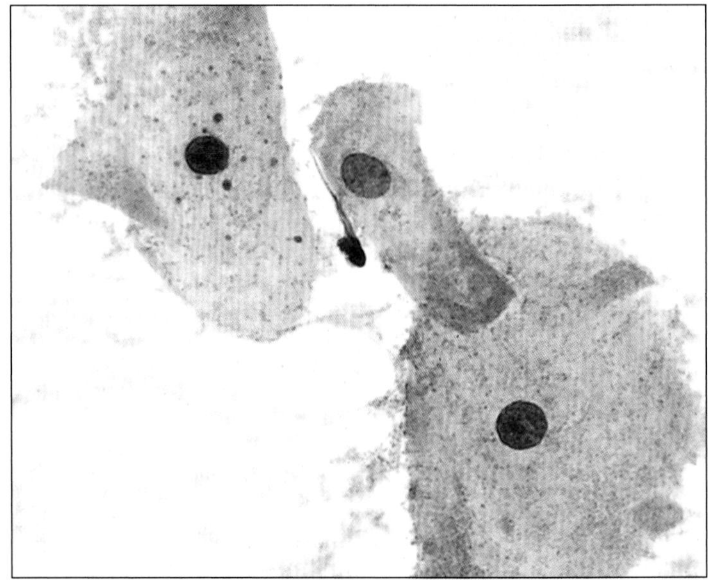

240. A 44-year-old woman, on day 18 of her menstrual cycle, presents for an annual Papanicolaou smear. Cytology suggests:

A. normal findings for clinical history
B. endometrial hyperplasia
C. endometrial adenocarcinoma
D. reparative/regenerative endocervical cells

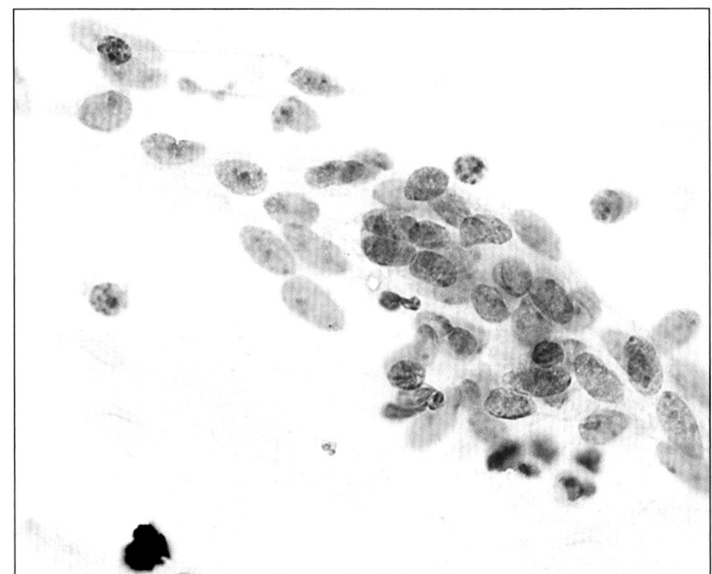

241. These cells are observed from a 65-year-old woman with recent onset of bleeding. The most appropriate diagnosis is:

A. endometrial adenocarcinoma, grade I
B. endometrial adenocarcinoma, grade III
C. mixed müllerian tumor, homologous type
D. mixed müllerian tumor, heterologous type

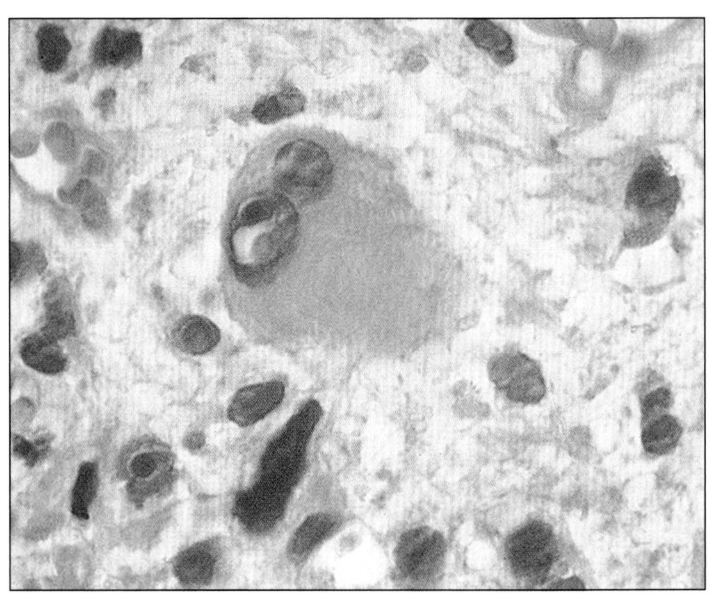

242. Which of the following is associated with these cytologic findings?

A. production of lactic acid
B. *Trichomonas vaginalis*
C. intracellular diplococcus
D. alkaline pH

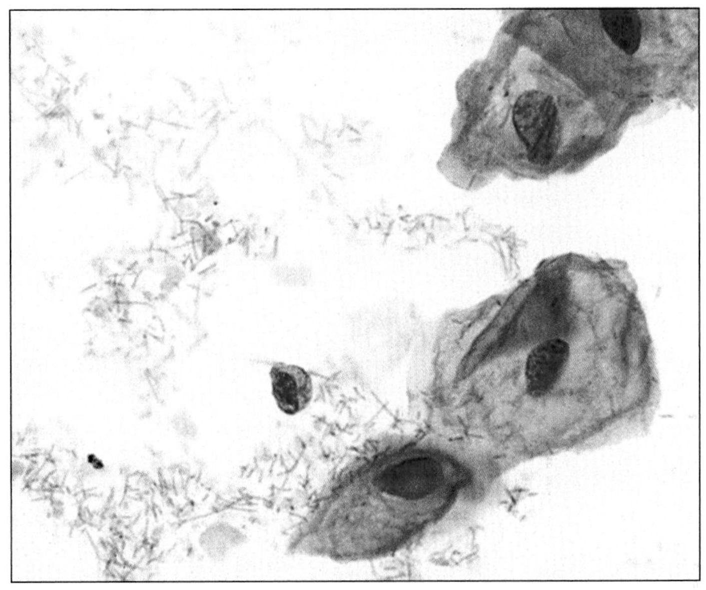

243. These cells are from a 62-year-old woman with recent complaints of vaginal bleeding. The diagnosis that correlates best with her clinical history is:

A. normal endocervical cells
B. endometrial adenocarcinoma, grade I
C. metastatic serous cystadenocarcinoma of the ovary
D. endometrial hyperplasia, suggest further evaluation

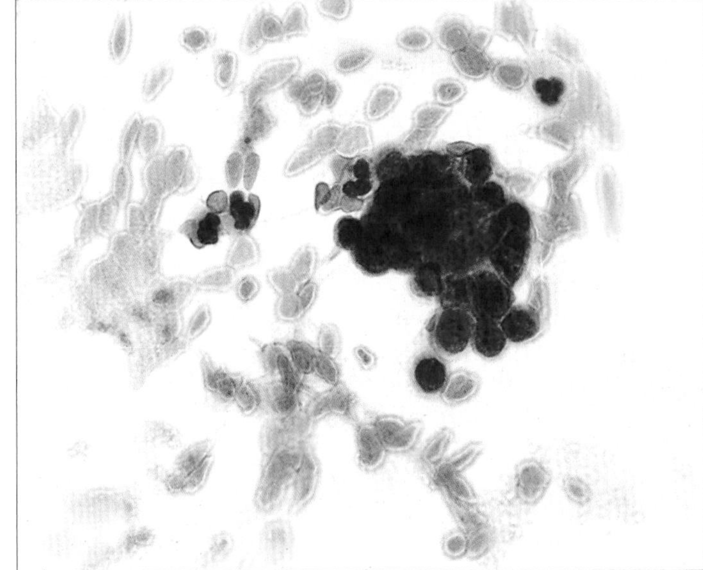

244. Which of the following terms best describes the depicted cellular findings?

A. air-dried
B. karyolytic
C. karyorrhectic
D. karyopyknotic

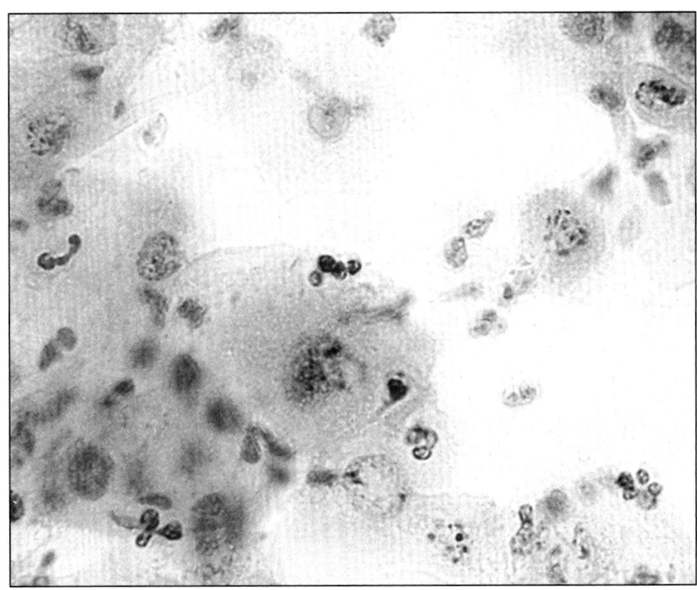

245. This cellular smear represents a cervical scrape and an endocervical brushing from a 33-year-old woman on day 12 of her menstrual cycle. This is diagnostic of infection with:

A. *Lactobacillus acidophilus*
B. *Chlamydia trachomatis*
C. *Gardnerella vaginalis*
D. *Actinomyces* sp.

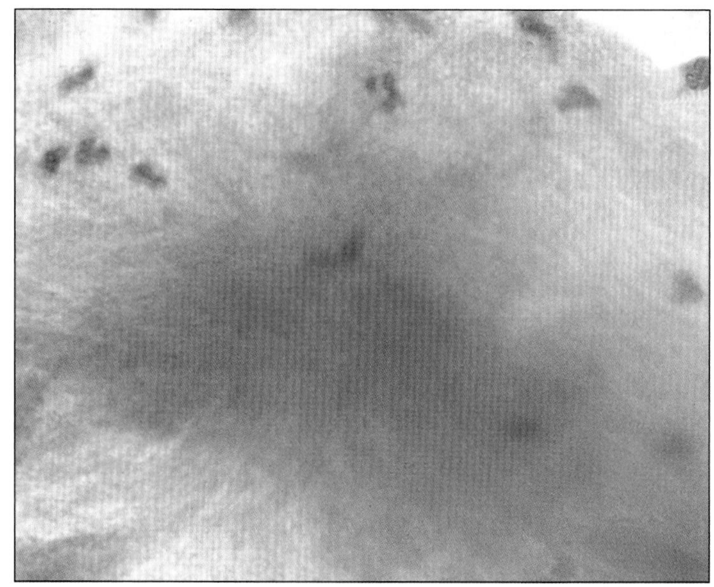

246. These cells are observed in a 44-year-old patient with dyschezia and dyspareunia. A CAT scan reveals a 3-cm lesion in the smooth muscular area of the uterus. A fine needle aspiration (FNA) was performed. The diagnosis is:

A. adenomyosis
B. metastatic cervical carcinoma
C. leiomyoma
D. leiomyosarcoma

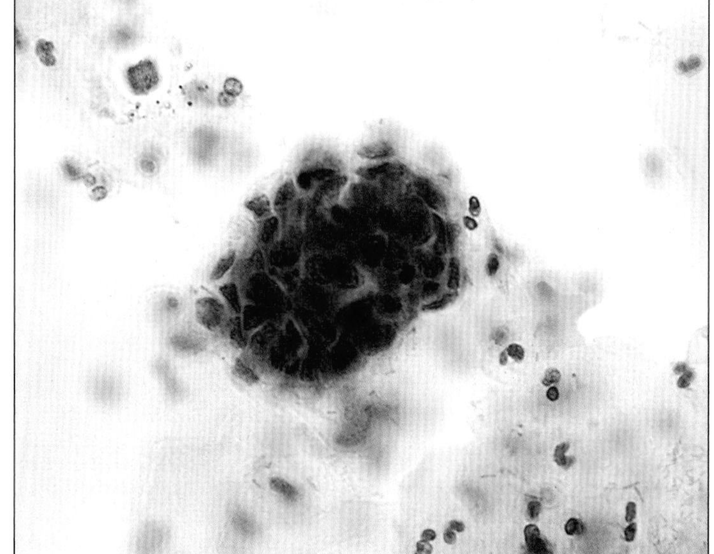

247. These cytologic findings are from a 34-year-old woman in her third trimester. What is the most appropriate clinical recommendation?

A. check placenta at delivery to rule out choriocarcinoma
B. deliver via cesarean
C. treat patient with penicillin
D. advise patient of the possibility of endometrial adenocarcinoma

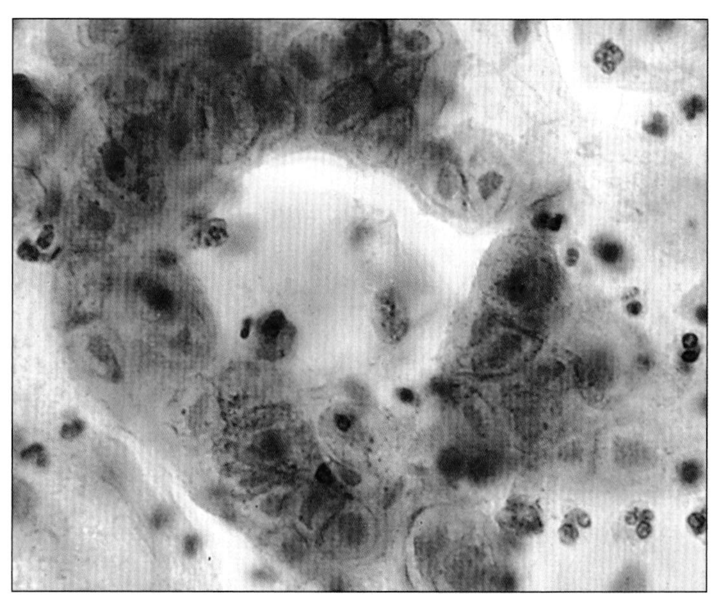

248. **Which clinical profile is associated with these cellular findings?**

A. endometritis
B. infection by a high-risk human papillomavirus viral subtype
C. unopposed estrogen stimulation
D. increased number of sexual partners

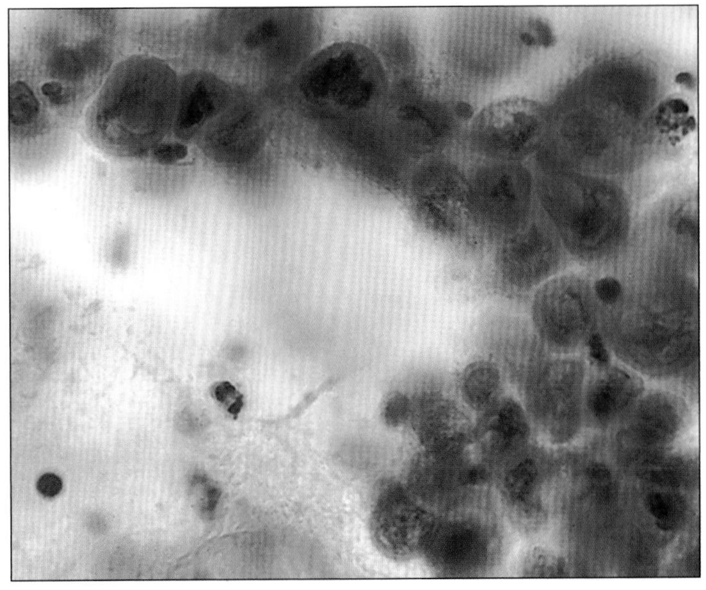

249. **A 36-year-old woman presents with infertility, menorrhagia, and recent onset of incontinence. A pelvic CT scan reveals a 2-cm mass involving the uterine wall with direct extension into the left ureter. Represented is an endometrial aspirate. The diagnosis is:**

A. endometrial stromal sarcoma
B. endometrial adenocarcinoma, grade III
C. mixed müllerian tumor, heterologous type
D. leiomyosarcoma

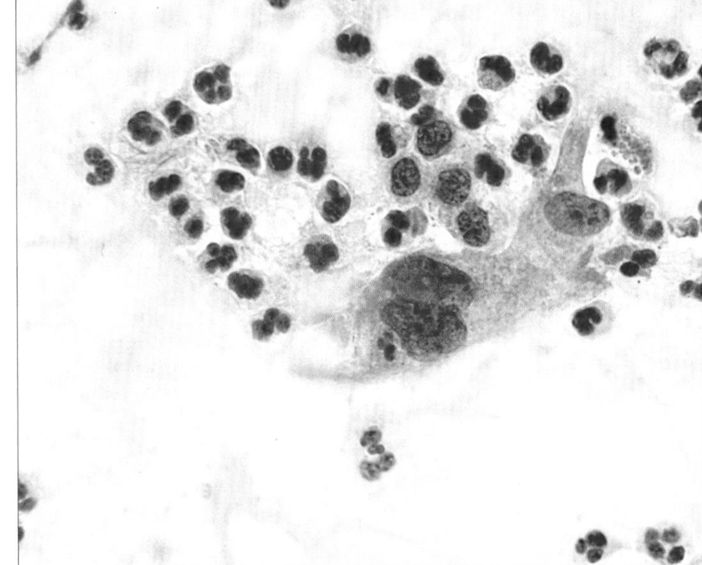

250. **The clinical findings associated with this vaginal/cervical scrape specimen are:**

A. frothy, yellow-green discharge/strawberry cervix
B. white, curd-like discharge/normal cervix
C. absence of discharge/leukoplakia on cervix
D. menorrhagia/exophytic mass

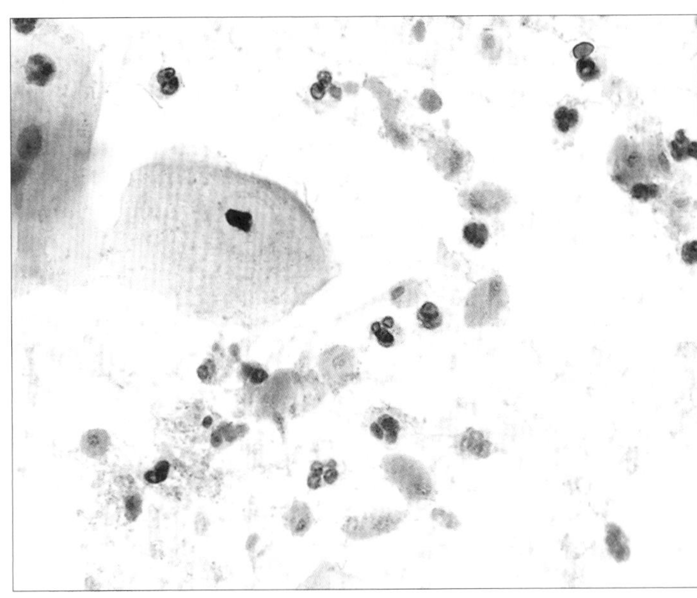

251. The cells of this lateral vaginal wall scraping are compatible with which of the following conditions?

A. Stein-Leventhal syndrome
B. granulosa-theca cell tumor
C. hepatic insufficiency
D. Turner syndrome

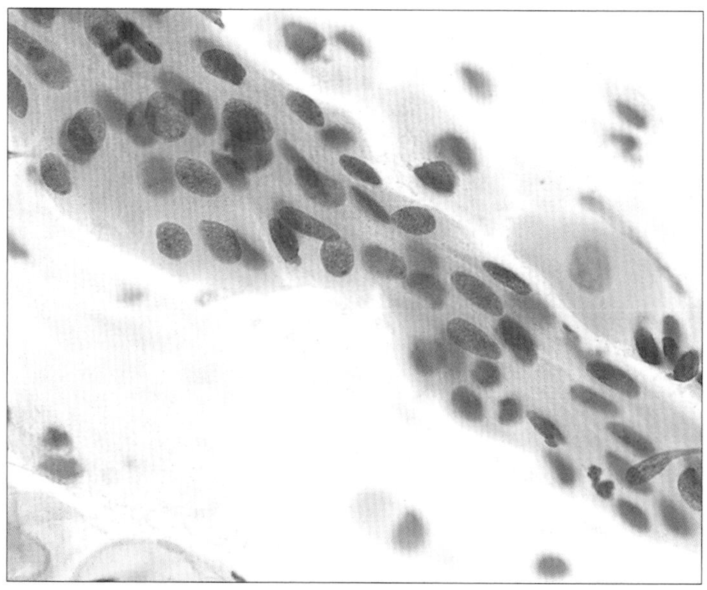

252. The diagnostic criteria that differentiate these cells from those of carcinoma in situ are:

A. finely granular, evenly distributed chromatin
B. nucleoli, diathesis, irregular chromatin distribution
C. hyperchromasia, regular chromatin distribution
D. koilocytic changes, parakeratosis

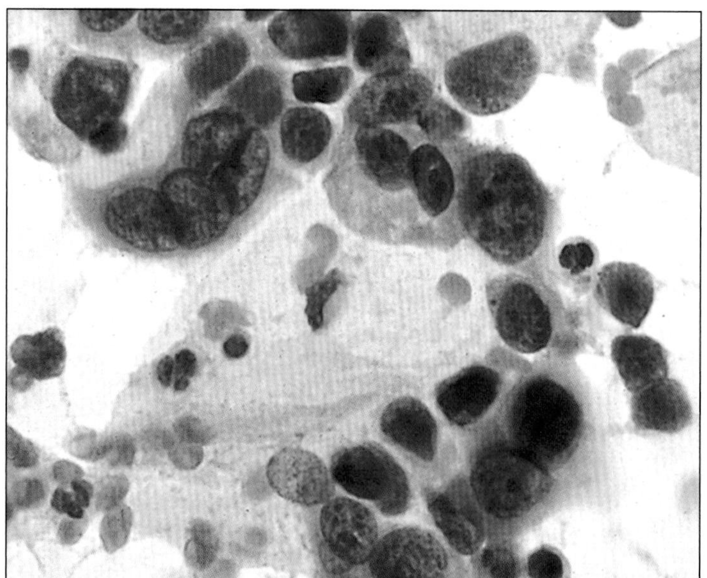

253. These cells are from a 34-year-old woman. Based on the morphologic findings, what is their likely source?

A. endometrium
B. internal cervical os
C. endocervical canal
D. vagina

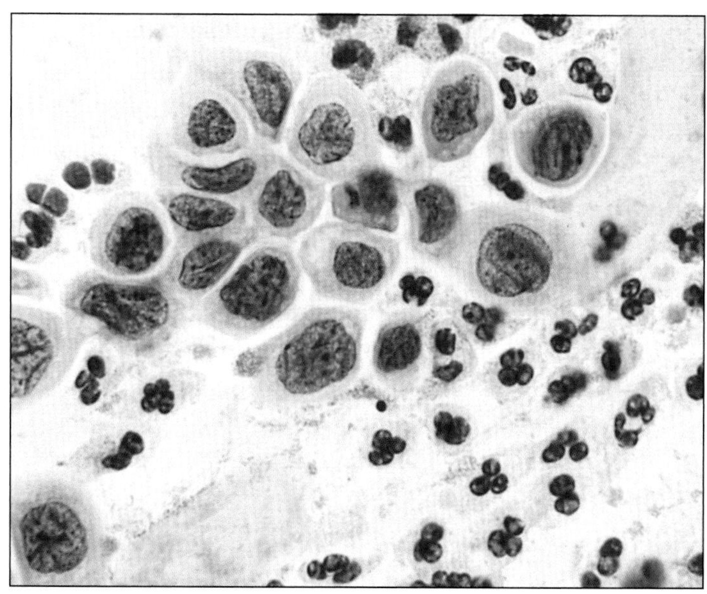

254. These cells are observed in a vaginal/cervical/endocervical sample taken from an 18-year-old woman. The findings are most consistent with:

A. LSIL, mild nonkeratinizing dysplasia
B. atypical glandular cells of undetermined significance (AGUS)
C. LSIL, mild metaplastic dysplasia
D. squamous atypia/mature metaplastic ASC-US (mimicking mature native squames)

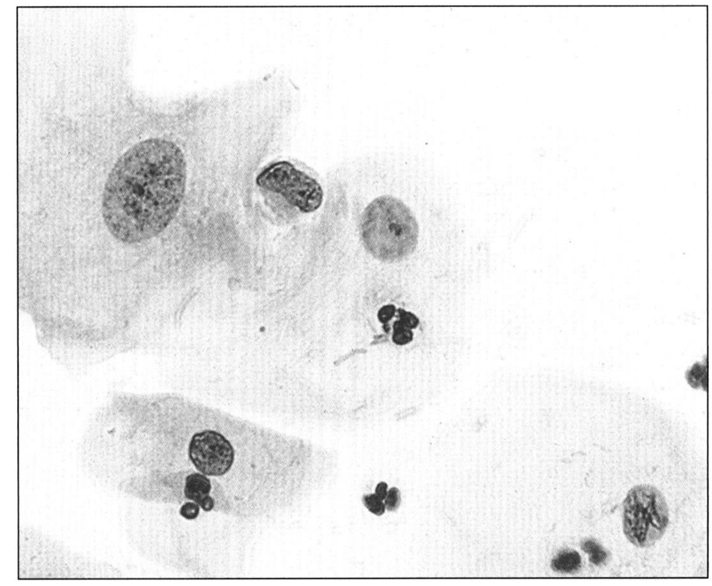

255. Compared with cells of other lesions arising within the cervix, the mitotic rate of this cell type is considered:

A. high
B. low
C. variable
D. equal

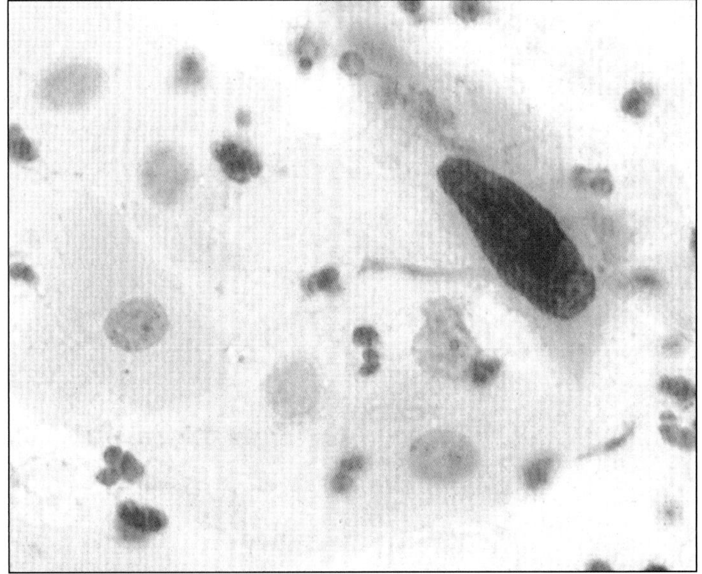

256. A 26-year-old woman was treated with electrocautery for a cervical intraepithelial neoplasia (CIN II) 6 months before collection of these cells. The cells were collected on day 16 of a normal 30-day estrous cycle. The cellular changes are suggestive of:

A. residual dysplasia, not otherwise specified
B. invasive squamous cell carcinoma
C. CIN II
D. reparative/regenerative changes secondary to therapy

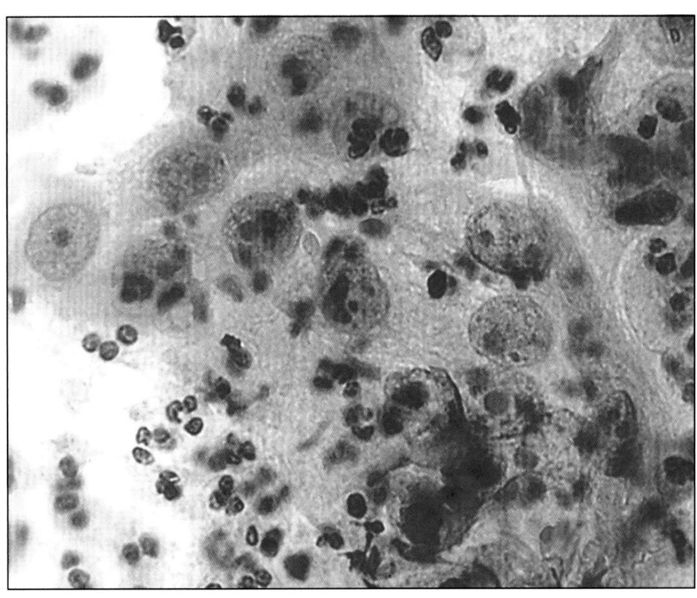

257. **These cellular findings are representative of:**

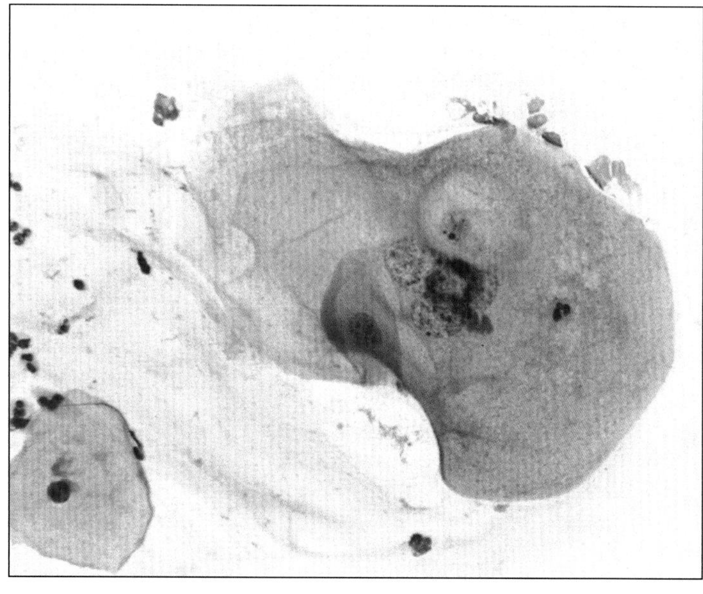

A. HSIL
B. radiation-induced cell changes
C. squamous cell carcinoma
D. parakeratosis

258. **A 33-year-old woman presents with dysfunctional uterine bleeding. These cells were collected with conventional cervical/endocervical brushings. The findings are most consistent with:**

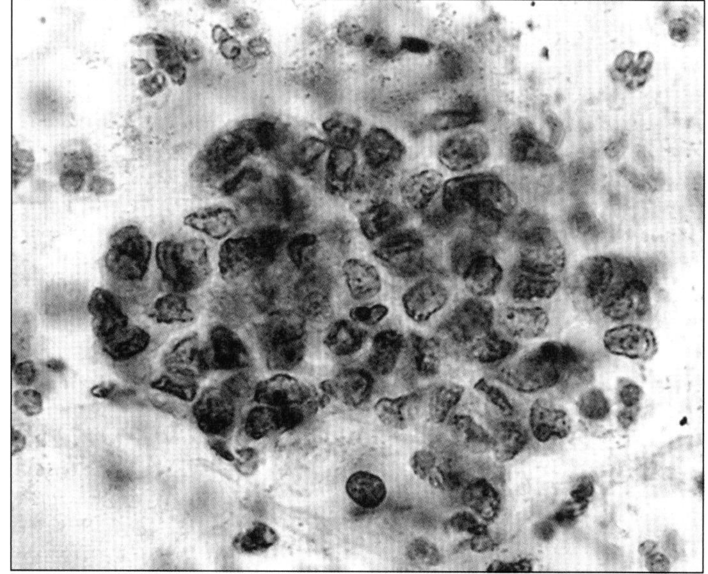

A. endometrial adenocarcinoma, grade I
B. endometrial polyp
C. normal endometrial cells, possibly associated with endometrial hyperplasia
D. endometrial adenocarcinoma, grade IV

259. **What percentage of the epithelial thickness is replaced in situ given these cytologic findings?**

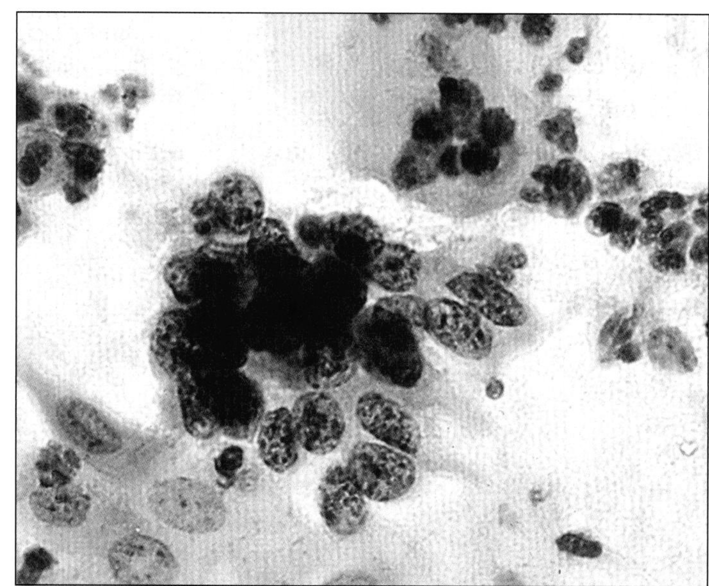

A. 25%
B. 50%
C. 75%
D. 100%

260. These cells represent a cervical/endocervical smear from a 66-year-old woman. The cytology represents:

A. atypia of atrophy
B. *Chlamydia trachomatis* infection
C. LSIL, koilocytosis associated with HPV
D. navicular cells

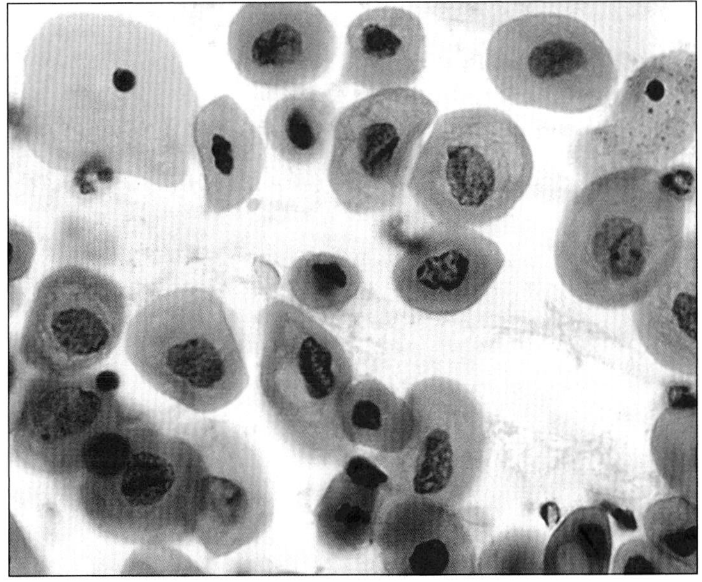

261. These cells are from a 40-year-old woman, grava 8, para 4, abortus 4, LMP 9 days ago. The findings are consistent with:

A. normal endometrial cells
B. atypical endometrial hyperplasia
C. reactive/reparative endocervical cells
D. endometrial adenocarcinoma

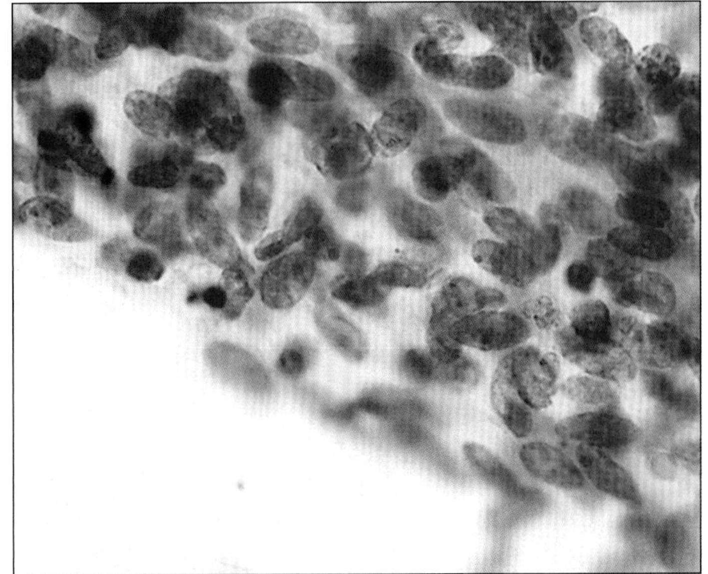

262. These cells are derived from a vaginal/cervical/ endocervical scraping taken from a 31-year-old woman, last menstrual period 12 days ago. The findings are most consistent with:

A. HSIL, moderate nonkeratinizing dysplasia
B. LSIL, mild nonkeratinizing dysplasia
C. HSIL, moderate metaplastic dysplasia
D. LSIL, mild metaplastic dysplasia

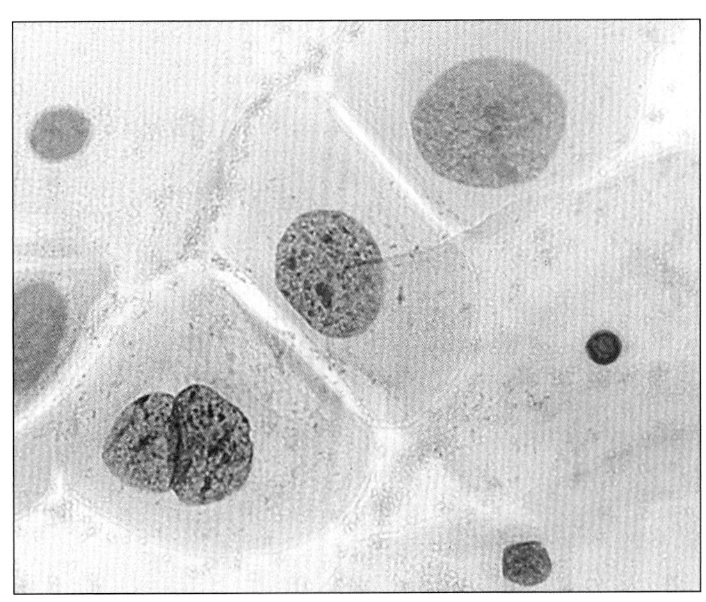

263. These cells would most likely originate from the:

A. ectocervix
B. mature metaplastic transformational zone
C. immature metaplastic transformational zone
D. endocervical glandular epithelium

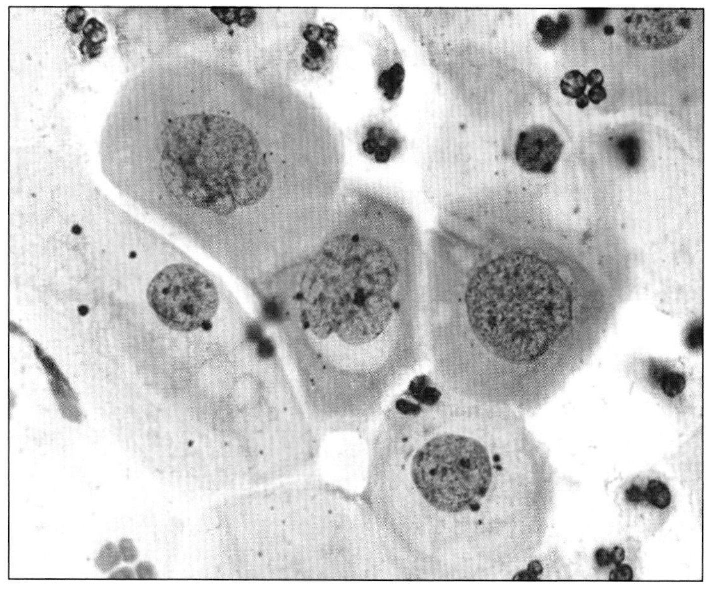

264. The hallmark for diagnosing the lesion represented is the presence of:

A. fine chromatin
B. hyperchromasia
C. irregular chromatin
D. cytoplasmic streaming

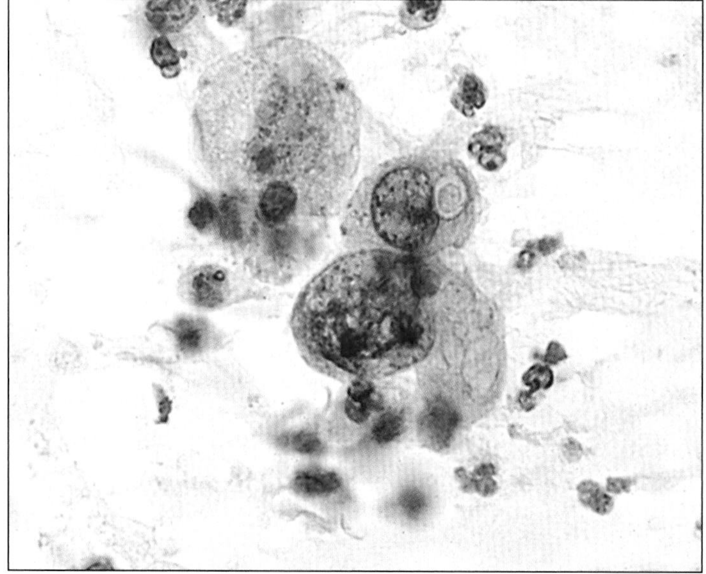

265. These cells represent a cervical specimen from a 48-year-old woman with an anterior lip cervical lesion. The findings are most consistent with:

A. squamous cell carcinoma, keratinizing type
B. HSIL, moderate dysplasia, keratinizing type
C. dyskeratosis associated with HPV
D. poorly differentiated squamous cell carcinoma

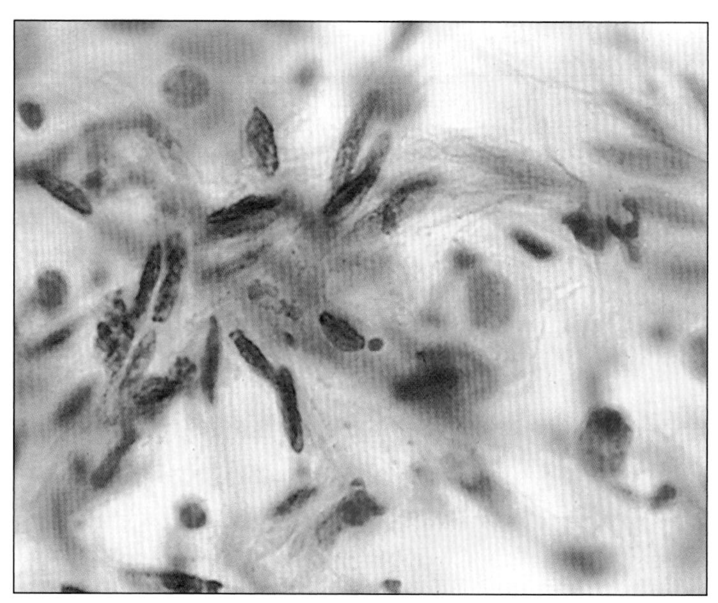

266. What feature becomes less predictable as the depicted lesion becomes poorly differentiated?

A. pleomorphism
B. anisocytosis
C. anisonucleosis
D. macronucleoli

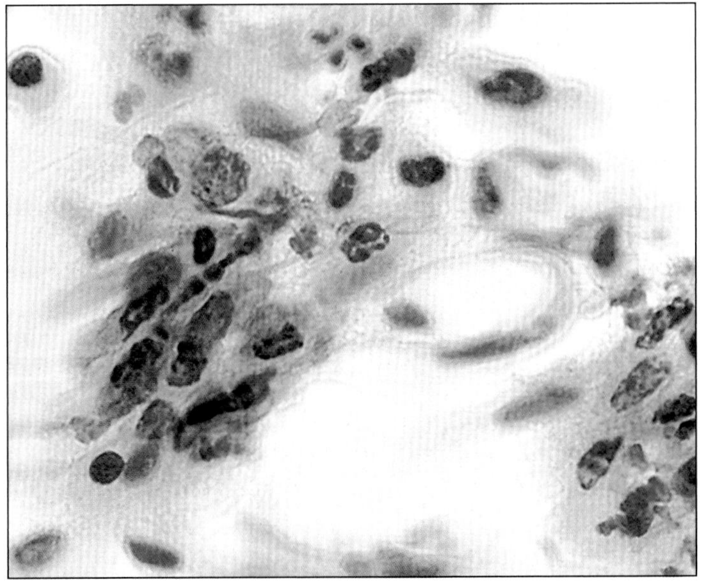

267. These cells are found 6 months after irradiation therapy for stage IB squamous cell carcinoma of the uterine cervix. Their presence indicates:

A. hyperkeratosis, a benign cellular change related to the irradiation therapy
B. a hyperdifferentiation that places the patient at a higher risk for post-irradiation dysplasia
C. normal findings
D. unrelated to the history

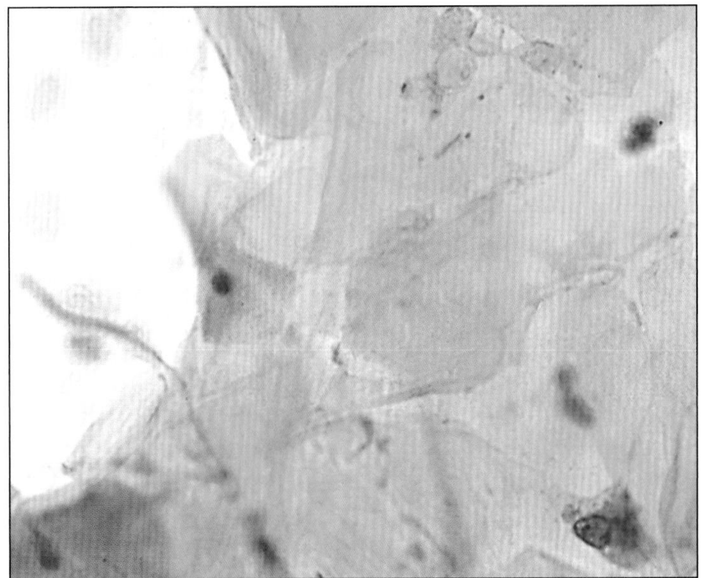

268. These cells are best differentiated from an intraepithelial squamous lesion by:

A. strips of pseudostratified or "feathering" epithelium in glandular lesions
B. elevated nuclear-to-cytoplasmic (N/C) ratios in squamous lesions
C. increased hyperchromasia in squamous lesions
D. the presence of nucleoli in squamous lesions

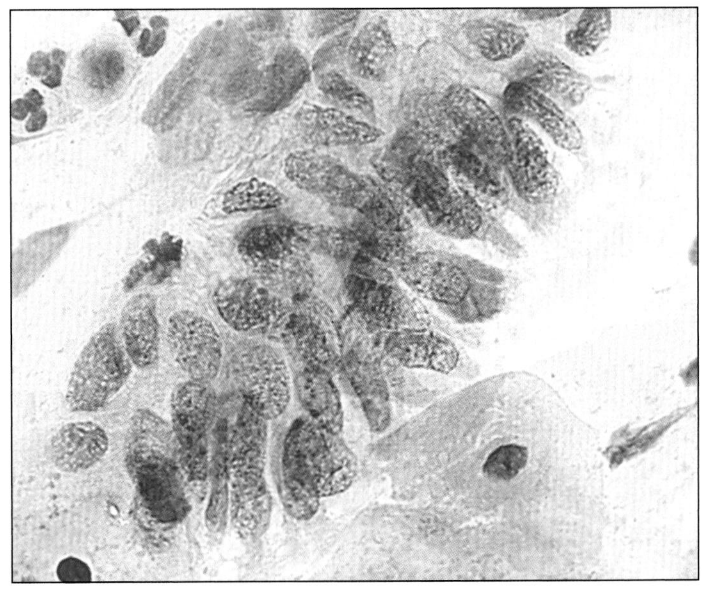

269. One of the best criteria for distinguishing these cells from their immediate precursor is:

A. coarse chromatin
B. diathesis
C. nucleoli
D. hyperchromasia

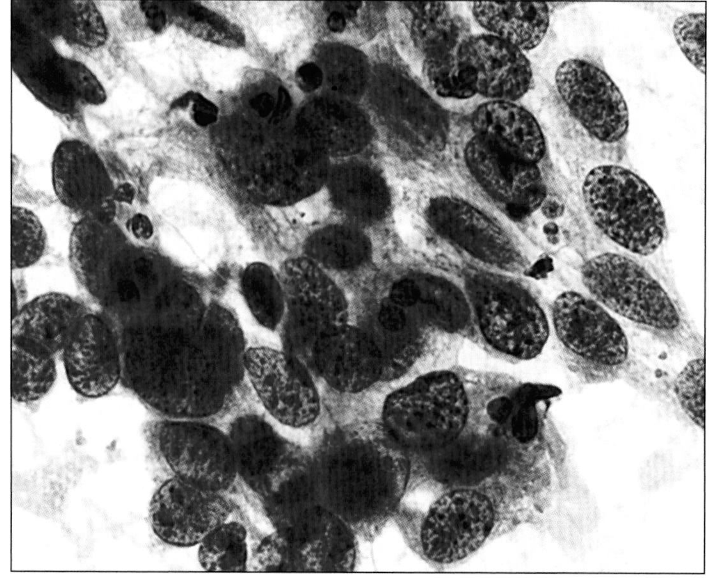

270. How common is the lesion shown relative to a nonkeratinizing squamous lesion?

A. it is more common
B. it is less common
C. they have about the same frequency
D. itt cannot be determined with the information provided

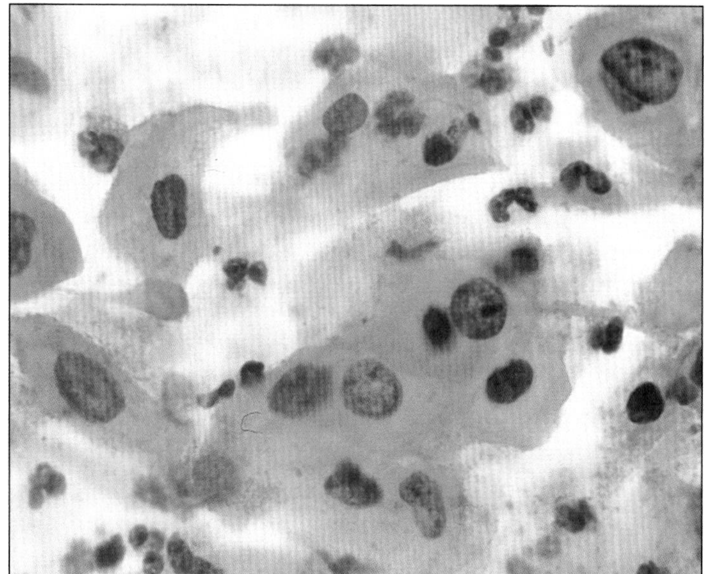

271. Which of the following criteria are helpful in establishing the diagnosis in this photomicrograph?

A. predominantly single cells
B. low nuclear-to-cytoplasmic (N/C) ratio
C. hyperchromatic crowded groups
D. rosettes, acinar morphology, feathering cytoplasmic borders

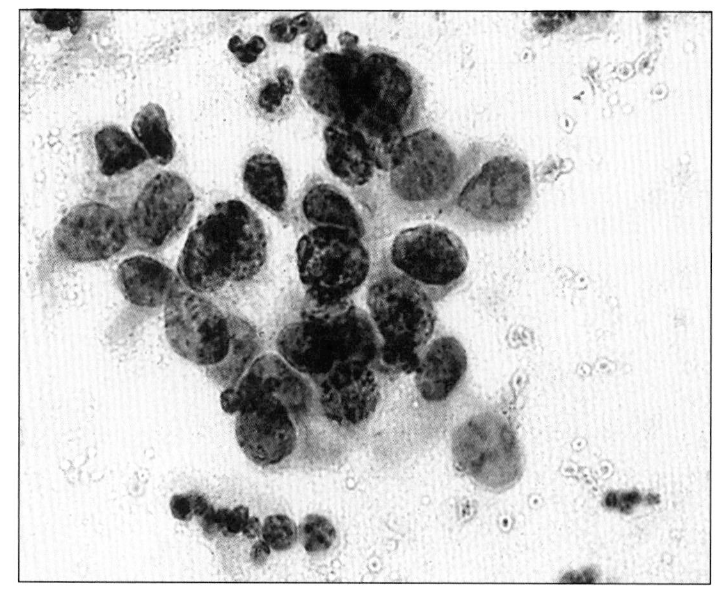

272. **These cells are from a 35-year-old patient with a history of normal Papanicolaou smears. The cellular findings are suggestive of:**

A. reserve cell hyperplasia
B. small cell carcinoma in situ
C. reactive endocervical cells
D. endocervical adenocarcinoma in situ

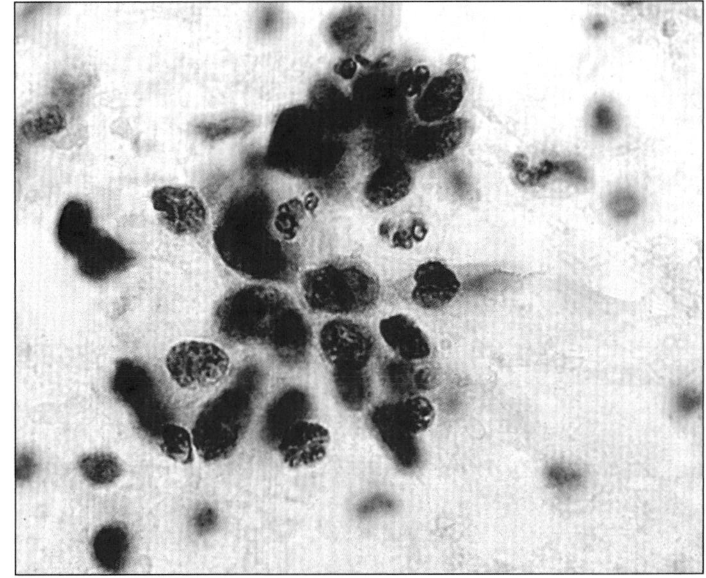

273. **These cells are observed in a 32-year-old woman, 6 months postpartum, with a history of HPV infection. The findings are most consistent with:**

A. LSIL, mild dysplasia with associated HPV infection
B. parakeratosis
C. dyskeratotic cells related to HPV infection
D. atrophic vaginitis

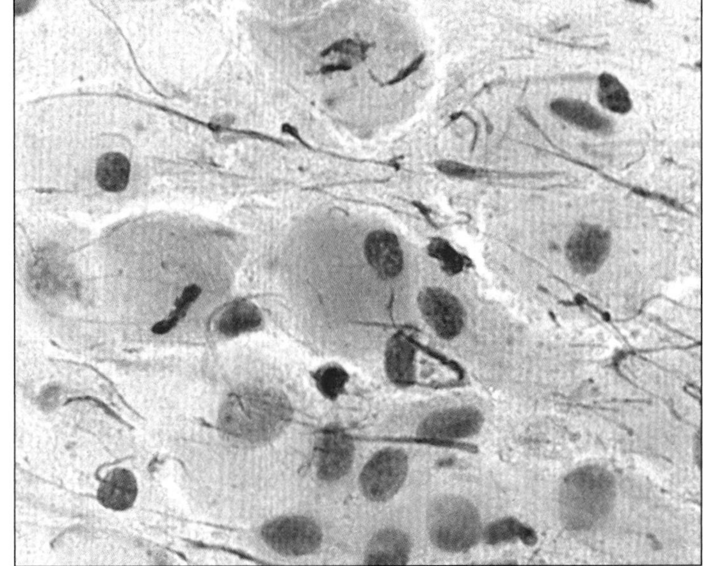

274. **The origin of these cells in a cervical/vaginal smear taken from a 44-year-old patient is most likely:**

A. vaginal, immature metaplastic
B. vaginal, endocervical
C. ectocervical, immature metaplastic
D. ectocervical, mature metaplastic

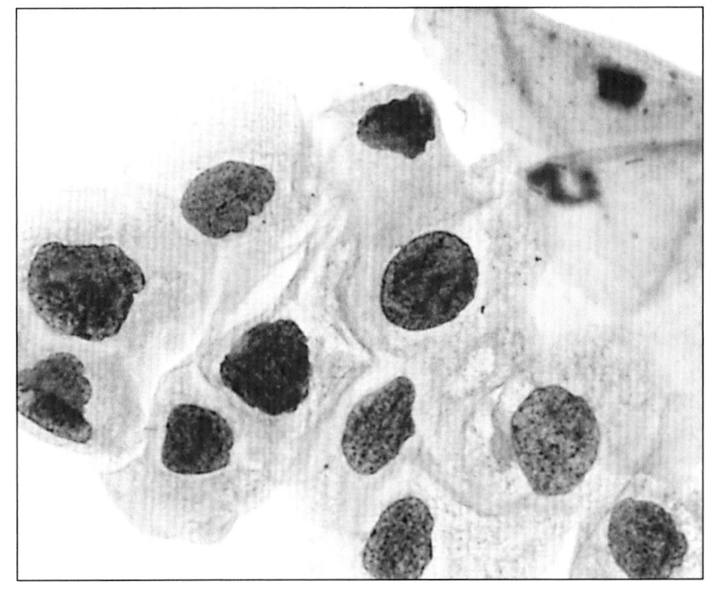

275. Cytologically, this tissue section is best characterized as:

A. possessing macronucleoli
B. pleomorphic, caudate, spindled
C. possessing large, round-to-oval cells with anisocytosis
D. isodiametric

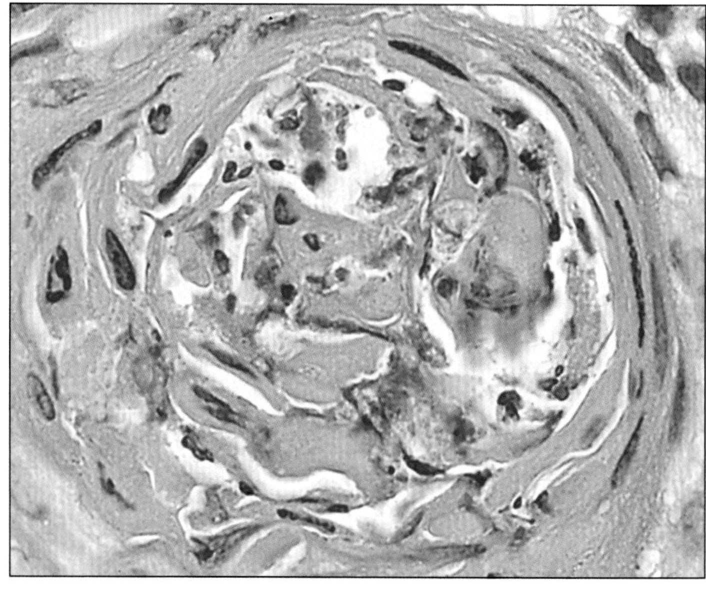

276. What histologic growth pattern may be associated with these cellular findings?

A. endophytic
B. verrucous
C. flat
D. inverted

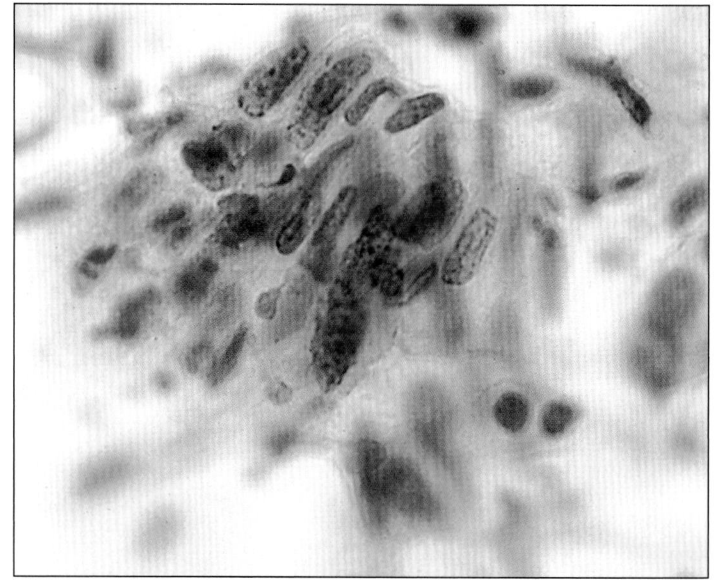

277. Based on these cytologic findings, is it possible to predict the histologic growth pattern of the lesion?

A. yes
B. no
C. not sure based on these cellular changes

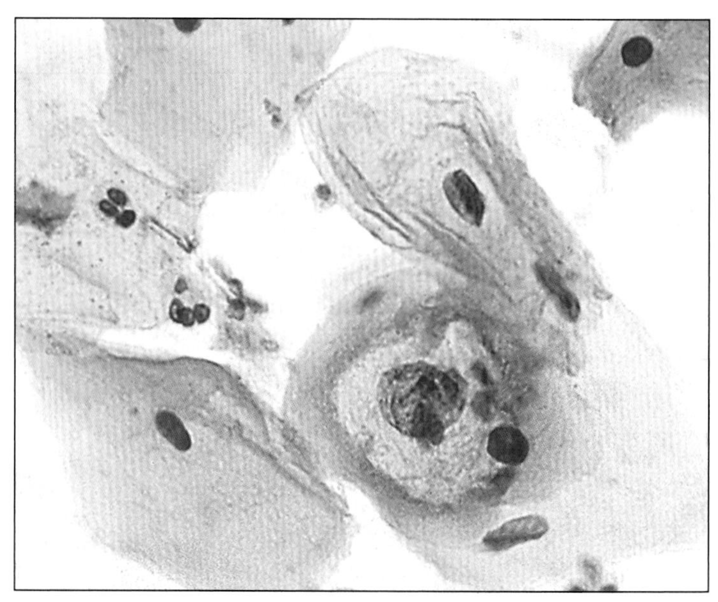

278. These cells, representative of a cervical scraping and an endocervical brushing, are diagnostic of:

A. cervical intraepithelial lesion, grade III
B. small cell squamous cell carcinoma
C. nonkeratinizing squamous carcinoma, moderately differentiated
D. mixed mesodermal tumor, homologous variety

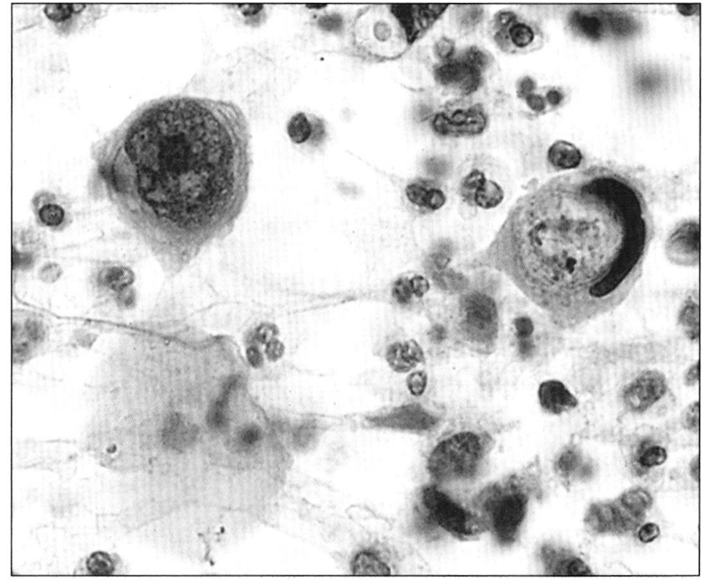

279. These cells are found in a 26-year-old patient, LMP 8 days ago. The findings are consistent with:

A. follicular cervicitis
B. pseudoparakeratosis/microglandular hyperplasia
C. degenerated neutrophils
D. small cell histiocytes

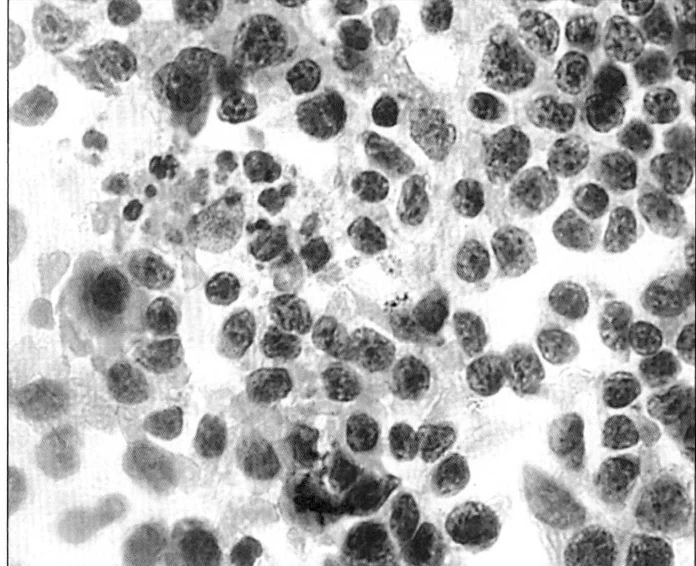

280. These cells represent a cervical scraping from a 33-year-old woman with a friable lesion within the endocervical canal. The findings are consistent with:

A. reactive/reparative reaction
B. carcinoma in situ, large cell type
C. sarcoma, NOS
D. squamous cell carcinoma, nonkeratinizing type

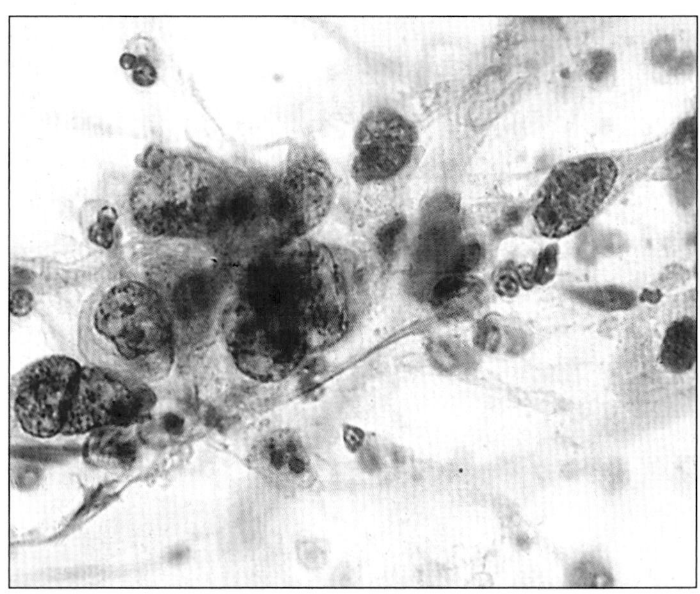

281. **These cells are from a patient, after radiation therapy for squamous cell carcinoma, grade I. She recently underwent hormonal therapy for vaginal atrophy. The diagnosis is most consistent with:**

A. folic acid deficiency
B. atrophic vaginitis
C. benign radiation-induced cellular changes
D. post-irradiation dysplasia

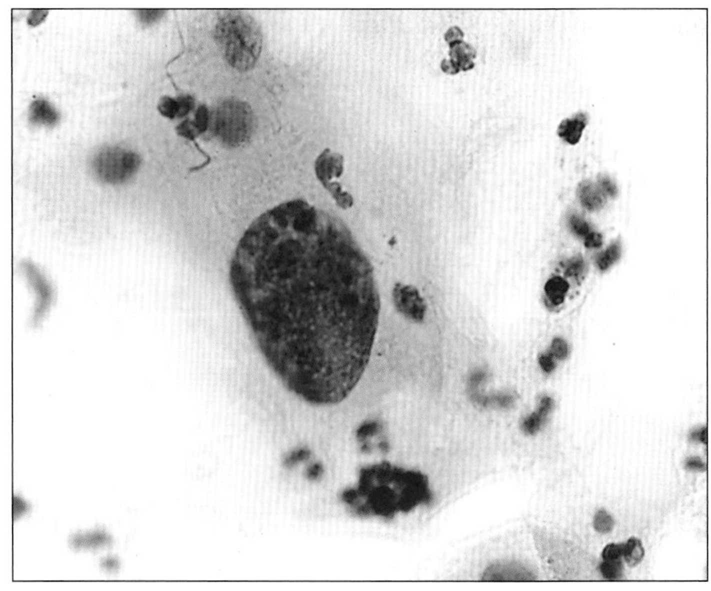

282. **These cells represent an endocervical aspirate from a 52-year-old woman with a recent history of vaginal bleeding. The cells are consistent with a diagnosis of:**

A. degenerated endocervical cells
B. endometrial hyperplasia
C. nonkeratinizing squamous cell carcinoma
D. small cell neuroendocrine carcinoma

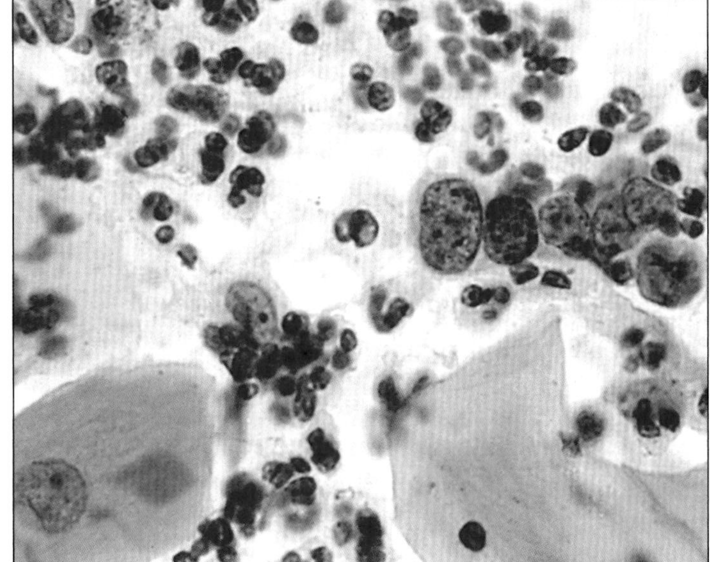

283. **These cellular changes are diagnostic of:**

A. benign radiation cellular changes
B. autolysis
C. cellular degeneration, secondary to inflammation
D. post-irradiation dysplasia

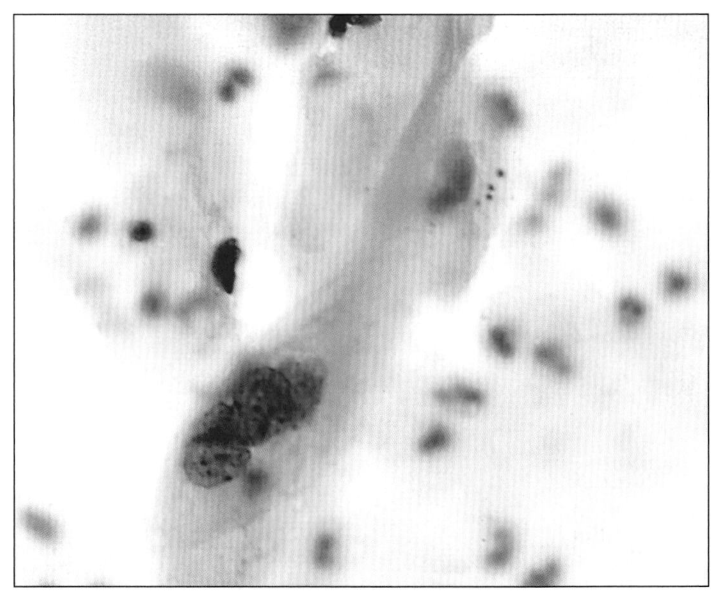

284. A 55-year-old patient, status post–total abdominal hysterectomy and bilateral tubal ligation and 6 weeks post irradiation for stage IIB squamous cell carcinoma of the uterine cervix, presents for a follow-up Papanicolaou smear. These cells are suggestive of:

A. residual carcinoma
B. negative for squamous intraepithelial lesion with radiation-induced cellular changes
C. post-irradiation dysplasia
D. ASC-US

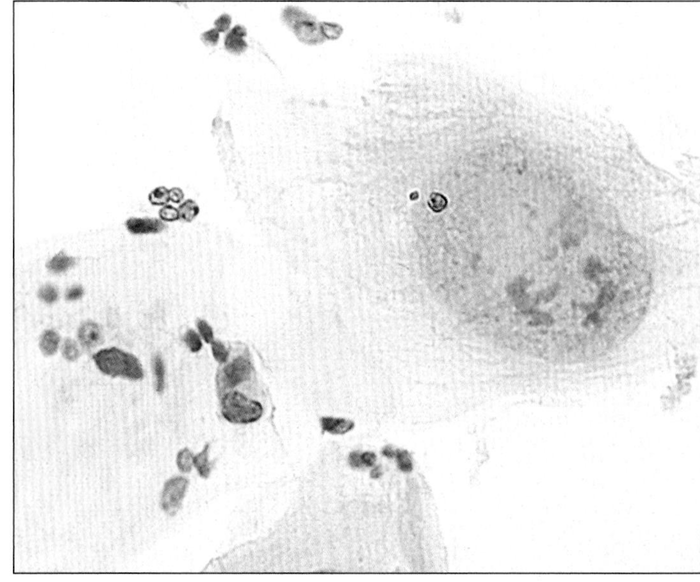

285. These cells are found in a vaginal cuff sample taken from a patient who had undergone irradiation therapy for squamous cell carcinoma of the cervix. The cellular findings suggest a diagnosis of:

A. post-irradiation dysplasia
B. residual carcinoma
C. reparative/regenerative changes
D. parakeratosis

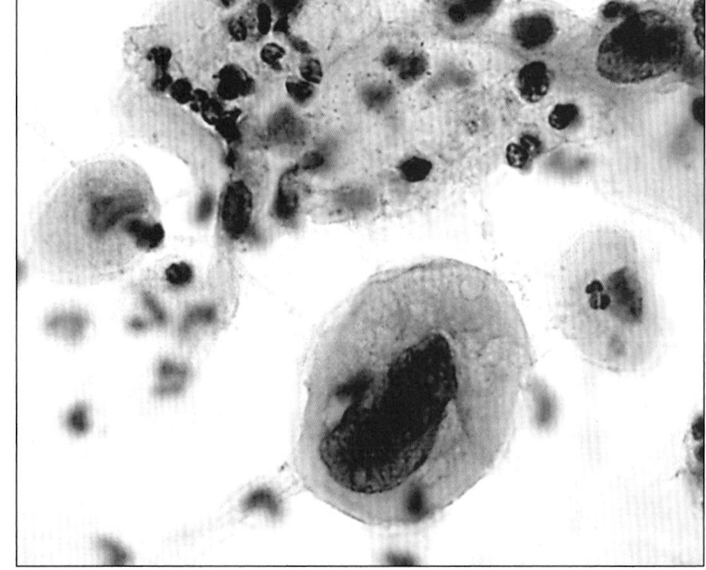

286. The cellular aggregate shown is most commonly described as:

A. a sheet
B. syncytial-like
C. a cluster
D. a rosette

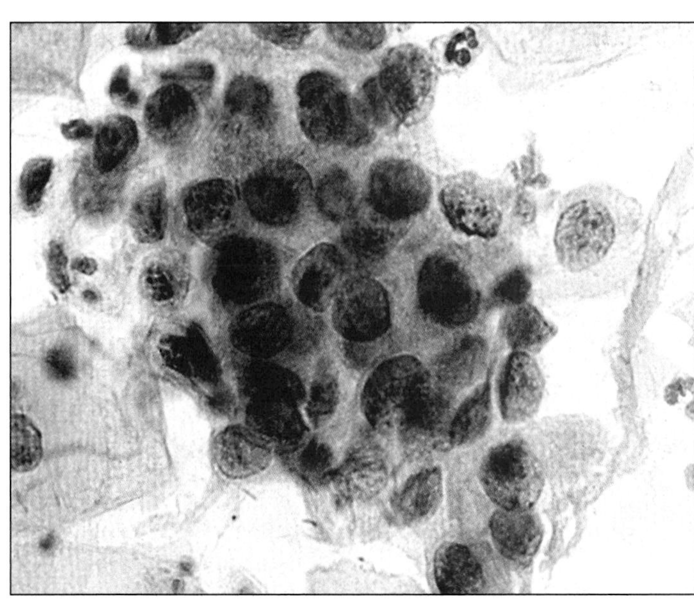

287. **These cells are normally located:**

A. in a prepubescent girl
B. at the internal cervical os
C. within the vagina
D. in the transformation zone

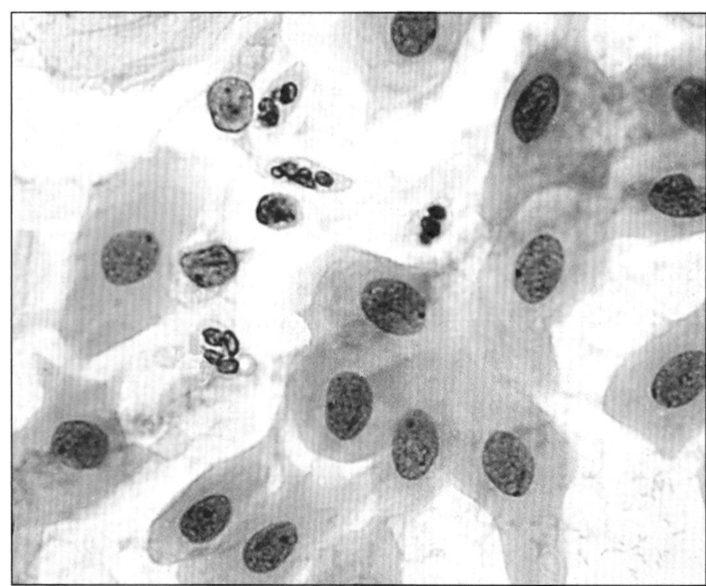

288. **These cells are from an ectocervical scrape and endocervical brushing. The findings depicted represent:**

A. malignant lymphoma
B. toxoplasmosis
C. chronic follicular cervicitis
D. acute inflammatory process

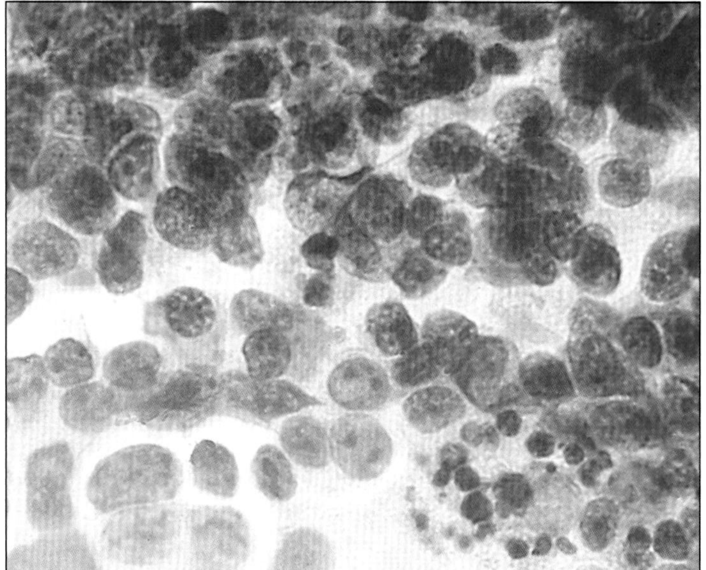

289. **Which of the following may be associated with these cells obtained from a vaginal/cervical scrape of a 42-year-old woman?**

A. invasive squamous cell carcinoma
B. endocervical dysplasia
C. severe cervicitis
D. pemphigus vulgaris

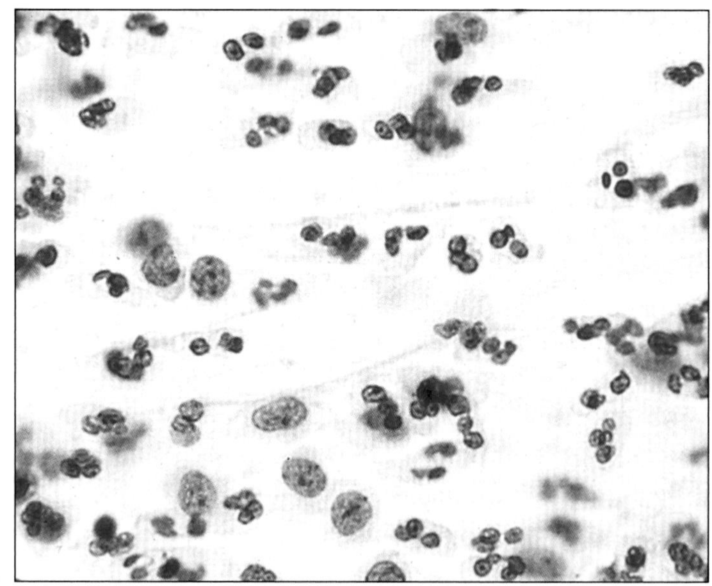

290. A 35-year-old diabetic woman presents in the second trimester of pregnancy. Which of the following correlates with the cytologic findings represented in this vaginal smear?

A. normal cytologic pattern for pregnancy
B. possible fetal death in utero
C. vaginal infection
D. folic acid deficiency

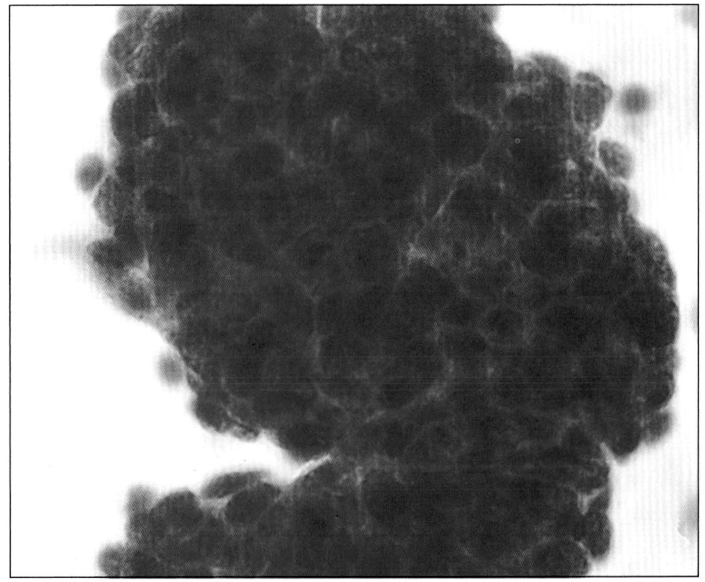

291. The background in the depicted cellular process may be described as:

A. a tumor diathesis
B. clean—no tumor diathesis
C. severe acute inflammation
D. cytolysis

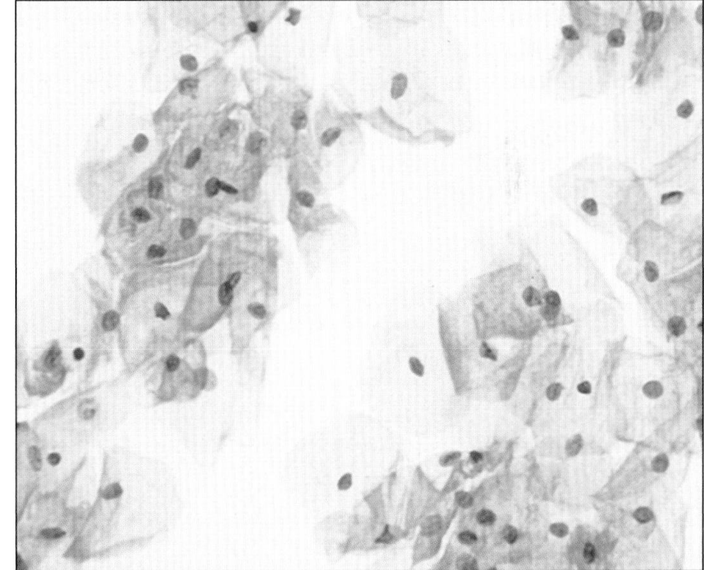

292. These cells are diagnostic of:

A. microglandular hyperplasia
B. parakeratosis
C. dyskeratosis
D. low-grade squamous intraepithelial lesion (LSIL)

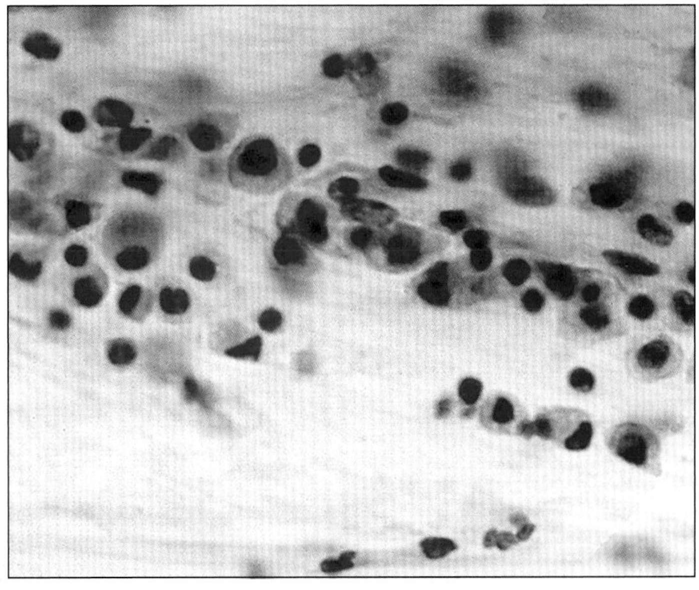

293. This vaginal smear is from a 42-year-old infertile patient. A diagnostic tool useful in evaluating the hormonal status of infertile patients is:

A. lateral vaginal wall smear (taken from the upper third)
B. lateral vaginal wall smear (taken from the lower third)
C. serum levels
D. cervical smear

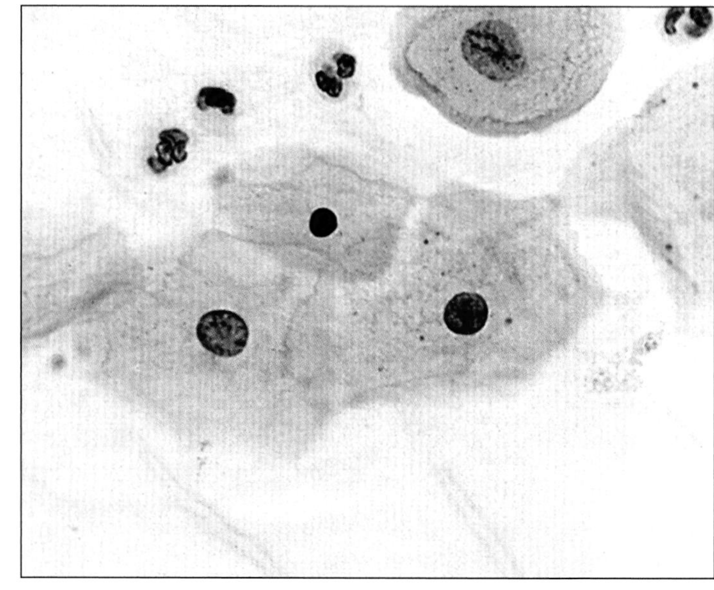

294. Which clinical condition may be associated with these cytologic findings from a vaginal smear from a 35-year-old woman?

A. Cushing syndrome
B. Stein-Leventhal syndrome
C. follicular persistency
D. hepatic insufficiency

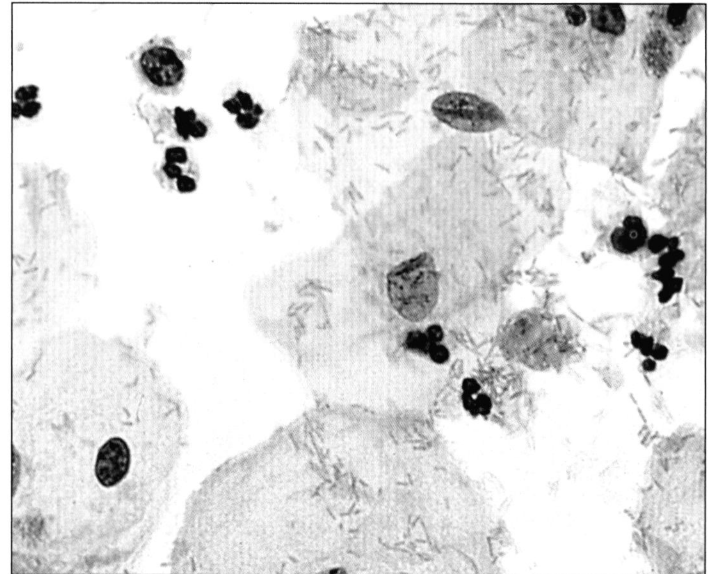

295. These cells are found in a cervical scrape and endocervical brushing from a 26-year-old woman with a history of cauterization for an abnormal Papanicolaou smear. The diagnosis is consistent with:

A. reparative/regenerative process
B. low-grade squamous intraepithelial lesion (LSIL)
C. high-grade squamous intraepithelial lesion (HSIL)
D. invasive squamous cell carcinoma

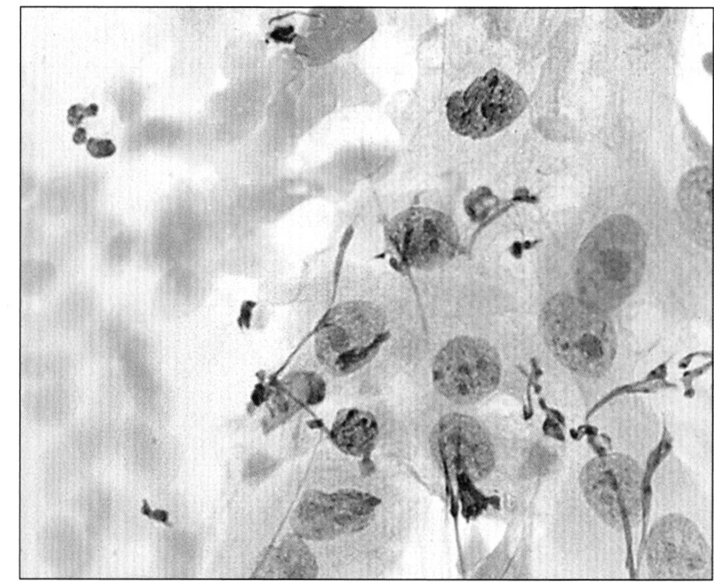

296. These cells are from a cervical scrape and endocervical brushing specimen from a 28-year-old woman suffering from a chronic skin disease. The diagnosis is:

A. pilomatrixoma
B. amelanotic melanoma
C. pemphigus vulgaris
D. basal cell carcinoma

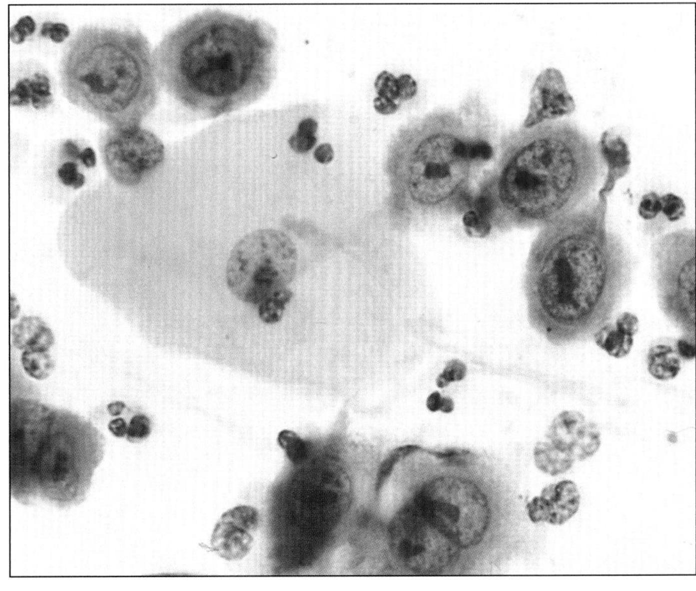

297. A 22-year-old woman presents with secondary amenorrhea. Clinical findings reveal that the patient suffers from Stein-Leventhal syndrome. Based on these cellular findings, the hormonal analysis:

A. correlates with history
B. does not correlate with history

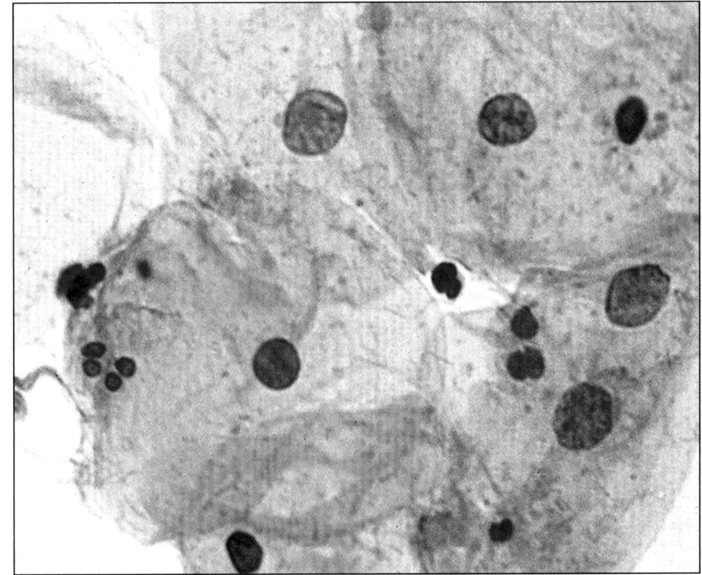

298. These cells represent a cervical/endocervical smear from a 43-year-old woman. The diagnosis is:

A. squamous cell carcinoma, keratinizing variety
B. LSIL, keratinizing variety
C. HSIL, keratinizing variety
D. parakeratosis

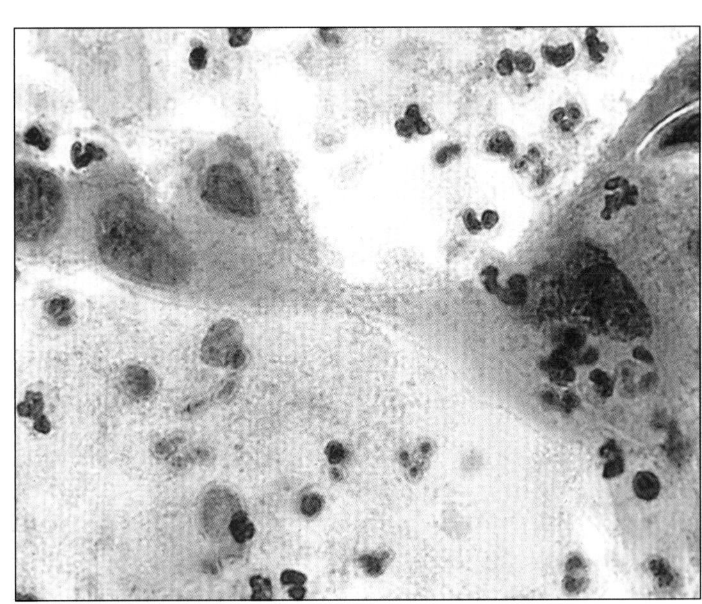

299. **These cytologic findings represent a vaginal/cervical smear from a 28-year-old asymptomatic woman. The diagnosis is consistent with:**

A. glycogenated cells
B. ASC-US
C. LSIL, HPV
D. HSIL

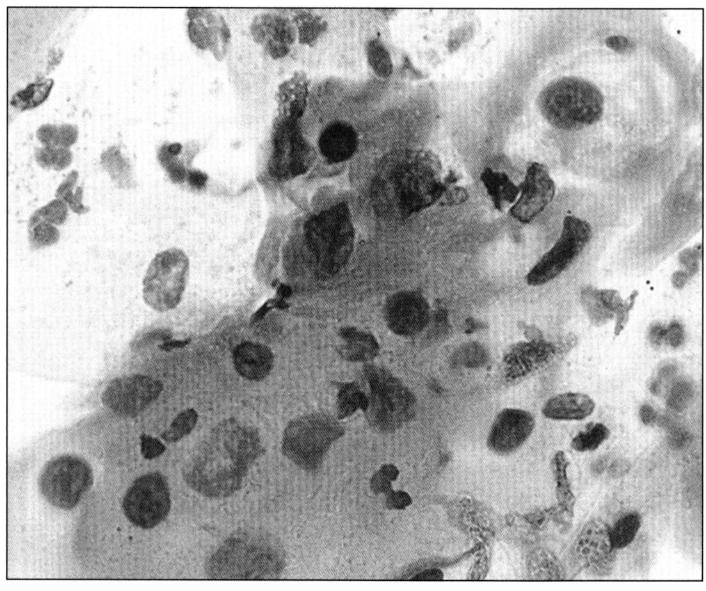

300. **Which clinical condition may be associated with this vaginal smear pattern?**

A. del Castillo syndrome
B. precocious puberty
C. granulosa-theca cell tumor
D. advanced cirrhosis of the liver

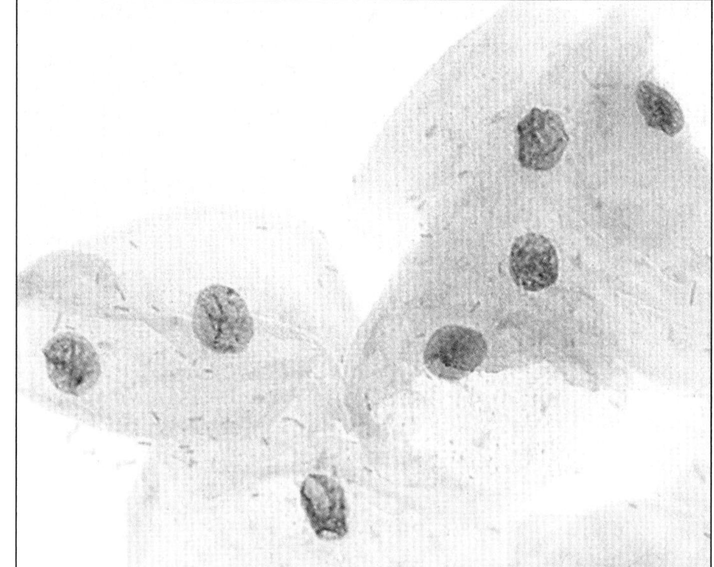

301. **A 16-year-old patient presents with primary amenorrhea. Primary clinical findings suggest feminizing testicular syndrome. A smear is performed for hormonal analysis. Based on the cellular findings, one would conclude:**

A. the hormonal analysis is compatible with history
B. the hormonal analysis is not compatible with history

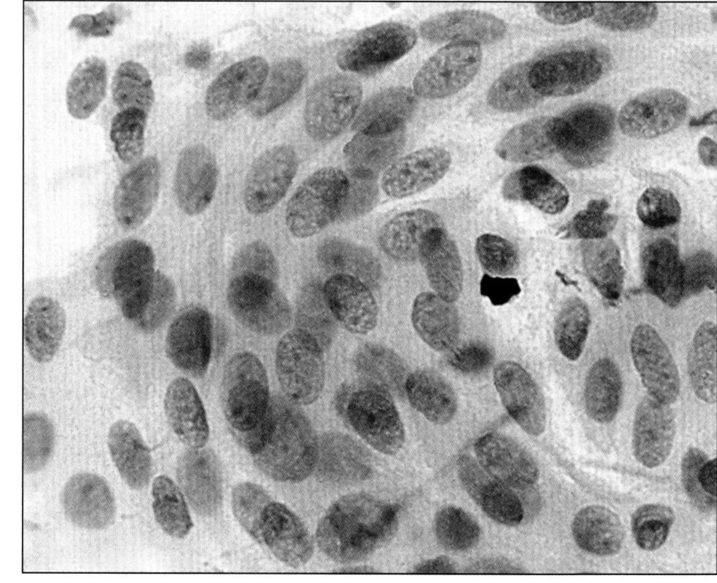

302. Which of the following might subsequently develop based on these cytologic findings?

A. keratinizing dysplasia
B. high-grade intraepithelial lesion, metaplastic dysplasia
C. atypical reserve cell hyperplasia
D. small cell carcinoma in situ

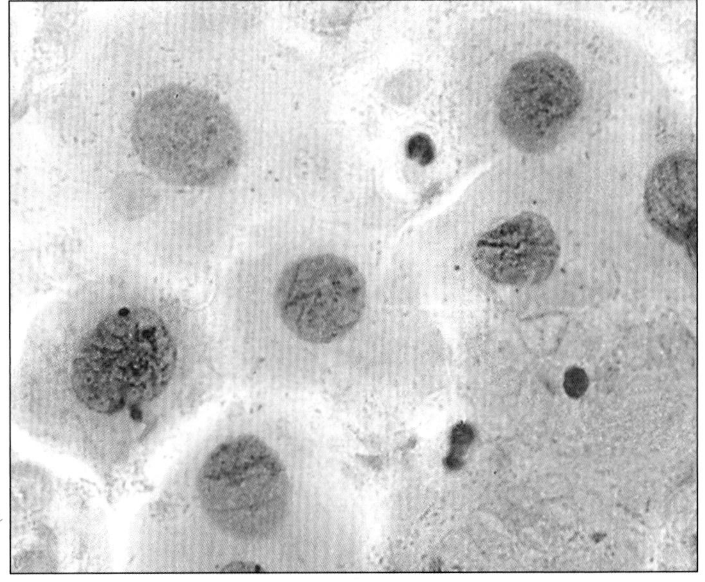

303. These cytologic findings from a vaginal smear are compatible with:

A. masculinizing ovarian tumor
B. patient with amenorrhea with galactorrhea
C. Chiari-Frommel syndrome
D. granulosa-theca cell tumor

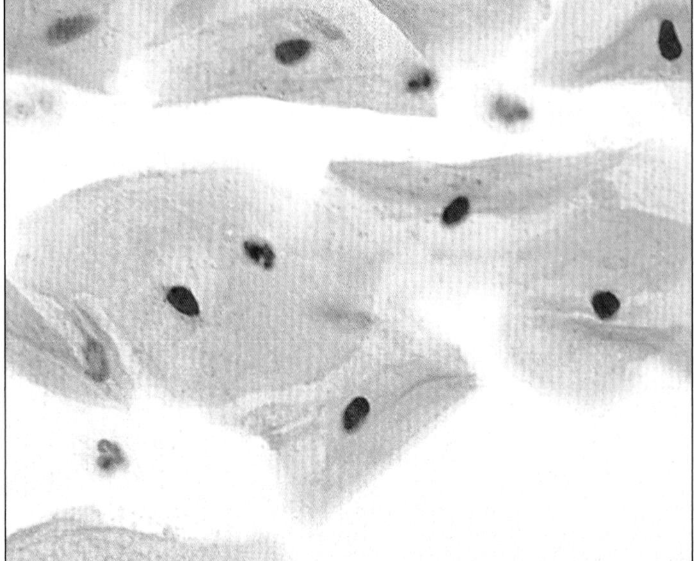

304. A 22-year-old postpartum (1 week) patient presents to her physician with vaginal bleeding. A Pap smear is performed. The findings are consistent with:

A. HPV-associated dyskeratosis
B. reparative/regenerative process
C. endometrial stromal cells
D. syncytiotrophoblasts

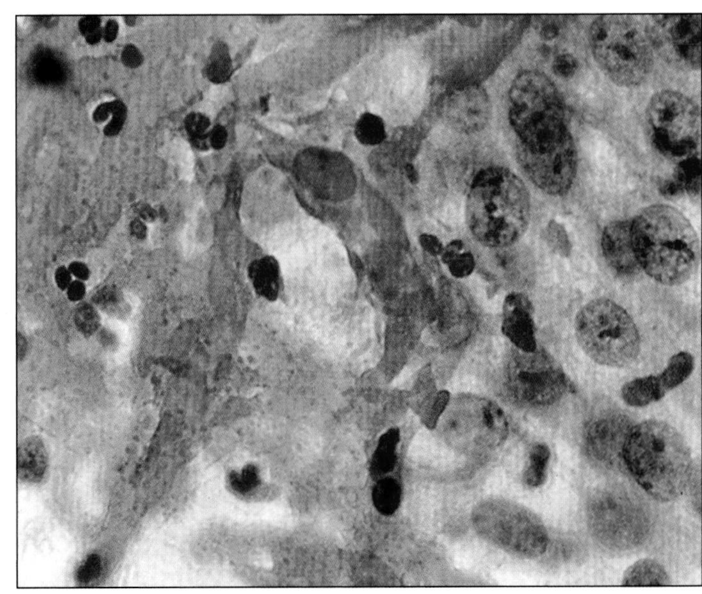

305. **These cells represent a cervical scrape and endocervical brushing in a 23-year-old woman. These cells are:**

A. endometrial stromal cells
B. endocervical glandular cells
C. immature metaplastic cells
D. mature metaplastic cells

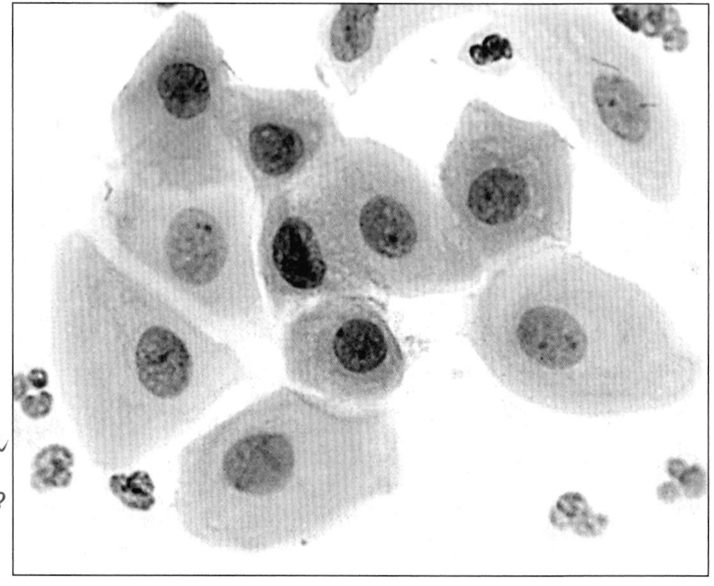

306. **An 18-year-old woman presents with primary amenorrhea and webbing of the neck. These cells are from a vaginal smear. The hormonal analysis is compatible with a clinical diagnosis of:**

A. feminizing testicular syndrome/androgen insensitivity syndrome
B. Stein-Leventhal syndrome
C. Turner syndrome
D. polycystic ovaries

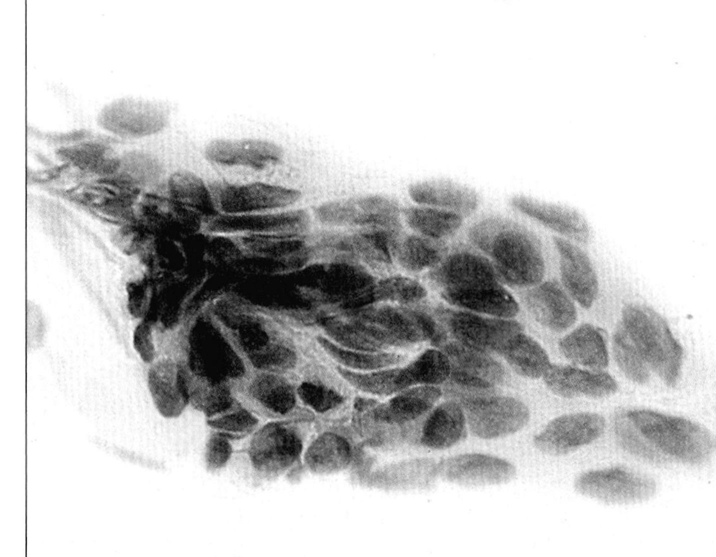

307. **Which of the following criteria would help to classify these cells as metastatic rather than primary?**

A. presence of columnar configuration
B. absence of a diathesis
C. cytoplasmic texture
D. nuclear characteristics

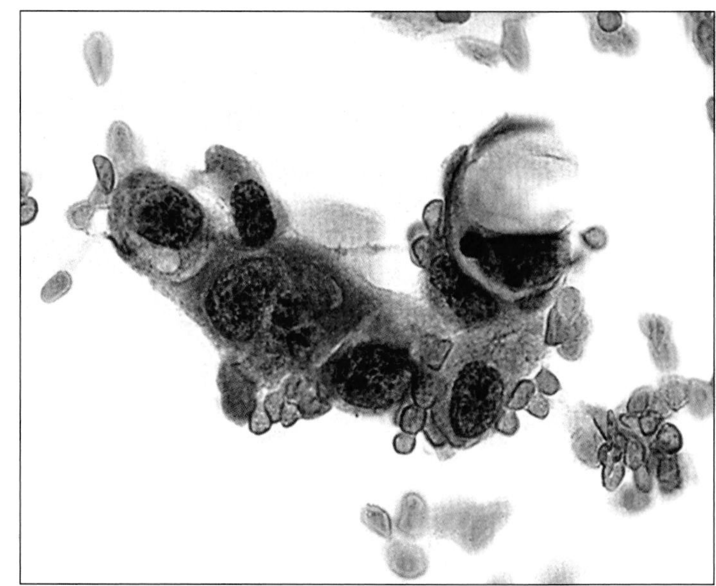

308. **What clinical condition may be associated with this vaginal smear taken from a 30-year-old woman (taken 8 weeks after her last menstrual period)?**

A. follicular cytosis
B. ovarian eunuchoidism
C. Turner syndrome
D. Chiari-Frommel syndrome

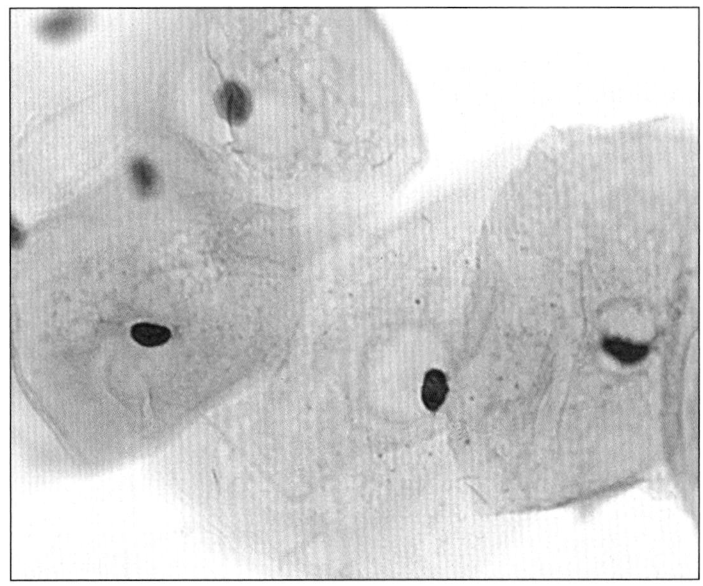

309. **The most important criterion for distinguishing these cells from mild dysplasia is the:**

A. nuclear-to-cytoplasmic ratio
B. hyperchromasia
C. nucleoli
D. nuclear membrane

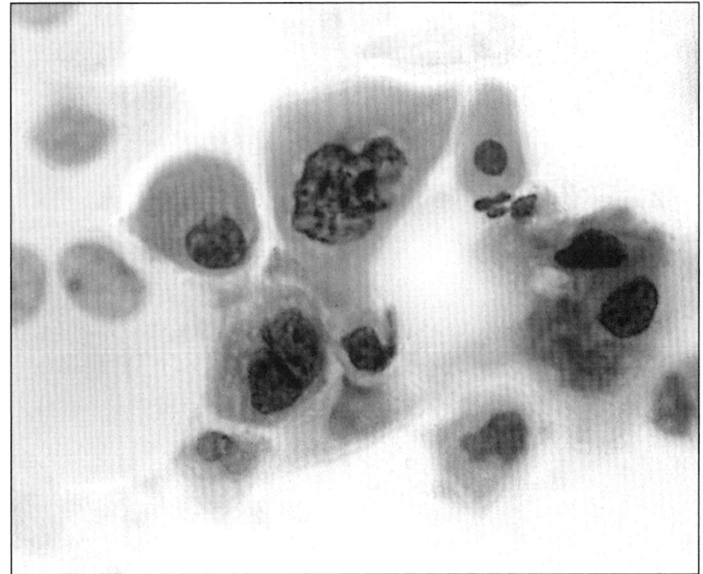

310. **These cells are from a cervical scrape and an endocervical brushing from a 41-year-old woman who presented for an annual Papanicolaou smear. These cells suggest a diagnosis of:**

A. mild nonkeratinizing dysplasia, LSIL
B. moderate nonkeratinizing dysplasia, HSIL
C. severe nonkeratinizing dysplasia, HSIL
D. carcinoma in situ, intermediate cell type, HSIL

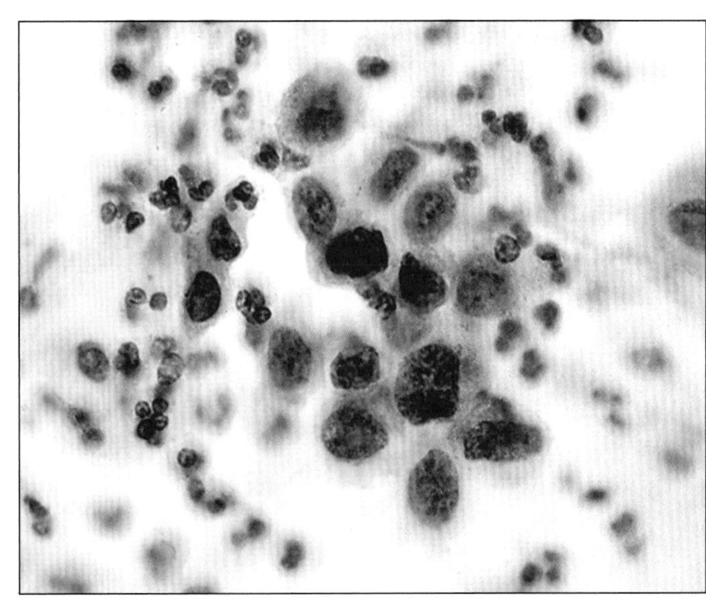

311. These cells are identified in a cellular sample obtained by an ectocervical scrape and endocervical aspiration from a 44-year-old woman. The diagnosis is:

A. normal immature squamous metaplasia
B. low-grade squamous intraepithelial lesion
C. high-grade squamous intraepithelial lesion
D. birth-control pill changes

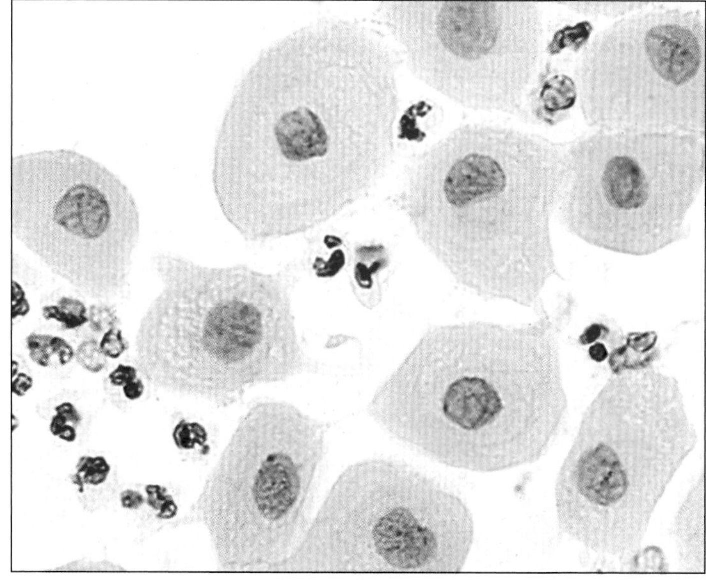

312. One criterion used to distinguish these cells from their precursor lesion includes the presence of:

A. diathesis
B. coarse, irregular chromatin
C. nucleoli
D. coarse, regular chromatin

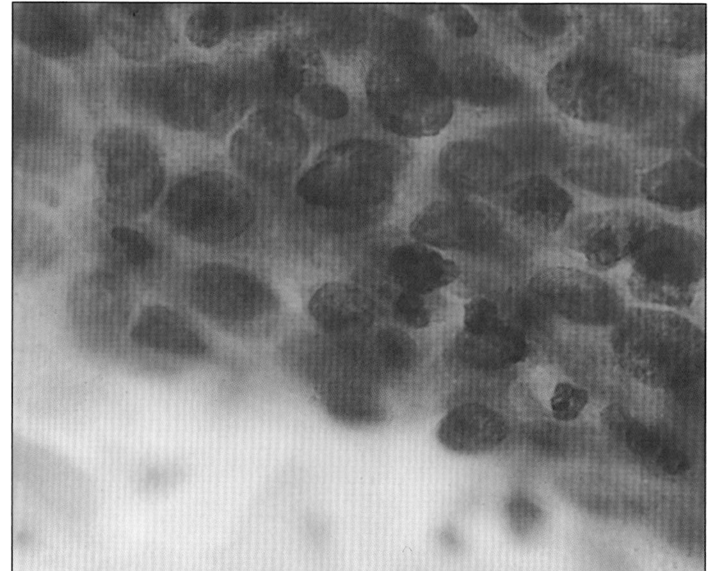

313. Which of the following papillomavirus types is etiologically related to these cells?

A. HPV-11
B. HPV-16
C. HPV-6
D. HPV-2

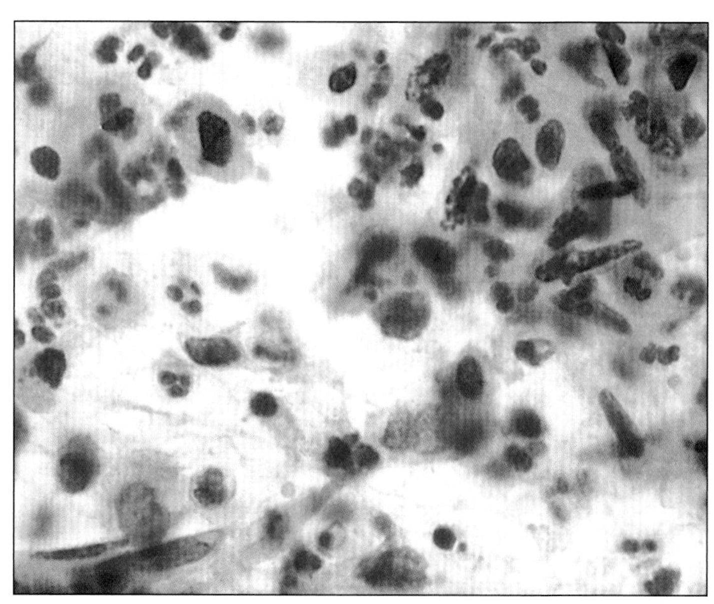

314. **These cells were taken from a 21-year-old woman who presented with a fungating mass protruding from the anterior cervical lip. Cervical scrapings suggest a diagnosis of:**

A. squamous cell carcinoma, large cell variety
B. HSIL, consistent with carcinoma in situ
C. HSIL, consistent with moderate dysplasia
D. LSIL, consistent with HPV

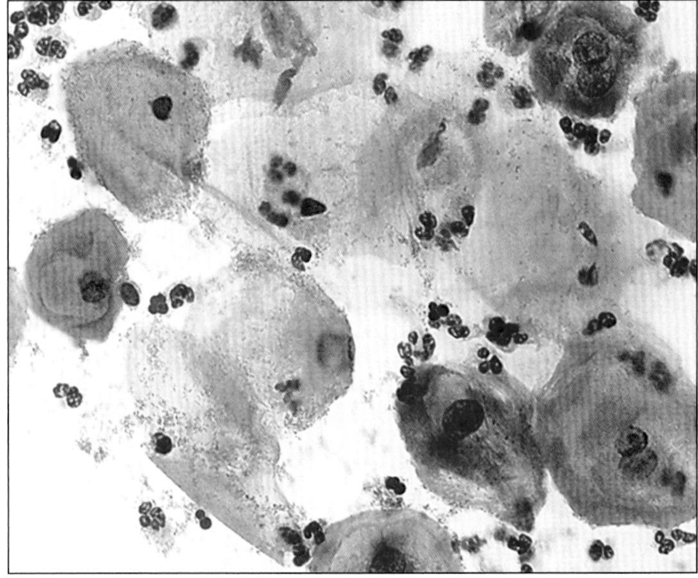

315. **An 18-year-old woman presents with primary amenorrhea. Which clinical condition may be associated with the cellular findings?**

A. congenital absence of the uterus
B. Chiari-Frommel syndrome
C. ovarian eunuchoidism
D. gonadal dysgenesis

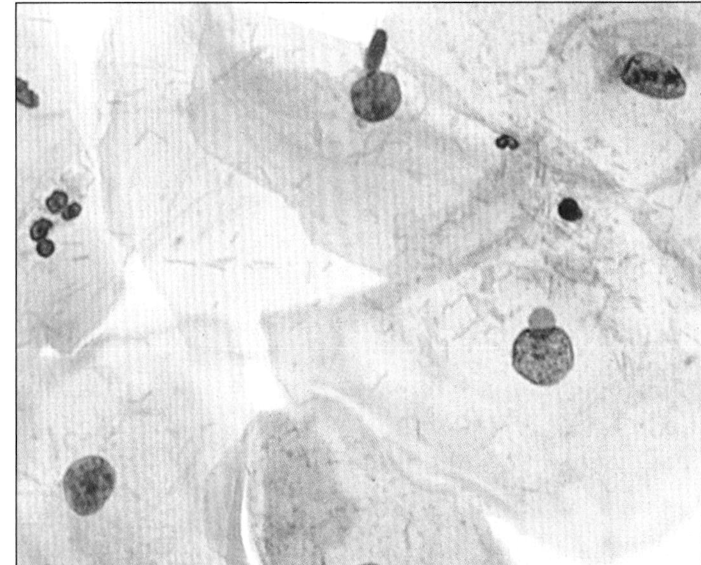

316. **These cells represent a cervical/endocervical scraping taken from a 33-year-old woman. The diagnosis is:**

A. negative for squamous intraepithelial lesion
B. ASC-US, dyskeratocytes (pleomorphic parakeratosis) most likely associated with HPV infection
C. LSIL, mild dysplasia, keratinizing type
D. HSIL, severe dysplasia, keratinizing type

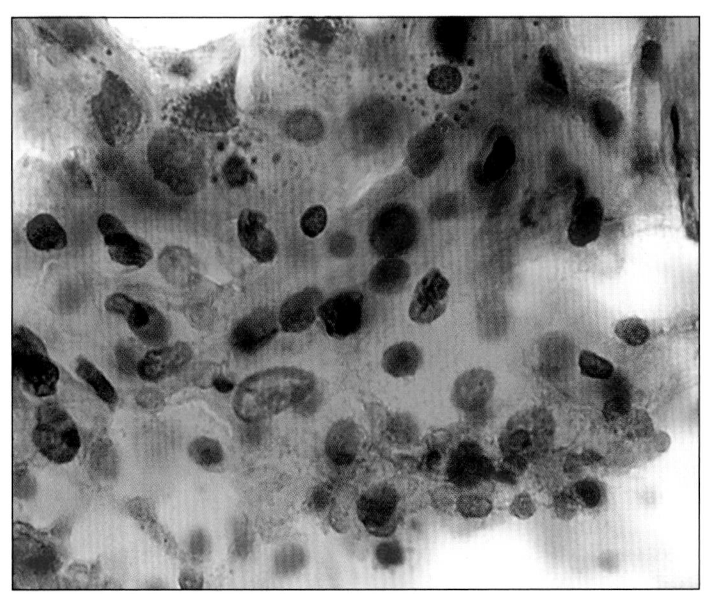

317. **Which of the following is commonly associated with these cells?**

A. Arias-Stella reaction
B. hyperkeratosis
C. reserve cell hyperplasia
D. follicular cervicitis

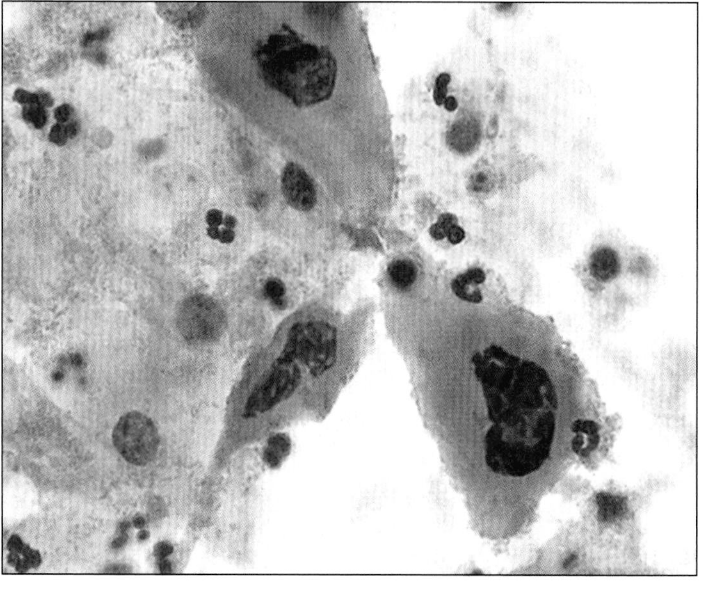

318. **Based on these histologic tissue findings, the appropriate diagnosis is:**

A. mild dysplasia, LSIL
B. severe dysplasia, HSIL
C. squamous metaplasia
D. reactive/reparative changes

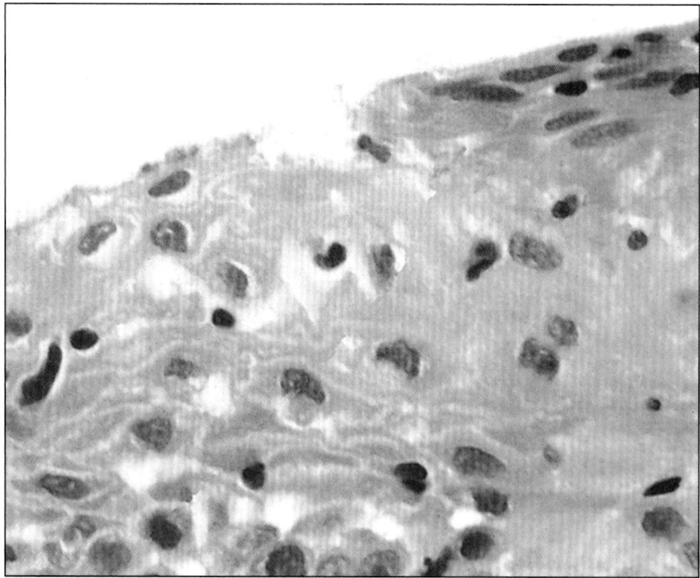

319. **These cells are from an endocervical aspirate from a 32-year-old woman with a recent history of conization for endocervical adenocarcinoma in situ. The cellular findings:**

A. are representative of recurrent disease
B. would mandate a biopsy
C. are consistent with a reparative/regenerative process, endocervical origin
D. are consistent with invasive adenocarcinoma, endocervical type

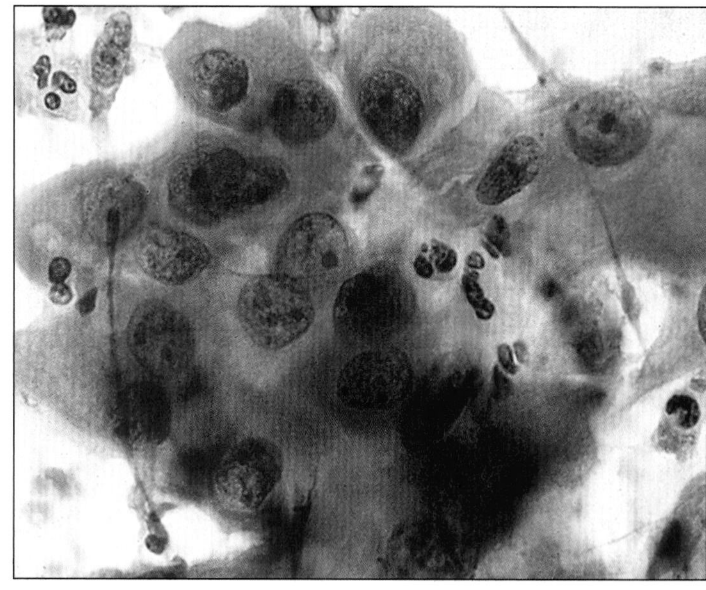

320. These cells are from an asymptomatic patient presenting for a routine Papanicolaou smear. The diagnosis is:

A. squamous atypia/mature metaplastic ASC-US (mimicking mature native squames)
B. moderate metaplastic dysplasia (HSIL)
C. herpes genitalis
D. human papillomavirus infection

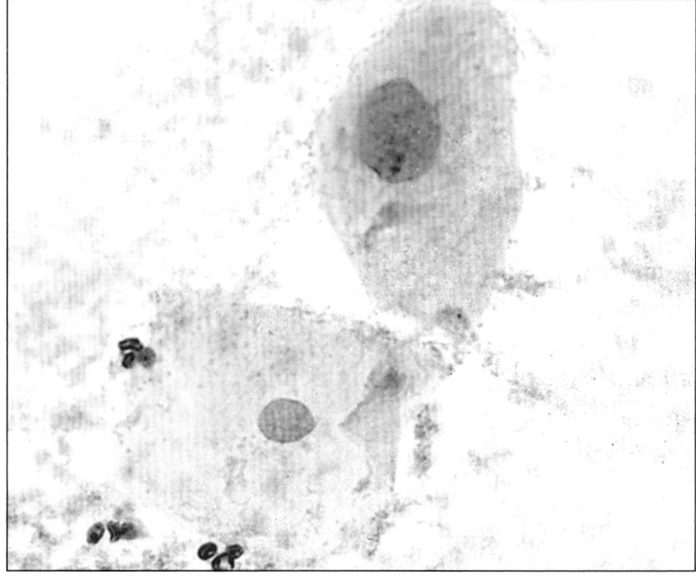

321. These cells represent a cervical/endocervical smear from a 43-year-old asymptomatic woman with no previous abnormal cytologic findings. The diagnosis is:

A. endocervical adenocarcinoma, well differentiated
B. AGUS, endocervical glandular dysplasia
C. tubal metaplasia
D. endocervical adenocarcinoma, poorly differentiated

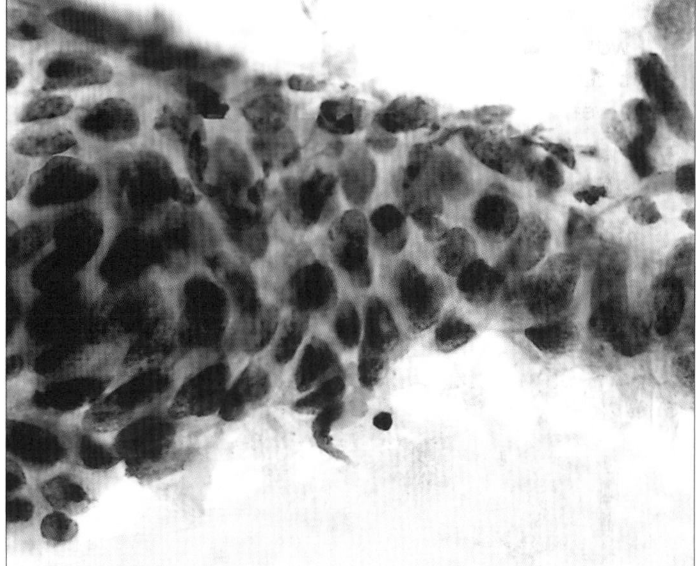

322. These cells represent a cervical/endocervical brushing from a 19-year-old woman. The diagnosis is:

A. reactive/reparative changes
B. adenocarcinoma, endocervix
C. AGUS, endocervical glandular dysplasia
D. ASC-US

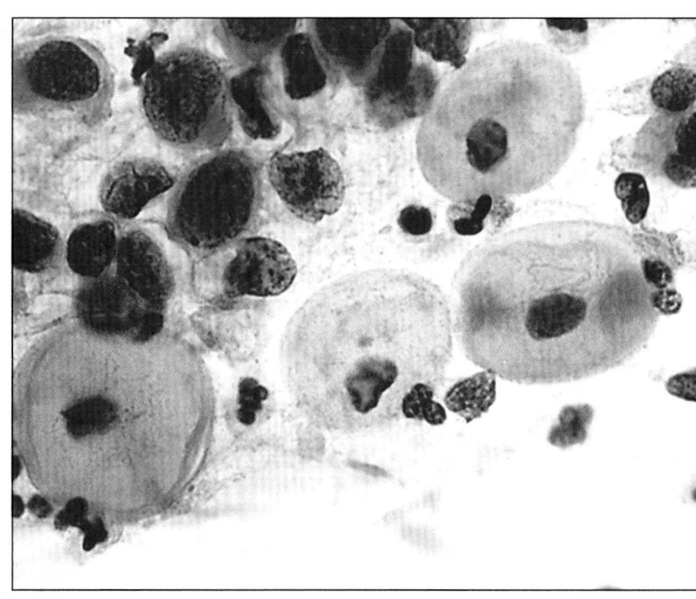

323. These cells are from a cervical/endocervical brushing from a 28-year-old woman, LMP 12 days ago. The diagnosis is:

A. reactive/reparative endocervical cells
B. squamous carcinoma in situ
C. squamous cell carcinoma, nonkeratinizing
D. adenocarcinoma in situ, endocervix

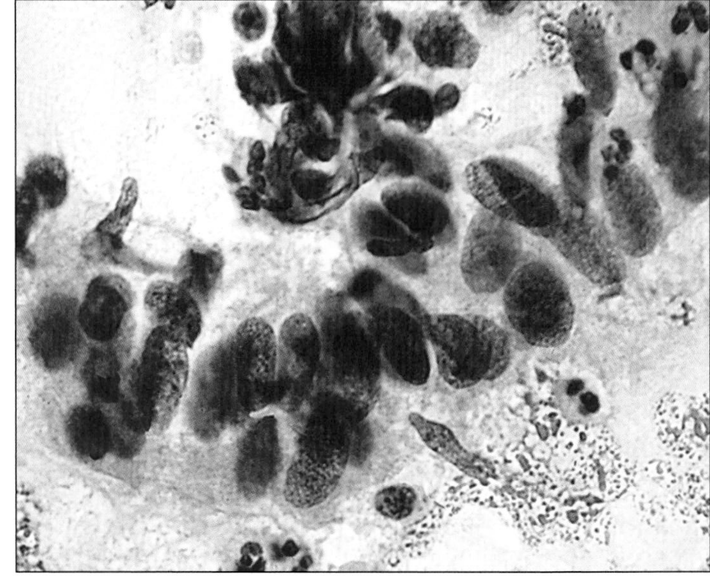

324. These cells are seen from a 57-year-old nulliparous woman with a history of obesity and postmenopausal bleeding. A vaginal/cervical/endocervical smear reveals:

A. atypical endometrial hyperplasia
B. low-grade squamous intraepithelial lesion
C. mixed mesodermal tumor, homologous
D. papillary serous adenocarcinoma, endometrium

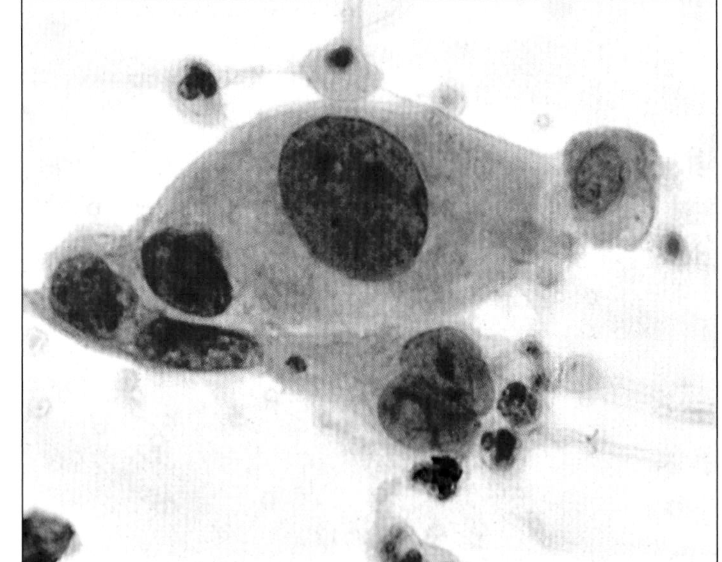

325. These cells were identified in a cellular sample obtained by an endometrial aspiration from a postmenopausal patient. The findings represent:

A. rhabdomyosarcoma
B. leiomyosarcoma
C. osteosarcoma
D. endometrial stromal sarcoma

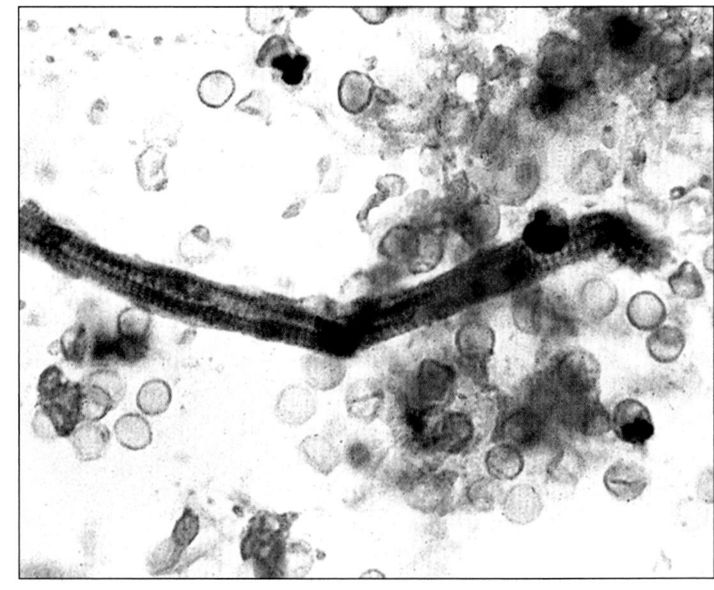

326. **These cellular findings represent a vaginal/cervical/endocervical (VCE) sample taken from a 25-year-old asymptomatic woman presenting for a routine annual Papanicolaou smear. The findings are most consistent with:**

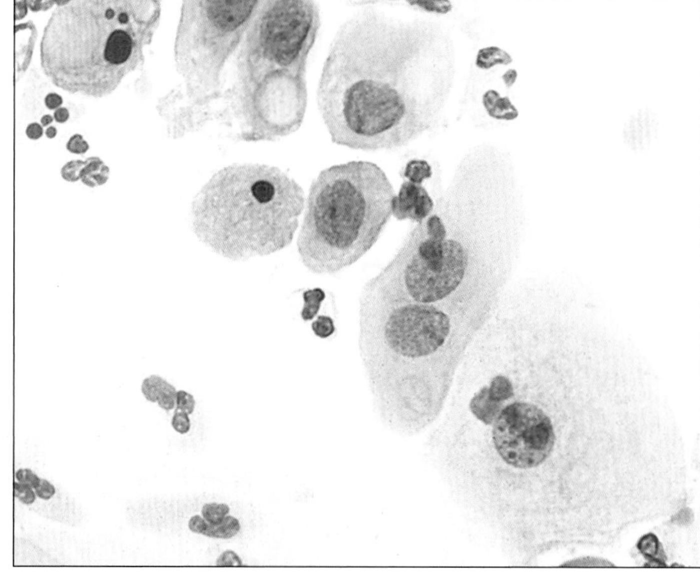

A. reactive/reparative squamous cells
B. ASC-US: atypical squamous metaplasia/immature metaplastic variety
C. LSIL, mild dysplasia
D. normal squamous cells

327. **The presence of these structures in a Papanicolaou smear indicates:**

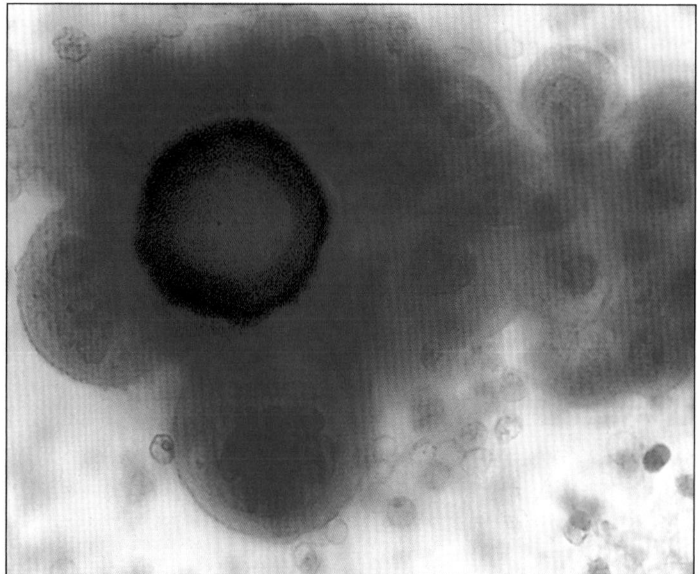

A. a malignant ovarian process
B. a benign ovarian process
C. a malignant metastatic process
D. nonspecific findings

328. **Culdocentesis and laparoscopic findings reveal the following structures in the presence of a malignant ovarian tumor. The most likely diagnosis is:**

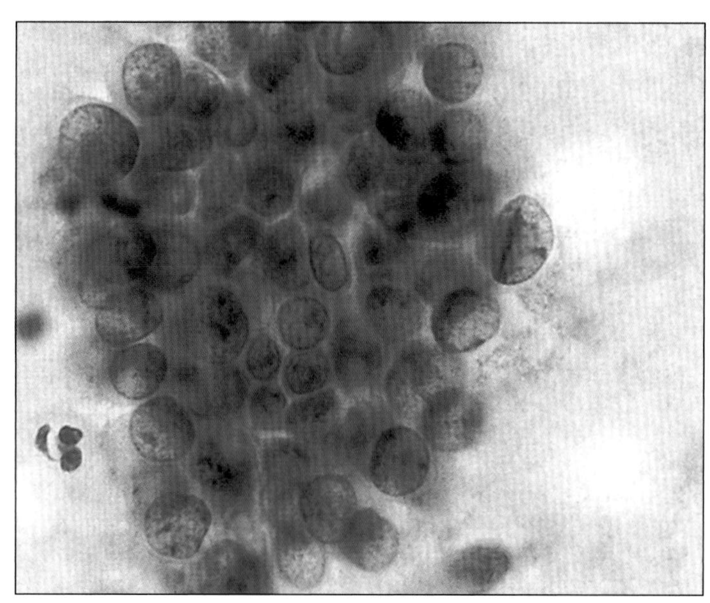

A. papillary serous cystadenocarcinoma
B. mucinous cystadenocarcinoma
C. endometrioid-type adenocarcinoma
D. Brenner tumor

329. A 44-year-old woman presents with a decrease in weight, abdominal distention, ascites, and malaise. A routine Papanicolaou smear reveals:

A. normal endometrial cells
B. tubal metaplasia
C. papillary serous cystadenocarcinoma, ovarian
D. nonkeratinizing squamous cell carcinoma

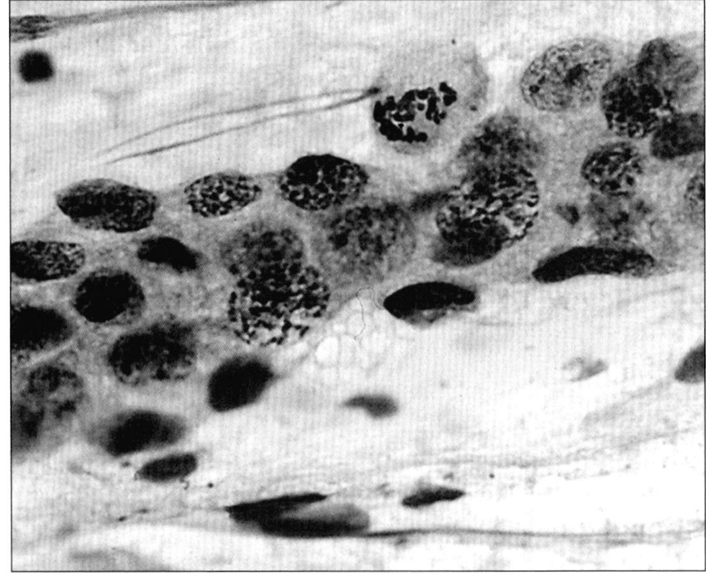

330. A 41-year-old patient suffering from oligomenorrhea presents for a Papanicolaou smear. Clinically, an ectocervical lesion is identified. A cervical scraping and endocervical brushing are performed. Based on the cellular findings, the diagnosis is:

A. nonkeratinizing squamous cell carcinoma
B. keratinizing squamous cell carcinoma
C. endocervical adenocarcinoma
D. LSIL, consistent with mild dysplasia

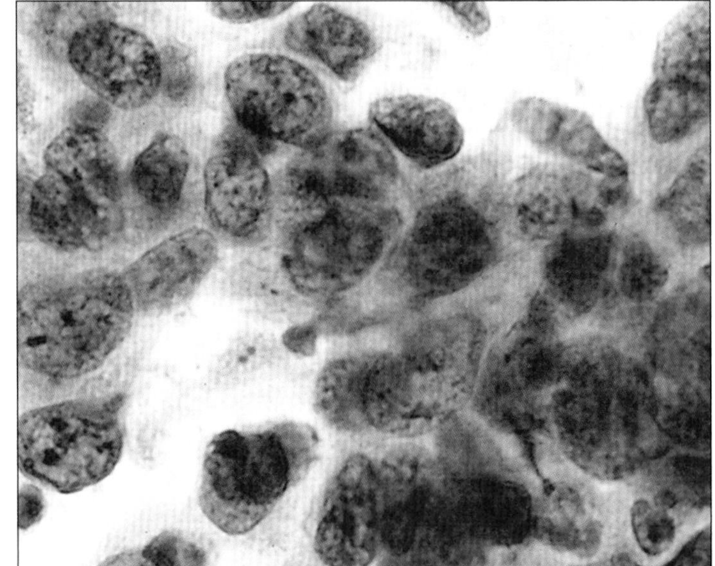

331. These cells are observed in a cervical/endocervical smear from a 58-year-old patient. The diagnosis is:

A. nonkeratinizing squamous cell carcinoma
B. ovarian adenocarcinoma
C. endocervical adenocarcinoma
D. mixed müllerian tumor

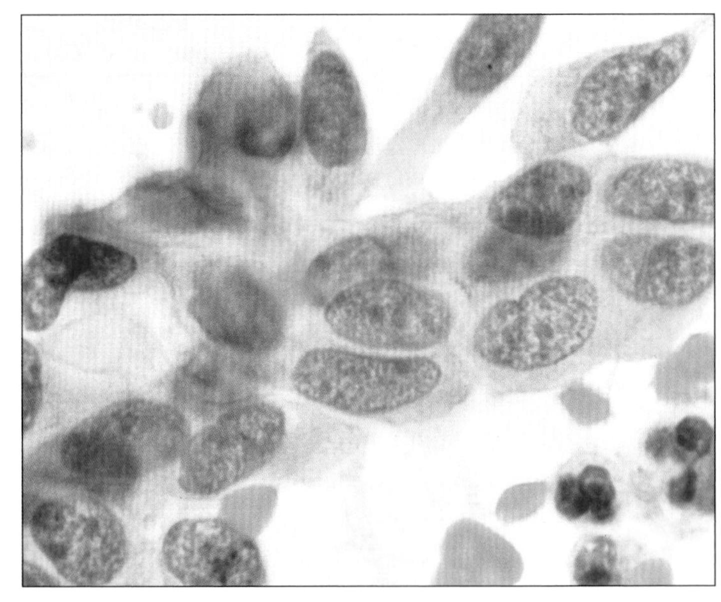

332. These cells are from a vaginal smear from a 61-year-old post-menopausal woman with a history of ovarian disease. The findings are consistent with:

A. adenocarcinoma, ovarian
B. poorly differentiated endocervical carcinoma
C. poorly differentiated squamous cell carcinoma
D. endometrial polyp

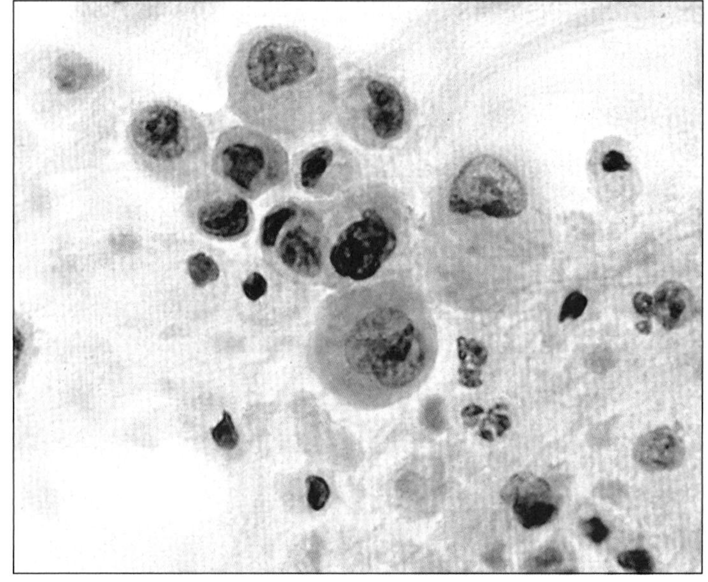

Female Reproductive Tract *Answer Key*

1. **B** secretory

The secretory or luteal phase lasts 14 days due to a programmed life/death span of 14 days for the corpus luteum/ corpus albicans.

2. **A** luteinizing hormone

Luteinizing hormone (LH) and follicle stimulating hormone (FSH) are pituitary gonadotropins associated with the menstrual cycle. Estrogen and progesterone are produced within the ovary as a result of these pituitary gonadotropins.

DeMay RM, The Art & Science of Cytopathology.
Intermediate predominant maturation index, p. 69.

3. **A** reserve cells

Reserve cells usually occur high in the endocervical canal. The presence of these cells occurs normally in response to squamous differentiation, but they may also serve as the stem cell for initiation of pre-neoplastic conditions. Histiocytic in appearance, they may be linked to endocervical mucosal cells, be associated with squamous metaplastic cells, or lie singularly.

DeMay RM, The Art & Science of Cytopathology.
Reserve cell hyperplasia, p. 71.

4. **C** 14

The surge of luteinizing hormone (LH) occurs at ovulation.

DeMay RM, The Art & Science of Cytopathology.
Superficial predominant maturation index, p. 69.

5. **D** no pathologic information

Mitotic figures are normal findings in benign, reactive/ reparative, premalignant, or malignant processes. Their presence merely infers metabolic activity, protein synthesis, and cell viability. Abnormal mitotic figures, however, may be occasionally found in association with premalignant or malignant processes.

DeMay RM, The Art & Science of Cytopathology.
The nucleus, p. 43.

6. **A** hyperkeratosis

Hyperkeratosis is a condition of overall greater epithelial thickness (hyperdifferentiation). A stratum corneum (anucleate squames) replaces the normally nonkeratinized superficial cells/ layer. Leukoplakia, clinically defined as a white patch, is the gross pathologic counterpart of hyperkeratosis acanthosis. This condition denotes the hard cornified visible area located either on the ectocervix or vagina.

DeMay RM, The Art & Science of Cytopathology.
Hyperkeratosis, pp. 72–73.

7. **C** large cells with multiple, tightly clustered nuclei

The presence of syncytiotrophoblasts found in vaginal/ cervical smears of pregnant patients may indicate a threatened abortion. In addition, increased superficial cell maturation is also considered an indication of abnormal pregnancy.

DeMay RM, The Art & Science of Cytopathology.
Trophoblasts, p. 134.

8. **C** vaginal adenosis

Vaginal adenosis is defined as the presence of ectopic glandular epithelium or squamous metaplastic cells within the normally gland-free or squamous-lined vagina. Their presence is increased in those patients who were exposed to diethylstilbestrol (DES) in utero.

DeMay RM, The Art & Science of Cytopathology.
Metaplastic reactions, p. 70.

9. **B** 14

Serum estrogen levels peak at ovulation (generally day 14).

DeMay RM, The Art & Science of Cytopathology.
Superficial predominant maturation index, p. 69.

10. **A** Sertoli-Leydig cell tumors

Sertoli-Leydig cell tumors, masculizing tumors of the ovarian stroma, produce increased serum androgen levels, which in turn create atrophic vaginal smear patterns.

DeMay RM, The Art & Science of Cytopathology.
Intermediate predominant maturation index, p. 69.

11. **A corpus luteum**

The corpus luteum degenerates to become a corpus albicans, and this ischemic structure allows for reinitiation of menstruation.

12. **B inverse**

As the serum estrogen levels increase, the follicular cells have increased sensitivity to follicle stimulating hormone (FSH). The direct feedback to the pituitary gland decreases the levels of FSH in the bloodstream.

DeMay RM, The Art & Science of Cytopathology.
Superficial predominant maturation index, p. 69.

13. **C oral contraceptives**

Synonyms include birth control pill changes, pseudoparakeratosis (pseudokeratosis) and microglandular hyperplasia. These cells represent degenerating forms of hyperplastic endocervical glandular mucosa. The finding has been associated with patients taking oral contraceptives, late luteal phase, and late pregnancy. They are benign cellular findings; however, the differentiation from true parakeratosis is imperative. Cells from microglandular hyperplasia generally have eosinophilic or basophilic cytoplasm, contain eccentric nuclei, or resemble reactive endocervical cells, whereas true parakeratosis represents a keratinizing process (orangeophilia) with centrally located pyknotic nuclei in polygonal "waxy" cytoplasm (possibly with accompanying HPV changes).

DeMay RM, The Art & Science of Cytopathology.
Microglandular endocervical hyperplasia, p. 122.

14. **A menses**

The corpus albicans in the late secretory phase of the menstrual cycle represents an ischemic corpus luteum. Subsequently, when ischemia of the endometrium occurs, the menstrual cycle is reinitiated.

Strayer DS, et al. Clinicopathologic foundations of medicine. Rubin's Pathology. Lippincott Williams & Wilkins, 2007.

15. **B FSH**

The development of the primitive primordial follicles of the ovary is related to the release of follicle stimulating hormone (FSH) from the pituitary gland.

DeMay RM, The Art & Science of Cytopathology.
Superficial predominant maturation index, p. 69.

16. **D 100/0/0**

Turner syndrome patients are ahormonal due to ovarian agenesis. A predominant population of basal to parabasal cells would be characteristic of the disease. Answers A, B, and C are all associated with hyperestrinism. Deep parabasal cells in sheets may represent an atrophic smear taken from a post pubertal patient with hyperestrinism. Conditions such as Turner syndrome may explain these findings. Turner syndrome is a nondisjunction of the X-chromosome. These patients are described as sex chromatin negative, or 45XO. Occasionally, mosaicism may be found. These patients have a low hairline, pigmented nevi, and increased carrying angle of their arms. Ovarian agenesis leaves streaks of connective tissue instead of viable ovaries. The vaginal smear pattern is atrophic.

DeMay RM, The Art & Science of Cytopathology.
Hormonal cytology, p. 68.

17. **A increased vascularization near the basal lamina in women with intermediate cell atrophy**

The increased vascularization may increase the permeability of the circulating endogenous androgens, which affects the overlying mucosa, creating an intermediate cell level of atrophy.

DeMay RM, The Art & Science of Cytopathology.
Intermediate cell maturation index, p. 69.

18. **B 75/25/0**

Parabasal or mixed intermediate cell patterns may be found in vaginal smears taken from postmenopausal patients. In addition, intermediate cell predominance may be observed in these patients (in the absence of hormonal therapy) due to endogenous androgens from the ovarian stroma or the adrenal cortex.

DeMay RM, The Art & Science of Cytopathology.
Parabasal predominant maturation index (atrophy), p. 69.

19. **C *Trichomonas vaginalis* infection**

Patients with vaginal infections should not have hormone analyses performed due to the false sensitivity of this test. Inflammatory agents such as *Candida* sp. or *Trichomonas vaginalis* often present with a false increased cellular maturation.

DeMay RM, The Art & Science of Cytopathology.
Superficial predominant maturation index, p. 69.

20. **A** increased estrogenic effect

An increased maturation index may be seen in patients with advanced liver cirrhosis due to the inability of the diseased liver to degrade estrogen, thus throwing it back into the bloodstream where estrogen-sensitive tissues respond by maturing or differentiating.

DeMay RM, The Art & Science of Cytopathology.
Superficial predominant maturation index, p. 69.

21. **D** cannot be determined based on the above clinical information

It is impossible to determine the vaginal smear pattern of a patient with secondary amenorrhea unless clinical history is provided.

DeMay RM, The Art & Science of Cytopathology.
Hormonal cytology, p. 67.

22. **A** may overlie and/or be associated with a possible lesion

Hyperkeratosis is a condition of overall greater epithelial thickness (hyperdifferentiation). A stratum corneum (anucleate squames) replaces the normally nonkeratinized superficial cells/layer. Hyperkeratosis and parakeratosis may overlie a serious abnormality such as infection by human papillomavirus (HPV), dysplasia, or even invasive carcinoma. The diagnosis is important and should be correlated with the surrounding cytologic findings.

DeMay RM, The Art & Science of Cytopathology.
Keratotic reactions, pp. 72–74.

23. **D** 75/25/0

In addition to hypothyroidism, other conditions that create parabasal predominant maturation indices include androgenic therapy, intrauterine fetal demise, hypopituitarism (starvation), and cervicovaginal ulceration.

DeMay RM, The Art & Science of Cytopathology.
Parabasal predominant maturation index (atrophy), pp. 68–69.

24. **A** increases cellular maturation

Increased maturation may result due to administration of this anti-estrogen due to its ability to bind to estrogen receptors of hormonally receptive cells, such as squamous mucosal cells.

DeMay RM, The Art & Science of Cytopathology.
Superficial predominant maturation index, pp. 69–70.

25. **C** immature metaplastic cells

Immature metaplasia is usually parabasal in size with basophilic cytoplasm, well-defined borders, and vesicular nuclei. Often a pavement configuration, remnants of cobblestone patterns, or the "cookie cutter" look is seen. These cells may possess spine-like or "spider cell" cytoplasmic processes when forcibly removed, or have ectoplasm/endoplasm rims when exfoliated. Squamous metaplasia, a common protective reaction found in mature cycling females, is a result of transformation of one adult type of epithelial tissue to another adult epithelial tissue via reserve cell hyperplasia. Squamous metaplasia is often associated with trauma, inflammation, or other endocrine disturbances. Squamocolumnar junctions, abrupt junctions occurring in young children, do not have associated transitional or transformational metaplastic zones.

DeMay RM, The Art & Science of Cytopathology.
Immature squamous metaplasia, p. 72.

26. **A** *Torulopsis glabrata* lacks hyphae

Torulopsis or *Candida glabrata* presents as yeast forms (stones) without the pseudohyphae (sticks). Sticks and stones are both seen with *Candida albicans;* however, culture analysis is preferred if speciation is necessary.

DeMay RM, The Art & Science of Cytopathology.
Fungi, p. 56, and Specific infections, p. 112.

27. **C** parakeratosis

Parakeratosis, an abortive attempt at keratinization, may overlie a serious abnormality such as infection by human papillomavirus (HPV), dysplasia, or even invasive carcinoma. The diagnosis is important and should be correlated with the surrounding cytologic findings. The finding of parakeratosis should be discriminated from related changes occurring in dyskeratocytes/atypical parakeratosis (atypical squamous cells suggestive of an HPV infection). Dyskeratosis or atypical parakeratosis is considered an ASC-US under the 2001 Bethesda terminology and not specific for the determination of an HPV infection. Only the presence of koilocytes is a sensitive diagnostic indicator of HPV.

DeMay RM, The Art & Science of Cytopathology.
Keratotic reactions, pp. 72–74.

28. **B** decreased maturation to the intermediate cell level

The overriding effects of progesterone on an estrogen-primed epithelium should allow for decreased maturation to the intermediate cell level.

DeMay RM, The Art & Science of Cytopathology.
Hormonal cytology, pp. 67–70.

29. **A** pituitary hypogonadism

Pituitary hypogonadism is usually related to trauma or damage to the gland. The degree of pituitary damage is related to its ability to release FSH. Deficient FSH levels lead to an inadequate estrogen balance; therefore, these patients will have a vaginal smear pattern that is parabasal to intermediate cell maturation.

Keebler CM, Somrak TM, The Manual of Cytotechnology.
Endocrinopathies, pp. 74–78.

30. **C** coarse, irregular chromatin in carcinoma

Sheets of cells with well-defined cytoplasmic borders, preserved nuclear polarity, predictable nuclear features, fine regular chromatin patterns, micro- to macronucleoli, and characteristic cytoplasmic streaming are diagnostic of reparative processes. This process is often associated with trauma, cervicitis, and inflammatory etiology. Although anisocytosis and anisonucleosis are common morphologic features seen with atypical reparative processes, predictability is maintained between cell groupings. In squamous carcinomas lack of predictability and single scattered cells with coarse irregular chromatin and hyperchromasia are predominant. In addition, the background of reparative/regenerative conditions is clean and free of necrosis. Malignancy-associated cellular backgrounds are generally composed of diathesis consisting of old and fresh blood, degenerated surrounding tissue, necrotic tumor cells, and assorted white blood cells.

DeMay RM, The Art & Science of Cytopathology.
Reparative/regeneration, pp. 115–116.

31. **C** follicular cervicitis

Chronic follicular cervicitis is a diffuse or localized lymphocytic infiltration as identified in cervical/vaginal smears. Small (mature) and large (immunoblastic) lymphocytes, plasma cells, and tingible body macrophages (intracytoplasmic inclusions) are necessary for the establishment of this diagnosis. The diagnosis of follicular cervicitis must be discriminated from other benign conditions including microglandular hyperplasia, degenerating neutrophils, and small cell histiocytes.

DeMay RM, The Art & Science of Cytopathology.
Specific infections (other manifestations of inflammation), pp. 113–114.

32. **A** superficial predominance, intermediate cells without folding or clustering

Stein-Leventhal syndrome is associated with a thickening of the tunica albuginea of the ovary, resulting in inability to expel the ovum. Patients with this condition are often overweight and have secondary amenorrhea. Vaginal smear patterns in these patients show generally intermediate to superficial cell maturation.

Keebler CM, Somrak TM, The Manual of Cytotechnology.
Endocrinopathies, pp. 74–78.

33. **D** pemphigus vulgaris

A bullous disease of the skin, pemphigus vulgaris is a condition that destroys the tonofilaments of the squamous mucosa, thus producing a sloughing of the skin. Reactive/reparative cells with bullet-shaped nucleoli are generally found, as are fine, even chromatin patterns. Clinical history is essential to rule out a possible adenocarcinoma. Tzanck tests are negative.

DeMay RM, The Art & Science of Cytopathology.
Benign lesions, pp. 331–332.

34. **A** folic acid

Folic acid deficiency (FAD) is a common water-soluble vitamin deficiency state among pregnant women. FAD is related to deficient ingestion, absorption and the increased demands of folic acid required during pregnancy. Folic acid deficiency produces cytomegaly (an increase in the cell volume without cytokinesis) and karyomegaly, changes similar to those seen in radiation cellular injury. Multinucleation and nuclei with fine regular chromatin are observed. Cytoplasmic vacuolization may mimic a "swiss cheese" effect, indicating the cells' degenerative qualities.

DeMay RM, The Art & Science of Cytopathology.
Vitamin deficiency states, p. 116.

35. **D** reparative/regenerative process

Sheets of cells with well-defined cytoplasmic borders, preserved nuclear polarity, predictable nuclear features, fine regular chromatin patterns, micro- to macronucleoli, and characteristic cytoplasmic streaming are diagnostic of repair. This process is often associated with trauma, cervicitis, and inflammatory etiology. The background of reparative/regenerative conditions is clean and free of necrosis. Malignancy-associated cellular backgrounds are generally composed of diathesis consisting of old and fresh blood, degenerated surrounding tissue, necrotic tumor cells, and assorted white blood cells.

DeMay RM, The Art & Science of Cytopathology.
Repair/regeneration, pp. 115–116.

36. **B** macrocytic changes, polychromasia

The cytological changes associated with radiation include cytomegaly (macrocytic changes) and karyomegaly. The maintenance of normal nuclear-to-cytoplasmic ratios and the evidence of cytoplasmic vacuolization (related to degeneration) are characteristic of these cells. The nuclei associated with radiation cell changes are often degenerative or preserved and multinucleated, while the cytoplasmic staining is polychromatic and amphophilic.

DeMay RM, The Art & Science of Cytopathology
Radiation cytology, p. 118.

37. A serous

Two-thirds of serous surface mesothelial tumors of the ovary may be bilateral. Cytological identification reveals papillary fragments and possible psammoma bodies.

DeMay RM, The Art & Science of Cytopathology.
Adenocarcinoma, p. 273.

38. D nonglycogenated areas that do not stain with iodine

The Schiller test uses iodine to help identify abnormal lesions within the female reproductive tract by outlining nonglycogenated areas.

DeMay RM, The Art & Science of Cytopathology.
Intermediate cells, p. 67.

39. A *Lactobacillus acidophilus*

Bacillus vaginalis, or *Lactobacillus acidophilus*, is considered normal vaginal flora that flourishes under progesterone-stimulated conditions (intermediate cell maturation). Lactic acid is produced and an acidic pH is maintained under normal conditions (pH 3.8–4.5). Döderlein bacilli predominate in the secretory phases of the menstrual cycle.

DeMay RM, The Art & Science of Cytopathology.
Inflammation and inflammatory change, p. 109.

40. C expression of HPV 16, 18 viral DNA

High-risk viral types (HPV 16, 18) integrate their viral genes into the host cellular DNA, creating malignant transformation.

DeMay RM, The Art & Science of Cytopathology.
Microbiology and molecular biology of HPV, pp. 103–108.

41. B mature cystic teratoma

A benign (mature) cystic teratoma, or dermoid cyst, is an ovarian tumor found generally in young females that is composed of germ cell tissues such as epithelial sebaceous glands, hair, sweat glands, or intestinal epithelium.

DeMay RM, The Art & Science of Cytopathology.
Teratoma, p. 1162.

42. A all cases of atypical squamous cells of undetermined significance (ASC-US) are considered part of the 5-year retrospective review process

CLIA '88 mandates a retrospective review of the patient's previous smears be performed if the current cytological findings are a high-grade intraepithelial lesion or worse. The intent of the requirement is to rule out the possibility of missed abnormal cells in cases previously diagnosed as negative for squamous intraepithelial lesion; however, if abnormal cells are detected in a previous case falsely diagnosed as "benign," documentation is required so that appropriate quality assurance measures may be employed to help avert a future false negative occurrence; however, because of the equivocal nature and poor interobserver reproducibility with the diagnosis of ASC-US, these diagnoses are not considered part of the 5-year retrospective review process.

Keebler CM, Somrak TM, The Manual of Cytotechnology.
Organization and inspection, pp. 334–343.

43. C endometrial hyperplasia

An increase in estrogen, unopposed estrogen stimulation, or pathological entities such as granulosa-theca cell tumors may be predisposing conditions for endometrial hyperplasia. Other risk factors for premalignant corpus disease include obesity, hypertension, nulliparity, and diabetes mellitus. Patients with these clinical histories are at a higher risk for developing invasive endometrial adenocarcinoma.

DeMay RM, The Art & Science of Cytopathology.
Abnormal shedding of endometrial cells, pp. 124–125.

44. A presence of granular cytoplasm and columnar cellular shape

The number of cells found in well-differentiated endocervical adenocarcinoma (ECA) is typically greater than that found in endometrial adenocarcinomas (EMA). Cell sizes associated with ECA are larger, contain more abundant cytoplasm, retain columnar configuration, and have finely granular, irregularly distributed chromatin with micronucleoli. EMAs are diffusely vacuolated and often contain engulfed polymorphonuclear cells, the opposite of the granular cytoplasm generally found in lesions arising from the endocervical glands. Endometrial adenocarcinoma cytologically presents with fewer numbers of cells on the slide (as opposed to endocervical adenocarcinomas), cell clusters with scalloping borders and three-dimensional tissue fragments, high nuclear-to-cytoplasmic ratios, and frothy, delicate, lacy, vacuolated cytoplasm. One of the key differential features between this lesion and endocervical adenocarcinoma is the cytoplasmic texture. Finally, the presence of a watery diathesis with associated lipophages may be helpful in discriminating endometrial adenocarcinomas from other epithelial malignancies.

DeMay RM, The Art & Science of Cytopathology.
Differential diagnosis of endocervical and endometrial adenocarcinoma, p. 129.

45. B endometrial carcinoma + osteosarcoma

A heterologous mixed müllerian tumor is diagnosed by the identification of well-differentiated endometrial adenocarcinoma plus a non-indigenous sarcomatous element. These heterologous connective tissue malignancies may include osteosarcoma, chondrosarcoma, or rhabdomyosarcoma.

DeMay RM, The Art & Science of Cytopathology.
Sarcomas, p. 136–137

46. B adjunctive methods that currently lack the specificity needed to determine the progression rate of any one lesion

To date, molecular determination of HPV is unable to provide predictable factors that can distinguish progression or regression of precancerous cervical lesions. Current studies focus on the interruption of antioncogenes such as p53 and the retinoblastoma gene.

DeMay RM, The Art & Science of Cytopathology.
Prognosis, pp. 106–109.

47. B mesoderm

The vagina, uterus, and ovaries are formed chiefly from embryological mesoderm.

DeMay RM, The Art & Science of Cytopathology.
Diagnostic map F8.1, p. 290.

48. B nonkeratinizing dysplasia, severe (high-grade squamous intraepithelial lesion)

Severe nonkeratinizing dysplasia cytologically presents as small immature metaplastic cells with hyperchromasia, high N/C ratios, and a thin rim of cytoplasm. The absence of coarse or irregular chromatin, nucleoli, and/or diathesis should help discriminate these cells from a carcinoma in situ or an invasive malignancy.

DeMay RM, The Art & Science of Cytopathology.
CIN mimicking immature squamous metaplasia, pp. 77–78. (+).
SC CA = coarse chromatin + nucleoli

49. B poorly differentiated type

Poorly differentiated endometrial adenocarcinomas (PDA), in contrast with well-differentiated lesions (most common), do not follow the typical natural history of hyperestrinism and endometrial hyperplasia. Instead, PDAs arise spontaneously in the atrophic epithelium of older, postmenopausal females, and are preceded only by an endometrial adenocarcinoma in situ.

DeMay RM, The Art & Science of Cytopathology. (ϕ HP)
Endometrial adenocarcinoma, pp. 125–127.

50. B pleomorphism

Pleomorphism is the single most important criterion in establishing a diagnosis of a keratinizing process.

DeMay RM, The Art & Science of Cytopathology.
Squamous cell carcinoma, pp. 83–84, and Keratinizing squamous cell carcinoma, p. 85.

51. D Bowen disease

Bowen disease is a synonym for carcinoma in situ of the vulva. This disease should not be confused with Paget disease, a malignant glandular tumor of extra mammary origin, or Gartner disease, remnants of the Wolffian duct.

Strayer DS, et al. Clinicopathologic foundations of medicine. Rubin's Pathology. Lippincott Williams & Wilkins, 2007.

52. A reserve cell hyperplasia

Reserve cells usually occur high in the endocervical canal. These cells occur normally in response to squamous differentiation, but they may also serve as the stem cell for initiation of preneoplastic conditions. Histiocytic in appearance, they may be linked to endocervical mucosal cells, be associated with squamous metaplastic cells, or lie singularly. (*)

DeMay RM, The Art & Science of Cytopathology.
Reserve cell hyperplasia, p. 71.

53. C smudged nuclear features and cave-like perinuclear vacuoles

The histologic diagnosis of human papillomavirus infection of the cervix is based on the presence of superficial dyskeratosis or abnormal parakeratosis, middle layers of koilocytes (containing smudged nuclear chromatin and cytoplasmic margination), and deeper layers containing normal-appearing parabasal and basal cells. Mitoses are frequently identified.

DeMay RM, The Art & Science of Cytopathology.
Condyloma and the human papilloma virus infection, pp. 85–87.

54. A Gartner cysts

Gartner cysts are remnants of the mesonephric system found within the lateral vaginal walls.

Strayer DS, et al. Clinicopathologic foundations of medicine. Rubin's Pathology. Lippincott Williams & Wilkins, 2007.

55. C pyknosis, karyorrhexis, karyolysis

Nuclear shrinking (pyknosis) is often followed by a rupture of the nuclear membrane (karyorrhexis) with subsequent dissolution of the nuclear material (karyolysis).

DeMay RM, The Art & Science of Cytopathology.
Inflammatory change, p. 110.

56. B HPV 6, HPV 11

Human papilloma virus types 6 and 11 are considered low-risk virotypes with episomal replication, an inability to transform cellular DNA in situ.

DeMay RM, The Art & Science of Cytopathology.
Microbiology and molecular biology of HPV, pp. 103–108.

57. D normochromasia, cytoplasmic streaming

Reparative/regenerative changes must be discriminated from low-grade epithelial lesions or those of more significance. Sheets of cells with distinct cytoplasmic borders and/or cytoplasmic streaming may be helpful in establishing the benign nature of these cells. Additional criteria include preserved nuclear polarity, predictable nuclear features, and fine regular chromatin patterns, micro- to macronucleoli. This process is often associated with trauma, cervicitis, and inflammatory etiology.

DeMay RM, The Art & Science of Cytopathology.
Repair/regeneration (atypical repair), pp. 115–116.

58. B diabetes mellitus

Pregnancy, patients with diabetes mellitus, or those taking birth control pills have an increased susceptibility for *Candida* sp. infections.

DeMay RM, The Art & Science of Cytopathology.
Specific infections, pp. 111–112.

59. B bicornate uterus

A malfusion of the müllerian ducts may result in a dual-horned uterus (one with two cavities).

Strayer DS, et al. Clinicopathologic foundations of medicine. Rubin's Pathology. Lippincott Williams & Wilkins, 2007.

60. B *Trichomonas vaginalis* infection

Trichomonas vaginalis infection appears clinically as petechial hemorrhagic mucosa, often referred to as a strawberry cervix.

DeMay RM, The Art & Science of Cytopathology.
Specific infections, p. 111.

61. A reactive trophoblasts

This bacterial-related endometritis may occur post-abortion or postpartum. Cytology reveals reactive trophoblasts, red and white blood cells, and multinucleated histiocytes.

DeMay RM, The Art & Science of Cytopathology.
Puerperal endometritis, p. 135.

62. D hematoidin crystals

Hematoidin crystals are associated with the degradation of hemoglobin secondary to hemorrhage. In contrast to true hematoidin cockleburs, hematoidin crystals are less common and are cytologically identified as radiate, spherical, or rhomboid structures. In addition, these entities are generally smaller than true cockleburs and possess crystalline rays that are fine (instead of club-like).

DeMay RM, The Art & Science of Cytopathology.
Cockleburs, p. 135.

63. A increased deposition of glycogen in the cytoplasm

Glycogen is gradually deposited within the cytoplasm of squamous cells during the proliferative phase of the menstrual cycle.

DeMay RM, The Art & Science of Cytopathology.
Hormonal cytology, pp. 67–68.

64. B glycogenated navicular cells

"Boat," or navicular cells, are glycogenated cells associated with an increase in progesterone. These cells are normally found during pregnancy or the secretory phase of the menstrual cycle.

DeMay RM, The Art & Science of Cytopathology.
Intermediate cells, pp. 66–67.

65. A dilatation and curettage to rule out hyperplasia of the endometrium

The presence of endometrial cells out of cycle may be associated with abnormal proliferation of glandular tissue such as endometrial hyperplasia, atypical hyperplasia, or an invasive malignant lesion. Dilatation and curettage is often necessary to rule out a disease process.

DeMay RM, The Art & Science of Cytopathology.
Abnormal shedding of endometrial cells, pp. 124–125.

66. C cockleburs

Hematoidin cockleburs may be seen in late pregnancy, patients taking birth control pills, or those using an IUD. The cytology reveals radiate arrays of golden refractile crystals with club-shaped spokes surrounded by histiocytes. These structures do not possess the visible central filaments associated with actinomycotic sulfur granules.

DeMay RM, The Art & Science of Cytopathology.
Cockleburs, p. 135.

67. B nulliparous

Several factors may contribute to the development of endometrial adenocarcinoma, including granulosa-theca cell tumors of the ovary, obesity, diabetes, unopposed estrogen stimulation, nulliparity, hypertension, and menopause.

DeMay RM, The Art & Science of Cytopathology.
Endometrial adenocarcinoma, p. 125.

68. A oncogene activation secondary to HPV

As indicated in the previous question, high-risk viral types have been associated with the development of cervical cancer. In this sequence of events, the E1-E2 region (early genes) are disrupted, interfering with the ability of the virus to transcribe its late genes, thus creating a biologic dead end for the viral life cycle. However, without transcription of these late genes, the feedback mechanism that controls the transcription of the E6-E7 genes (the viral region that codes for proteins that regulate viral growth) is lost. E6-E7 genes may bind antioncogenes or tumor suppressor genes such as p53 or Rb (retinoblastoma), which serve as protective genes that prevent transcription of cancer-causing oncogenes.

DeMay RM, The Art & Science of Cytopathology.
Microbiology and molecular biology of HPV, pp. 103–108.

69. A produced by the corpus luteum in early pregnancy

The emergence of human chorionic gonadotropin is important in maintaining the corpus luteum of pregnancy for 3 months until the placenta has developed.

DeMay RM, The Art & Science of Cytopathology.
Hormonal cytology of pregnancy, p. 113.

70. C paramesonephric

The paramesonephric ducts are responsible for the development of the female genital system. The mesonephric system develops the external male genitalia.

Strayer DS, et al. Clinicopathologic foundations of medicine. Rubin's Pathology. Lippincott Williams & Wilkins, 2007.

71. C syncytiotrophoblasts

The presence of large, poorly preserved, multinucleated cells, often with degenerated nuclei, may represent syncytiotrophoblasts of the placenta. These cells when identified in a pregnant woman may suggest a threatened abortion. The emergence of an estrogenic stimulation upon the vagina mucosa may be a concomitant finding.

DeMay RM, The Art & Science of Cytopathology.
Trophoblasts, p. 134.

72. D gastrointestinal epithelium

Radiosensitive tissues are considered those that will suffer severe damage when exposed to 2,500 roentgens or less. Cells of bone marrow origin, gastrointestinal epithelium, and germ cells are considered highly radiosensitive.

Qui W, Carson-Walter E, Liu H, et al. Puma regulates intestinal progenitor cell radiosenstivity and gastrointestinal syndrome. Cell Stem Cell. 2008;2:576-583.

73. A basophilic watery diathesis

A watery vaginal discharge associated with endometrial adenocarcinoma is represented by a finely granular, basophilic diathesis. Choice B represents a squamous cell carcinoma, choice C represents a poorly differentiated lesion, and choice D may represent a poorly differentiated papillary serous carcinoma.

DeMay RM, The Art & Science of Cytopathology.
Cytology of endometrial hyperplasia and neoplasia, p. 126.

74. C granulosa-theca cell tumor

Granulosa-theca cell tumors are benign estrogen-producing tumors that, unless removed, may predispose the patient to endometrial adenocarcinoma. Their presence has also been linked to precocious puberty. An increase in estrogen, unopposed estrogen stimulation, or pathological entities such as granulosa-theca cell tumors may be predisposing conditions for endometrial hyperplasia. Other risk factors for premalignant corpus disease include obesity, hypertension, nulliparity, and diabetes mellitus.

DeMay RM, The Art & Science of Cytopathology.
Endometrial adenocarcinoma, pp. 125–126.

75. A ovarian

The diagnosis of papillary serous adenocarcinoma of the ovary in a pap smear is centered around the finding of three-dimensional aggregates with hyperchromatic nuclei and finely granular, irregularly distributed chromatin with a cervical/endocervical/endometrial biopsy negative and colposcopy negative examination. The presence of papillary groups of malignant cells and psammoma bodies may help in identifying these lesions as ovarian origin, but are not specific findings. A history of ascites is helpful. Mucinous adenocarcinomas of the ovary present with signet ring morphology and may recapitulate signet ring endometrial adenocarcinomas. Clinical history is paramount in establishing an ovarian primary tumor. A tumor diathesis is usually absent in cases of metastatic carcinoma unless the lesion has seeded at the secondary site.

DeMay RM, The Art & Science of Cytopathology.
Metastasis, p. 137.

76. A colon for malignancy

The diagnosis of metastatic colon cancer in gynecological specimens is related to the presence of abundant abnormal palisading cells with basophilic granular cytoplasm and cigar-shaped nuclei. Presence of finely granular, regularly distributed chromatin is important in the diagnosis of this disease. A diathesis may be visualized if the tumor has metastasized by direct extension or seeded within the vagina. The diagnosis of this lesion may be difficult to distinguish from endocervical adenocarcinoma; therefore, a history of normal pelvic examinations may be necessary.

DeMay RM, The Art & Science of Cytopathology.
Metastasis, p. 137.

77. D tubal metaplasia

Tubal metaplasia (TM) is a benign condition that may be confused with a true abnormal process such as adenocarcinoma in situ of the endocervix (AIS), with the exception that TM presents with cilia and/or terminal bars/webs. Crowded sheets of glandular cells and anisokaryosis are common findings, mimicking the feathering effect seen in AIS.

DeMay RM, The Art & Science of Cytopathology.
Tubal metaplasia, p. 132.

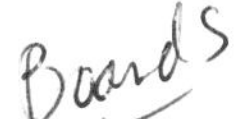

78. B serous adenocarcinoma, ovarian

Psammoma bodies are three-dimensional structures with concentric ringing containing calcified secretions of mucus. These structures are often found associated with papillary lesions of the ovary, including papillary serous adenocarcinoma. However, these are nonspecific findings and are not pathognomonic of malignancy.

DeMay RM, The Art & Science of Cytopathology.
Adenocarcinoma, p. 273.

79. C ovary

The diagnosis of papillary serous adenocarcinoma of the ovary in a pap smear is centered around the finding of three-dimensional aggregates with hyperchromatic nuclei and finely granular, irregularly distributed chromatin with a cervical/endocervical/endometrial biopsy negative and colposcopy negative examination. The presence of papillary groups of malignant cells and psammoma bodies may help in identifying these lesions as ovarian origin, but are not specific findings. A history of ascites is helpful.

DeMay RM, The Art & Science of Cytopathology.
Adenocarcinoma, p. 273.

80. C round-to-oval

Vulvar epithelial neoplasia (VIN) has been associated with exposure to the human papillomavirus. These lesions may cytologically be identified using criteria similar to those necessary to diagnose nonkeratinizing cervical lesions. Round to oval cells with high nuclear-to-cytoplasmic ratios, hyperchromasia, and finely granular, evenly distributed chromatin are suggestive of a high grade VIN.

Keebler CM, Somrak TM, The Manual of Cytotechnology.
Non-neoplastic vulvar intraepithelial neoplasia, p. 150.

81. C columnar configuration and granular cytoplasm are observed in endocervical adenocarcinoma

The number of cells found in well-differentiated endocervical adenocarcinoma (ECA) are typically greater than those found in endometrial adenocarcinomas (EMA). Cell sizes associated with ECA are larger, contain more abundant cytoplasm, retain columnar configuration, and have finely granular, irregularly distributed chromatin with micronucleoli. EMAs are diffusely vacuolated and often contain engulfed polymorphonuclear cells, the opposite of the granular cytoplasm generally found in lesions arising from the endocervical glands. Finally, the presence of a watery diathesis with associated lipophages may be helpful in discriminating endometrial adenocarcinomas from other epithelial malignancies.

DeMay RM, The Art & Science of Cytopathology.
Differential diagnosis of endocervical and endometrial carcinoma, p. 129.

82. D *Haemophilus ducreyi*

Gram-negative bacilli found in the cytoplasm of leukocytes may suggest the diagnosis of *Haemophilus ducreyi*. Isolation of the bacillus in culture is imperative.

Keebler CM, Somrak TM, The Manual of Cytotechnology.
Infectious diseases, pp. 148–149.

83. C leiomyosarcoma

Cytology reveals spindle cells with pleomorphic features, giant cells, isolated, fibrillar cytoplasm, and oval nuclei. The chromatin is finely granular, irregularly distributed, and may or may not contain nuclei. Leiomyosarcomas represent the most common sarcomatous lesion of the uterus. These lesions represent a malignant transformation of the indigenous smooth muscle elements.

DeMay RM, The Art & Science of Cytopathology.
Sarcomas, pp. 136–137.

84. **A** dyskeratosis

Dyskeratocytes are small cells with pleomorphic orangeophilic cytoplasm and smudged irregular nuclei. These cells may also be larger in size, making their differentiation from keratinizing dysplasia virtually impossible. Keratinizing or pleomorphic dysplasia (CIN mimicking keratosis) cytologically presents with well-defined borders, dense refractile cytoplasm, and hyperchromatic, coarse, irregular chromatin or India ink pyknosis. These cells may often stain orangeophilic. However, the degree of pleomorphism is more important when establishing the severity of keratinizing dysplasia. Associated changes include hyperkeratosis, parakeratosis, and dyskeratosis. Dyskeratocytes, or pleomorphic parakeratosis, are classified as atypical squamous cells of undetermined significance under the Bethesda System. Their presence is suggestive but not pathognomonic for human papillomavirus (HPV) infection.

DeMay RM, The Art & Science of Cytopathology.
Diagnosis of condyloma in the Pap smear (dyskeratosis), pp. 87–88.

85. **A** atypia of atrophy and maturity

The presence of bare nuclei seen in postmenopausal patients may be autolytic cells associated with atrophy or degenerated endocervical cell nuclei. Endocervical nuclei are oval in shape possessing well-preserved or degenerative chromatin. They may lie free or be trapped in streams of mucin. Atypia of atrophy represent low-level parabasal-to-basal cells and often may mimic more significant disorders such as carcinoma in situ or endocervical dysplasia. These cells are basal-to-parabasal cells in syncytial-like arrangements or hyperchromatic crowded groups (HCGs) found among a granular precipitate containing degenerated epithelial cells and scattered red and white blood cells. The chromatin, if visible, is fine and evenly distributed. More commonly, the chromatin of these atypical cells is poorly preserved, smudged and indistinct. Clinical history should be evaluated before rendering a diagnosis.

DeMay RM, The Art & Science of Cytopathology.
Atypia of atrophy and maturity, pp. 116–117.

86. **C** endometrial biopsy to rule out cystic hyperplasia

An increase in estrogen, unopposed estrogen stimulation, or pathological entities such as granulosa-theca cell tumors may be predisposing conditions for endometrial hyperplasia. Other risk factors for premalignant corpus disease include obesity, hypertension, nulliparity, and diabetes mellitus. Patients with these clinical histories are at higher risk for developing invasive endometrial adenocarcinoma. The presence of normal endometrial cells at times other than days 1–14 of the menstrual cycle may be related to a hyperplastic endometrium. Cytologic features are those of normal endometrial cells. A tumor diathesis is absent. Endometrial cells identified outside of the proliferative phase of the menstrual cycle (days 14-28) are considered abnormal in the absence of clinical history. Normal-appearing endometrial cells may be associated with hyperplasia, a predisposing condition for endometrial adenocarcinoma. An endometrial biopsy is often necessary to rule out a disease process.

DeMay RM, The Art & Science of Cytopathology.
Cytology of endometrial hyperplasia and neoplasia, pp. 126–127.

87. **C** degenerated parabasal cells of atrophy

Sheets of lower-level parabasal-to-basal cells with autolytic features, degenerating karyolytic cells ("blue blobs"), and the finding of pyknotic parabasal cells with eosinophilic cytoplasm (often referred as "mummified cells") are characteristic of deep atrophy as found in postmenopausal or postpartum patients. Care should be taken to discriminate these findings from more significant conditions such as parakeratosis or dyskeratosis, lesions associated with true keratinizing processes.

DeMay RM, The Art & Science of Cytopathology.
Atypia of atrophy and maturity, pp. 116–117.

88. **D** malignant lymphoma

Malignant lymphoma may mimic follicular cervicitis (FC); however, the findings of a polytypic cell population, which includes lymphocytes (mature, immunoblasts), plasma cells, and tingible body macrophages, are indicative of FC. In contrast, classic malignant lymphoma presents as a monomorphic population of immature lymphocytes. Furthermore, lymphoma presents with a gross cervical abnormality and generally an established history.

DeMay RM, The Art & Science of Cytopathology.
Specific infections (other manifestations of inflammation), pp. 113–114.

89. **B** sheets of cells without single cells in repair

Sheets of cells with well-defined cytoplasmic borders, preserved nuclear polarity, predictable nuclear features, fine regular chromatin patterns, micro- to macronucleoli, and characteristic cytoplasmic streaming are diagnostic of repair. This process is often associated with trauma, cervicitis, and inflammatory etiology.

DeMay RM, The Art & Science of Cytopathology.
Repair/regeneration, pp. 115–116.

90. **D** mucinous endometrial adenocarcinoma

These well-differentiated endometrial adenocarcinomas resemble intestinal-type adenocarcinomas. The cytology reveals mucin intracytoplasmically and contained within the background.

DeMay RM, The Art & Science of Cytopathology.
Cytology of endometrial hyperplasia and neoplasia, p. 127.

91. C a squamous metaplastic component

These cells are round to oval in shape, possesses acidophilic cytoplasm, and resemble oncocytes found in the salivary glands or thyroid. They are thought to be of squamous metaplastic origin and may cover the surface of normal or cancerous cells within the uterus. Their presence is necessary in establishing a diagnosis of adenoacanthoma. The clinical management of pure endometrial adenocarcinoma and adenoacanthoma is essentially the same.

DeMay RM, The Art & Science of Cytopathology.
Cytology of endometrial hyperplasia and neoplasia, p. 127.

92. C AGUS/endocervical dysplasia

Endocervical cells with slightly enlarged hyperchromatic nuclei with inconspicuous nucleoli, loss of polarity, and rosette formations are helpful in establishing a diagnosis of atypical glandular cells of undetermined significance (AGUS), in this case, referred to as endocervical columnar dysplasia (ECD). Its differential diagnosis is endocervical adenocarcinoma in situ (AIS); however, ECD has fine, regular chromatin whereas endocervical AIS contains coarse chromatin features. The identification of endocervical adenocarcinoma is grounded upon the findings of increased endocervical nuclear size, stratification of the cells, a feathering and splattering effect, frequent nucleoli, and the presence of finely granular, irregularly distributed chromatin. Columnar-shaped morphology is maintained in these malignancies. Endocervical adenocarcinoma must be discriminated from atypical glandular cells of undetermined significance, endocervical origin. These "endocervical dysplasias" do not have classic malignant chromatin features of adenocarcinoma and do not present with true tissue fragments.

DeMay RM, The Art & Science of Cytopathology.
Early endocervical glandular neoplasia, pp. 129–131.

93. B endocervical adenocarcinoma

The identification of endocervical adenocarcinoma is grounded upon the findings of increased endocervical nuclear size, stratification of the cells, a feathering and splattering effect, frequent nucleoli, and the presence of finely granular, irregularly distributed chromatin. Columnar-shaped morphology is maintained in these malignancies. Endocervical adenocarcinoma must be discriminated from atypical glandular cells of undetermined significance, endocervical origin. "Endocervical dysplasias" do not have classic malignant chromatin features of adenocarcinoma and do not present with true tissue fragments. The presence of columnar morphology in the presence of obvious malignant criteria may help one to distinguish endocervical adenocarcinomas from those of endometrial origin. Other criteria that help discriminate the cells of endocervical adenocarcinoma (EA) from endometrial adenocarcinoma (EM) include the presence of rosettes versus cell balls and elongated, hyperchromatic, multinucleated cells with prominent multiple nucleoli vs. rounded, finely granular chromatin and conspicuous nucleoli. EA possesses a granular cytoplasmic texture, whereas EM lesions have a lacy, frothy, vacuolated cytoplasmic texture. Lastly, EA tends to stain eosinophilic while EM is generally basophilic.

DeMay RM, The Art & Science of Cytopathology.
Endocervical carcinoma, pp. 127–128.

94. C large, distended vacuoles

Patients with an intrauterine device (IUD) may often present with proliferative or secretory endometrial cells that are reactive in nature. These cells are often single or in clusters, have large distended vacuoles, and contain fiely granular, evenly distributed chromatin.

DeMay RM, The Art & Science of Cytopathology
IUD Changes, pp. 131-132.

95. D endometrial polyps

Endometrial polyps have not been established as precursor lesions within the morphogenesis or development of endometrial adenocarcinoma.

DeMay RM, The Art & Science of Cytopathology.
Cytology of endometrial hyperplasia and neoplasia, pp. 126–127

96. D mucinous cystadenocarcinoma/ovary

Mucinous adenocarcinomas of the ovary present with signet ring morphology and may recapitulate signet ring endometrial adenocarcinomas. Clinical history is paramount in establishing an ovarian primary tumor. A tumor diathesis is usually absent in cases of metastatic carcinoma unless the lesion has seeded at the secondary site.

DeMay RM, The Art & Science of Cytopathology.
Adenocarcinoma, p. 273.

97. A hyperkeratosis, plasma cells

Lichen sclerosus is a dermatologic hyperplastic disease that primarily affects postmenopausal females. The cytological diagnosis requires the presence of hyperkeratosis, plasma cells, and mixed inflammatory cells. Parakeratotic cells may also be seen.

Keebler CM, Somrak TM, The Manual of Cytotechnology.
Non-neoplastic epithelial disorders, p. 150.

98. A granular cell tumor (myoblastoma)

Granular cell tumors represent a small percentage of the primary vulval tumors. These lesions cytologically yield large cells containing intracytoplasmic eosinophilic granules and finely granular, eccentrically placed nuclei. The finding of a submucosal mass with overlying pigmented mucosa on the labia majora is essential in establishing the diagnosis of this neoplasm.

Keebler CM, Somrak TM, The Manual of Cytotechnology.
Benign tumors, p. 150.

99. A children

Children are generally at a higher risk for gonorrhea infections due to the fragility of the vulval and vaginal mucosa.

Keebler CM, Somrak TM, The Manual of Cytotechnology.
Infectious diseases, p. 148.

100. C fine needle aspiration

The diagnosis of Bartholin gland infections may require access via aspiration due to their submucosal location.

Keebler CM, Somrak TM, The Manual of Cytotechnology.
Infectious diseases, p. 149.

101. A an increase in sheets over gland formation

As adenocarcinoma of the endometrium becomes less differentiated, the ability to cytologically diagnose the presence of glandular formation is diminished. These cells are predominantly found in sheets, as single cells, or in syncytia. Obvious malignant morphology is present, such as an increase in size and number of nucleoli, coarse irregular chromatin, and anisonucleosis. It is important to correctly identify the nature and texture of the cytoplasm as adenocarcinoma rather than of squamous origin. Poorly differentiated glandular lesions lack the ability to form glandular groupings as seen in well-differentiated tumors.

DeMay RM, The Art & Science of Cytopathology.
Endometrial adenocarcinoma, pp. 125–127.

102. C serous adenocarcinoma of the ovary

The diagnosis of papillary serous adenocarcinoma of the ovary in a Pap smear is centered on the finding of three-dimensional aggregates with hyperchromatic nuclei and finely granular, irregularly distributed chromatin with a cervical/endocervical/endometrial biopsy negative and colposcopy negative examination. The presence of papillary groups of malignant cells and psammoma bodies may help in identifying these lesions as ovarian origin, but are not specific findings. A history of ascites is helpful.

DeMay RM, The Art & Science of Cytopathology.
Adenocarcinoma, p. 273.

103. A increase

As adenocarcinoma of the endometrium becomes less differentiated, the ability to cytologically diagnose the presence of glandular formation is diminished. These cells are predominantly found in sheets, as single cells, or in syncytia. Obvious malignant morphology is present, such as an increase in size and number of nucleoli, coarse irregular chromatin, and anisonucleosis. It is important to correctly identify the nature and texture of the cytoplasm as adenocarcinoma rather than of squamous origin. Poorly differentiated glandular lesions lack the ability to form glandular groupings as seen in well-differentiated tumors.

DeMay RM, The Art & Science of Cytopathology.
Cytology of endometrial hyperplasia and neoplasia, pp. 125–127.

104. A folic acid deficiency

Folic acid deficiency (FAD) produces cytomegaly (an increase in the cell volume without cytokinesis) and karyomegaly, changes similar to those seen in radiation cellular injury. Multinucleation and nuclei with fine regular chromatin are observed. Cytoplasmic vacuolization may mimic a "swiss cheese" effect, indicating the cells' degenerative qualities. Folic acid deficiency (FAD) is a common water-soluble vitamin deficiency state among pregnant women. FAD is related to deficient ingestion, absorption and the increased demands of folic acid required during pregnancy.

DeMay RM, The Art & Science of Cytopathology.
Vitamin deficiency states, p. 116.

105. A Donovan bodies, *Calymmatobacterium granulomatis*

Donovan bodies represent histiocytic inclusions or gram-negative bacilli, also identified as *Calymmatobacterium granulomatis*. The morphologic identification of Donovan bodies is based on their "safety pin" appearance. Special staining with Romanowsky may be necessary to establish this diagnosis.

Keebler CM, Somrak TM, The Manual of Cytotechnology.
Infectious diseases, p. 149.

106. B del Castillo syndrome

Patients with del Castillo syndrome may have previously taken birth control pills, and a milky discharge may be elaborated from the breast. The pituitary gland shuts down the production of follicle-stimulating hormone and luteinizing hormone. Therefore, these patients are atrophic.

Keebler CM, Somrak TM, The Manual of Cytotechnology.
Endocrinopathies, pp. 74–78.

107. A mosaic patterns

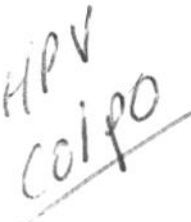

Mosaic patterns and punctuated mucosa are colposcopic findings associated with HPV.

DeMay RM, The Art & Science of Cytopathology.
Clinical considerations (delineation), pp. 139–140.

108. B koilocytosis

Diagnosis of human papillomavirus infection is made based on the presence of koilocytes with or without associated dyskeratosis and/or immature metaplastic infected cells. The cytomorphologic diagnosis provides no information on whether the viral type is low risk (episomal) or high risk (transforming); therefore, risk prediction is not possible. Sophisticated molecular tests, including polymerase chain reaction and Southern blot analysis, may be employed to help decipher the biology of the disease. The 2001 Bethesda System classifies condyloma acuminata (human papillomavirus [HPV]) as a low-grade squamous epithelial lesion. The pathognomonic cell for establishing an HPV infection is the koilocyte. This cell possesses large perinuclear halos (often referred to as cytoplasmic margination or large halo) or crater-like morphology. The nuclei may be well-preserved with fine even chromatin or hyperchromatic and smudged, representing a degenerative quality.

DeMay RM, The Art & Science of Cytopathology.
Diagnosis of condyloma in the Pap smear, pp. 87–88.

109. C an abrupt increase in squamous cell maturation

Patients who have an abrupt rise in maturation or hyperdifferentiation of the squamous mucosa after receiving radiation therapy for squamous carcinoma are at an increased risk for recurrence. Other key indicators include the presence of spindle cells and tissue necrosis.

DeMay RM, The Art & Science of Cytopathology.
Radiation cytology (persistent vs recurrent carcinoma), pp. 119–120.

110. A LEEP/LLETZ

In most instances, treatment for high grade lesions includes cryotherapy, laser ablation, endocervical curettage, large loop excision of the transformation zone (LLETZ), loop electrosurgical excision procedure (LEEP), or a cold knife conization.

DeMay RM, The Art & Science of Cytopathology.
Clinical management, pp. 139–140.

111. A changes associated with *Trichomonas* infections

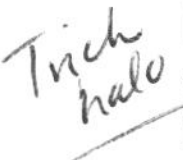

Perinuclear (inflammatory) halos may be found within squamous cells associated with *Trichomonas* or other inflammatory infections. These inflammatory halos are related to alcoholic fixation of an inflamed nucleus, whereas true koilocytic halos are large "cave-like" halos that are at least the width of an intermediate cell nucleus or larger.

DeMay RM, The Art & Science of Cytopathology.
Diagnosis of condyloma in the Pap smear (differential diagnosis of condyloma), p. 88.

112. A parabasal cell predominance

Patients suffering from anorexia nervosa commonly have markedly atrophic vaginal smear patterns due to pituitary inhibition, which in turn, results in its inability to release FSH and LH.

Keebler CM, Somrak TM, The Manual of Cytotechnology.
Endocrinopathies, pp. 74–78.

113. D high-risk HPV types inducing exophytic lesions

Exophytic lesions are those that create condylomatous or papillary lesions. These histologic HPV types are more often associated with low-risk viral types 6 and 11. High-risk viral types have been associated with the development of cervical cancer. In this sequence of events, the E1-E2 region (early genes) are disrupted, interfering with the ability of the virus to transcribe its late genes, thus creating a biologic dead end for the viral life cycle. However, without transcription of these late genes, the feedback mechanism that controls the transcription of the E6-E7 genes (the viral region that codes for proteins that regulate viral growth) is lost. E6-E7 genes may bind anti-oncogenes or tumor suppressor genes such as p53 or Rb (retinoblastoma), which serve as protective genes that prevent transcription of cancer-causing oncogenes.

DeMay RM, The Art & Science of Cytopathology.
Microbiology and molecular biology of HPV, pp. 103–104.

114. D 8 weeks post-irradiation

Should malignant cells with radiation changes be found 8 weeks post-irradiation therapy, it is considered persistent. However, should malignant cells without radiation effect be found 8 weeks post-irradiation therapy, it is considered recurrent malignancy.

DeMay RM, The Art & Science of Cytopathology.
Persistent vs recurrent carcinoma, pp. 119–120.

115. A endocervical reserve cell

The stem cell (if initiated) for nonkeratinizing, metaplastic squamous, and small cell lesions of the uterine cervix is the endocervical reserve cell. Mature metaplastic epithelium may give rise to nonkeratinizing dysplasia, immature squamous metaplasia may give rise to metaplastic dysplasia, and atypical reserve cells may give rise to small cell squamous carcinoma.

DeMay RM, The Art & Science of Cytopathology.
Reserve cell hyperplasia, p. 71.

116. A macrocytes, kite, polka dot, and balloon cells

Markedly enlarged cells (macrocytes), the presence of nuclear smudging without cave-like cytoplasmic margination, and cells with long cytoplasmic tails (kite cells) are nonspecific cells associated with HPV infection. Other minor changes include cells with small globules of condensed cytoplasm (polka dot cells), tone cells, cracked cells, and squamous cells that resemble adipocytes possessing clear cytoplasm and peripherized nuclei (balloon cells). These nonclassical, minor, or "soft" criteria may serve as antecedent cytomorphological changes to a "classical" (koilocytic) HPV diagnosis.

DeMay RM, The Art & Science of Cytopathology.
Diagnosis of condyloma in the Pap smear, p. 88.

117. D intermediate-like cells in cobblestone pattern

Answer D suggests a mature metaplastic cell. Syncytial-like aggregates, hyperchromatic crowded "chaotic" groups with indistinct cell borders are associated with squamous carcinoma in situ.

DeMay RM, The Art & Science of Cytopathology.
Carcinoma in situ, pp. 76–79. Cytoplasm and nucleus, yin and yang of diagnosing dysplasia, pp. 90–94.

118. A large, round-to-oval stripped nuclei

These nuclei are often variable in size and contain "washed out" nuclear chromatin and prominent nucleoli. Their presence represents recurrence and may predate the findings of classic adenocarcinoma, which presents in clusters and glandular formations.

DeMay RM, The Art & Science of Cytopathology.
Radiation cytology (persistent vs recurrent carcinoma), pp. 119–120.

119. A flat

HPV viral types 16 and 18 are more commonly associated with planum (flat) cervical lesions and occur in mature metaplastic epithelium. The acuminatum variety (cauliflower-like) is associated with keratinized lesions.

DeMay RM, The Art & Science of Cytopathology.
Condyloma and human papillomavirus infection, pp. 85–86.

120. B intermediate cell predominance

Long-term, low-dose estrogen replacement produces intermediate level maturation instead of the superficial level maturation associated with short-term estrogen therapy.

DeMay RM, The Art & Science of Cytopathology.
Intermediate predominant maturation index, p. 69.

121. D pseudokeratosis

Synonyms include birth control pill changes, microglandular hyperplasia, and pseudoparakeratosis (pseudokeratosis). These cells represent degenerating forms of hyperplastic endocervical glandular mucosa. The finding has been associated with patients taking oral contraceptives, late luteal phase, and late pregnancy. They are benign cellular findings; however, the differentiation from true parakeratosis is imperative. Cells from microglandular hyperplasia generally have eosinophilic or basophilic cytoplasm, contain eccentric nuclei, or resemble reactive endocervical cells, whereas parakeratosis represents a true keratinizing process (orangeophilia) with centrally located pyknotic nuclei in polygonal "waxy" cytoplasm (possibly with accompanying HPV changes).

DeMay RM, The Art & Science of Cytopathology.
Microglandular endocervical hyperplasia, p. 122.

122. A smaller than the original tumor cells

The small cell sizes associated with recurrent carcinoma are due in part to their anaplastic nature. These cells may also lack the pleomorphism commonly associated with the primary diagnosis of cervical carcinoma. In comparison, an indication of post irradiation dysplasia of the cervix (small cell type) may be the presence of small cells with high N/C ratios and hyperchromatic nuclei. The nuclear chromatin pattern is often too dense to interpret. small cell type post-irradiation dysplasia is more likely to be found in older age groups. These cells mimic small cell carcinoma in situ; however, any grade of post-irradiation dysplasia recurring before 3 years post-irradiation therapy carries a poor prognosis.

DeMay RM, The Art & Science of Cytopathology.
Radiation cytology (persistent vs recurrent carcinoma), pp. 119–120.

123. B abnormal cells replacing the full thickness of the squamous mucosa, no differentiation at the surface

Carcinoma in situ of the cervix replaces the full epithelial thickness of the squamous mucosa with primitive cells, resulting in a total loss of cellular maturation throughout the epithelial strata.

DeMay RM, The Art & Science of Cytopathology.
The cytoplasm, pp. 91–92.

124. C dyskeratocytes

These pleomorphic cells with elongated nuclei, often described as dyskeratocytes or pleomorphic parakeratosis, are classified as atypical squamous cells of undetermined significance under the Bethesda System. Their presence is suggestive but not pathognomonic for human papillomavirus (HPV) infection.

DeMay RM, The Art & Science of Cytopathology.
Diagnosis of condyloma in the Pap smear (dyskeratocytes), pp. 87–88.

125. C increased nuclear to cytoplasmic area in high-grade lesions

One of the most important criteria for distinguishing low-grade squamous epithelial lesions from those of high-grade variety is the nuclear-to-cytoplasmic ratio. As the N/C ratio increases, so does the severity of dysplasia.

DeMay RM, The Art & Science of Cytopathology.
Cytoplasm and nucleus, yin and yang of diagnosing dysplasia, pp. 90–95.

126. D high-grade squamous intraepithelial neoplasia, carcinoma in situ

Abnormal cells lacking nuclear polarity, containing hyperchromatic nuclei with fine-to-coarse and even chromatin and arranged in single cells or syncytia, are suggestive of an in situ lesion. The differential diagnosis between squamous and endocervical in situ lesions depends on many features, including the cell shape (columnar-endocervical) and/or accompanying dysplasia (squamous). Feathering or splattering cytoplasmic processes are often associated with endocervical lesions. One of the hallmarks of squamous carcinoma in situ is its coarse, regular chromatin distribution. Chromatin patterns found in dysplasia are typically finely granular and evenly distributed. Syncytial-like aggregates, hyperchromatic crowded "chaotic" groups with indistinct cell borders are associated with squamous carcinoma in situ. Distinguishing these aggregates from true papillary tissue fragments with community borders, well-formed glandular structures, or HCGs with feathery edges may help in differentiating glandular lesions from those of squamous origin.

DeMay RM, The Art & Science of Cytopathology.
Carcinoma in situ, pp. 76–79, Cytoplasm and nucleus, yin and yang of diagnosing dysplasia, pp. 90–94.

127. B CIN III

Cervical intraepithelial neoplasia (CIN) is a diagnostic classification system that has three classifications: CIN I (mild dysplasia or low-grade intraepithelial lesion), CIN II (moderate dysplasia or high-grade intraepithelial lesion), and CIN III (severe dysplasia, carcinoma in situ, or high-grade intraepithelial lesion).

DeMay RM, The Art & Science of Cytopathology.
Carcinoma in situ, pp. 76–79.

128. A diathesis, increased cellular pleomorphism in carcinoma

A diathesis is defined as the tissue necrosis associated with an invasive malignancy. The debris includes hemolyzed red blood cells, degenerated epithelial cells, and inflammatory cells in a granular or "sandy" background.

DeMay RM, The Art & Science of Cytopathology.
Keratinizing squamous cell carcinoma, p. 85.

129. A *Chlamydia trachomatis*

This obligate intracellular bacterium is the most common cause of nongonococcal cervicitis. Cytologic changes are nonspecific and may range from cytoplasmic inclusions with fine vacuolization that do not displace the nucleus or cytoplasm (nebular bodies) to dysplastic mimicking morphology. Because these findings are neither sensitive nor specific, cytology should not be the method of detection.

DeMay RM, The Art & Science of Cytopathology.
Chlamydia trachomatis, pp. 112–113.

130. A karyomegaly and macrocytosis

Benign radiation changes include vacuolization of the cytoplasm, macrocytosis, amphophilia, nucleomegaly, and well-preserved nuclear-to-cytoplasmic ratios. Nuclear pyknosis and karyorrhexis are degenerative changes associated with benign radiation changes.

DeMay RM, The Art & Science of Cytopathology.
Radiation cytology, pp. 118–119.

131. A irradiation

Benign radiation changes include vacuolization of the cytoplasm, macrocytosis, amphophilia, nucleomegaly, and well-preserved nuclear-to-cytoplasmic ratios. Nuclear pyknosis and karyorrhexis are degenerative changes associated with benign radiation changes.

DeMay RM, The Art & Science of Cytopathology.
Radiation cytology, pp. 118–120.

132. B squamous cell carcinoma, keratinizing type

These cells are demonstrating cellular pleomorphism, orangeophilia, and irregular, hyperchromatic, opaque nuclei. The background contains a granular diathesis. The presence of single cells with these characteristics is diagnostic of a squamous cell carcinoma. Keratinizing squamous carcinomas generally originate on the anterior cervical lip. The single or syncytial-like pleomorphic-to-bizarre tadpole or spindle cell formations are the trademarks of this lesion. The cells may stain orangeophilic or cyanophilic; however, eosinophilia is more often seen. Pyknotic hyperchromatic nuclei are more commonly due to its degenerative features; however, when better preserved, the chromatin is considered coarsely granular and irregularly distributed with nucleoli. A granular diathesis may or may not be present due to the exophytic nature of this lesion. Pearl formations, parakeratosis, and hyperkeratosis may accompany the malignant cells.

DeMay RM, The Art & Science of Cytopathology.
Keratinizing squamous cell carcinoma, p. 85.

133. D atypical reserve cell hyperplasia

Immature metaplastic cells may give rise (if initiated) to metaplastic dysplasias, whereas mature metaplastic cells are linked to nonkeratinizing dysplasia. Atypical reserve cell hyperplasia is related to the development of small cell lesions, and small cell carcinomas in situ give rise to small cell carcinomas.

DeMay RM, The Art & Science of Cytopathology.
Metaplastic lesions (CIN mimicking reserve cell hyperplasia), p. 77.

134. B reserve cells

Replication of the virus begins in the reserve cell or squamous basal cell.

DeMay RM, The Art & Science of Cytopathology.
Prognosis, pp. 106–107.

135. B nonkeratinizing squamous cell carcinoma

Single cells, syncytial fragments, and naked nuclei exhibiting hyperchromasia and coarse irregular chromatin with macronucleoli are diagnostic criteria of nonkeratinizing squamous cell carcinoma of the uterine cervix. A tumor diathesis is more commonly seen with nonkeratinizing carcinomas than in keratinizing malignancies.

DeMay RM, The Art & Science of Cytopathology.
Nonkeratinizing squamous cell carcinoma, pp. 84–85.

136. D early region 6, 7

These early genomic regions are found within cervical carcinomas and their metastases. High-risk viral types have been associated with the development of cervical cancer. In this sequence of events, the E1-E2 region (early genes) are disrupted, interfering with the ability of the virus to transcribe its late genes, thus creating a biologic dead end for the viral life cycle. However, without transcription of these late genes, the feedback mechanism that controls the transcription of the E6-E7 genes (the viral region that codes for proteins that regulate viral growth) is lost. E6-E7 genes may bind antioncogenes or tumor suppressor genes such as p53 or Rb (retinoblastoma), which serve as protective genes that prevent transcription of cancer-causing oncogenes.

DeMay RM, The Art & Science of Cytopathology.
Microbiology and molecular biology of HPV. pp. 103–104.

137. B folic acid deficiency

Folic acid deficiency (FAD) produces cytomegaly (an increase in the cell volume without cytokinesis) and karyomegaly, changes similar to those seen in radiation cellular injury. Multinucleation and nuclei with fine regular chromatin are observed. Cytoplasmic vacuolization may mimic a "swiss cheese" effect, indicating the cells' degenerative qualities. Folic acid deficiency (FAD) is a common water-soluble vitamin deficiency state among pregnant women. FAD is related to deficient ingestion, absorption and the increased demands of folic acid required during pregnancy.

DeMay RM, The Art & Science of Cytopathology.
Radiation cytology (persistent vs. recurrent carcinoma), pp. 119–120, and Vitamin deficiency states, p. 116.

138. C keratinizing processes, nonspecific

Pearl formations, parakeratosis, and hyperkeratosis often accompany keratinizing processes.

DeMay RM, The Art & Science of Cytopathology.
Parakeratosis, pp. 73–74.

139. A small cell neuroendocrine carcinoma, cervix

Small cell lesions arise from atypical reserve cells, foregoing the morphological spectrum associated with dysplastic lesions arising from the mature and immature metaplastic zones. Small cell neuroendocrine carcinoma is a highly malignant neuroendocrine neoplasm that is ultrastructurally part of the amine precursor uptake and decarboxylation (APUD) tumors due to its cytoplasmic evidence of androgenic amines (membrane-bound membrane granules). These cells contain hyperchromatic stippled chromatin, coarse clumping, nuclear molding, scanty cytoplasm, and micronucleoli. They have characteristic vertebral column formation, microbiopsy aggregates, cords, nests, or ribbons. I n 1/3 of the cases, neuroendocrine differentiation may be demonstrated by immunocytochemical staining with chromogranin, neuron-specific enolase, or synaptophysin. Neuroendocrine differentiation (argyrophilia) may also be demonstrated. Small cell carcinomas may be poorly differentiated squamous lesions or neuroendocrine tumors, both of which arise within the endocervical canal. Poorly differentiated squamous carcinomas are composed of small cells with high N/C ratios, uniform cellular sizes with well-defined borders, coarse chromatin with nucleoli, but little-to-absent "crush" artifact. An abnormal host response or necrotic tumor diathesis often accompanies these squamous lesions. The oval nature of the nuclei in small cell squamous carcinoma reflects its high mitotic rate.

DeMay RM, The Art & Science of Cytopathology.
Small cell squamous carcinoma, p. 84.

140. D nucleic acid analysis

Hybrid Capture 2 (Digene Corp) is the only commercially approved in vitro HPV virotyping test for determining low- or high-risk infections. The test uses microplates for capturing RNA hybrids and has an analytical sensitivity of 1.0 pg/mL (5,000 HPV genomes per test). The test is approved direct to vial or can be tested off liquid-based medium (ThinPrep Pap Test only as of March 2002).

DeMay RM, The Art & Science of Cytopathology.
Methods of detection of HPV infection, pp. 86–87 and Microbiology and molecular biology, pp. 103–104.

141. A synaptophysin

Small cell neuroendocrine carcinoma is a highly malignant neuroendocrine neoplasm that is ultrastructurally part of the amine precursor uptake and decarboxylation (APUD) tumors due to its cytoplasmic evidence of androgenic amines (membrane-bound membrane granules). These cells contain hyperchromatic stippled chromatin, coarse clumping, nuclear molding, scanty cytoplasm, and micronucleoli. They have characteristic vertebral column formation, microbiopsy aggregates, cords, nests, or ribbons. In 1/3 of the cases, neuroendocrine differentiation may be demonstrated by immunocytochemical staining with chromogranin, neuron-specific enolase, or synaptophysin. Neuroendocrine differentiation (argyrophilia) may also be demonstrated.

DeMay RM, The Art & Science of Cytopathology.
Small cell cervical cancers, p. 136.

142. C immunohistochemistry

Immunocytochemistry may be helpful in differentiating metastatic lesions. Special staining with chromogranin (neuroendocrine lesions), S-100 (melanoma), leukocyte common antigen (lymphoma), and alpha-fetoprotein (GI tract lesions) are some examples of its utility.

DeMay RM, The Art & Science of Cytopathology.
Metastasis, p. 137.

143. A greater

Immature metaplastic cells may give rise (if initiated) to metaplastic dysplasias, a variant that more commonly progresses to cancer (untreated) than nonkeratinizing dysplasia.

DeMay RM, The Art & Science of Cytopathology.
Metaplastic lesions, pp. 77–78.

144. A 1

Intestinal or mucinous endometrial adenocarcinoma usually presents as a grade I (well-differentiated) lesion. The cells contain abundant mucin secretion as represented by the distended cytoplasmic vacuolization. The differential diagnosis is mucinous adenocarcinoma of the ovary, but the presence of a pale sticky diathesis will help establish this lesion as primary.

DeMay RM, The Art & Science of Cytopathology.
Cytology of endometrial hyperplasia and neoplasia, p. 127.

145. A diathesis-related changes with malignancies involving direct extension

Metastatic carcinomas usually lack a notable diathesis unless tumor seeding has occurred within the ectopic area.

DeMay RM, The Art & Science of Cytopathology.
Metastasis, p. 137.

146. C few "atypical" cells, associated benign epithelial elements

This degenerative artifactual change may show hyperchromatic crowded groups; however, these groups are generally sparse when compared with true neoplasia. Furthermore, cellular crowding is less pronounced as compared with neoplasia, and the chromatin is fine and regular. Mitotic figures are rare. Ciliated cells may be seen in conjunction with benign endometrial or endocervical elements.

DeMay RM, The Art & Science of Cytopathology.
Differential diagnosis of atypical glandular (endocervical) cells, pp. 132–133.

147. D carcinoma in situ

Syncytial-like aggregates, hyperchromatic crowded "chaotic" groups with indistinct cell borders, are associated with squamous carcinoma in situ. Distinguishing these aggregates from true papillary tissue fragments with community borders, well-formed glandular structures, or HCGs with feathery edges may help in differentiating glandular lesions from those of squamous origin.

DeMay RM, The Art & Science of Cytopathology.
Carcinoma in situ, p. 76, and The secrets of diagnosing dysplasia and carcinoma in situ, pp. 93–94.

148. B eighth week of gestation

Vaginal adenosis is defined as the presence of ectopic glandular epithelium or squamous metaplastic cells within the normally gland-free or squamous-lined vagina. Their presence is increased in those patients who were exposed to diethylstilbestrol (DES) in utero.

DeMay RM, The Art & Science of Cytopathology.
Metaplastic reactions, p. 70.

149. A *Vorticella* sp.

In addition to *Vorticella,* other examples of uncommon protozoa include *Entamoeba histolytica* and *Balantidium coli.* Answers B, C, and D represent contaminants of vaginal smears.

Keebler CM, Somrak TM, The Manual of Cytotechnology.
Microbiologic classification, p. 90.

150. B *Staphylococcus aureus*

Staphylococcus aureus, as identified by culture, is the most common cause of toxic shock syndrome in females.

Keebler CM, Somrak TM, The Manual of Cytotechnology.
Microbiologic classification, p. 88.

151. B myofibroblasts

Fibroblasts are common findings represented in cervical/vaginal specimens from patients who have received radiation for epithelial malignancies. Ulceration or epithelial fragility secondary to radiation is responsible for their presence. Differentiation from recurrent squamous carcinoma (SC) is based on the findings of single cells without opaque/nuclear hyperchromasia or coarse, irregular chromatin. In addition, the cytoplasm of fibroblasts is described as sparse, wispy, or vacuolated, whereas cells from SC typically possess abundant pleomorphic and/or orangeophilic dense cytoplasm.

DeMay RM, The Art & Science of Cytopathology.
Other manifestations of inflammation, pp.115–116.

152. D *Turbatrix aceti*

Turbatrix aceti is an uncommon vinegar eel, which may be found in smears from patients who douche with vinegar-based solutions.

Keebler CM, Somrak TM, The Manual of Cytotechnology.
Microbiologic classification, p. 90.

153. B rhabdomyosarcoma

Rhabdomyosarcoma is a heterologous sarcoma of the uterus that presents itself cytologically similar to leiomyosarcoma; however, this malignancy represents a striated muscle rather than a smooth muscle origin. The findings of "strap cells" are diagnostic of malignant blasts; however, strap cells represent only 1% of the total malignant population. It is important, however, to find these striations to help elucidate the origin of these cells. Multinucleated tumor giant cells are also observed with these malignancies. A heterologous mixed müllerian tumor is diagnosed by the identification of well-differentiated endometrial adenocarcinoma plus a nonindigenous sarcomatous element. Heterologous connective tissue malignancies may include osteosarcoma, chondrosarcoma, or rhabdomyosarcoma.

DeMay RM, The Art & Science of Cytopathology.
Sarcomas, pp. 136–137.

154. B poorly differentiated, delicate cytoplasm, prominent nucleoli

Clear cell adenocarcinomas of the endometrium are poorly differentiated tumors, which may have glycogenated cytoplasm. Classic malignant nuclear features are represented.

DeMay RM, The Art & Science of Cytopathology.
Cytology of endometrial hyperplasia and neoplasia, p. 127.

155. B small cell carcinoma

Small cell neuroendocrine carcinoma is a highly malignant neuroendocrine neoplasm that is ultrastructurally part of the amine precursor uptake and decarboxylation (APUD) tumors due to its cytoplasmic evidence of androgenic amines (membrane-bound membrane granules). These cells contain hyperchromatic stippled chromatin, coarse clumping, nuclear molding, scanty cytoplasm, and micronucleoli. They have characteristic vertebral column formation, microbiopsy aggregates, cords, nests, or ribbons. In 1/3 of the cases, neuroendocrine differentiation may be demonstrated by immunocytochemical staining with chromogranin, neuron-specific enolase, or synaptophysin. Neuroendocrine differentiation (argyrophilia) may also be demonstrated.

DeMay RM, The Art & Science of Cytopathology.
Small cell cervical cancers, p. 136.

156. A CIS involves the underlying gland-like spaces

Glandular or microacinar differentiation within the syncytial-like aggregates may be seen if the squamous carcinoma in situ extends into the endocervical glands.

DeMay RM, The Art & Science of Cytopathology.
Differential diagnosis of atypical glandular (endocervical) cells (squamous carcinoma in situ), p. 133, Carcinoma in situ, p. 76, and Early endocervical glandular neoplasia, pp. 129–130.

157. A secretory adenocarcinoma

Secretory adenocarcinoma of the endometrium cytologically recapitulates well-differentiated adenocarcinoma features, making these two conditions extremely difficult to differentiate using conventional cytopathology. With few exceptions, the cytologic manifestations do not reveal the secretory nature of these cells. Glycogen-positive cytoplasm is a feature of these tumors, but cytoplasmic vacuolization may not be a reliable distinguishing feature due to the shared morphology with mucinous adenocarcinomas of the endometrium. On the other hand, serous lesions often lack a tumor diathesis or the mucinous background associated with mucinous adenocarcinomas.

DeMay RM, The Art & Science of Cytopathology.
Endometrial adenocarcinoma, p. 127.

158. C micronucleoli, diathesis

Microinvasive carcinomas of the cervix may be discriminated from carcinoma in situ by the presence of irregular chromatin distribution and micronucleoli. The cells are isolated, have syncytial-like arrangement, or are arranged in hyperchromatic crowded groups. The background contains a diathesis in up to 35% of the cases.

DeMay RM, The Art & Science of Cytopathology.
Microinvasive squamous cell carcinoma, pp. 80–83.

159. A radiation

Granulomatous cervicitis may be related to tuberculosis, sutures, radiation, granuloma inguinale, lymphogranuloma venereum, schistosomiasis, syphilis, and possibly chlamydia. The cytologic identification of this nonspecific condition is dependent upon the findings of foreign body giant cells (often with intracytoplasmic antigenic substance), epithelioid cells, and an inflammatory background.

DeMay RM, The Art & Science of Cytopathology.
Granulation tissue, pp. 114–115.

160. B multinucleated giant histiocyte

Multinucleated histiocytes are often identified in vaginal smears taken from postmenopausal patients. Their presence is a normal finding in conjunction with epithelial atrophy.

DeMay RM, The Art & Science of Cytopathology.
Other manifestations of inflammation, p. 114.

161. B vitamins A, B, and C deficiency

Other cofactors may include smoking, cervical trauma, cytomegalovirus, chlamydia, smoking, steroids, pregnancy (immunodeficiency), decreased cellular immunity, or genetic susceptibility.

DeMay RM, The Art & Science of Cytopathology.
Possible cofactors in cervical carcinogenesis, pp. 105–106.

162. D squamous cell carcinoma, keratinizing type

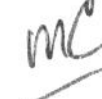

Primary carcinoma of the vulva, a disease predominantly affecting elderly women, is cytologically diagnosed as keratinizing or pleomorphic squamous carcinoma. Cytoplasmic pleomorphism, India ink nuclei, decreased polarity, and coarse irregular chromatin are cytologic hallmarks of this disease.

Keebler CM, Somrak TM, The Manual of Cytotechnology.
Malignant tumors, p. 151.

163. C Bartholin gland adenocarcinoma

Bartholin gland adenocarcinomas are submucosal lesions that cytologically present as typical mucous glands possessing classic malignant criteria. Aspiration cytology may be necessary to diagnose this rare tumor.

Keebler CM, Somrak TM, The Manual of Cytotechnology.
Malignant tumors, p. 152.

164. A serous cystadenocarcinoma

The diagnosis of papillary serous adenocarcinoma of the ovary in a Pap smear is centered on the finding of three-dimensional aggregates with hyperchromatic nuclei and finely granular, irregularly distributed chromatin with a cervical/endocervical/endometrial biopsy negative and colposcopy negative examination. The presence of papillary groups of malignant cells and psammoma bodies may help in identifying these lesions as ovarian origin, but are not specific findings. A history of ascites is helpful.

DeMay RM, The Art & Science of Cytopathology.
Adenocarcinoma, p. 273.

165. B endometrial stromal sarcoma

Endometrial stromal sarcoma is a homologous sarcoma found as small cells or groups with high N/C ratios and coarse hyperchromatic nuclei. The cytoplasmic morphology recapitulates that of benign endometrial superficial stromal cells.

DeMay RM, The Art & Science of Cytopathology.
Sarcomas, p. 137.

166. D Sertoli-Leydig cell tumor

The presence of psammoma bodies may be associated with most papillary lesions of the female genital tract. Endometrial adenocarcinomas, tubal malignancies, and reactive endometrium secondary to IUD implants may produce psammoma bodies in vaginal/cervical smears. The finding of these entities is not pathognomonic for malignancy.

DeMay RM, The Art & Science of Cytopathology.
Psammoma bodies, p. 139.

167. B little pleomorphism

Adenocarcinoma in situ of the endocervix is identified cytologically with hyperchromasia, predictable nuclear sizes, loss of polarity, and irregular nuclear sizes and shapes, all in the presence of feathering effects. Large numbers of atypical cells will be found in comparison with normal endocervical cells. Abnormal cells lacking nuclear polarity, containing hyperchromatic nuclei with fine to coarse and even chromatin, and arranged in single cells or syncytia, are suggestive of an in situ lesion. The differential diagnosis between squamous and endocervical in situ lesions depends on many features, including the cell shape (columnar-endocervical) and/or accompanying dysplasia (squamous). Feathering or splattering cytoplasmic processes are often associated with endocervical lesions.

DeMay RM, The Art & Science of Cytopathology.
Early endocervical glandular neoplasia, pp. 129–130.

168. B not before 6–8 weeks post administration

The acute phase of post irradiation consists of an admixture of necrotic tumor cells, white blood cells, and regenerative/reparative changes amongst a diathesis-laden background. Due to the smear's degenerative nature and the lingering malignant cells, effective analysis of these smears is best at least 6 to 8 weeks post irradiation. Should malignant cells with radiation changes be found 8 weeks post irradiation therapy, it is considered persistent. However, should malignant cells without radiation effect be found 8 weeks post irradiation therapy, it is considered recurrent malignancy.

DeMay RM, The Art & Science of Cytopathology.
Radiation cytology, p. 118.

169. A atypical glandular cells (AGUS) often accompany squamous dysplasia

The presence of atypical (dysplastic) endocervical glandular cells found in concert with squamous dysplasia is not an unusual finding, primarily due to their shared HPV etiology.

DeMay RM, The Art & Science of Cytopathology.
Early endocervical glandular neoplasia, pp. 129–130.

170. A Paget disease

The diagnosis of extramammary Paget disease of the vulva is based on the clinical manifestation of erythematous lesions. The presence of signet ring cells with frankly malignant nuclear criteria is helpful in establishing the primary diagnosis. Should Paget cells contain intracytoplasmic granules, the differential diagnosis of malignant melanoma might be difficult. Immunocytochemical staining with S100 may be helpful in discriminating melanomas from extramammary adenocarcinomas.

Keebler CM, Somrak TM, The Manual of Cytotechnology.
Malignant tumors, p. 151.

171. C atypical glandular cells of undetermined significance, favor neoplastic

Adenocarcinoma in situ of the endocervix is identified cytologically with hyperchromasia, predictable nuclear sizes, loss of polarity, and irregular nuclear sizes and shapes, all in the presence of feathering effects. Large numbers of atypical cells will be found in comparison with normal endocervical cells. Abnormal cells lacking nuclear polarity, containing hyperchromatic nuclei with fine to coarse and even chromatin, and arranged in single cells or syncytia, are suggestive of an in situ lesion. The differential diagnosis between squamous and endocervical in situ lesions depends on many features, including the cell shape (columnar-endocervical) and/or accompanying dysplasia (squamous). Feathering or splattering cytoplasmic processes are often associated with endocervical lesions.

DeMay RM, The Art & Science of Cytopathology.
Early endocervical glandular neoplasia, pp. 129–130.

172. C granular

One of the key differential features between endometrial adenocarcinoma and endocervical adenocarcinoma is the cytoplasmic texture. Endocervical adenocarcinoma tends to have granular cytoplasm.

DeMay RM, The Art & Science of Cytopathology.
Endocervical carcinoma, pp. 127–128.

173. D Arias-Stella reaction

Arias-Stella changes involve endometrial and endocervical cells and are seen in late pregnancy (high levels of HCG/prolonged progesterone stimulation). The endocervical cells possess pale PAS + cytoplasm and hyperchromatic nuclei with macronucleoli. Intranuclear cytoplasmic inclusions may also be seen. This "atypical reparative" morphology needs to be discriminated from clear cell adenocarcinoma; however, correlation of these changes with the clinical history will help define these changes as benign.

DeMay RM, The Art & Science of Cytopathology.
Arias-Stella reaction, p. 134.

174. A cells with columnar morphology arranged into rosettes and crowded sheets with holes for endocervical adenocarcinoma compared with round, plump cells arranged into balls and molded groups for endometrial adenocarcinoma

The number of cells found in well-differentiated endocervical adenocarcinoma (ECA) is typically greater than that found in endometrial adenocarcinomas (EMA). Cells associated with ECA are larger, contain more abundant cytoplasm, retain columnar configuration, and have finely granular, irregularly distributed chromatin with micronucleoli. EMAs are diffusely vacuolated and often contain engulfed polymorphonuclear cells, the opposite of the granular cytoplasm generally found in lesions arising from the endocervical glands. Endometrial adenocarcinoma cytologically presents with fewer numbers of cells on the slide (as opposed to endocervical adenocarcinomas), cell clusters with scalloping borders and three-dimensional tissue fragments, high nuclear-to-cytoplasmic ratios, and frothy, delicate, lacy, vacuolated cytoplasm. One of the key differential features between this lesion and endocervical adenocarcinomas is the cytoplasmic texture. Endocervical adenocarcinoma, as indicated earlier, tends to have granular cytoplasm. Finally, the presence of a watery diathesis with associated lipophages may be helpful in discriminating endometrial adenocarcinomas from other epithelial malignancies.

DeMay RM, The Art & Science of Cytopathology.
Differential diagnosis of endocervical and endometrial carcinoma, p. 129.

175. A prolonged progesterone stimulation

Arias-Stella changes involve endometrial and endocervical cells and are seen in late pregnancy (high levels of HCG/prolonged progesterone stimulation). The endocervical cells possess pale PAS + cytoplasm and hyperchromatic nuclei with macronucleoli. Intranuclear cytoplasmic inclusions may also be seen. This "atypical reparative" morphology needs to be discriminated from clear cell adenocarcinoma; however, correlation of these changes with the clinical history will help define these changes as benign.

DeMay RM, The Art & Science of Cytopathology.
Arias-Stella reaction, p. 134.

176. D malignant melanoma

Melanoma typically presents in single cells, aggregates, or as spindle cells with bizarre malignant nuclear features, macronucleoli, intranuclear cytoplasmic inclusions, and possibly intracytoplasmic golden brown pigment. Due to the fact that these diseases may be amelanotic, it may be helpful to confirm this disease process with S-100, HMB-45, Melan A or MITF (microphthalmia-associated transcription factor)—all which preferentially react with melanoma cells.

Wang JF, Sarma DP, and Ulmer P. Diagnostic dilemma: HMB-45 and Melan-A negative tumor, can it be still a melanoma?: MITF (Microphthalmia-associated transcription factor) stain may confirm the diagnosis. The Internet Journal of Dermatology. 2007. Volume 5 Number 1.

177. A increase in single cells, loosely arranged cell groups, macronucleoli, and diathesis present in endocervical adenocarcinoma

Endocervical adenocarcinoma must be discriminated from adenocarcinoma in situ. Endocervical adenocarcinoma in situ does not have the classic malignant chromatin features of adenocarcinoma and does not present in true tissue fragments, but rather with feathering cytoplasmic effects.

DeMay RM, The Art & Science of Cytopathology.
Early endocervical glandular neoplasia, pp. 129–131.

178. A chromatin is fine-to-moderately granular and cells present with minimal anisocytosis and lack pseudostratification in endocervical glandular dysplasia

Endocervical cells with slightly enlarged hyperchromatic nuclei with inconspicuous nucleoli, loss of polarity, and rosette formations are helpful in establishing a diagnosis of atypical glandular cells of undetermined significance, in this case, referred to as endocervical columnar dysplasia (ECD). Its differential diagnosis is endocervical adenocarcinoma in situ (AIS); however, ECD has fine, regular chromatin, whereas endocervical AIS contains coarse chromatin features and cellular pseudostratification (trailing, splattering, feathering patterns).

DeMay RM, The Art & Science of Cytopathology.
Early endocervical glandular neoplasia, pp. 129–130.

179. B vacuolated cytoplasm, finely granular chromatin with macronucleoli in endometrial adenocarcinoma

Due to the lack of differentiation found in large cell/poorly differentiated squamous carcinomas, it if often difficult to distinguish these lesions from poorly differentiated adenocarcinoma (PDA). PDA, however, may present with vacuolated cytoplasm and finely granular chromatin, whereas large cell squamous lesions contain densely granular cytoplasm and coarse, irregular chromatin patterns. Special stains are ineffective due to the fact that many PDAs are non-mucus-secreting lesions.

DeMay RM, The Art & Science of Cytopathology.
Cytology of endometrial hyperplasia and neoplasia, p. 126.

180. C embryonal rhabdomyosarcoma

Embryonal rhabdomyosarcoma is considered an uncommon vaginal lesion affecting young girls (generally less than 5 years of age). Clinically, these patients present with grape-like neoplasms protruding from the vagina. The cytological identification of small single cells, clusters, and cells with elongated tadpole-like morphology with broad bands ("strap cells") is helpful in identifying this lesion. Tissue biopsy confirmation is essential.

Keebler CM, Somrak TM, The Manual of Cytotechnology.
Embryonal rhabdomyosarcoma, p. 154.

181. B 20

The development of vaginal adenocarcinoma arising in patients exposed to diethylstilbestrol (DES) in utero usually occurs in the third decade. The precursor lesion is vaginal adenosis. Clear cell adenocarcinoma presents as a typical mucinous adenocarcinoma containing enlarged nuclei and hypochromatic irregularly distributed chromatin. The presence of "hobnail cells," in which the nuclei are peripherally oriented toward the glandular lumen, may be helpful in identifying this malignancy.

Keebler CM, Somrak TM, The Manual of Cytotechnology.
Clear cell adenocarcinoma, p. 155.

182. C "hobnail" serous adenocarcinoma, endometrium

Serous or "hobnail" adenocarcinoma of the endometrium is a poorly differentiated endometrial lesion. Cells found in papillary clusters with associated psammoma bodies scattered among a necrotic background may be helpful in discriminating these lesions from serous adenocarcinoma of the ovary, due to the clean background associated with metastatic tumors.

DeMay RM, The Art & Science of Cytopathology.
Papillary serous adenocarcinoma, p. 127.

183. D primary endometrioid endocervical adenocarcinoma

Primary endometrioid endocervical adenocarcinoma (EEA) may mimic true endometrial adenocarcinoma (EA) with the exception that many of the cells of endometrioid endocervical adenocarcinoma have columnar morphology as well as endometrioid features. In addition, EEA presents with an increased number of malignant cells when compared with EA. Care should be taken to rule out the possibility of an endometrial adenocarcinoma that directly extends into the cervical os.

DeMay RM, The Art & Science of Cytopathology.
Endocervical carcinoma, p. 128.

184. D bowenoid papulosis

Bowenoid papulosis is often referred to as carcinoma in situ of the vulva. Human papillomavirus exposure has been implicated as causative etiology in its histiogenesis, usually affecting young females. Cytologic criteria for diagnosing bowenoid papulosis are similar to those of cervical carcinoma in situ.

Keebler CM, Somrak TM, The Manual of Cytotechnology.
Bowenoid papulosis, p. 150.

185. A a spore form predominates in this species

Torulopsis glabrata has uninterrupted outer walls as well as budding encapsulated yeast, whereas *Candida* sp. possess pseudohyphae.

DeMay RM, The Art & Science of Cytopathology.
Fungi, p. 56.

186. A elementary bodies

This obligate intracellular bacterium (*Chlamydia trachomatis*) is the most common cause of nongonococcal cervicitis. Cytologic changes are nonspecific and may range from cytoplasmic inclusions with fine vacuolization that do not displace the nucleus or cytoplasm (nebular bodies) to dysplastic mimicking morphology. Because these findings are neither sensitive nor specific, cytology should not be the method of detection.

DeMay RM, The Art & Science of Cytopathology.
Chlamydia trachomatis, pp. 112–113.

187. D diathesis changes associated with an invasive primary malignancy

A diathesis is defined as the tissue necrosis associated with an invasive malignancy. The debris includes hemolyzed red blood cells, degenerated epithelial cells, and inflammatory cells scattered in a granular or "sandy" background. Care must be taken not to confuse this process with normal necrobiosis or coccoid bacteria, which often accompany *Trichomonas vaginalis.*

DeMay RM, The Art & Science of Cytopathology.
Squamous cell carcinoma, p. 83.

188. A increased risk of fetal infection, possibly resulting in death in utero

Cells with large, basophilic inclusions suggestive of an "owl's eye" are diagnostic of infection with cytomegalovirus. Occasionally, eosinophilic intracytoplasmic inclusions are found. The diagnosis is imperative in pregnant females due to the increased risk of abortion or development of severe physical and mental malformities in the fetus.

DeMay RM, The Art & Science of Cytopathology.
Viruses, p. 54.

189. D *Trichomonas vaginalis*

Leptothrix vaginalis are long hair-like structures that tend to aggregate in the presence of *Trichomonas vaginalis.*

DeMay RM, The Art & Science of Cytopathology.
Specific infections, p. 111.

190. D adenosis

The presence of glandular or squamous metaplastic epithelium in the vagina (normally lined by native squamous epithelium) is diagnostic of vaginal adenosis. This condition has been linked to in utero exposure to diethylstilbestrol (DES).

DeMay RM, The Art & Science of Cytopathology.
Endocervical cells, p. 121.

191. A these cells are indicative of infection by human papillomavirus

Parakeratosis is considered ASC-US under the Bethesda terminology and not specific for the determination of an HPV infection. Only the presence of koilocytes is a specific diagnostic indicator of HPV.

DeMay RM, The Art & Science of Cytopathology.
Keratotic reactions, pp. 72–74.

192. B cytomegalovirus

Cells with large, basophilic inclusions suggestive of an "owl's eye" are diagnostic of an infection with cytomegalovirus. Occasionally, eosinophilic intracytoplasmic inclusions are found. The correct diagnosis is imperative in pregnant females due to the increased risk of abortion or development of severe physical and mental malformities in the fetus.

DeMay RM, The Art & Science of Cytopathology.
Viruses, p. 54

193. B use of birth control pills

Candida sp. is a common yeast found in pregnancy, late luteal phase, birth control pill users, patients with diabetes mellitus, immunosuppression, or those taking broad spectrum antibiotics. The characteristic pseudohyphae structures ("sticks") and/or the presence of small spores ("stones") are necessary to establish the diagnosis.

DeMay RM, The Art & Science of Cytopathology.
Hormonal cytology, p. 69.

194. A hyperkeratosis

Leukoplakia, clinically defined as a white patch, is the gross pathologic counterpart of hyperkeratosis acanthosis. This condition denotes the hard, cornified visible area located either on the ectocervix or vagina.

DeMay RM, The Art & Science of Cytopathology.
Keratotic reactions, pp. 72–73.

195. C *Geotrichum candidum*

Geotrichum candidum appears as a large fungal structure that often branches at 90-degree angles. Diagnosis is confirmed by the evaluation of true hyphae (not pseudohyphae as in *Candida albicans*) and/or arthrospores.

DeMay RM, The Art & Science of Cytopathology.
Fungi, p. 56.

196. B postmenopausal patient with adrenal hyperplasia

An intermediate cell/level vaginal epithelial maturation will predominate in patients taking exogenous androgens. Answer A will create superficial cell/level maturation while answers C and D are associated with deep parabasal level dematuration.

DeMay RM, The Art & Science of Cytopathology.
Hormonal cytology, p. 69.

197. D suggestive of pollen

Pollen is often found in cervical smears due to aerial contamination from plant sources within the laboratory or physician's office. These structures present as transparent oval structures with a refractile glassy capsule and a thick cell wall with spikes.

DeMay RM, The Art & Science of Cytopathology.
Arthropods and contaminants, p. 58.

198. A may mask an underlying pathologic condition

Parakeratosis, an abortive attempt at keratinization, may overlie a serious abnormality such as infection by human papillomavirus (HPV), dysplasia, or even invasive carcinoma. The diagnosis is important and should be correlated with the surrounding cytologic findings. The finding of parakeratosis should be discriminated from related changes occurring in dyskeratocytes, atypical squamous cells suggestive of an HPV infection.

DeMay RM, The Art & Science of Cytopathology.
Keratotic reactions, pp. 72–74.

199. A benign protective reaction

Hyperkeratosis is a condition of overall greater epithelial thickness (hyperdifferentiation). A stratum corneum (anucleate squames) replaces the normally nonkeratinized superficial cell layer.

DeMay RM, The Art & Science of Cytopathology.
Keratotic reactions, pp. 72–73.

200. C vaginal acidity

Döderlein bacillus, or *Lactobacillus acidophilus,* is considered normal flora of the vagina. Its production of lactic acid serves as an endogenous inhibitor of microbial growth by maintaining a low pH. The organism is commonly seen in the latter half of the menstrual cycle (days 15–28), at which time glycogenated cells predominate. These organisms produce lactic acid by destroying the intermediate cells, thus creating cytolysis.

DeMay RM, The Art & Science of Cytopathology.
Bacteria, p. 54.

201. B use of intrauterine devices

Actinomyces sp. is a filamentous bacillus that branches at acute angles and clumps together to form structures known as "sulfur granules." These entities may be found in patients who have intrauterine devices (IUD).

DeMay RM, The Art & Science of Cytopathology.
Specific infections, p. 112.

202. A atrophy

Sheets of lower level parabasal-to-basal cells with autolytic features and degenerating karyolytic cells or "blue blobs," and the finding of pyknotic parabasal cells with eosinophilic cytoplasm, often referred to as "mummified cells," are characteristic of deep atrophy, which is often found in postmenopausal or post-partum patients. Care should be taken to discriminate these findings from more significant conditions such as parakeratosis or dyskeratosis, lesions which are associated with true keratinizing processes.

DeMay RM, The Art & Science of Cytopathology.
Hormonal cytology, pp. 68–69.

203. C lubricant jelly

Lubricant jelly often appears in the background of cervical smears as a blue to purple haze or tint. Differential diagnosis would include "sticky" mucus from the endocervical canal; however, mucin usually stains eosinophilic. Clinicians should apply warm water instead of lubricant to the speculum before performing a Pap smear.

DeMay RM, The Art & Science of Cytopathology.
Arthropods and contaminants, p. 58.

204. C late secretory

The predominance of intermediate cells and cytolysis suggests an increased progesterone stimulation, which in turn produces epithelial dedifferentiation of the vaginal mucosa. The presence of Döderlein bacillus will often accompany these cytologic findings.

DeMay RM, The Art & Science of Cytopathology.
Hormonal cytology, pp. 67–69.

205. D herpesvirus

The presence of "ground glass" chromatin, chromatinic margination, multinucleation, and nuclear molding, with or without intranuclear eosinophilic Cowdry Type A inclusions, suggests a diagnosis of herpesvirus. Grossly, these lesions appear as erythematous papules or ulcerations. They must be distinguished from other multinucleated cells found within smears.

DeMay RM, The Art & Science of Cytopathology.
Specific infections, p. 112.

206. B it is impossible to predict the progression rate of the lesion

Diagnosis of human papillomavirus infection is based on the presence of koilocytes with or without associated dyskeratosis and/or immature metaplastic infected cells. The cytomorphologic diagnosis provides no information on whether the viral type is low risk (episomal) or high risk (transforming); therefore, risk prediction is not possible. Sophisticated molecular tests, including polymerase chain reaction and Southern blot analysis, may be employed to help decipher the biology of the disease.

DeMay RM, The Art & Science of Cytopathology.
Natural history of squamous intraepithelial lesions, pp. 100–109.

207. A diabetes mellitus

Patients with diabetes mellitus are at an increased risk for endogenous and exogenous vaginal infections. Fungal infections, such as the *Candida* infection shown here, are common.

DeMay RM, The Art & Science of Cytopathology.
Specific infections, pp. 111–112.

208. D too long between application of mounting medium and coverslipping

Improper coverslipping may lead to "corn flaking" or brown artifact, which is most likely caused by the drying of the mounting medium before the coverslip has been placed. Gill indicates an increased occurrence with the required small fume hoods (personal communication). Conversely, water in the xylene will cause a milky haze to appear on the slide, not a brown artifact.

DeMay RM, The Art & Science of Cytopathology.
Hyperkeratosis, p. 73.

209. A perimenarche

Three cell patterns (ie, superficial, intermediate, and parabasal) found simultaneously in vaginal smears are often associated with perimenarchal early squamous maturation. Parabasal cells are generally not observed in mature cycling females (as in answers B and C) and the presence of a large population of superficial cells (estrogenic stimulation, answer D) is a contraindication in postmenopausal females unless the patient is under the administration of short-term exogenous estrogen therapy, or if found with other pathologic disorders such as endometrial adenocarcinomas or granulosa-theca cell tumors of the ovary.

DeMay RM, The Art & Science of Cytopathology.
Hormonal cytology, pp. 67–69.

210. A 0/50/50

In this example, there is a 50% admixture of superficial (pyknotic) cells and intermediate (vesicular) cells.

Keebler CM, Somrak TM, The Manual of Cytotechnology.
Endocrinopathies, pp. 74–78.

211. B menopausal patient on high-dose, short-term estrogen therapy

Short-term estrogen therapy in many atrophic patients will create a hyperdifferentiation of the squamous mucosa of the vagina, the result being a richly estrogen-primed epithelium. A predominant population of superficial cells will be observed when hormonal smears are performed on these patients. Answers A, C, and D are associated with intermediate cell/level maturation.

DeMay RM, The Art & Science of Cytopathology.
Hormonal cytology, pp. 69-70.

212. B vaginal adenosis

Squamous metaplasia should not be observed in mucosa of the vagina. These findings suggest possible DES exposure in utero. The presence of glandular or squamous metaplastic epithelium in the vagina (normally lined by native squamous epithelium) is diagnostic of vaginal adenosis.

DeMay RM, The Art & Science of Cytopathology.
Metaplastic reactions, p. 70.

213. A 18-year-old woman with primary amenorrhea

The cellular pattern, consistent with deep parabasal cells in sheets, may represent an atrophic smear taken from a post-pubertal patient with hyperestrinism. Conditions such as Turner syndrome may explain these findings.

DeMay RM, The Art & Science of Cytopathology.
Hormonal cytology, pp. 68–69.

214. C alkalinity

When the pH of the vagina rises, organisms such as *Candida* sp. tend to proliferate. Changes in the hormonal status, administration of birth control pills, pregnancy, and antibiotic therapy are other situations in which these organisms tend to flourish. The characteristic pseudohyphae structures and/or the presence of small spores are necessary to establish the diagnosis.

DeMay RM, The Art & Science of Cytopathology.
Fungi, p. 56.

215. B molluscum contagiosum

This disease, related to the poxvirus and sexually transmitted in cases of vaginal infections, presents clinically as papillomatous skin lesions. Cytological identification of parabasal cells with large eosinophilic intracytoplasmic inclusions and degenerated (often karyolytic) nuclei are important for the diagnosis of molluscum contagiosum.

DeMay RM, The Art & Science of Cytopathology.
Viruses, p. 54.

216. B good prognostic information

The cytologic picture is consistent with that of pregnancy or progesterone-stimulated epithelium. The administration of estrogen has no effect upon a progesterone-primed epithelium; therefore, no cytohormonal deviation will be found in a normal pregnancy. Should a hormonal imbalance exist, the estrogen test would promote cellular maturation.

DeMay RM, The Art & Science of Cytopathology.
Hormonal cytology, p. 69.

217. C treat and repeat due to presence of microbiologic agent

The presence of *Trichomonas vaginalis* precludes the possibility of rendering a hormonal evaluation due to the pseudoeosinophila (a false estrogenic maturation) that is associated with its presence.

DeMay RM, The Art & Science of Cytopathology.
Specific infections, p. 111.

218. D late proliferative phase of the menstrual cycle

Answer D indicates a hyperestrogenic pattern which should predominate in a normal mature cycling female prior to ovulation. Estrogen primed epithelium should consist of a superficial cell/level maturation, whereas the hormonal pattern depicted in this photomicrograph is consistent with a progesterone-stimulated mucosa, such as the maturation levels found in answers A, B, and C.

DeMay RM, The Art & Science of Cytopathology.
Hormonal cytology, p. 69.

219. A pleomorphism/caudate shape/opaque, irregular chromatin distribution

The cytologic attributes described represent squamous cell carcinoma. Answer B represents an adenocarcinoma, answer C is diagnostic of immature metaplastic cells, and answer D represents a diagnosis of reparative/reactive changes.

DeMay RM, The Art & Science of Cytopathology.
Keratinizing squamous cell carcinoma, p.85.

220. C adenocarcinoma in situ/carcinoma in situ

Abnormal cells lacking nuclear polarity, containing hyperchromatic nuclei with fine to coarse and even chromatin, and arranged in single cells or syncytia are suggestive of an in situ lesion. The differential diagnosis between squamous and endocervical in situ lesions depends on many features, including the cell shape (columnar-endocervical) and/or accompanying dysplasia (squamous). Feathering or splattering cytoplasmic processes are often associated with endocervical lesions.

DeMay RM, The Art & Science of Cytopathology.
Carcinoma in situ, p. 76, and Early endocervical neoplasia, pp. 129–131.

221. D squamous cell carcinoma, keratinizing type

These cells are demonstrating cellular pleomorphism, orangeophilia, and irregular, hyperchromatic, opaque nuclei. The background contains a granular diathesis. The presence of single cells with these characteristics is diagnostic of a squamous cell carcinoma.

DeMay RM, The Art & Science of Cytopathology.
Keratinizing squamous cell carcinoma, p. 85.

222. C endometrial adenocarcinoma

Stein-Leventhal disease (SLD) is associated with hyperestrinism. Endometrial adenocarcinoma (EA), a disease more commonly found in peri- and postmenopausal women, has been linked to excessive or unopposed estrogen levels. Patients with SLD are at a greater risk for carcinogenic development. The cells of EA are found in clusters, have nuclei similar to that of an intermediate squamous cell, and possess irregular chromatin, macronucleoli, and anisokaryosis. Often, a watery diathesis is present.

DeMay RM, The Art & Science of Cytopathology.
Endometrial adenocarcinoma, pp. 125–127.

223. D chronic lymphocytic cervicitis

Chronic lymphocytic cervicitis is associated with findings of small and large lymphocytes (immunoblasts), plasma cells, and tingible body macrophages. The cellular findings are always single cells without cohesiveness. In contrast, small cell neuroendocrine carcinoma maintains nuclear molding, vertebral column formation, and coarse chromatin patterns.

DeMay RM, The Art & Science of Cytopathology.
Specific infections (other manifestations of inflammation), pp. 113–114.

224. D unsatisfactory for evaluation because of drying artifact

Air drying or inadequate fixation often creates cellular ballooning, karyorrhexis, karyolysis, and cytolytic features, thus preventing evaluation of the cellular sample.

DeMay RM, The Art & Science of Cytopathology.
Specimen adequacy, pp. 148–150.

225. B pouch of Douglas

The pouch of Douglas, also referred as the cul-de-sac, contains cells indigenous to body cavities such as mesenchymal elements.

DeMay RM, The Art & Science of Cytopathology.
Culdocentesis, pp. 285–286.

226. A radiation changes

Radiation changes include cytomegaly with proportionate karyomegaly, normal nuclear-to-cytoplasmic ratios, and hypochromatic nuclei. Recurrent squamous carcinoma possesses true hyperchromasia and intact coarse irregular chromatin, often in the presence of accompanying diathesis.

DeMay RM, The Art & Science of Cytopathology.
adiation cytology, pp. 118–119.

227. C endocervical area

Endocervical cells possess well-defined borders with honeycombing, picket fence, or single columnar cell forms. The nuclei are vesicular and often contain micronucleoli. These cells must be distinguished from endometrial cells, which present in three-dimensional clusters or as single cells with frothy cytoplasm.

DeMay RM, The Art & Science of Cytopathology.
Metaplastic reactions, pp. 71–72.

228. C endometrium

Normal endometrial glandular cells often occur in three-dimensional ("double contour") cell balls, but often occur singly. The cells present with round to oval (often degenerated) nuclei and scanty ill-defined basophilic cytoplasm.

DeMay RM, The Art & Science of Cytopathology.
Endometrial cells, p. 123.

229. C mucinous cystadenocarcinoma, ovarian primary

The finding of large cells with distended, vacuolated cytoplasm, anisonucleosis, irregular nuclear membranes, irregular chromatin, hyperchromasia, macronucleoli, and signet ring morphology from a female with a peritoneal effusion suggests mucinous adenocarcinoma of the ovary. Special staining for mucin is necessary to confirm the diagnosis. Differential diagnoses include metastatic gastrointestinal tract malignancies (especially poorly differentiated adenocarcinoma of the stomach) and primary mucinous adenocarcinoma of the endometrium.

DeMay RM, The Art & Science of Cytopathology.
Adenocarcinoma, p. 273.

230. A erosion

The presence of endocervical components on the ectocervical region suggests a rolling out of these cells during processes such as erosion. This may occur as a normal process during menarche or as a result of pathogenic infection.

DeMay RM, The Art & Science of Cytopathology.
Endocervical cells, p. 121.

231. B adenocarcinoma, fallopian tube

These cells possess typical features of an adenocarcinoma: three-dimensional clusters, anisokaryosis, irregular chromatin, and nucleoli. The clinical feature of a profuse watery discharge and the negative clinical indicators suggest fallopian tube adenocarcinoma.

DeMay RM, The Art & Science of Cytopathology.
Some miscellaneous findings in the pap smear, pp. 137–138.

232. C LSIL; ablation without histologic confirmation is considered unacceptable

All low-grade lesions (HPV changes, mild dysplasia/CIN I) should be histologically confirmed to rule out a more invasive process.

DeMay RM, The Art & Science of Cytopathology.
Recommendations, p. 153, and Clinical management, pp. 139–140.

233. C endometrial adenocarcinoma, grade I

The depicted cells are diagnostic of well-differentiated endometrial adenocarcinoma, grade I. These cells demonstrate cellular clusters with nuclear overlapping, anisonucleosis, irregular chromatin, and macronucleoli. A granular basophilic (watery) diathesis as well as the presence of old and fresh blood is often associated with these tumors.

DeMay RM, The Art & Science of Cytopathology.
Endometrial adenocarcinomas, pp. 125–127.

234. C navicular cells

Often referred as "boat-shaped," these glycogenated cells are indicative of a progesterone-stimulated epithelium. They must be differentiated from koilocytes infected by HPV, which have true cytoplasmic margination (cave-like), rasinoid nuclei, smudged degenerative chromatin, or well-preserved nuclei with binucleation.

DeMay RM, The Art & Science of Cytopathology.
Hormonal cytology, p. 69.

235. D endometrial adenocarcinoma

The presence of endometrial cells in a postmenopausal female raises suspicion of a possible endometrial neoplasm. These cells demonstrate cellular clusters with overlapping nuclei, anisonucleosis, irregular chromatin, and macronucleoli. A granular basophilic (watery) diathesis as well as the presence of old and fresh blood is often associated with these tumors.

DeMay RM, The Art & Science of Cytopathology.
Endometrial adenocarcinoma, pp. 125–127.

236. D immature metaplastic

Immature metaplasia is usually parabasal in size with basophilic cytoplasm, well-defined borders, and vesicular nuclei. Often a pavement configuration, remnants of cobblestone patterns (not unlike those of Charleston's streets) or the "cookie cutter" look is seen. These cells may possess spine-like or "spider cell" cytoplasmic processes when forcibly removed, or have ectoplasm/endoplasm rims when exfoliated.

DeMay RM, The Art & Science of Cytopathology.
Metaplastic reactions, pp. 71–72.

237. C possible exposure to diethylstilbestrol (DES) in utero

Vaginal adenosis is defined as the presence of ectopic glandular epithelium or squamous metaplastic cells within the normally gland-free or squamous-lined vagina. The presence of these cells is increased in those patients who were exposed to diethylstilbestrol (DES) in utero.

DeMay RM, The Art & Science of Cytopathology.
Metaplastic reactions, p. 70.

238. A endometrial stromal cells, in cycle

The photomicrograph represents normal stromal cells from the endometrial cavity. These cells, both deep (stratum spongiosa) and superficial (stratum compacta), are normally present in the first half of the menstrual cycle. Deep stromal cells possess spindle-shaped cytoplasm with oval nuclei whereas superficial stromal cells generally contain reniform, kidney bean- or boomerang-shaped nuclear features and frothy cytoplasm.

DeMay RM, The Art & Science of Cytopathology.
Endometrial cells, p. 123.

239. A within normal limits, negative for squamous intraepithelial lesion

Normal cellular elements from squamous and endocervical origin are necessary for a cell sample to be considered negative for squamous intraepithelial lesion.

DeMay RM, The Art & Science of Cytopathology.
General categorization, p. 150.

240. B endometrial hyperplasia

The presence of normal endometrial cells at times other than days 1–14 of the menstrual cycle may be related to a hyperplastic endometrium. Cytologic features are those of normal endometrial cells. Atypical (complex) endometrial hyperplasia may be difficult to distinguish from a frankly invasive malignant process. Tissue confirmation is strongly suggested, especially in those women approaching menopause.

DeMay RM, The Art & Science of Cytopathology.
Cytology of endometrial hyperplasia and neoplasia, pp. 124–126.

241. C mixed müllerian tumor, homologous type

The identification of endometrial carcinoma with concomitant leiomyosarcoma or endometrial stromal sarcoma is necessary to establish the diagnosis of a homologous mixed müllerian tumor.

DeMay RM, The Art & Science of Cytopathology.
Sarcomas, p. 137.

242. A production of lactic acid

Döderlein bacillus, or *Lactobacillus acidophilus,* is considered normal flora of the vagina. Its production of lactic acid serves as an endogenous inhibitor of microbial growth by maintaining a low pH. The organism is commonly seen in the latter half of the menstrual cycle (days 15–28), at which time glycogenated cells predominate. These organisms produce lactic acid by utilizing the glycogen in intermediate cells, thus creating cytolysis.

DeMay RM, The Art & Science of Cytopathology.
Inflammation and inflammatory change, p. 109.

243. **B** endometrial adenocarcinoma, grade I

Well-differentiated endometrial adenocarcinomas (Type I) often appear in patients with a history of hyperestrinism and endometrial hyperplasia. These lesions have enlarged nuclei, irregularly aggregated chromatin, and slight nucleolar enlargement. Neutrophils may be present within the cytoplasm of these neoplastic cells. A watery diathesis, presenting as a finely granular, basophilic diathesis, often accompanies the malignant cellular components.

DeMay RM, The Art & Science of Cytopathology.
Endometrial adenocarcinoma, pp. 125–127.

244. **C** karyorrhectic

Chromatinic nuclear membranes and broken or interrupted nuclear membranes are associated with karyorrhexis. Other types of nuclear degeneration include karyopyknosis (condensed) and karyolysis (dissolution).

DeMay RM, The Art & Science of Cytopathology.
Inflammation and inflammatory change, p. 110.

245. **D** *Actinomyces* sp.

Actinomyces sp. is a filamentous bacillus that branches at acute angles and clumps together to form structures known as "sulfur granules." These entities are often associated with patients who have intrauterine devices (IUD).

DeMay RM, The Art & Science of Cytopathology.
Specific infections, p. 112.

246. **A** adenomyosis

The presence of ectopic normal endometrial glands embedded within the smooth muscular layer of the uterus is diagnostic of adenomyosis. Cytologic features are those of normal endometrial cells. Endometriosis may be intramural, submucosal, or subserosal.

DeMay RM, The Art & Science of Cytopathology.
Endometrial cells, p. 122.

247. **B** deliver via cesarean

The cytologic findings are consistent with a herpetic infection. In this example, the fetus is at an increased risk of infection due to exposure to the mother's infected birth canal. Neonatal infection can be life-threatening.

DeMay RM, The Art & Science of Cytopathology.
Specific infections, p. 112.

248. **C** unopposed estrogen stimulation

Endometrial adenocarcinoma has been linked to increased exposure or unopposed estrogen. Estrogen most likely acts as a promoter in the development of this disease.

DeMay RM, The Art & Science of Cytopathology.
Endometrial cells, pp. 124–125.

249. **D** leiomyosarcoma

These cells suggest a sarcomatous neoplasm, most consistent with a leiomyosarcoma. Cytology reveals spindle cells with pleomorphic features, giant cells, and isolated cells with fibrillar cytoplasm and oval nucleoli. The chromatin is finely granular, irregularly distributed and may or may not contain nucleoli. Leiomyosarcomas represent the most common sarcomatous lesion of the uterus. These lesions represent a malignant transformation of the indigenous smooth muscle elements.

DeMay RM, The Art & Science of Cytopathology.
Sarcomas, p. 137.

250. **A** frothy, yellow-green discharge/strawberry cervix

Trichomonas vaginalis parasites are transmitted through sexual contact. Cytologically they appear as small gray to blue, faint-staining, pear-shaped structures with eccentric nuclei. Flagella are rare unless preparation is with cellular suspension process. These organisms are often accompanied by coccoid bacteria and *Leptothrix.*

DeMay RM, The Art & Science of Cytopathology.
Specific infections, p. 111.

251. **D** Turner syndrome

Turner syndrome patients are ahormonal due to ovarian agenesis. A predominant population of basal to parabasal cells would characterize the vaginal smear pattern. Answers A, B, and C are all associated with hyperestrinism.

DeMay RM, The Art & Science of Cytopathology.
Hormonal cytology, p. 68.

252. **B** nucleoli, diathesis, irregular chromatin distribution

These cells represent nonkeratinizing squamous cell carcinoma, a neoplasm that must be differentiated from that of its precursor, carcinoma in situ (CIS). CIS usually possesses regular chromatin, lacks nucleoli and has a clean "diathesis-free" background.

DeMay RM, The Art & Science of Cytopathology.
Nonkeratinizing squamous cell carcinoma, pp. 84–85.

253. B internal cervical os

These cells are diagnostic of a high-grade squamous intraepithelial lesion of metaplastic origin. Metaplastic dysplasia arises from immature metaplastic areas within the endocervical canal, in contrast to nonkeratinizing dysplasias, which arise from mature areas of metaplasia, distal to the ectocervix.

DeMay RM, The Art & Science of Cytopathology.
Metaplastic lesions (CIN mimicking reserve cell hyperplasia), p. 77.

254. D squamous atypia/mature metaplastic ASC-US (mimicking mature native squames)

The diagnosis of atypical squamous cells of undetermined significance (ASC-US) should be rendered when the cells lack the specific features necessary to diagnosis dysplasia, including hyperchromasia and increased N/C ratios. Cells diagnostic of ASC-US or squamous atypia (mature metaplastic derivative) typically have slightly increased nuclear sizes (2–3 times that of a normal intermediate cell nucleus) and hypochromasia. In the absence of true inflammatory sequelae this diagnosis may be necessary. The diagnosis of ASC-US is considered a slight risk for the subsequent development of HPV or dysplasia.

DeMay RM, The Art & Science of Cytopathology.
Atypical squamous cells of undetermined significance, pp. 94–97.

255. B low

Keratinizing and nonkeratinizing squamous carcinomas have a low mitotic rate in comparison with that of small cell squamous carcinomas.

DeMay RM, The Art & Science of Cytopathology.
Squamous cell carcinoma, pp. 83–84, and Keratinizing squamous cell carcinoma, p. 85.

256. D reparative/regenerative changes secondary to therapy

Reparative changes secondary to cauterization must be discriminated from true dysplastic or invasive squamous processes. As described earlier, reparative/regenerative cells often contain macronucleoli, respectable polarity, and/or cytoplasmic streaming. The predictability of these cells is important in establishing their benignity. A necrotic background may be found secondary to cauterization, especially if smears are performed shortly after therapy.

DeMay RM, The Art & Science of Cytopathology.
Repair/regeneration, pp. 115–116.

257. B radiation-induced cell changes

The cytologic changes associated with radiation include cytomegaly (macrocytic changes) and karyomegaly. The maintenance of normal nuclear-to-cytoplasmic ratios and the evidence of cytoplasmic vacuolization (related to degeneration) are characteristic of these cells. The nuclei associated with radiation cell changes are often degenerative or preserved and multinucleated, while the cytoplasmic staining is polychromatic and amphophilic.

DeMay RM, The Art & Science of Cytopathology.
Radiation cytology, pp. 118–119.

258. C normal endometrial cells, possibly associated with endometrial hyperplasia

Endometrial cells identified outside of the proliferative phase of the menstrual cycle (days 14–28) are considered abnormal in the absence of appropriate clinical history. Normal endometrial cells may be associated with hyperplasia, a predisposing condition for endometrial adenocarcinoma.

DeMay RM, The Art & Science of Cytopathology.
Endometrial cells (abnormal shedding of endometrial cells), pp. 122–125.

259. D 100%

Carcinoma in situ of the cervix replaces the full epithelial thickness of the squamous mucosa with primitive cells, resulting in a total loss of cellular maturation throughout the epithelial strata.

DeMay RM, The Art & Science of Cytopathology.
The cytoplasm, pp. 91–92.

260. A atypia of atrophy

Atypical cells associated with atrophy are basal-to-parabasal cells in single syncytial-like arrangements or hyperchromatic crowded groups (HCGs) found amongst a granular precipitate containing degenerated epithelial cells and scattered red and white blood cells. The chromatin, if visible, is fine and evenly distributed. More commonly, the chromatin of these atypical cells is poorly preserved, smudged, and indistinct. In comparison with dysplasia or cancer, the chromatin of truly dysplastic lesions is described as distinct and "crisp," whereas malignant lesions generally possess coarsely granular, irregularly distributed chromatin.

DeMay RM, The Art & Science of Cytopathology.
Atypia of atrophy and maturity, pp. 116–117.

261. A normal endometrial cells

The finding of normal endometrial cells within the proliferative phase of the menstrual cycle is common. Parenchymal epithelial cells may present in three-dimensional clusters or as single cells with normally high N/C ratios, nuclear hypochromasia, finely granular, evenly distributed chromatin, and micronuclei. Stromal cells are often seen between days 6 and 10. Deep stromal cells are fibroblastic, whereas superficial stromal cells resemble histiocytes (with reniform nuclei).

DeMay RM, The Art & Science of Cytopathology.
Endometrial cells, pp. 122–124.

262. A HSIL, moderate nonkeratinizing dysplasia

Nonkeratinizing dysplasias are the most common morphological variant of dysplasia and less apt to progress to more invasive processes. The nuclei of these cells are large compared with immature metaplastic dysplasia, the texture of the cytoplasm is translucent, and the nuclear-to-cytoplasmic ratios increase correspondingly with the degree of severity.

DeMay RM, The Art & Science of Cytopathology.
Morphogenesis, pp. 75–76, and CIN mimicking mature squamous metaplasia, pp. 78–79.

263. C immature metaplastic transformational zone

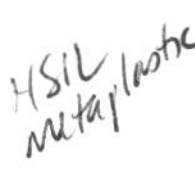

These cells are diagnostic of a high-grade squamous intraepithelial lesion of metaplastic origin. Metaplastic dysplasia arises from immature metaplastic areas within the endocervical canal, in contrast to nonkeratinizing dysplasias, which arise from mature areas of metaplasia, distal to the ectocervix.

DeMay RM, The Art & Science of Cytopathology.
Metaplastic lesions (CIN mimicking immature squamous metaplasia), pp. 77–78.

264. C irregular chromatin

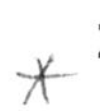

These cells are diagnostic of nonkeratinizing squamous cell carcinoma. Important features that are helpful in establishing the diagnosis of this lesion are the presence of irregularly distributed chromatin, nucleoli, and a diathesis—three key features absent in squamous carcinoma in situ.

DeMay RM, The Art & Science of Cytopathology.
Squamous cell carcinoma (nonkeratinizing carcinoma), pp. 83–84.

265. A squamous cell carcinoma, keratinizing type

Keratinizing squamous carcinomas generally originate on the anterior cervical lip. The single or syncytial-like pleomorphic-to-bizarre tadpole or spindle cell formations are the trademarks of this lesion. The cells may stain orangeophilic or cyanophilic; however, eosinophilia is more often seen. A granular diathesis may or may not be present due to the exophytic nature of this lesion. Pearl formations, parakeratosis, and hyperkeratosis may accompany the malignant cells.

DeMay RM, The Art & Science of Cytopathology.
Squamous cell carcinoma, pp. 83–84, and Keratinizing squamous cell carcinoma, p. 85.

266. A pleomorphism

The more undifferentiated or anaplastic the squamous lesion becomes, the more likely the cells will begin to recapitulate each other and become more "clone"-like. In keratinizing malignancies, pleomorphism will decrease with an increasing tumor grade.

DeMay RM, The Art & Science of Cytopathology.
Small cell squamous carcinoma, p. 84, and Small cell cervical cancers. p. 136

267. B a hyperdifferentiation that places the patient at a higher risk for post-irradiation dysplasia

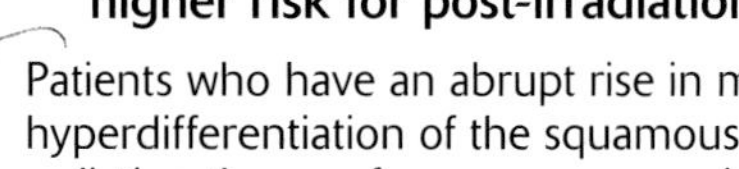

Patients who have an abrupt rise in maturation or hyperdifferentiation of the squamous mucosa after receiving radiation therapy for squamous carcinoma are at an increased risk for recurrence. Other key indicators include the presence of spindle cells and tissue necrosis.

DeMay RM, The Art & Science of Cytopathology.
Radiation cytology, pp. 118–120.

268. A strips of pseudostratified or "feathering" epithelium in glandular lesions

The diagnosis of endocervical adenocarcinoma in situ (AIS) may often be difficult to differentiate from squamous carcinoma in situ (CIS) with the exception that AIS often possesses feathering or pseudostratified syncytial-like fragments, stratified strips, or rosettes. The maintenance of columnar morphology may also be a key feature in establishing the diagnosis of an atypical endocervical process.

DeMay RM, The Art & Science of Cytopathology.
Early endocervical glandular neoplasia, pp. 129–131

269. A coarse chromatin

Cells with coarse even chromatin patterns arranged within syncytial-like aggregates amongst a "clean" background are diagnostic of squamous carcinoma in situ. These cells must be discriminated from their precursor lesion—severe dysplasia—a process that possesses finely granular, evenly distributed chromatin.

DeMay RM, The Art & Science of Cytopathology.
Carcinoma in situ, p. 76, and CIN mimicking mature squamous metaplasia (large cell carcinoma), p. 79.

270. B it is less common

Immature metaplastic dysplasia is less frequent than nonkeratinizing squamous dysplasias, which arise from mature metaplastic epithelium.

DeMay RM, The Art & Science of Cytopathology.
Keratinizing lesions, p. 79.

271. D rosettes, acinar morphology, feathering cytoplasmic borders

The diagnosis of endocervical adenocarcinoma in situ (AIS) may often be difficult to differentiate from squamous carcinoma in situ (CIS) with the exception that AIS often possesses feathering or pseudostratified syncytial-like fragments, stratified strips, or rosettes. The maintenance of columnar morphology may also be a key feature in establishing the diagnosis of an atypical endocervical process.

DeMay RM, The Art & Science of Cytopathology.
Early endocervical glandular neoplasia, pp. 129–130.

272. B small cell carcinoma in situ

The presence of small cell carcinoma in situ may be difficult to distinguish from frankly invasive small cell carcinoma in endocervical smears. The absence of a necrotic diathesis as well as the presence of coarse regular chromatin may help confirm small cell carcinoma in situ. Small cell lesions arise from atypical reserve cells, foregoing the morphological spectrum associated with dysplastic lesions arising from the mature and immature metaplastic zones.

DeMay RM, The Art & Science of Cytopathology.
CIN mimicking reserve cell hyperplasia (small cell carcinoma in situ), p. 77.

273. D atrophic vaginitis

Sheets of lower level parabasal-to-basal cells with autolytic features and degenerating karyolytic cells ("blue blobs"), and the finding of pyknotic parabasal cells with eosinophilic cytoplasm, often referred to as "mummified cells," are characteristic of deep atrophy, as may be found in postmenopausal or postpartum patients. Care should be taken to discriminate these findings from more significant conditions such as parakeratosis or dyskeratosis, lesions associated with true keratinizing processes.

DeMay RM, The Art & Science of Cytopathology.
The cells, p. 66, and Atypia of atrophy and maturity, pp. 116–117.

274. D ectocervical, mature metaplastic

These cells represent a moderate nonkeratinizing dysplasia, a high-grade squamous intraepithelial lesion. Their origin is distal to the ectocervical canal within areas of mature metaplastic epithelium. The clinical course for nonkeratinizing dysplasia is generally less severe.

DeMay RM, The Art & Science of Cytopathology.
Morphogenesis, pp. 75–76.

275. B pleomorphic, caudate, spindled

This tissue section reveals a keratinizing squamous carcinoma of the cervix. Histopathologic findings include pleomorphism, orangeophilia, pearl formation, and stromal invasion.

DeMay RM, The Art & Science of Cytopathology.
Squamous cell carcinoma, pp. 83–84, and Keratinizing squamous cell carcinoma, p. 85.

276. B verrucous

Pleomorphic or keratinizing squamous carcinoma generally occurs as an exophytic (verrucous) lesion. The lesion may be papillary, cauliflower-form, or everted.

DeMay RM, The Art & Science of Cytopathology.
Squamous cell carcinoma, pp. 83–84, and Keratinizing squamous cell carcinoma, p. 85.

277. B no

Although the presence of koilocytes is a specific cytologic criterion for the detection of HPV, the specific histologic pattern cannot be predicted with cytology. HPV may manifest itself histologically as papillomatous, flat, or inverted. In addition, cytologic identification of HPV is neither sensitive nor specific in determining whether the patient is infected with a "low" or "high" risk viral type, nor can it help in predicting the possibility of progression to dysplasia or cancer.

DeMay RM, The Art & Science of Cytopathology.
Condyloma and human papilloma virus infection, pp. 85–86.

278. C nonkeratinizing squamous carcinoma, moderately differentiated

Moderately differentiated squamous carcinomas of the cervix present with classic malignant morphology. Numerous populations of single cells and/or syncytial aggregates with large nuclear sizes, coarse irregular chromatin patterns, and macronucleoli scattered amongst a granular diathesis validate the diagnosis. Stripped nuclei are often found in association with the above criteria.

DeMay RM, The Art & Science of Cytopathology.
Nonkeratinizing squamous cell carcinoma, pp. 84–85.

279. A follicular cervicitis

The diagnosis of follicular cervicitis must be discriminated from other benign conditions including microglandular hyperplasia, degenerating neutrophils, and small cell histiocytes. When establishing a diagnosis of follicular cervicitis, the presence of small mature lymphocytes and large immunoblasts in an admixture of plasma cells and tingible body macrophages identifies this process.

DeMay RM, The Art & Science of Cytopathology.
Specific infections (other manifestations of inflammation), pp. 113–114.

280. D squamous cell carcinoma, nonkeratinizing type

Single cells, syncytial fragments, and naked nuclei exhibiting hyperchromasia and coarse irregular chromatin with macronucleoli are diagnostic criteria of nonkeratinizing squamous cell carcinoma of the uterine cervix. A tumor diathesis is more commonly seen in nonkeratinizing carcinomas than in keratinizing malignancies.

DeMay RM, The Art & Science of Cytopathology.
Nonkeratinizing squamous cell carcinoma, pp. 84–85.

281. D post-irradiation dysplasia

An indication of post irradiation dysplasia of the cervix may be the presence of dysplastic cells with high N/C ratios and hyperchromatic nuclei. The nuclear chromatin pattern is often too dense to interpret. Small cell type post-irradiation dysplasia is more likely to be found in older age groups. These cells mimic small cell carcinoma in situ; however, any grade of post irradiation dysplasia recurring within 3 years carries a poor prognosis.

DeMay RM, The Art & Science of Cytopathology.
Radiation cytology, pp. 118–119.

282. D small cell neuroendocrine carcinoma

Small cell carcinomas may be poorly differentiated squamous lesions or neuroendocrine tumors, both of which arise within the endocervical canal. Poorly differentiated squamous carcinomas are composed of small cells with high N/C ratios, uniform cellular sizes with well-defined borders, coarse chromatin with nucleoli, but little-to-absent "crush" artifact. An abnormal host response or necrotic tumor diathesis often accompanies these squamous lesions. Conversely, and as depicted in this photomicrograph, neuroendocrine small cell tumors reveal fine chromatin, inconspicuous nucleoli, and distinguished vertebral-like arrangements and nuclear molding, recapitulating their lung counterparts. These cells contain hyperchromatic stippled chromatin, coarse clumping, nuclear molding, scanty cytoplasm, and micronucleoli. They have characteristic vertebral column formation, microbiopsy aggregates, cords, nests, or ribbons. In 1/3 of the cases, neuroendocrine differentiation may be demonstrated by immunocytochemical staining with chromogranin, neuron-specific enolase, or synaptophysin. Neuroendocrine differentiation (argyrophilia) may also be demonstrated.

DeMay RM, The Art & Science of Cytopathology.
Small cell squamous carcinoma, p. 84.

283. A benign radiation cellular changes

The cells depicted in this photomicrograph are consistent with the benign cellular changes associated with radiation cell injury. The cytological changes associated with radiation include cytomegaly (macrocytic changes) and karyomegaly. The maintenance of normal nuclear-to-cytoplasmic ratios and the evidence of cytoplasmic vacuolization (related to degeneration) are characteristic of these cells. The nuclei associated with radiation cell changes are often degenerative or preserved and multinucleated, while the cytoplasmic staining is polychromatic and amphophilic. Recurrent squamous carcinoma possesses true hyperchromasia and intact coarse irregular chromatin, often in the presence of accompanying diathesis.

DeMay RM, The Art & Science of Cytopathology.
Radiation cytology, pp. 118–119.

284. B negative for squamous intraepithelial lesion with radiation-induced cellular changes

Benign radiation changes include vacuolization of the cytoplasm, macrocytosis, amphophilia, nucleomegaly, and well-preserved nuclear-to-cytoplasmic ratios. Nuclear pyknosis and karyorrhexis are degenerative changes associated with benign radiation changes. The cytoplasmic staining is polychromatic and amphophilic.

DeMay RM, The Art & Science of Cytopathology.
Radiation cytology, pp. 118–119

285. A post-irradiation dysplasia

The cytology of post-irradiation dysplasia mirrors that found in ordinary dysplasia. The large-cell type is generally seen in younger women, whereas a small cell type may be more common in older women.

DeMay RM, The Art & Science of Cytopathology.
Radiation cytology, pp. 118–120.

286. B syncytial-like

Syncytial-like aggregates, or hyperchromatic crowded "chaotic" groups (HCGs), with indistinct cell borders are associated with squamous carcinoma in situ. Distinguishing these aggregates from true papillary tissue fragments with community borders, well-formed glandular structures, or HCGs with feathery edges may help in differentiating glandular lesions from those of squamous origin.

DeMay RM, The Art & Science of Cytopathology.
Carcinoma in situ, p. 76, Intermediate carcinoma in situ, p. 78, Large cell carcinoma in situ, p. 79, The secrets of diagnosing dysplasia and carcinoma in situ, pp. 93–94, and Differential diagnosis of atypical glandular (endocervical) cells, p. 133.

287. D in the transformation zone

Squamous metaplasia, a common protective reaction found in mature cycling females, is a result of transformation of one adult type of epithelial tissue to another adult epithelial tissue via reserve cell hyperplasia. The finding of parabasal to intermediate cells in pavement or "cobblestone" configuration, either in pools or as single cells, is diagnostic. Squamous metaplasia is often associated with trauma, inflammation, or other endocrine disturbances. Squamocolumnar junctions, abrupt junctions occurring in young children, do not have associated transitional or transformational metaplastic zones.

DeMay RM, The Art & Science of Cytopathology.
Metaplastic reactions, pp. 71–72.

288. C chronic follicular cervicitis

Chronic follicular cervicitis is a diffuse or localized lymphocytic infiltration as identified in cervical/vaginal smears. Small (mature) and large (immunoblastic) lymphocytes, plasma cells, and tingible body macrophages (intracytoplasmic inclusions) are necessary to establish this diagnosis.

DeMay RM, The Art & Science of Cytopathology.
Specific infections (other manifestations of inflammation), pp. 113–114.

289. C severe cervicitis

These cells are representative of a severe inflammatory exudate associated with acute inflammations. A hypercellular population of polymorphonuclear neutrophils is seen.

DeMay RM, The Art & Science of Cytopathology.
Specific infections, pp. 113–114.

290. B possible fetal death in utero

A pure population of superficial cells suggests an estrogenic effect that is contraindicative for a normal pregnancy.

Keebler CM, Somrak TM, The Manual of Cytotechnology.
Endocrinopathies, pp. 74–78.

291. B clean—no tumor diathesis

The background in this benign condition is clean and free of necrosis. Malignancy-associated cellular backgrounds are generally composed of diathesis consisting of old and fresh blood, degenerated surrounding tissue, necrotic tumor cells, and assorted white blood cells.

DeMay RM, The Art & Science of Cytopathology.
Carcinoma in situ, p. 76.

292. A microglandular hyperplasia

Synonyms include birth control pill changes and pseudoparakeratosis (pseudokeratosis). These cells represent degenerated forms of hyperplastic endocervical glandular mucosa. The findings are often associated with patients taking oral contraceptives, late luteal phase, and late pregnancy. They are benign cellular findings; however, the differentiation from true parakeratosis is imperative. Cells from microglandular hyperplasia generally have eosinophilic or basophilic cytoplasm, contain eccentrically located nuclei, or resemble reactive endocervical cells. Parakeratosis represents a true keratinizing process (orangeophilia) with centrally located pyknotic nuclei in polygonal "waxy" cytoplasm (possibly with accompanying HPV changes).

DeMay RM, The Art & Science of Cytopathology.
Microglandular hyperplasia, p. 112.

293. C serum levels

A serum analysis is considered the gold standard for determining hormonal levels.

Keebler CM, Somrak TM, The Manual of Cytotechnology.
Endocrinopathies, pp. 74–78.

294. A Cushing syndrome

Cushing syndrome is a physiological condition related to an overproduction of cortisol by the adrenal gland. This effect may be secondary to hyperplasia, pheochromocytoma, or adrenal cortical adenoma. Afflicted women present with buffalo obesity, a moon-shaped face, and hirsutism. The vaginal smear pattern is generally intermediate maturation but may be atrophic.

Keebler CM, Somrak TM, The Manual of Cytotechnology.
Endocrinopathies, pp. 74–78.

295. A reparative/regenerative process

Squamous reparative/regenerative changes must be discriminated from low-grade squamous epithelial lesions or those of more significance. Sheets of cells with distinct cytoplasmic borders and/or cytoplasmic streaming may be helpful in establishing the benign nature of these cells. Normal N/C ratios, normochromasia, and nucleoli are also helpful diagnostic features.

DeMay RM, The Art & Science of Cytopathology.
Repair/regeneration, pp. 115–116.

296. C pemphigus vulgaris

A bullous disease of the skin, pemphigus vulgaris is a condition that destroys the squamous tonofilaments, producing a sloughing of the skin. Reactive/reparative cells with bullet-shaped nucleoli are generally found amongst fine, even chromatin patterns. Clinical history is essential to rule out a possible abnormality. Tzanck tests are negative.

DeMay RM, The Art & Science of Cytopathology.
Benign lesions, pp. 331–332.

297. A correlates with history

Stein-Leventhal syndrome is associated with a thickening of the tunica albuginea of the ovary, resulting in the inability to expel the ovum. Patients with this condition are often overweight and have secondary amenorrhea. Vaginal smear patterns in these patients show intermediate to superficial cell maturation.

Keebler CM, Somrak TM, The Manual of Cytotechnology.
Endocrinopathies, pp. 74–78.

298. C HSIL, keratinizing variety

Keratinizing or pleomorphic dysplasia (CIN mimicking keratosis) cytologically presents with well-defined borders, dense refractile cytoplasm, and hyperchromatic, fine to coarse, regular chromatin or India ink pyknosis. These cells may often stain orangeophilic. The degree of pleomorphism is most important when establishing the severity of keratinizing dysplasia. Associated changes include hyperkeratosis, parakeratosis, and dyskeratosis.

DeMay RM, The Art & Science of Cytopathology.
Keratinizing lesions, p. 79.

299. C LSIL, HPV

The identification of koilocytes are compulsory findings for establishing the diagnosis of HPV. The 2001 Bethesda System classifies condyloma acuminata (human papilloma virus [HPV]) as a low-grade squamous epithelial lesion.

DeMay RM, The Art & Science of Cytopathology.
Diagnosis of condyloma in the Pap smear, pp. 87–88.

300. A del Castillo syndrome

Patients with del Castillo syndrome present with a milky discharge in the absence of recent delivery. These patients may have previously taken birth control pills and a milky breast discharge may be elaborated. The pituitary gland shuts down the production of follicle-stimulating hormone and luteinizing hormone. Therefore, the hormonal pattern of these patients is atrophic.

Keebler CM, Somrak TM, The Manual of Cytotechnology.
Endocrinopathies, pp. 74–78.

301. B the hormonal analysis is not compatible with history

Patients with feminizing testicular syndrome are responsive to the endogenous effects of estrogens; therefore, a hormonal analysis would show a maturation pattern consisting of mixed intermediate and superficial cells. Instead, this photomicrograph reveals a deep atrophic condition, suggesting male pseudohermaphroditism.

Keebler CM, Somrak TM, The Manual of Cytotechnology.
Endocrinopathies, pp. 74–78.

302. B high-grade intraepithelial lesion, metaplastic dysplasia

Immature metaplastic cells may give rise (if initiated) to metaplastic dysplasias, whereas mature metaplastic cells are linked to nonkeratinizing dysplasia. Atypical reserve cell hyperplasia is related to the development of small cell lesions (answer C), and small cell carcinoma in situ gives rise to small cell carcinoma (answer D).

DeMay RM, The Art & Science of Cytopathology.
Morphology of dysplasia and carcinoma in situ, pp. 75–79, The cytoplasm, pp. 91–92, and The nucleus, pp. 92–94.

303. D granulosa-theca cell tumor

Feminizing tumors, such as granulosa-theca cell tumors, overproduce estrogen, hence typically increased maturation on the vaginal smear. These tumors may be related to precocious puberty as well as endometrial adenocarcinoma.

Keebler CM, Somrak TM, The Manual of Cytotechnology.
Endocrinopathies. pp. 74–78.

304. B reparative/regenerative process

These cells are representative of squamous reparative/regenerative changes. Sheets of cells with well-defined cytoplasmic borders, preserved nuclear polarity, predictable nuclear features, fine regular chromatin patterns, micro- to macronucleoli, and characteristic cytoplasmic streaming are diagnostic of repair. This process is often associated with trauma, cervicitis, and inflammatory etiology. The background of reparative/regenerative conditions is clean and free of necrosis.

DeMay RM, The Art & Science of Cytopathology.
Repair/regeneration, pp. 115–116.

305. D mature metaplastic cells

Nonkeratinizing dysplasias (CIN mimicking mature squamous metaplasia) arise from mature metaplastic areas of the transformational zone.

DeMay RM, The Art & Science of Cytopathology.
Metaplastic reactions, p. 72.

306. C Turner syndrome

Turner syndrome is a nondisjunction of the X-chromosome. These patients are described as sex chromatin negative, or 45XO. Occasionally, mosaicism may be found. These patients have a low hairline, pigmented nevi, and increased carrying angle of their arms. Ovarian agenesis leaves streaks of connective tissue instead of viable ovaries. The vaginal smear pattern is atrophic.

Keebler CM, Somrak TM, The Manual of Cytotechnology.
Endocrinopathies, pp. 74–78.

307. B absence of a diathesis

Metastatic carcinomas usually lack a notable diathesis unless tumor seeding has occurred within the ectopic area.

DeMay RM, The Art & Science of Cytopathology.
Metastasis, p. 137.

308. A follicular cytosis

Follicular cystosis is associated with ovarian follicle persistence, thus forming cystic structures. The increase in endogenous estrogen produces a vaginal smear pattern with a predominant superficial cell pattern.

Keebler CM, Somrak TM, The Manual of Cytotechnology.
Endocrinopathies, pp. 74–78.

309. A nuclear-to-cytoplasmic ratio

One of the most important criteria for distinguishing low-grade squamous epithelial lesions from those of high-grade variety is the nuclear-to-cytoplasmic ratio. As the N/C ratio increases, so does the severity of dysplasia. The cells depicted in this photomicrograph represent a moderate dysplastic process.

DeMay RM, The Art & Science of Cytopathology.
Atypical squamous cells of undetermined significance, pp. 94–97.

310. C severe nonkeratinizing dysplasia, HSIL

Severe nonkeratinizing dysplasia cytologically presents as small immature metaplastic cells with hyperchromasia, high N/C ratios, and a thin rim of cytoplasm. The absence of coarse and irregular chromatin, nucleoli and/or diathesis should help discriminate these cells from a carcinoma in situ or an invasive malignancy.

DeMay RM, The Art & Science of Cytopathology.
Morphology of dysplasia and carcinoma in situ, pp. 75–79, The cytoplasm, pp. 91–92, and The nucleus, pp. 92–94.

311. A normal immature squamous metaplasia

Immature metaplastic cells or "spider cells" are found proximal to the endocervical glandular mucosa. Their nuclei often appear darker due to the increased nucleoprotein and dark cytoplasmic nature. A one-to-one staining N/C ratio may aid the cytologist in defining these cells as normal.

DeMay RM, The Art & Science of Cytopathology.
Metaplastic reactions, pp. 71–72.

312. D coarse, regular chromatin

One of the hallmarks of carcinoma in situ is its coarse, regular chromatin distribution. Chromatin patterns found in dysplasia are typically finely granular and evenly distributed.

DeMay RM, The Art & Science of Cytopathology.
Morphology of dysplasia and carcinoma in situ, pp. 75–79, The cytoplasm, pp. 91–92, and The nucleus, pp. 92–94

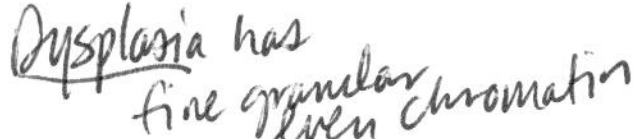

313. B HPV-16

Using molecular biological techniques, the presence of HPV 16, 18, 31, 33, 35, and 39 and other viral sequences has been shown to transform keratinocyte cancer cell lines in vitro and to be integral in the etiology of squamous carcinoma of the uterine cervix.

DeMay RM, The Art & Science of Cytopathology.
Prognosis, pp. 106–109.

314. D LSIL, consistent with HPV

The 2001 Bethesda System classifies condyloma acuminata (human papillomavirus [HPV]) as a low-grade squamous epithelial lesion. The pathognomonic cell for establishing an HPV infection is the koilocyte. This cell possesses large perinuclear halos (often referred to as cytoplasmic margination or large halo) or crater-like morphology. The nuclei may be well-preserved with fine even chromatin or hyperchromatic and smudged, representing a degenerative quality.

DeMay RM, The Art & Science of Cytopathology.
Morphology of dysplasia and carcinoma in situ, pp. 75–79, The cytoplasm, pp. 91–92, and The nucleus, pp. 92–94.

315. A congenital absence of the uterus

Patients with congenital absence of the uterus usually present with normal secretory patterns (normal ovaries). Although these patients lack menstrual cycles, the vaginal mucosa is hormonally receptive.

Keebler CM, Somrak TM, The Manual of Cytotechnology.
Endocrinopathies, pp. 74–78.

316. B ASC-US, dyskeratocytes (pleomorphic parakeratosis) most likely associated with HPV infection

These pleomorphic cells with elongated nuclei, often described as dyskeratocytes or pleomorphic parakeratosis, are classified as atypical squamous cells of undetermined significance under the Bethesda System. Their presence is suggestive but not pathognomonic for human papillomavirus (HPV) infection.

DeMay RM, The Art & Science of Cytopathology.
Atypical parakeratosis, p. 74.

317. B hyperkeratosis

Hyperkeratosis and parakeratosis are protective reactions often associated with keratinizing lesions such as this example of keratinizing dysplasia.

DeMay RM, The Art & Science of Cytopathology.
Keratinizing lesions, p. 79.

318. A mild dysplasia, LSIL

The histological findings in dysplasia show some degree of cellular abnormality throughout the entire epithelial thickness. In this example of mild dysplasia, the more primitive basal cells replace up to 25% of the lower epithelial surface, and more differentiated abnormal cells are seen in the upper 75% of the epithelial thickness. Nuclear sizes are variable, hyperchromasia is evident, and an increased mitotic activity may be observed.

DeMay RM, The Art & Science of Cytopathology.
Morphogenesis, pp. 75–79, The cytoplasm, pp. 91–92, The nucleus, pp. 92–94.

319. C are consistent with a reparative/regenerative process, endocervical origin

Reactive/reparative endocervical cells may at times be difficult to distinguish from endocervical atypia. These cells have normochromatic enlarged nuclei and possess well-defined borders and maintenance of polarity.

DeMay RM, The Art & Science of Cytopathology.
Repair/regeneration, pp. 115–116.

320. A squamous atypia/mature metaplastic ASC-US (mimicking mature native squames)

The diagnosis of atypical squamous cells of undetermined significance (ASC-US) is an alteration in the normal squamous nuclear size, possibly 2–3 times greater than that of a normal intermediate cell nucleus. The chromatin is finely granular, regularly distributed, and generally hypochromatic (normochromatic). A true ASC-US is a non-inflammatory related change that may be related to subclinical or early manifestations of the human papillomavirus infection or dysplasia. Illustrated is an example of squamous atypia occurring in mature metaplastic squamous cells. ASC-US may also involve immature squamous epithelial cells as well as basal and parabasal cells found in atrophic conditions.

DeMay RM, The Art & Science of Cytopathology.
Atypical squamous cells of undetermined significance, pp. 94–97.

321. C tubal metaplasia

Tubal metaplasia (TM) is a benign condition that may be confused with a true abnormal process, such as adenocarcinoma in situ of the endocervix (AIS), with the exception that TM presents with cilia and/or terminal bars/webs. Crowded sheets of glandular cells and anisokaryosis are common findings, mimicking the feathering effects seen in AIS.

DeMay RM, The Art & Science of Cytopathology.
Differential diagnosis of atypical glandular (endocervical) cells, p. 132, and Fallopian tube cells, pp. 137–138.

322. C AGUS, endocervical glandular dysplasia

Endocervical cells with slightly enlarged hyperchromatic nuclei with inconspicuous nucleoli, loss of polarity, and rosette formations are helpful in establishing a diagnosis of atypical glandular cells of undetermined significance (AGUS), in this case, referred to as endocervical columnar dysplasia (ECD). Its differential diagnosis is endocervical adenocarcinoma in situ (AIS); however, ECD has fine, regular chromatin, whereas endocervical AIS contains coarse chromatin features.

DeMay RM, The Art & Science of Cytopathology.
Early endocervical glandular neoplasia, pp. 129–131.

323. D adenocarcinoma in situ, endocervix

The diagnosis of endocervical adenocarcinoma in situ (AIS) may often be difficult to differentiate from squamous carcinoma in situ (CIS) with the exception that AIS often possesses feathering or pseudostratified syncytial-like fragments, stratified strips, or rosettes. The maintenance of columnar morphology may also be a key feature in establishing the diagnosis of an atypical endocervical process.

DeMay RM, The Art & Science of Cytopathology.
Early endocervical glandular neoplasia, pp. 129–131.

324. C mixed mesodermal tumor, homologous

The diagnosis of mixed mesodermal/müllerian tumor is determined by the cytologic identification of endometrial adenocarcinoma (usually well-differentiated) with a concomitant homologous or heterologous sarcomatous element. The findings represented by this photomicrograph indicate the sarcomatous element composed of isolated spindle cells with classic malignant criteria, suggesting leiomyosarcoma. Also identified are epithelial cells with enlarged nuclei, macronucleoli, and irregular chromatin.

DeMay RM, The Art & Science of Cytopathology.
Sarcomas, p. 136.

325. A rhabdomyosarcoma

Rhabdomyosarcoma is a heterologous sarcoma of the uterus that presents itself cytologically similar to leiomyosarcoma; however, this malignancy originates from striated muscle rather than smooth muscle. The findings of "strap cells" are diagnostic of malignant blasts; however, strap cells represent only 1% of the total malignant population. Multinucleated tumor giant cells also may be observed with these malignancies.

DeMay RM, The Art & Science of Cytopathology.
Sarcomas, p. 137.

326. B ASC-US: atypical squamous metaplasia/immature metaplastic variety

The diagnosis of atypical squamous cells of undetermined significance (ASC-US) includes an alteration in the normal squamous nuclear size, possibly 2–3 times greater than that of a normal intermediate cell nucleus. The chromatin is finely granular, regularly distributed, and generally hypochromatic (normochromatic). A true ASC-US is a non-inflammatory related change that may be related to subclinical or early manifestations of the human papillomavirus infection or dysplasia. ASC-US may also involve immature squamous epithelial cells as well as basal and parabasal cells found in atrophic conditions.

DeMay RM, The Art & Science of Cytopathology.
Atypical squamous cells of undetermined significance, pp. 94–97.

327. D nonspecific findings

Psammoma bodies are three-dimensional structures with concentric ringing containing calcified secretions of mucus. These structures are often found associated with papillary lesions of the ovary, including papillary serous adenocarcinoma. However, these are nonspecific findings and are not pathognomonic of malignancy.

DeMay RM, The Art & Science of Cytopathology.
Psammoma bodies, p. 139.

328. **A** papillary serous cystadenocarcinoma

The diagnosis of papillary serous adenocarcinoma of the ovary in a Pap smear is centered on the finding of three-dimensional aggregates with hyperchromatic nuclei and finely granular, irregularly distributed chromatin. Cervical/endocervical/ endometrial biopsies and colposcopy findings are negative. The presence of papillary groups of malignant cells and psammoma bodies may help in identifying these lesions as ovarian, but are not specific findings. A history of ascites is helpful.

DeMay RM, The Art & Science of Cytopathology.
Psammoma bodies, p. 139.

329. **C** papillary serous cystadenocarcinoma, ovarian

The diagnosis of papillary serous adenocarcinoma of the ovary in a Pap smear is centered around the finding of three-dimensional aggregates with hyperchromatic nuclei and finely granular, irregularly distributed chromatin. Cervical/ endocervical/endometrial biopsies and colposcopy findings are negative. The presence of papillary groups of malignant cells and psammoma bodies may help in identifying these lesions as ovarian, but are not specific findings. A history of ascites is helpful.

DeMay RM, The Art & Science of Cytopathology.
Adenocarcinoma, p. 273.

330. **C** endocervical adenocarcinoma

The cellular morphology suggests an endocervical adenocarcinoma. Cells with palisading features, overlapping nuclei, irregular chromatin, and columnar morphology demonstrate invasive endocervical morphology.

DeMay RM, The Art & Science of Cytopathology.
Endocervical carcinoma, pp. 127–129.

331. **C** endocervical adenocarcinoma

The presence of columnar morphology in the presence of obvious malignant criteria may help one to distinguish endocervical adenocarcinomas from those of endometrial origin. Other criteria that help discriminate the cells of endocervical adenocarcinoma (EA) from endometrial adenocarcinoma (EM) include the presence of rosettes versus cell balls and elongated, hyperchromatic, multinucleated cells with prominent multiple nucleoli vs. rounded, finely granular chromatin and conspicuous nucleoli. EA possesses a granular cytoplasmic texture whereas EM lesions have lacy, frothy, vacuolated cytoplasm. Last, EA tends to stain eosinophilic while EM shows generally basophilic cytoplasm.

DeMay RM, The Art & Science of Cytopathology.
Endocervical carcinoma, pp. 127–129.

332. **A** adenocarcinoma, ovarian

Mucinous adenocarcinomas of the ovary present with signet ring morphology and may recapitulate signet ring endometrial adenocarcinomas. Clinical history is paramount in establishing an ovarian primary tumor. A tumor diathesis is usually absent in cases of metastatic carcinoma unless the lesion has seeded at the secondary site. A vaginal smear, rather than a directed cervical smear and endocervical brushing, also helps rule out the other processes.

DeMay RM, The Art & Science of Cytopathology.
Adenocarcinoma, p. 273.

Chapter 3

Respiratory Tract

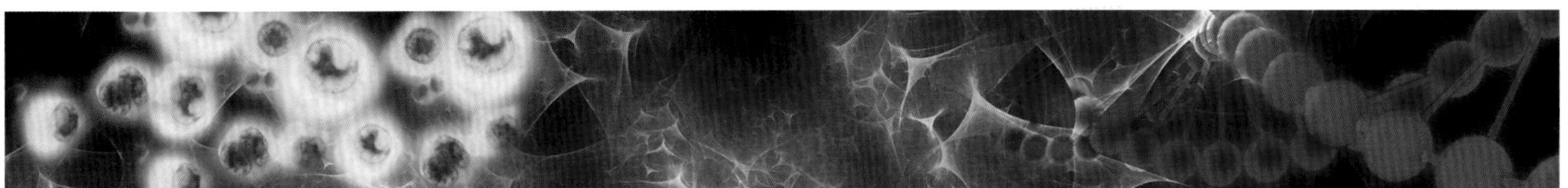

1. A 70-year-old man presents with hypertension and redness of the face, neck and arms. The patient complains of dyspnea and a loss of appetite. The patient has a 30-year history of smoking two packs per day. Emphysema was diagnosed 5 years previously. Sputum cytology analysis shows small cells in linear arrays caught in mucus strands with scanty cytoplasm. Hyperchromasia was present as well as a coarse chromatin pattern. Nuclear compression is present and nucleoli are inconspicuous. These cells represent:

   A. carcinoid tumor
   B. metastatic adenocarcinoma, prostate
   C. atypical reserve cells
   D. small cell carcinoma, oat cell variety

2. A 42-year-old man with a previous history of malignancy presents with sessile infiltrating growths in the major bronchi. A bronchial brush specimen reveals large cells arranged in nests. The cells possess large nuclei with frankly malignant nuclear features and intranuclear cytoplasmic inclusions. Immunoperoxidase stains with S-100 are positive. Based on the preceding criteria, the diagnosis is:

   A. melanoma
   B. hepatocellular carcinoma
   C. adenocarcinoma, bronchogenic
   D. mesothelioma

3. Large cells with multinucleation, nuclear molding, chromatin margination, and ground glass nuclei with intranuclear, eosinophilic inclusions found in a sputum specimen are diagnostic of:

   A. respiratory syncytial virus
   B. herpesvirus
   C. molluscum contagiosum
   D. cytomegalovirus

4. Cohesive groups and single cells exhibiting uniform polarity, high nuclear/cytoplasmic ratios, cytoplasmic ringing, prominent nucleoli, and coarse irregular chromatin scattered among a necrotic background are diagnostic of:

   A. well-differentiated squamous cell carcinoma, keratinizing
   B. poorly differentiated squamous cell carcinoma
   C. bronchogenic adenocarcinoma
   D. pulmonary hamartoma

5. All of the following are considered etiologic agents for the development of lung cancer, EXCEPT:

   A. radiation
   B. tobacco
   C. nickel
   D. microbacteria

6. A 65-year-old man presents with a 4 × 5-cm focal mass on chest x-ray. Bronchial brushing reveals large numbers of round-to-oval single cells lying singly and in sheet-like aggregates. The cells have elevated N/C ratios, large nucleoli, and granular to lacy cytoplasmic features. Special stains with mucicarmine are negative. Based on the cytologic features, the diagnosis is:

   A. large cell carcinoma
   B. adenocarcinoma, bronchogenic
   C. squamous cell carcinoma, well-differentiated type
   D. small cell carcinoma, oat cell type

7. A 66-year-old man on corticosteroid therapy for recent coronary bypass surgery presents with a solitary lesion within the left upper lung. Bronchial brushing reveals hyphae-like structures with dichotomous branching. Large exophytic structures are often found attached to the septa. The diagnosis is:

   A. *Actinomyces israelii*
   B. *Aspergillus fumigatus*
   C. *Nocardia asteroides*
   D. *Mucor* sp.

8. A 32-year-old man presents with pulmonary abscesses, enlargement of the mediastinal nodes, dry hacking cough, low grade fever, and chest pain. A blood-streaked sputum cytologically reveals numerous neutrophils as well as large multinucleated histiocytes. Special staining with PAS revealed many single, spherical structures with a thick refractile double-contoured cell wall, many of which had attached broad-based buds. The diagnosis is most consistent with:

   A. *Mycobacterium tuberculosis*
   B. *Pneumocystis carinii*
   C. *Blastomyces dermatitidis*
   D. *Cryptococcus neoformans*

9. A bronchial washing of a 2 × 3-cm mass reveals small, uniform appearing cells lacking cilia or terminal bars. Many of the cells appear in sheets, clusters, cords or nests. Nuclei are uniform and predictable in appearance with salt-and-pepper chromatin, and nucleoli are inconspicuous. The diagnosis is:

   A. reactive bronchial epithelial cells
   B. small cell carcinoma, oat cell type
   C. reserve cell hyperplasia
   D. carcinoid tumor

10. A 55-year-old woman presents with a history of tobacco abuse, malaise, and hemoptysis. Based on these clinical symptoms, one may suggest evaluation to rule out:

   A. disseminated microbiological infection
   B. viral pneumonia
   C. atypical squamous metaplasia
   D. invasive carcinoma

11. A 2 × 3-cm bronchial mass discovered in a 62-year-old man with a history of tobacco abuse was brushed using a flexible bronchoscope. The cells were papillary in configuration and possessed vacuolated cytoplasm. The nuclei were oval in shape and often lobulated. Single cells were interspersed among the fragments. The diagnosis is:

   A. adenocarcinoma, terminal bronchioloalveolar type
   B. adenocarcinoma, bronchogenic type
   C. large cell carcinoma, giant cell features
   D. mixed adenosquamous carcinoma

12. A 62-year-old woman presents with multiple lung lesions in the left and right lung. Abdominal ascites was noted at the time of examination. Bronchial brushing of the lung lesion reveals a large population of cells with hyperchromatic nuclei, fine irregular chromatin, prominent nucleoli, and tall columnar morphology in clusters as well as single cells. The most likely diagnosis/primary site for these cells is:

   A. reactive bronchial epithelial cells/lung
   B. adenocarcinoma/bronchioloalveolar variety
   C. angiosarcoma/breast
   D. adenocarcinoma/colon

13. A 56-year-old man with no history of a primary malignancy presents with a 3 × 4-cm mass in the left lower lobe of the lung. A bronchial washing shows orangeophilic pleomorphic cells with elongated opaque nuclear features and numerous pearl formations. Also present are acinar structures with single distended vacuoles and nuclei with slight hyperchromasia and prominent nucleoli. What diagnosis do you suspect and what special stain might prove useful in your determination?

A. poorly differentiated squamous carcinoma, immunoperoxidase positive for S-100
B. large cell carcinoma, mucicarmine negative
C. adenosquamous carcinoma, immunoperoxidase positive for keratin
D. metastatic medullary carcinoma of the thyroid, immunoperoxidase positive for calcitonin

14. A 31-year-old man presents with a spiking temperature and pneumonitis. A bronchioloalveolar lavage reveals a vast population of bronchial epithelial cells with enlarged cleared out nuclei exhibiting chromatinic margination. Large oval intranuclear and occasional small intracytoplasmic basophilic inclusions are seen. The diagnosis is consistent with:

A. metastatic melanoma
B. Hodgkin disease
C. cytomegalovirus
D. hemosiderin-laden macrophages

15. A sputum specimen reveals branching organisms with a central mass and peripheral filamentous mycelia. A large population of neutrophils are seen; however, dust cells are absent. Based on these cytologic findings, your recommendation is:

A. repeat sputum, *Actinomyces* sp. may represent tonsillar contamination
B. recommend removal of lung tissue to prevent further infection by *Aspergillus* sp.
C. repeat sputum, *Aspergillus* sp. may represent contamination
D. recommend GMS staining to confirm fungal infection

16. A 43-year-old man shows dense shadows on chest x-ray and diffuse interstitial pneumonia. Cytology reveals a large population of thick-walled organisms with a gelatinous capsule. Teardrop budding is frequent. The diagnosis is most consistent with:

A. *Pneumocystis carinii*
B. *Histoplasma capsulatum*
C. *Coccidioides immitis*
D. *Cryptococcus neoformans*

17. A 38-year-old man presents with difficulty in breathing and an elevated temperature. Chest x-ray reveals multiple nodules in both lungs. Sputum analysis reveals a heterogeneous population of normal lymphocytes, plasma cells, and large binucleated cells with coarse irregular chromatin features and macronucleoli. The diagnosis is:

A. plasma cell granulomas
B. sclerosing hemangiomas
C. chronic follicular bronchitis
D. Hodgkin disease

18. A 44-year-old Filipino man presents with a nonproductive cough and constriction and pain in the upper chest. Sputum cytology reveals spherical thick-walled structures resembling a pomegranate. Multiple spores are encapsulated within the structures. The diagnosis was confirmed with GMS. The diagnosis is:

A. *Coccidioides immitis*
B. *Histoplasma capsulatum*
C. *Nocardia asteroides*
D. *Allescheria boydii*

19. A 49-year-old woman with a previous history of a malignant disease presents with multiple lung nodules on chest x-ray. Bronchial brushings revealed small cells in ribbons or cords with hyperchromatic nuclei and frothy, lacy cytoplasm, often with intracytoplasmic alveoli. The diagnosis/primary site may be:

A. small cell carcinoma/lung
B. carcinoid tumor/lung
C. lobular adenocarcinoma/breast
D. adenocarcinoma/ovary

20. A 52-year-old man presents with emaciation, leukopenia, and pyrexia. Sputum analysis reveals numerous histiocytes containing intracellular multiple spherules possessing a refractile cell wall. GMS stains are positive. The diagnosis is:

A. *Pneumocystis carinii*
B. *Cryptococcus neoformans*
C. *Histoplasma capsulatum*
D. *Blastomyces dermatitidis*

21. A 55-year-old man presents with a productive cough and dysphagia. Sputum analysis reveals spindle-shaped cells in clusters with orangeophilic staining cytoplasm. The nuclear features are hyperchromatic with irregular nuclear borders and the chromatin is coarse. Bronchial washings and brushings are negative. The most likely diagnosis/primary site for these cells is:

A. squamous cell carcinoma/esophagus
B. leiomyosarcoma/colon
C. normal squamous metaplasia/lung
D. adenocarcinoma/prostate

22. A 61-year-old woman presents with chronic obstructive pulmonary disease and pneumonitis. A history of tuberculosis exposure was noted. Sputum analysis revealed small round cells in uniform clusters (20+ cells) exhibiting prominent nuclei with fine, irregular chromatin. Psammoma bodies were also present in a degenerative background. Based on this information, the diagnosis is consistent with:

A. adenocarcinoma, poorly differentiated lung
B. adenocarcinoma, terminal bronchioloalveolar
C. creola bodies
D. metastatic breast carcinoma, ductal

23. A 21-year-old AIDS patient presents with a productive cough and purulent sputum. Cytology reveals multiple transparent, thin filamentous branching structures with beaded hyphae. Special stains including acid-fast and Gram stains are positive. The diagnosis represents:

A. *Mycobacterium tuberculosis*
B. *Nocardia asteroides*
C. saprophytic Phycomycetes
D. *Geotrichum candidum*

24. Cytologic analysis of a bronchial brushing reveals elongated cells, variation in cellular size, refractile/glassy cytoplasm, and opaque India ink nuclei. These cells are arranged singly and in sheets. Orangeophilic whorls are present among a granular amorphous material. The best diagnosis is:

A. squamous cell carcinoma, nonkeratinizing
B. poorly differentiated squamous cell carcinoma
C. well-differentiated squamous cell carcinoma, keratinizing
D. reparative/regenerative process

25. A sputum specimen from a 70-year-old man with Goodpasture syndrome reveals a population of small cells with eccentrically located nuclei that are reniform in shape. The cytoplasm contains refractile eosinophilic pigment that often occludes the nuclear detail. The most likely diagnosis is:

A. a contaminant from the larynx
B. malignant melanoma
C. Clara cells
D. siderophages

26. A 6-year-old child with severe anemia, liver insufficiency, and dyspnea is diagnosed clinically with pulmonary hemosiderosis. Papanicolaou-stained bronchioalveolar lavage analysis would reveal histiocytes with:

A. brown-black pigment
B. distended clear vacuoles
C. refractile golden pigment
D. green pigment

27. A sputum specimen from a 55-year-old man with a tracheostomy tube reveals a scanty population of small keratinized cells. The nuclei are round-to-oval and possess fine, regular chromatin. The diagnosis is:

A. keratinizing squamous cell carcinoma
B. atypical squamous metaplasia
C. reserve cell hyperplasia
D. parakeratosis

28. **A Papanicolaou-stained bronchoalveolar lavage specimen yielded large groups of frothy, eosinophilic mats containing refractile, spherical-shaped structures interspersed among alveolar macrophages. These findings would suggest the investigator perform:**

A. mucicarmine staining for *Cryptococcus neoformans*
B. oil red O staining for lipid-laden macrophages, suggesting lipoid pneumonia
C. acid-fast stains for confirmation of *Nocardia asteroides*
D. GMS staining for confirmation of *Pneumocystis carinii*

29. **A Saccomanno-processed sputum specimen yields small cells with normal nuclear/cytoplasmic ratios and dense cyanophilic cytoplasm. The cells are found in sheets and as single cells. The cytologic findings are considered:**

A. pathognomonic of malignancy
B. diagnostic of a benign reparative process
C. suspicious for malignancy
D. bronchial metaplastic cells

30. **A sputum specimen reveals a biphasic population of round cells with uniform cell shape and round nuclei possessing fine, regular chromatin. Each of the cells lies singly. The cytologic findings are suggestive of:**

A. small cell carcinoma
B. small cell non-cleaved lymphoma
C. normal lymphocytes
D. creola bodies

31. **In sputum samples, cells demonstrating slight pleomorphism, moderate variation in size, a variable nuclear/cytoplasmic ratio, nuclear hyperchromasia, and finely granular, evenly distributed chromatin are suggestive of:**

A. reserve cell hyperplasia
B. large cell undifferentiated carcinoma
C. keratinizing squamous cell carcinoma
D. atypical squamous metaplasia

32. **Coiled structures composed of inspissated mucus often associated with bronchial obstruction are:**

A. corpora amylacea
B. creola bodies
C. Curschmann spirals
D. calcospherites

33. **What epithelia lines the larynx?**

A. simple squamous
B. nonkeratinizing stratified squamous
C. simple cuboidal
D. transitional

34. **A patient who is a known abuser of nose drops is at risk for developing:**

A. lipoid pneumonia
B. Barrett metaplasia
C. sarcoidosis
D. There is no known risk

35. **All of the following may yield abundant eosinophils in a pulmonary specimen, EXCEPT:**

A. *Strongyloides stercoralis*
B. Löffler pneumonia
C. asthma
D. inflammatory pseudotumor

36. **A 36-year-old man diagnosed as HIV-positive presents with an active *Mycobacterium tuberculosis* infection. Recent sputum analysis shows small cells with scanty cytoplasm and uniform cell size in tight compact sheets. The nuclei are small and dense. These cells represent:**

A. small cell carcinoma, oat cell type
B. intermediate cell carcinoma
C. atypical squamous metaplasia, severe
D. reserve cell hyperplasia

37. **Cells associated with viral infections and presenting with degenerative qualities and detached cilia represent:**

A. reactive bronchial cells
B. creola bodies
C. ciliocytophthoria
D. reserve cell hyperplasia

38. **Cells exhibiting eosinophilic cytoplasm containing refractile granules, squared-off cytoplasmic borders, and double, translucent, refractile cell walls, and dark/smudged nuclear morphology are diagnostic of:**

A. atypical squamous metaplasia
B. keratinizing squamous cell carcinoma
C. plant cells
D. reparative/regenerative cellular changes

39. **The findings of creola bodies, Charcot-Leyden crystals, eosinophils, and occasional Curschmann spirals are suggestive of:**

A. asthma
B. ciliocytophthoria
C. tuberculosis
D. Wegener granulomatosis

40. **A 4-month-old infant presents with difficulty in breathing and chronic vomiting. Chest x-ray reveals a diffuse infiltrate suggestive of pneumonia. A cytologic examination of the regurgitate reveals a large population of bronchial epithelial cells, a population of histiocytes with signet ring formation, and cells with multiple vacuolization. The most likely diagnosis is:**

A. *Histoplasma capsulatum*
B. lipid pneumonia
C. liposarcoma
D. metastatic neuroblastoma

41. **Which entity is etiologically related to malignant mesothelioma?**

A. ferruginous bodies
B. calcospherites
C. *Mycobacterium tuberculosis*
D. *Schistosoma haematobium*

42. **A 70-year-old man with a productive cough and a previous negative bronchoscopy presents with a sputum containing cells with large nuclei, corresponding increase in cytoplasm, and multinucleation. The nuclear chromatin is fine and regular. Many of the cells have macronucleoli and terminal bars. These cells are diagnostic of:**

A. reactive bronchial epithelial cells
B. atypical squamous metaplasia
C. nonkeratinizing squamous cell carcinoma
D. squamous metaplasia

43. **A 44-year-old woman with bronchiectasis submits material for sputum analysis. The sample yields cells in three-dimensional fragments, cells in papillary groups, and cells producing mucin and containing nucleoli. The peripheries of the fragments have intact cilia and/or terminal bars. The diagnosis is consistent with:**

A. well-differentiated bronchogenic adenocarcinoma
B. creola bodies
C. bronchioloalveolar adenocarcinoma
D. carcinoid tumor

44. **A common cell type associated with patients diagnosed with anthracosis is:**

A. carbon histiocyte
B. beryllium
C. starch
D. hemosiderin-laden macrophage

45. **A 55-year-old patient with a papillary neoplasm shows structures with concentrically laminated calcifying rings in a sputum specimen. These structures are:**

A. corpora amylacea
B. creola bodies
C. Curschmann spirals
D. psammoma bodies

46. **The "dysplasia" preceding keratinizing squamous cell carcinoma is:**

A. reserve cell hyperplasia
B. atypical bronchial hyperplasia
C. atypical squamous metaplasia
D. atypical reparative processes

47. A 65-year-old woman suffers from pulmonary edema. A population of concentrically laminated, non-calcifying structures are found in a sputum specimen prepared using the pick-and-smear method. These structures represent:

A. Curschmann spirals
B. corpora amylacea
C. calcospherites
D. keratinizing pearl associated with squamous carcinoma

48. Cells from a bronchial washing, prepared using membrane filtration, exhibit nuclear molding/compression, hyperchromatic nuclei, coarsely granular chromatin, and high nuclear/cytoplasmic ratios. The cells are organized into ribbons, nests, and vertebral column formation. The diagnosis is:

A. reserve cell hyperplasia
B. oat cell carcinoma
C. metastatic pancreatic carcinoma
D. bronchioloalveolar adenocarcinoma

49. **These cells represent a bronchial brushing obtained from a patient with a 3-cm central pulmonary mass. They are diagnostic of:**

A. large cell carcinoma
B. squamous cell carcinoma
C. adenocarcinoma, poorly differentiated
D. small cell carcinoma, intermediate cell type

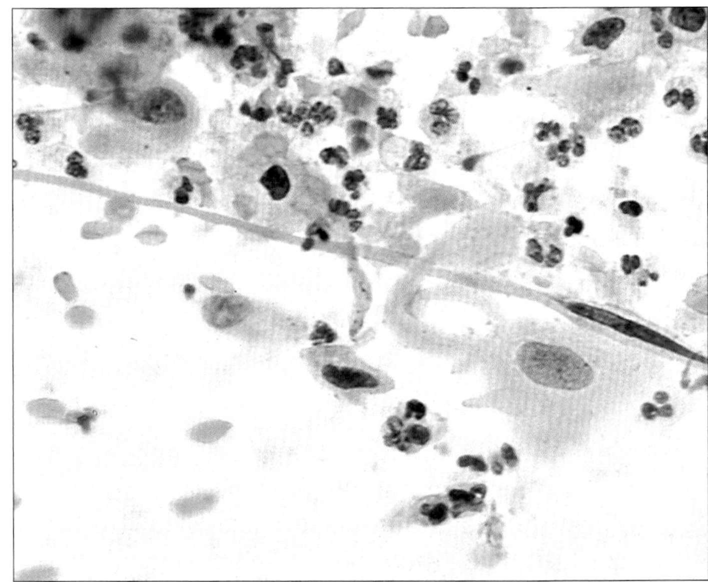

50. **A 55-year-old agriculture worker presents with rhinitis and recent weight loss. Sputum cytology reveals these structures. The cellular findings are:**

A. *Actinomyces israelii*
B. Phycomycetes
C. *Nocardia asteroides*
D. *Aspergillus* sp.

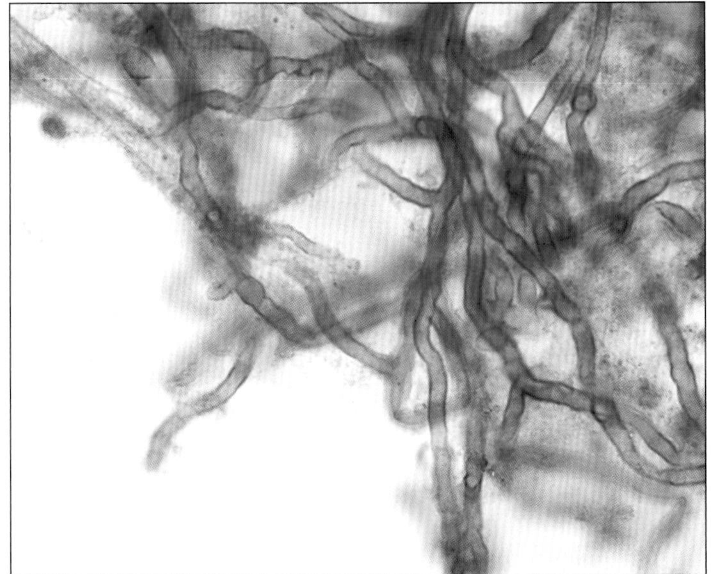

51. **These cells found in a sputum sample may be related to:**

A. bronchioloalveolar adenocarcinoma
B. asthma
C. well-differentiated bronchogenic adenocarcinoma
D. metastatic ductal carcinoma of the breast

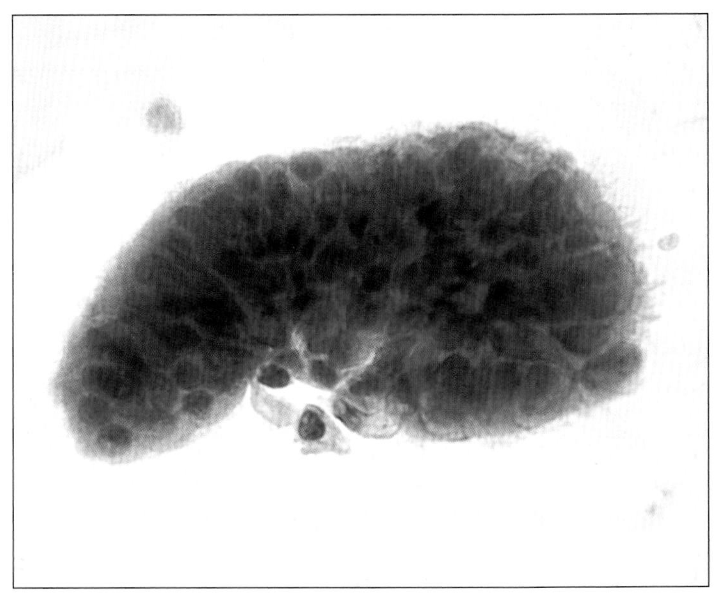

52. **A 68-year-old man presents with recent weight loss and a history of tobacco use. A coin lesion is observed on chest x-ray. These cells represent a sputum sample. The findings are consistent with:**

A. squamous cell carcinoma
B. neuroendocrine tumor
C. malignant lymphoma
D. reactive lymphocytes

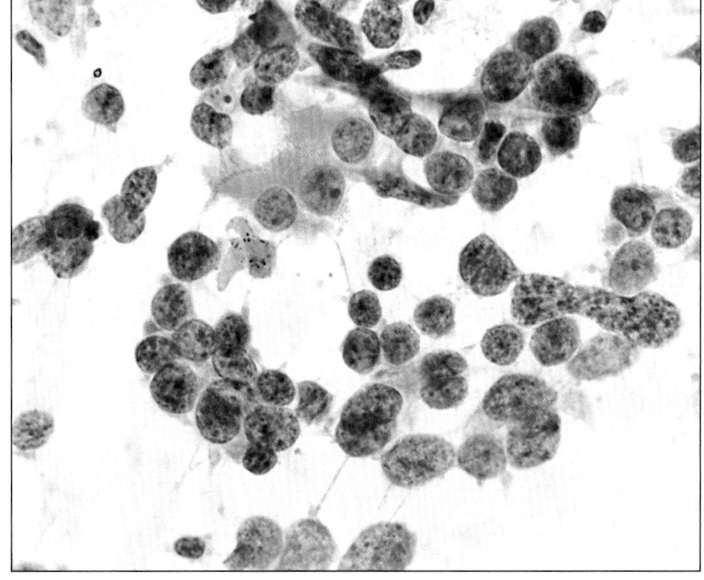

53. **These cells were identified in a sputum specimen from a patient with laryngitis and negative bronchoscopic findings. Their most likely origin is:**

A. lung
B. trachea
C. pharynx
D. oral cavity

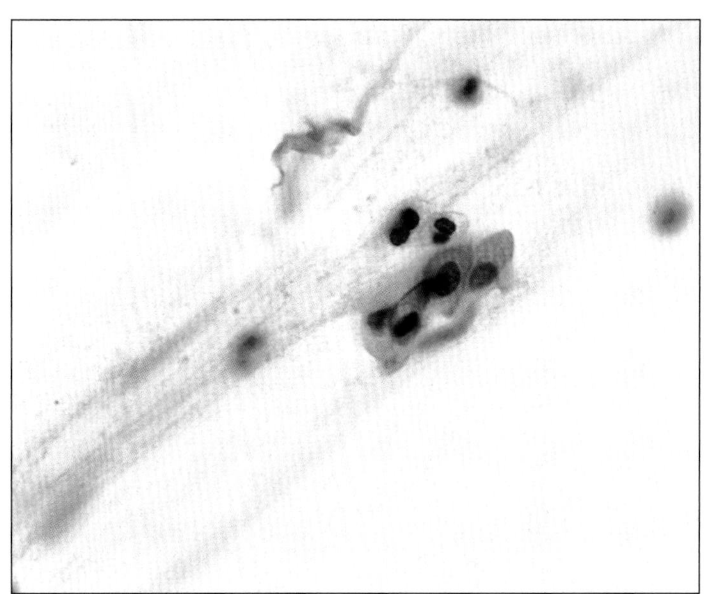

54. **A bronchial brushing from a 61-year-old man with a 2-cm coin lesion reveals these cells. The findings are most consistent with:**

A. large cell lymphoma
B. squamous cell carcinoma
C. small cell carcinoma
D. carcinoid tumor

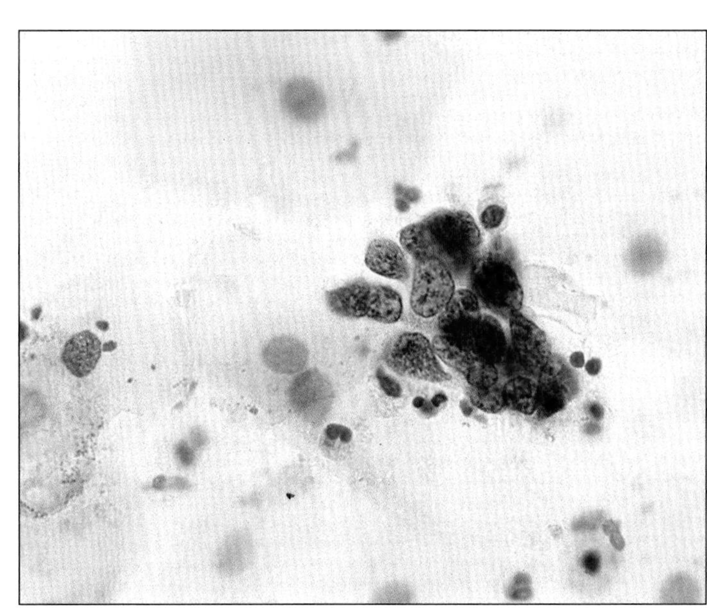

55. A 71-year-old physician recently diagnosed with renal carcinoma, status post excision and post chemotherapy, presents with a pulmonary infiltrate and a 3-cm lesion in the right middle lobe of the lung. A sputum evaluation is performed. These structures are found within alveolar macrophages and fluoresced with auramine-O. The findings are:

A. *Legionella* sp.
B. *Nocardia asteroides*
C. acid-fast bacilli, *Mycobacterium avium-intracellulare*
D. *Actinomyces israelii*

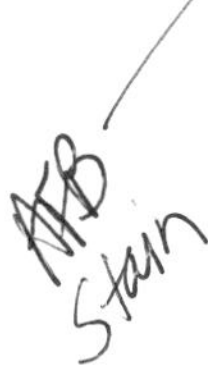

56. An immunosuppressed man with discrete multiple lesions on chest x-ray and a recent diagnosis of a granulomatous pulmonary condition presents for a repeat sputum analysis. The diagnosis is infection with:

A. *Strongyloides stercoralis*
B. *Echinococcus* sp.
C. *Alternaria* sp.
D. *Paragonimus westermani*

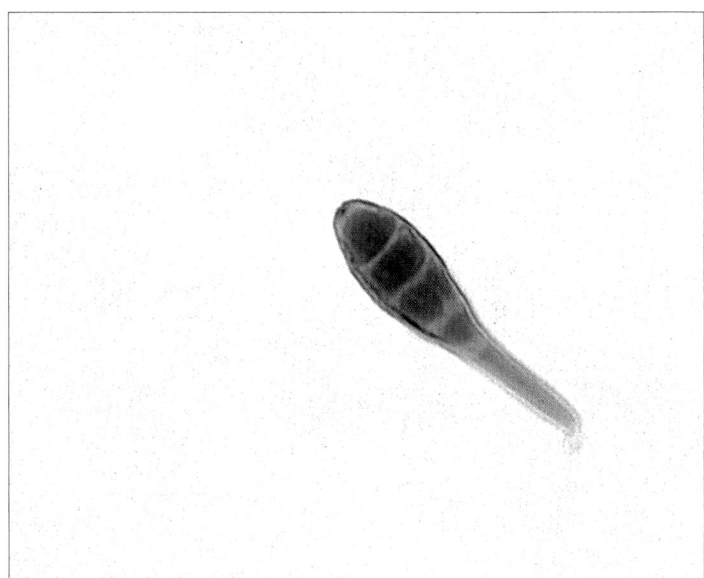

57. A 45-year-old man with a 2×3-cm mass located in the right middle lobe of the lung presents with a spiking fever and recent weight loss. Bronchial brushing reveals these cells, which are diagnostic of:

A. small cell carcinoma
B. carcinoid tumor
C. reactive lymphoid hyperplasia
D. non-Hodgkin lymphoma

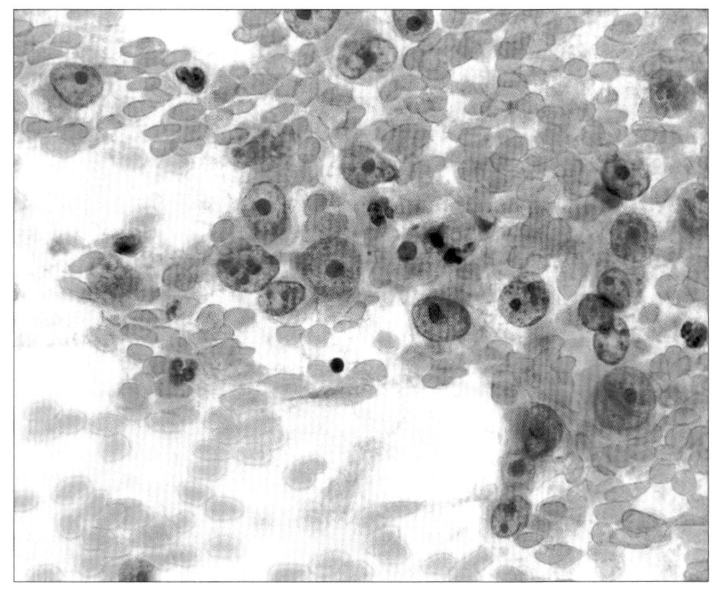

58. **These cells were obtained from a bronchial brushing from a 44-year-old man with a history of an autoimmune disease. The findings are consistent with:**

A. squamous cell carcinoma
B. sarcoma, not otherwise specified
C. epithelioid histiocytes
D. microfilaria

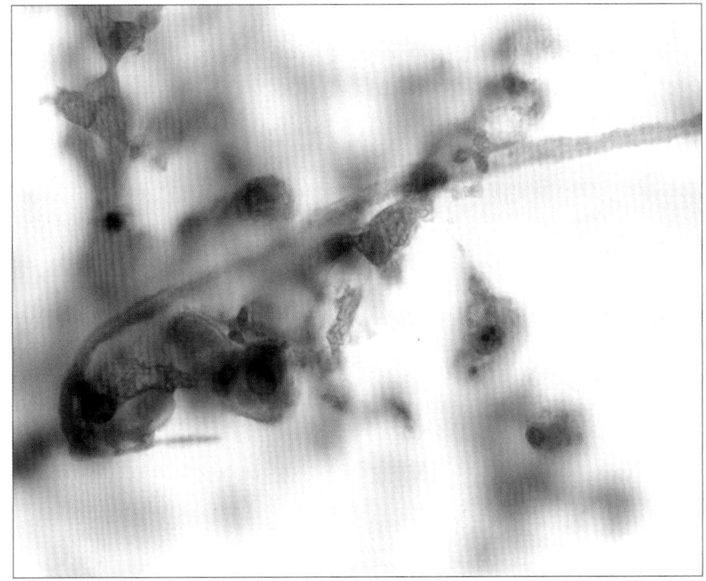

59. **These cells were found in a bronchial brushing from a 61-year-old woman with a history of tuberculosis now presenting with a peripheral lung mass. These cells:**

A. are associated with a chronic obstructive disease
B. are associated with amine precursor uptake and decarboxylase
C. arise from type II pneumocytes
D. stain positive with common leukocytic antigen

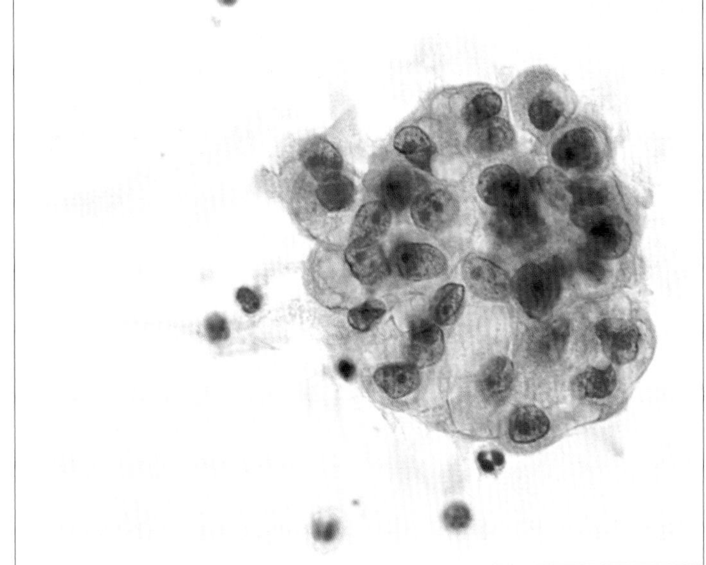

60. **A 44-year-old man presents with hemoptysis and enlarged axillary lymph nodes. Sputum analysis reveals these structures. The cytologic pattern depicted is compatible with infection by:**

A. *Blastomyces dermatitidis*
B. *Cryptococcus neoformans*
C. *Histoplasma capsulatum*
D. *Pneumocystis carinii*

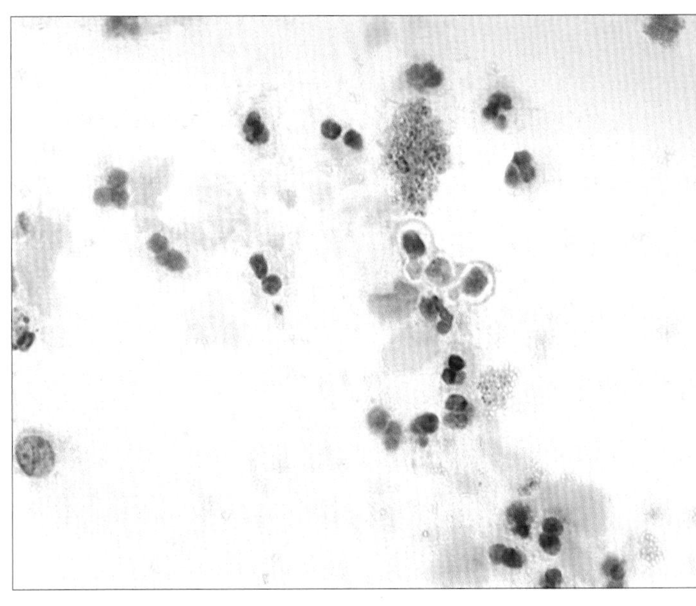

61. **The representative cells were found in an endobronchial brushing. Which of the following apply?**

A. small cell carcinoma; chromogranin (–)
B. carcinoid tumor; chromogranin (+)
C. squamous cell carcinoma; parathormone (+)
D. non-Hodgkin lymphoma; S-100 (+)

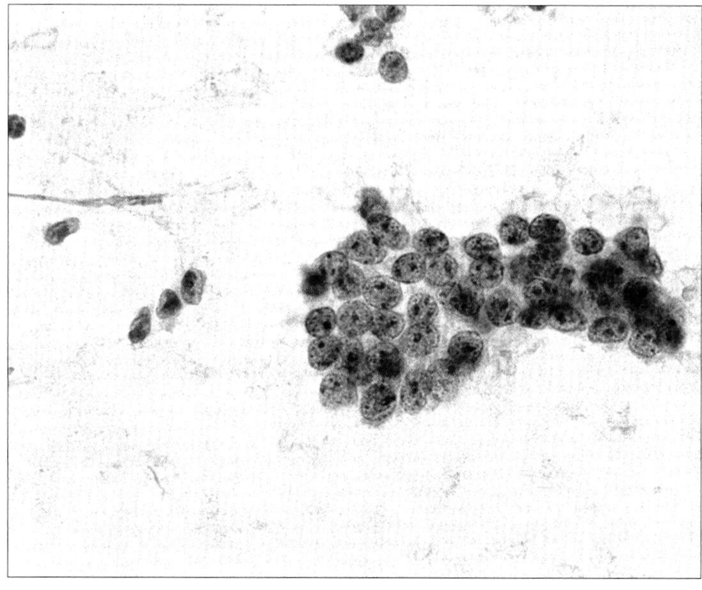

62. **A bronchopulmonary washing revealed the following cells. What immunocytochemical stain would be positive?**

A. keratin
B. chromogranin
C. common leukocytic antigen
D. alpha-fetoprotein

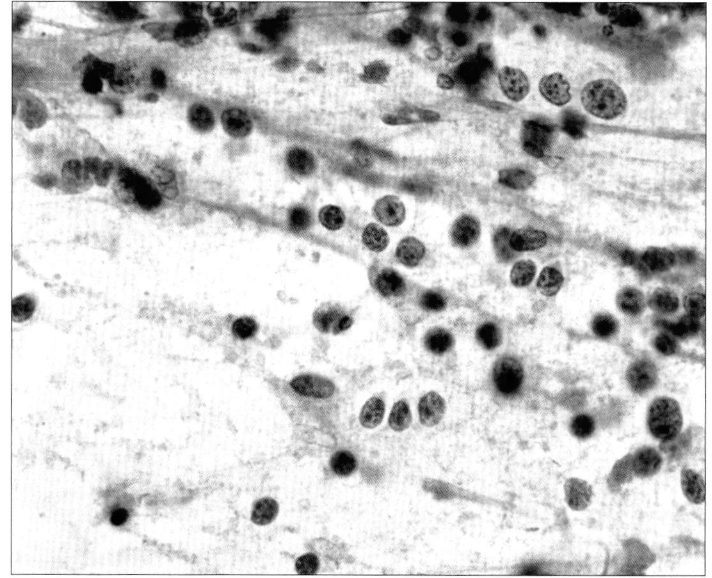

63. **These structures contain:**

A. glycoproteins (and calcify)
B. glycoproteins (and do not calcify)
C. phosphates (and calcify)
D. phosphates (and do not calcify)

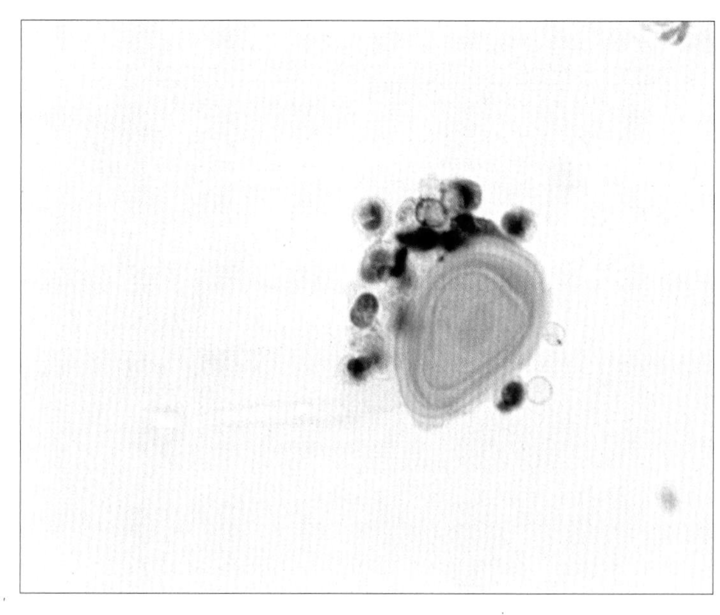

64. A 42-year-old man with a history of recurrent generalized infections presents with pneumonia. Laboratory findings include anemia, thrombocytopenia, and an elevated erythrocyte sedimentation rate (above 15 mm/h). The diagnosis is:

A. cytomegalovirus
B. herpes
C. respiratory syncytial virus
D. parainfluenza virus

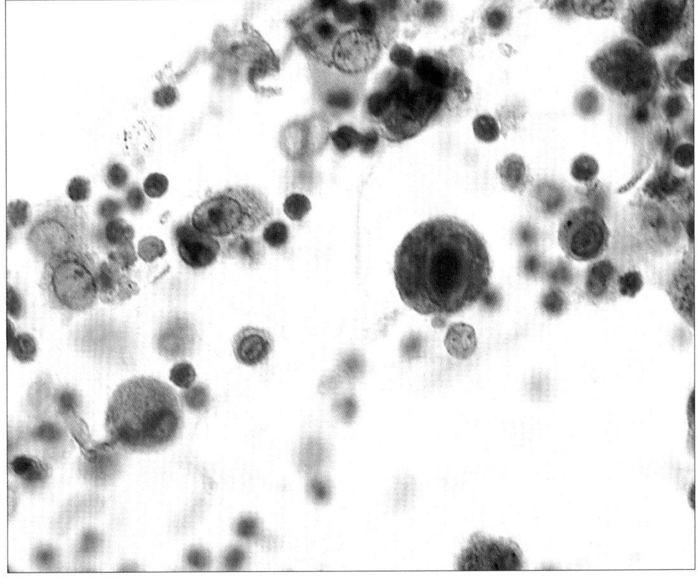

65. A purulent sputum sample from a diabetic patient with pneumonitis reveals these structures. The diagnosis is infection with:

A. *Candida* sp.
B. *Actinomyces israelii*
C. *Allescheria boydii*
D. *Aspergillis* sp.

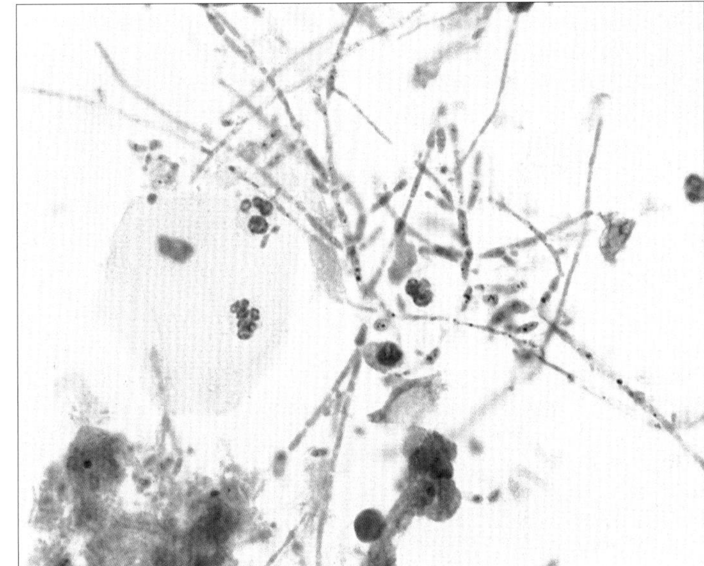

66. A elderly woman presents with pancytopenia, chorioretinitis, and endocarditis. Further examination reveals pneumonia. Sputum samples contain these entities. The cellular findings are:

A. *Cryptococcus neoformans*
B. *Histoplasma capsulatum*
C. *Blastomyces dermatitidis*
D. *Toxoplasma gondii*

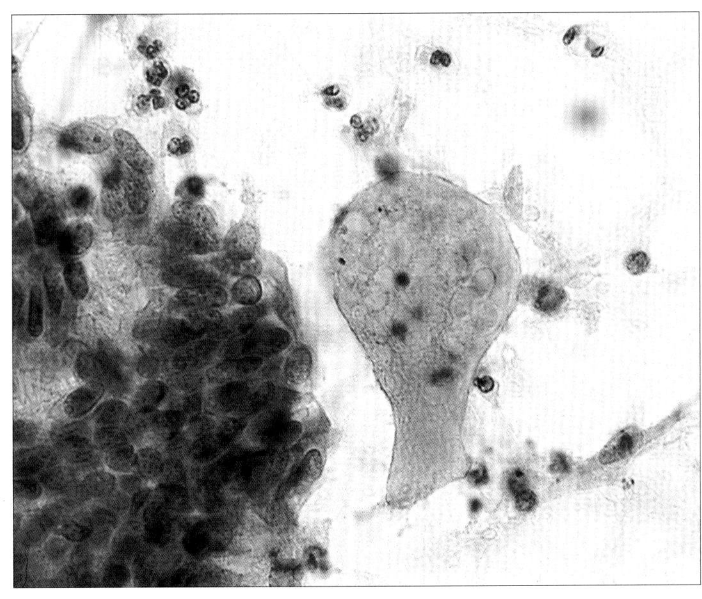

67. A 66-year-old man with a nonproductive cough and shortness of breath produces an induced sputum specimen. The process is consistent with:

A. *Histoplasma capsulatum*
B. *Pneumocystis carinii*
C. *Coccidioides immitis*
D. *Pseudallescheria boydii*

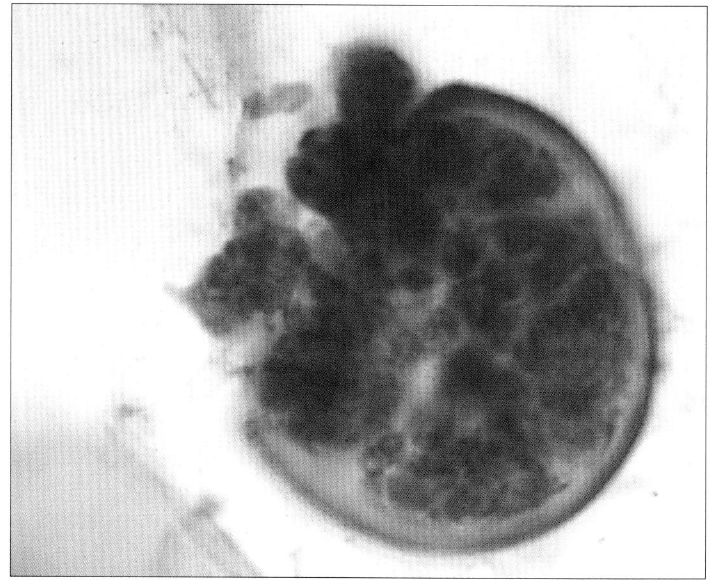

68. A 55-year-old woman with a history of endometrial adenocarcinoma presents to her physician complaining of difficulty in breathing. Chest x-ray reveals a diffuse pneumonitis. This bronchial brushing is consistent with:

A. metastatic endometrial adenocarcinoma
B. large cell undifferentiated carcinoma
C. reactive bronchial epithelial cells
D. reactive mesothelial cells

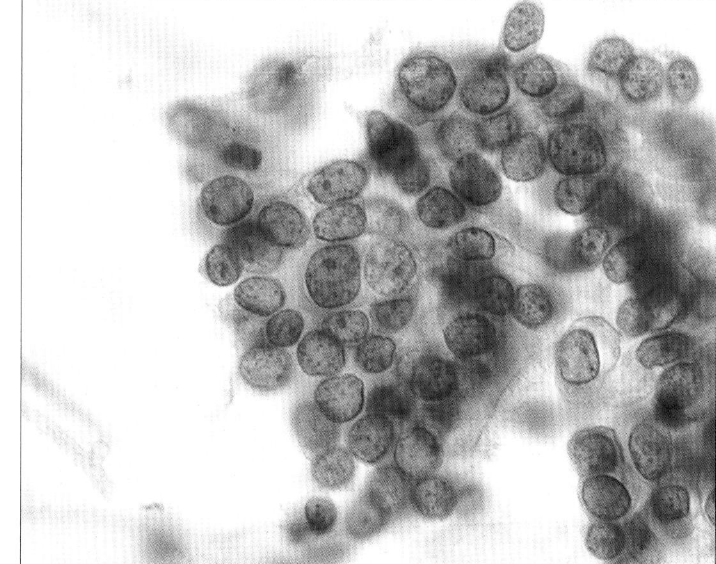

69. A 67-year-old man with advanced carcinoma of the lung presents with recent interstitial pneumonitis. The diagnosis is infection by:

A. *Candida* sp.
B. *Actinomyces* sp.
C. *Nocardia asteroides*
D. *Aspergillus* sp.

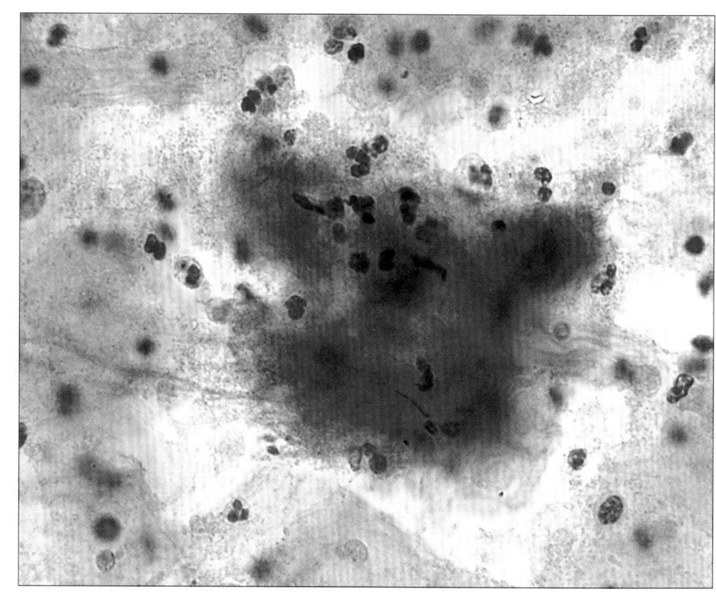

70. **These cells represent a bronchial brushing from a 55-year-old woman. The cellular findings are diagnostic of:**

A. bronchioloalveolar carcinoma
B. poorly differentiated squamous cell carcinoma
C. creola bodies associated with asthma
D. bronchogenic adenocarcinoma

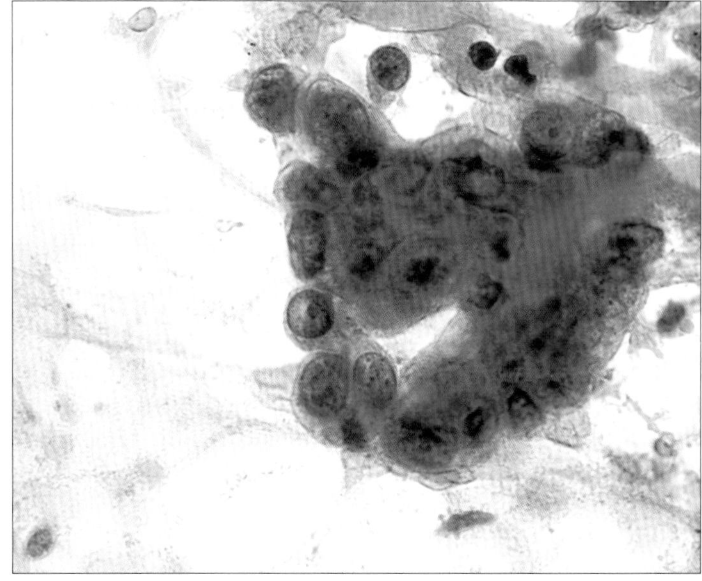

71. **These cells were found in a sputum specimen from a patient with a productive purulent cough. The cytologic diagnosis is:**

A. small cell carcinoma
B. carcinoid tumor
C. squamous metaplasia
D. reserve cell hyperplasia

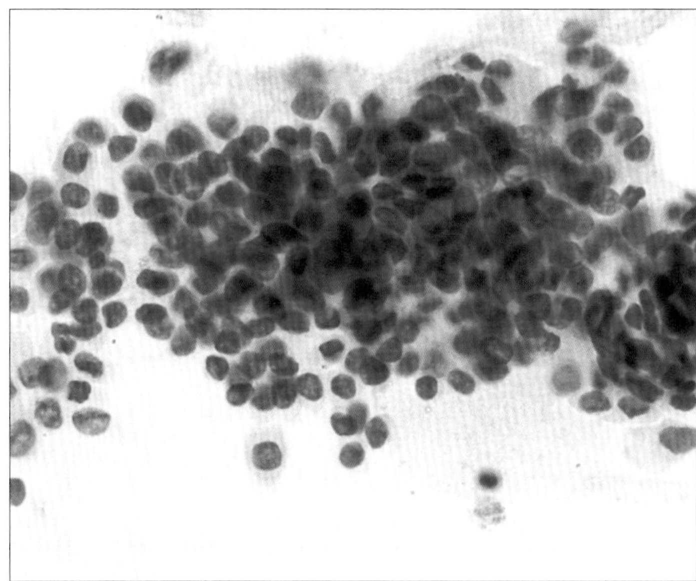

72. **The process identified represents a bronchial brushing from a 56-year-old man. The diagnosis is:**

A. hamartoma
B. reactive/reparative changes
C. metastatic colonic adenocarcinoma
D. granulomatous process

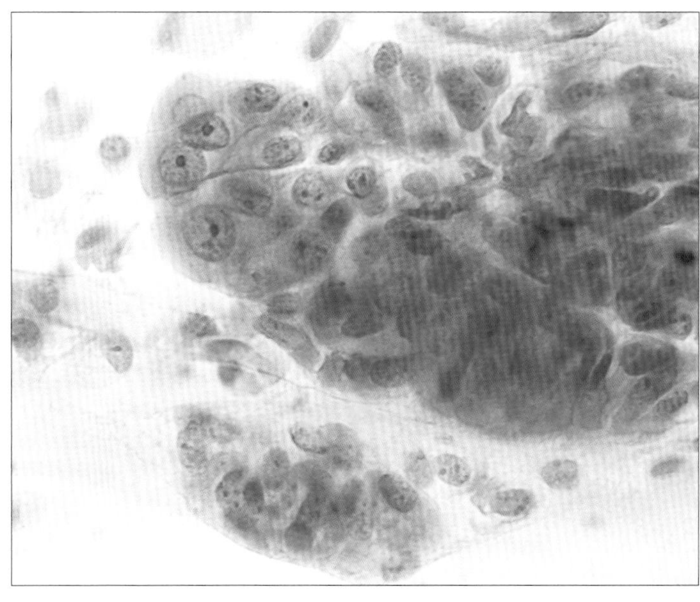

73. **These cells were taken from a 35-year-old man with hemoptysis and a 10-year history of occupational fume inhalation. The cellular findings are most compatible with:**

A. bronchogenic adenocarcinoma
B. atypical histiocytes
C. multinucleated bronchial cells
D. atypical bronchial cells

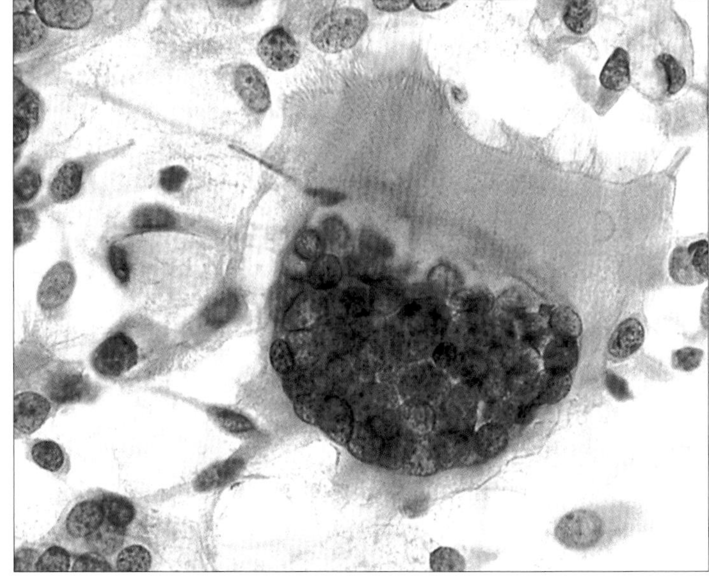

74. **These cells were obtained from a sputum sample of an elderly man with recent heart failure. The findings are consistent with:**

A. melanoma
B. bronchioloalveolar adenocarcinoma
C. siderophages
D. cytomegalovirus

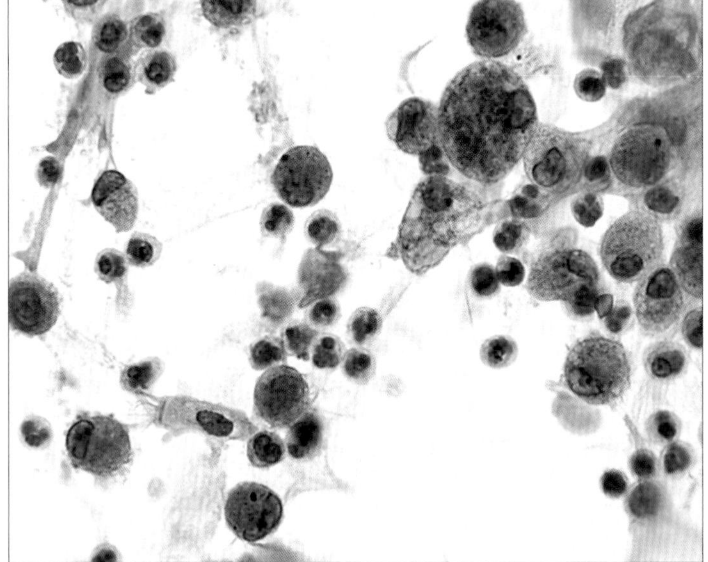

75. **When seen in pulmonary specimens, these cells represent:**

A. atypical metaplastic cells
B. normal metaplastic cells
C. pneumocytes, type II
D. alveolar macrophages

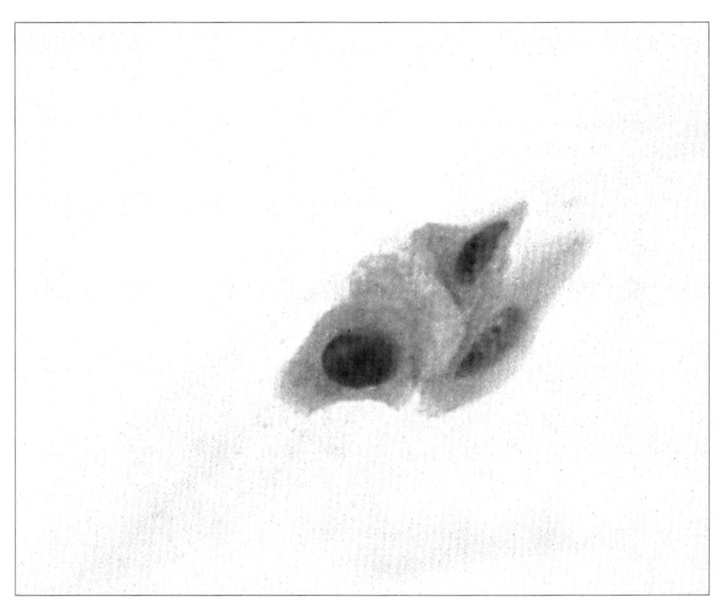

76. **A special stain often used to help identify these entities is:**

A. mucicarmine
B. oil red O
C. Sudan black
D. immunocytochemical antibodies against cytomegalovirus (CMV)

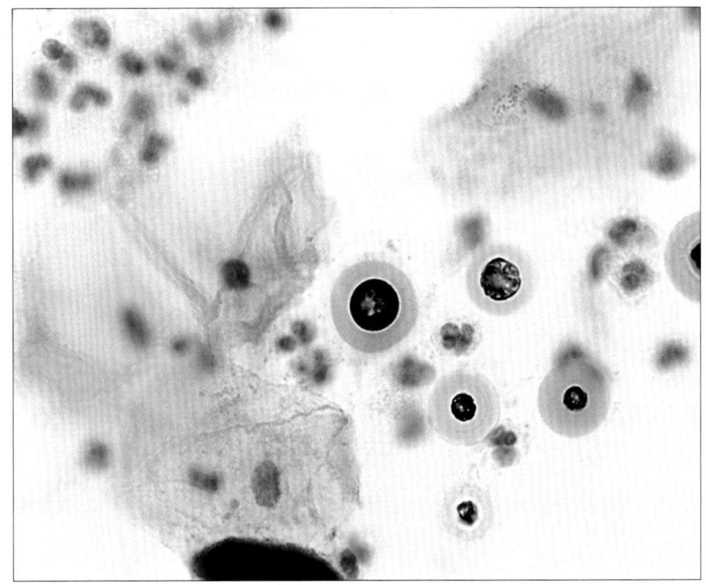

77. **The finding depicted in this sputum specimen is often associated with:**

A. tuberculosis
B. tumor diathesis
C. contamination
D. asthma

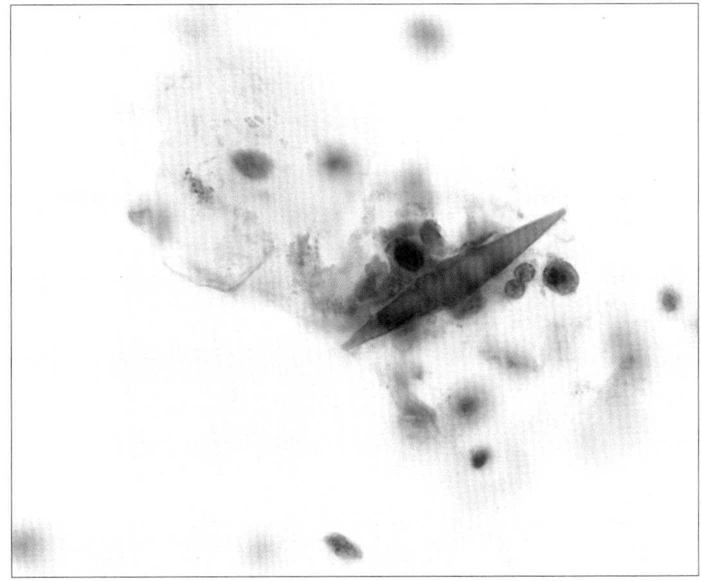

78. **These cells originate within:**

A. granulomas
B. bone marrow
C. the trachea
D. main stem bronchi

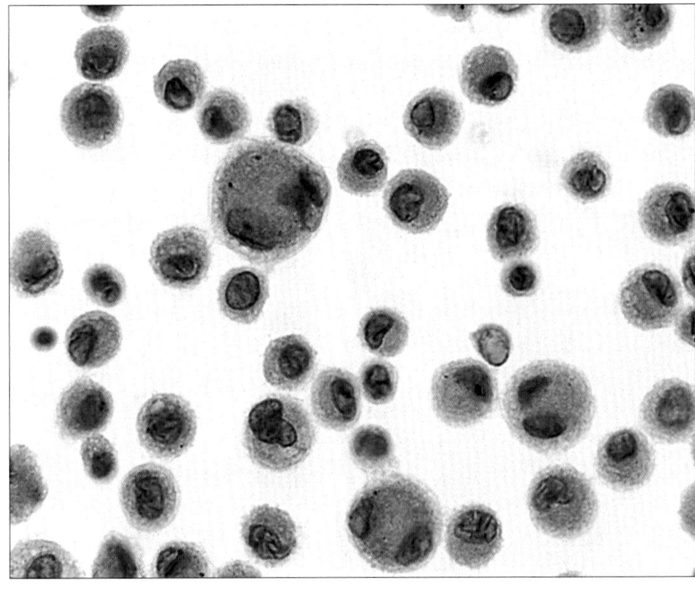

79. **A 35-year-old man complains of a dry, nonproductive cough and a 20-pound weight loss. Chest x-ray film reveals interstitial pneumonitis and a disseminated hilar infiltrate. Bronchial brush and alveolar washings are submitted for evaluation. GMS staining reveals:**

A. *Histoplasma capsulatum*
B. *Cryptococcus neoformans*
C. degenerated bronchial epithelial cells
D. *Pneumocystis carinii*

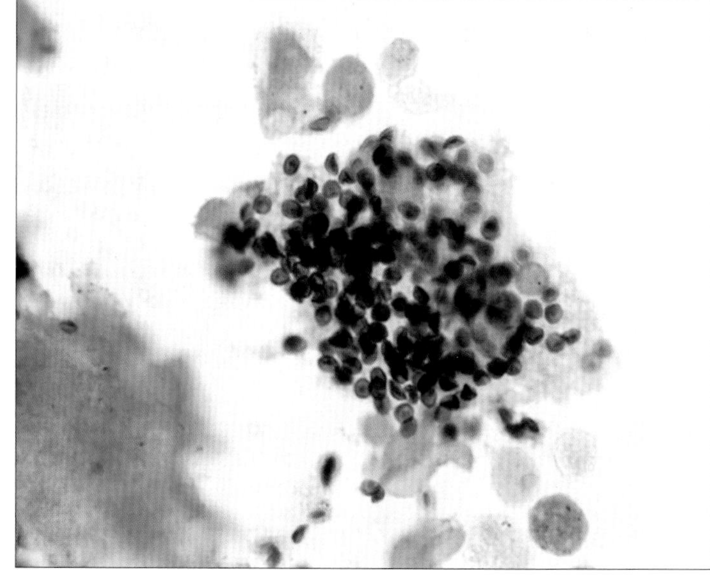

80. **A 44-year-old woman presents with a productive cough. Sputum analysis reveals these cells. Which of the following clinical histories apply?**

A. HIV
B. tuberculosis
C. smoking
D. nose inhalant abuse

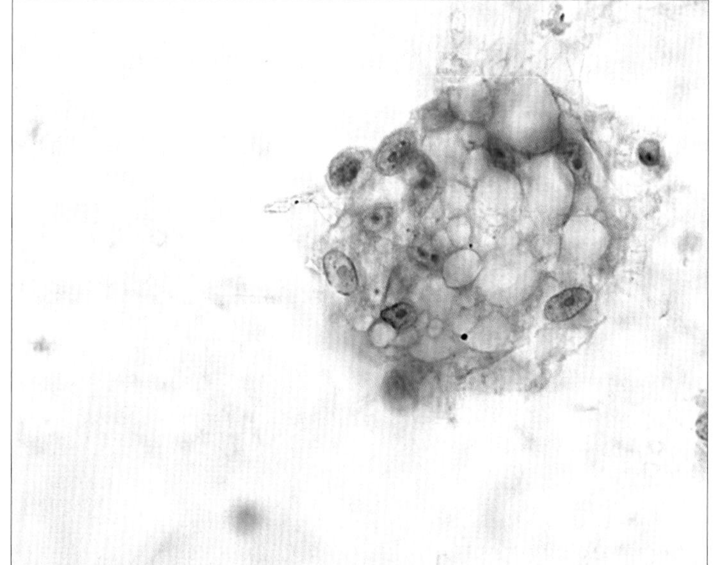

81. **A possible clinical explanation for these findings obtained from a sputum specimen is:**

A. right upper lobe mass
B. hypersensitivity reaction
C. history of bronchopulmonary silicosis
D. lipoid pneumonia

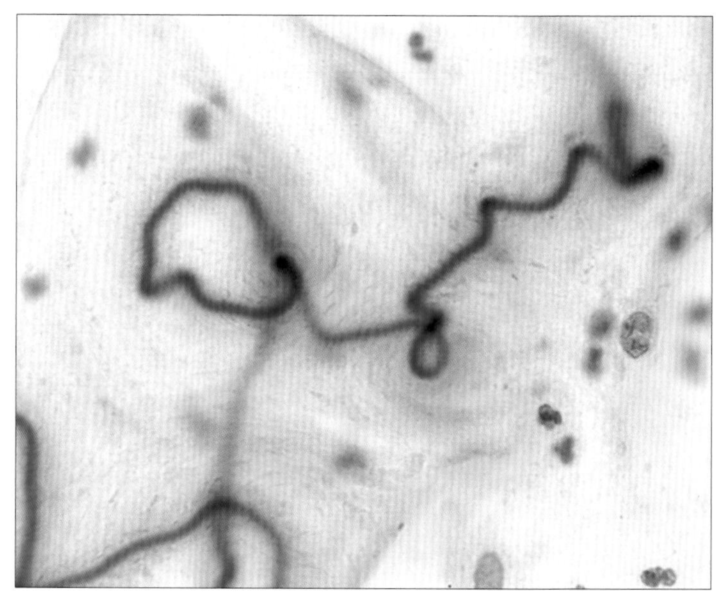

82. **These cells represent a sputum sample from a 55-year-old woman with a history of smoking. They are:**

A. lipophages
B. carbon histiocytes
C. siderophages
D. muciphages

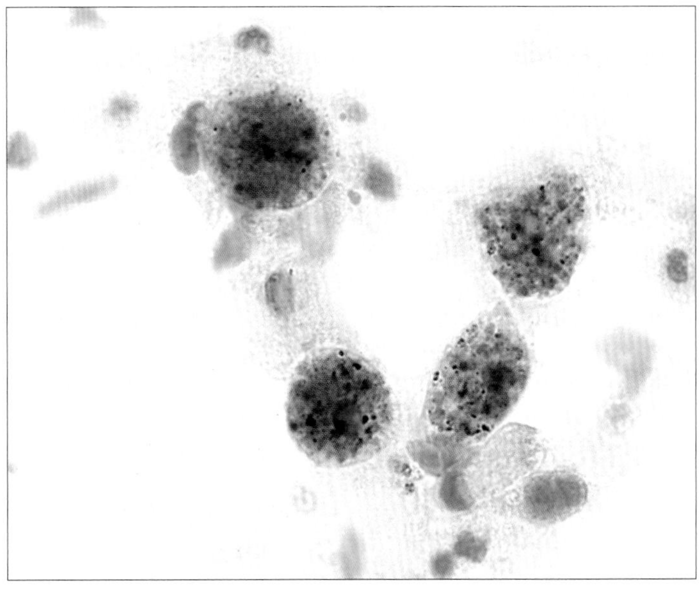

83. **A 21-year-old immunocompromised patient presents with shortness of breath. Sputum analysis reveals:**

A. cytomegalovirus
B. respiratory syncytial virus
C. herpesvirus
D. parainfluenza virus

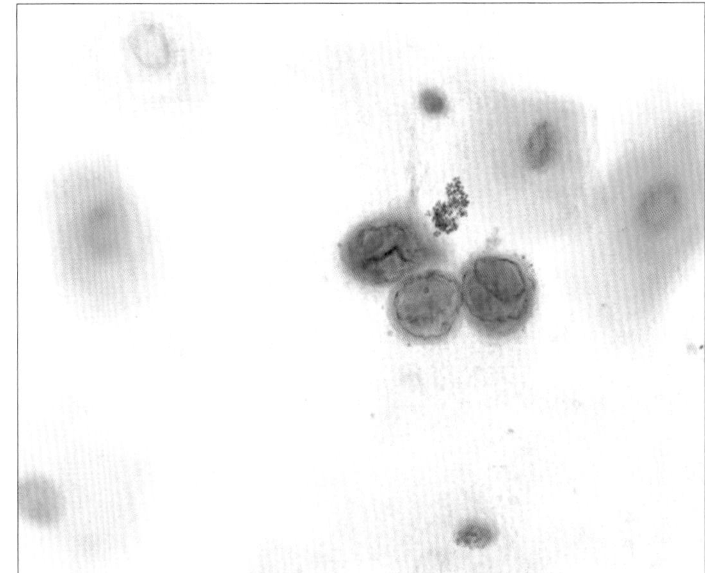

84. **These cells represent a sputum specimen from a 44-year-old man. The diagnosis is consistent with:**

A. viral infection
B. carcinoid tumor
C. alveolar proteinosis
D. reserve cell hyperplasia

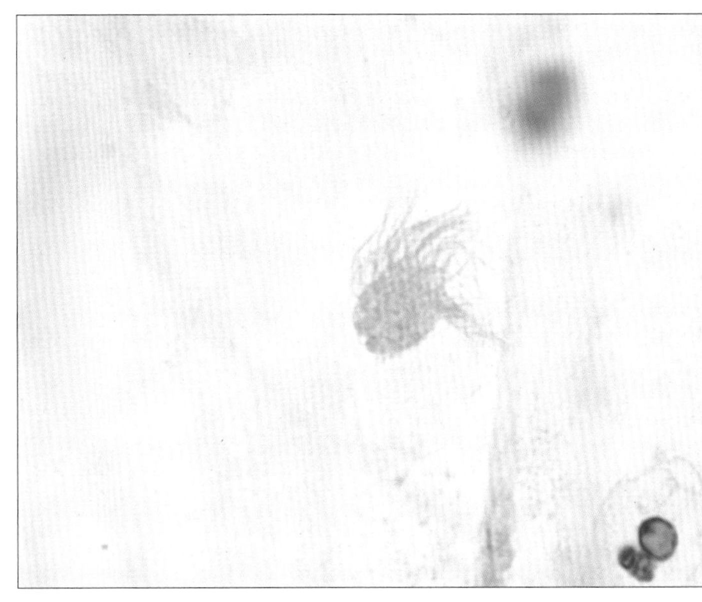

85. A patient who recently underwent surgery for squamous cell carcinoma of the lung presents with a small nodule on chest x-ray in the general area of the original tumor. Bronchial aspiration reveals epithelioid cells, giant cells, and these entities. The findings are most compatible with:

A. starch granulomatosis
B. *Cryptococcus neoformans*
C. *Blastomyces dermatitidis*
D. pollen contamination, suggest repeat bronchoscopy

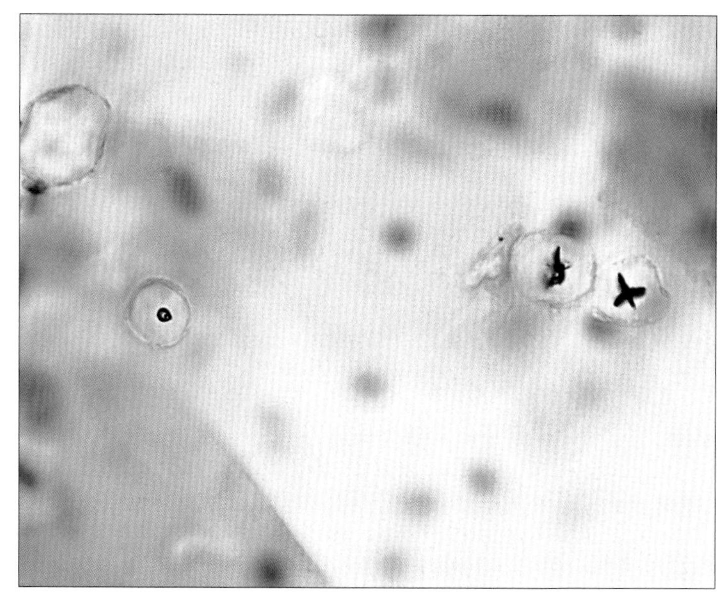

86. A 62-year-old woman presents with shortness of breath. A sputum sample is processed for cytology. The diagnosis is consistent with:

A. metastatic spindle cell sarcoma
B. metastatic rhabdomyosarcoma
C. primary neoplasm
D. striated muscle (meat) contamination, repeat sputum

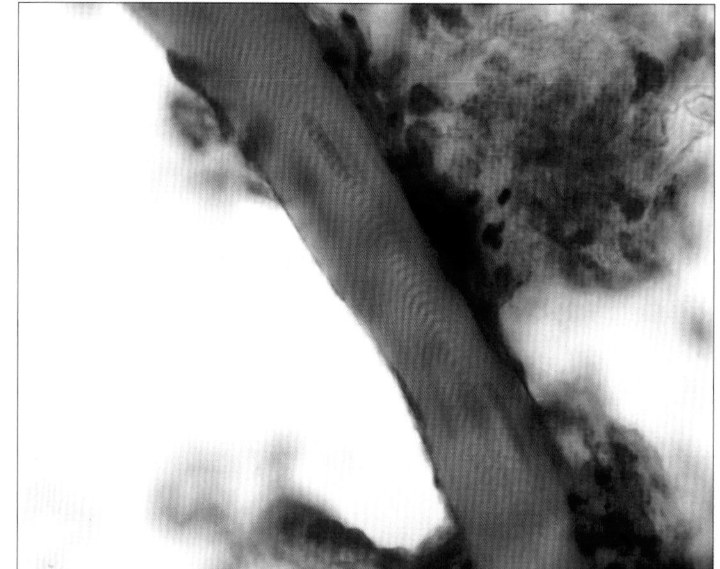

87. These cells represent a cytologic preparation of a sputum sample taken from a 62-year-old woman presenting with shortness of breath. The cytologic diagnosis may be related to:

A. large cell lymphoma
B. mesothelioma
C. lipoid pneumonia
D. asthma

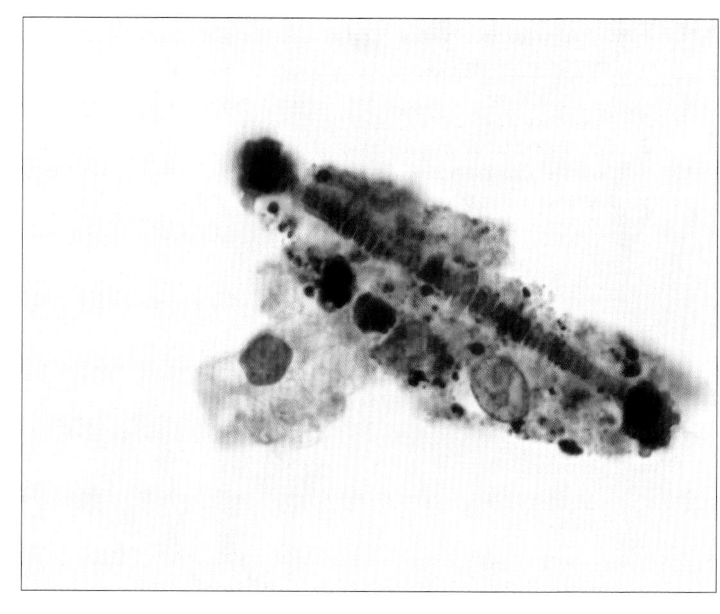

88. **These cells represent a bronchial brushing obtained from a 63-year-old man with a history of chronic obstructive pulmonary disease. The findings are most consistent with:**

A. metastatic colonic adenocarcinoma
B. carcinoid tumor
C. normal bronchial epithelial cells
D. nondiagnostic

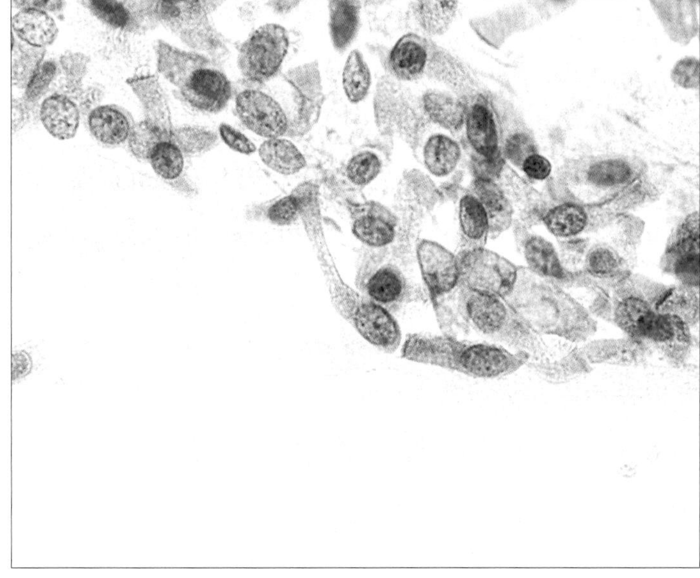

89. **A 55-year-old man with a lesion on chest x-ray and a nonproductive cough presents for an early-morning induced sputum specimen. These cells are diagnostic of:**

A. squamous cell carcinoma
B. vegetable cells
C. atypical squamous metaplasia
D. large cell undifferentiated carcinoma

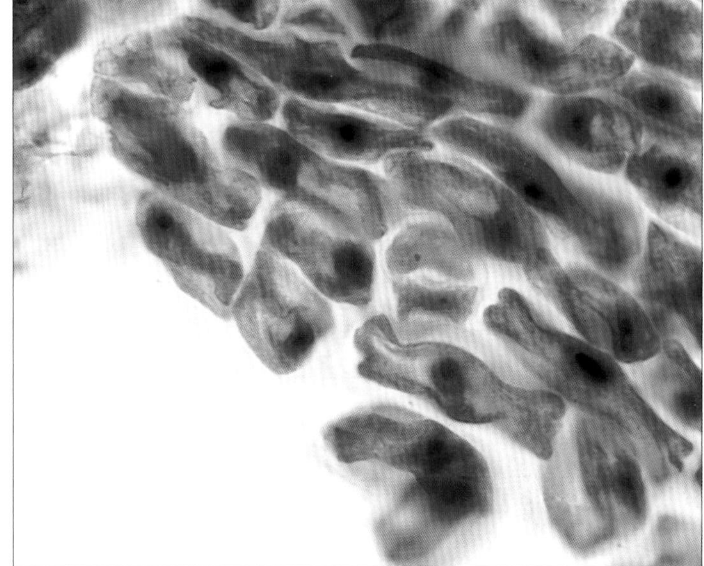

90. **These structures, found in a sputum specimen represent:**

A. a primary lung disease
B. *Cryptococcus neoformans*
C. pollen contamination
D. starch

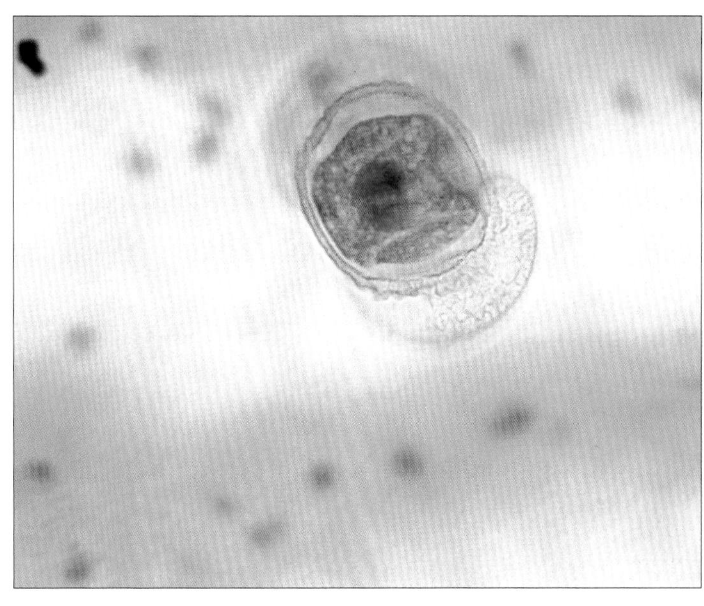

91. This bronchial brushing taken from a 55-year-old man with a history of a pulmonary disorder reveals:

A. adenocarcinoma
B. large cell carcinoma
C. reactive bronchial cells
D. viral infection, not otherwise specified

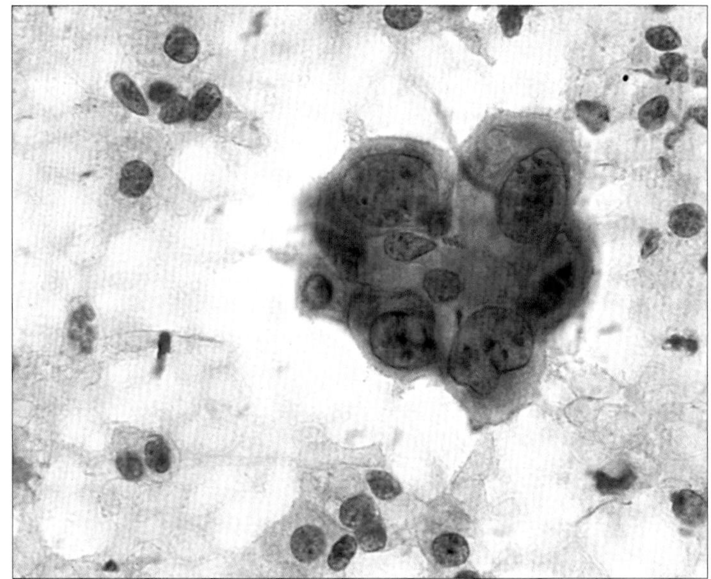

92. The cytologic findings represent a sputum specimen from a 2-week-old premature infant. The diagnosis is:

A. *Cryptococcus neoformans*
B. *Blastomyces dermatitidis*
C. *Pneumocystis carinii*
D. none of the above

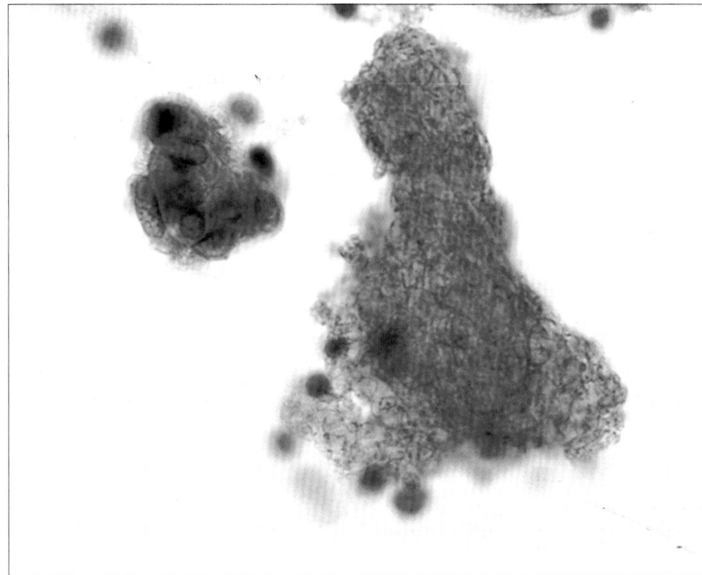

Respiratory Tract *Answer Key*

1. **D small cell carcinoma, oat cell variety**

Small cell carcinoma is a highly malignant neuroendocrine neoplasm that is ultrastructurally part of the amine precursor uptake and decarboxylation (APUD) tumors. These cells contain hyperchromatic stippled chromatin, coarse clumping, nuclear molding, scanty cytoplasm, and micronucleoli. They characteristically have vertebral column formation, microbiopsy aggregates, cords, nests, or ribbons. The oat cell type, which may represent a degenerated form of the tumor, typically is found in streams of mucin when evaluating the cells using the pick-and-smear or crush technique. The Saccomanno technique may not preserve the molding patterns as often. The intermediate cell small cell carcinoma represents both fusiform and polygonal variants, which are typically better preserved with open coarse chromatin patterns and enlarged cell areas. Immunocytochemical staining with chromogranin is helpful in establishing the neurosecretory nature of this tumor.

DeMay RM, The Art & Science of Cytopathology.
Small cell carcinoma, oat cell type, pp. 931–932.

2. **A melanoma**

Melanoma typically presents in single cells, aggregates, or as spindle cells with bizarre malignant nuclear features, macronucleoli, intranuclear cytoplasmic inclusions, and possibly intracytoplasmic golden brown pigment. Due to the fact that these diseases may be amelanotic, it may be helpful to confirm this disease process with S-100, HMB-45, Melan A or MITF (microphthalmia-associated transcription factor)—all which preferentially react with melanoma cells.

Jeff F. Wang, Deba P. Sarma, Pamela Ulmer: Diagnostic dilemma: HMB-45 and Melan-A negative tumor, can it be still a melanoma?: MITF (Microphthalmia-associated transcription factor) stain may confirm the diagnosis. The Internet Journal of Dermatology. 2007. Volume 5 Number 1.

3. **B herpesvirus**

Herpesvirus infections may be seen in immunocompromised hosts, including patients affected with concomitant HIV infections, patients receiving therapy for malignant disease, or those with other chronic debilitating disorders. Cytologic identification is based on the findings of multinucleated cells containing ground-glass nuclei, karyolytic chromatin, nuclear molding, and eosinophilic Cowdry Type A inclusions. Possible contamination from the oral cavity must be considered in the absence of clinically apparent infections.

DeMay RM, The Art & Science of Cytopathology.
Viruses, p. 54, and Specific infections (viral pneumonia), p. 223.

4. **B poorly differentiated squamous cell carcinoma**

Cells from poorly differentiated squamous lesions present as single cells and monolayer tissue fragments. Anisocytosis, dense basophilic, hard or waxy cytoplasm often with characteristic cytoplasmic ringing and coarse, irregular chromatin and macronucleoli may be present.

DeMay RM, The Art & Science of Cytopathology.
Nonkeratinizing "poorly differentiated" squamous cell carcinoma, p. 926.

5. **D microbacteria**

Tobacco smoke, radiation, radon gas, occupational exposure to certain metals such as nickel and chromate, asbestos, and environmental factors represent some of the etiologic agents associated with bronchogenic carcinoma.

DeMay RM, The Art & Science of Cytopathology.
Lung cancer, p. 958.

6. **A large cell carcinoma**

These highly malignant lesions tend to arise within the large bronchi, have idiopathic histogenesis, and are cytologically distinguished as cells arranged in syncytial groupings and in single cell fashion. The absence of true gland formation or the presence of keratinization (including cytoplasmic ringing) make this lesion a diagnosis by exclusion only. The nuclei are hyperchromatic, possessing coarsely granular, irregularly distributed chromatin, multiple irregular macronucleoli, with marked anisonucleosis. The cytoplasm tends to be basophilic and homogeneous. A variant of this lesion is the so-called giant-cell type, diagnosed primarily based on the macrocytosis.

DeMay RM, The Art & Science of Cytopathology.
Large cell carcinoma, pp. 930–931.

7. **B *Aspergillus fumigatus***

The cytologic presentation of thick-walled hyphae with dichotomous acute angled branching is characteristic of *Aspergillus* sp.

DeMay RM, The Art & Science of Cytopathology.
Fungi, p. 56, and Specific infections (miscellaneous infections), p. 223.

8. **C *Blastomyces dermatitidis***

Blastomyces dermatitidis is a yeast-like organism that cytologically presents as single organisms with thick-walled refractile cytoplasm. The organism reproduces by single broad-based budding, which characteristically differentiates it from *Cryptococcus neoformans*.

DeMay RM, The Art & Science of Cytopathology.
Fungi, p. 56, and Specific infections (miscellaneous infections), p. 223.

9. **D carcinoid tumor**

Carcinoid tumors are slow-growing neuroendocrine tumors that have association with small cell carcinoma etiology. The polyploid tumors cytologically present as small cells with high N/C ratios, hypochromatic, finely granular, evenly distributed chromatin patterns, with typical oat cell groupings of cords, nests, ribbons, and vertebral column formations. Reactive/reparative cells can be discriminated from these lesions based on the absence of terminal bars and/or cilia with carcinoid tumors. A radiographically detectable lesion and physiological changes are essential elements in diagnosing carcinoid lesions. Immunocytochemical staining with chromogranin will confirm its neuroendocrine origin. Atypical carcinoid, usually associated with the physiological carcinoid syndrome of right-sided fibrosis of the heart, cyanotic flushing of the skin, and liver metastasis, generally have classical neuroendocrine malignant features that may be difficult to distinguish from small cell carcinomas.

DeMay RM, The Art & Science of Cytopathology.
Carcinoids, pp. 233–234.

10. **D invasive carcinoma**

The peak incidence of lung cancer occurs at 60 years of age. Signs and symptoms often appear late in the course of the disease with weight loss, dyspnea, weakness, chest pain, hemoptysis, and coughing being most common.

DeMay RM, The Art & Science of Cytopathology.
Lung cancer, p. 958.

11. **B adenocarcinoma, bronchogenic type**

Bronchogenic adenocarcinomas cytologically present in three-dimensional acinar clusters and single cells and have hypochromatic/bland chromatin, or, if less well-differentiated, hyperchromasia. The presence of central macronucleoli is helpful in establishing this disease process. These true tissue fragments possess frothy cytoplasm, high N/C ratios, and uniform or lobulated nuclei.

DeMay RM, The Art & Science of Cytopathology.
Bronchogenic adenocarcinoma, pp. 928–929.

12. **D adenocarcinoma/colon**

The presence of tall columnar or "cigar-shaped" cells in aggregates with frankly malignant nuclear features, granular cytoplasm, or the presence of malignant signet ring cells may suggest a diagnosis of metastatic adenocarcinoma of the colon. Confirmation by surgical pathology of the primary lesion is critical.

DeMay RM, The Art & Science of Cytopathology.
Metastases, p. 235, and Adenocarcinoma, p. 355.

13. **C adenosquamous carcinoma, immunoperoxidase positive for keratin**

The diagnosis of adenosquamous carcinoma depends on the diligence of the cytologist in identifying both epidermal and glandular constituents.

DeMay RM, The Art & Science of Cytopathology.
Adenosquamous carcinoma, p. 933.

14. **C cytomegalovirus**

Large cells with intranuclear basophilic inclusions surrounded by halos resembling an "owl's eye" are diagnostic of cytomegalovirus.

DeMay RM, The Art & Science of Cytopathology.
Viruses, p. 54, and Specific infections (viral pneumonia), p. 223.

15. **A repeat sputum, *Actinomyces* sp. may represent tonsillar contamination**

Actinomyces sp., branching diphtheroid saprophytic organisms, produce sulfur granules that contain radiating bacillary fragments. Care must be taken to rule out possible contamination from the oral cavity or tonsils.

DeMay RM, The Art & Science of Cytopathology.
Bacteria, p. 55, and Specific infections (Candida, bacterial colonies), p. 223.

16. **D *Cryptococcus neoformans***

The presence of single yeast-like structures with mucinous capsules is diagnostic of *Cryptococcus neoformans.* These organisms reproduce by tear-drop budding. Special staining with mucicarmine will help elucidate the distinctive mucoid capsule.

DeMay RM, The Art & Science of Cytopathology.
Fungi, p. 56, and Specific infections (miscellaneous infections), p. 223.

17. **D Hodgkin disease**

The presence of a reactive polymorphic inflammatory background composed of eosinophils, neutrophils, plasma cells, and small round lymphocytes, in the presence of large cells with pale cyanophilic cytoplasm, mononuclear and binucleated "mirror image" irregularly lobulated nuclei, coarse irregular chromatin, and macronucleoli, is diagnostic of Reed-Sternberg cells and Hodgkin disease.

DeMay RM, The Art & Science of Cytopathology.
Malignant lymphoma, p. 234, and Hodgkin disease, pp.816–821.

18. A ***Coccidioides immitis***

Coccidioides immitis is associated with mild respiratory tract infections. The organisms are cytologically identified as spherical structures containing multiple endospores and revealing a pomegranate appearance.

DeMay RM, The Art & Science of Cytopathology.
Fungi, p. 56, and Specific infections (miscellaneous infections), p. 223.

19. C lobular adenocarcinoma/breast

Metastatic lobular carcinoma of the breast typically presents as single bland cells in vertebral column formations, often containing intracytoplasmic or intranuclear inclusions. Immunopositivity with E-cadherin (a cell-cohesion protein encoded by a gene on chromosome 16q22.1) may help discriminate between lobular and ductal carcinoma of the breast. Lobular carcinomas lack expression while ductal carcinomas typically express cytoplasmic E-cadherin.

DeMay RM, The Art & Science of Cytopathology.
Metastases, p. 235, and Lobular carcinoma, pp. 882–883.

Yeh I and Mies C. Application of Immunohistochemistry to Breast Lesions Archives of Pathology and Laboratory Medicine: (2007); Vol. 132, No. 3, pp. 349–358.

20. C ***Histoplasma capsulatum***

Histoplasma capsulatum is a reticuloendothelial organism cytologically presenting as small, thick refractile spherules with endospores that invariably must be identified as intracytoplasmic inclusions within histiocytes. Confirmation with GMS is imperative.

DeMay RM, The Art & Science of Cytopathology.
Fungi, p. 56, Specific infections (miscellaneous infections), p. 223.

21. A squamous cell carcinoma/esophagus

In the absence of a primary lung neoplasm, a diagnosis of metastatic squamous carcinoma should be considered, such as those originating in the oral cavity or esophagus.

DeMay RM, The Art & Science of Cytopathology.
Metastases, p. 235, and Squamous cell carcinoma, pp. 338–339.

22. B adenocarcinoma, terminal bronchioloalveolar

Bronchioloalveolar adenocarcinomas present cytologically in large tissue fragments, flower or petal-like acinar clusters with great depth of focus and mucinous or nonmucinous cytoplasm. The cells are typically uniform in size and shape and contain round-to-oval nuclei. These malignant cells are often accompanied by alveolar macrophages or rare psammoma bodies.

DeMay RM, The Art & Science of Cytopathology.
Bronchioloalveolar carcinoma, pp. 929–930.

23. B ***Nocardia asteroides***

The diagnosis of *Nocardia asteroides* may be confirmed by identifying the presence of delicate thin, transparent mycelium with beaded hyphae and lacking granule formation. Nocardia is a gram-positive organism that may also demonstrate acid-fast positivity should coccal forms be identified.

DeMay RM, The Art & Science of Cytopathology.
Bacteria, p. 55, Specific infections (miscellaneous infections), p. 223.

24. C well-differentiated squamous cell carcinoma, keratinizing

Pleomorphic cells with caudate or spindle formations with refractile cytoplasm, anisonucleosis, and opaque India ink nuclei are representative of squamous cell carcinoma. A necrotic background is helpful in establishing this lesion.

DeMay RM, The Art & Science of Cytopathology.
Keratinizing "well differentiated" squamous cell carcinoma, pp. 925–226.

25. D siderophages

The presence of hemosiderin-laden (iron positive) macrophages or siderophages is associated with blood within the alveolar septum. These cells may be secondary to hemorrhage, heart failure, necrosis, or pulmonary hemosiderosis.

DeMay RM, The Art & Science of Cytopathology.
Alveolar macrophages (siderophages), p. 216.

26. C refractile golden pigment

Iron stains will help confirm the presence of hemosiderin-laden macrophages; however, the diagnosis can only be suggested in light of the clinical findings.

DeMay RM, The Art & Science of Cytopathology.
Pneumoconiosis and miscellaneous disease (hemosiderosis), p. 224.

27. B atypical squamous metaplasia

Parakeratosis, as in the Pap smear, may be related to inflammation or precancerous lesions. These cells generally arise from the oral cavity or tracheobronchial tree. Care should be exercised to differentiate these small cells from a more serious process such as squamous cell carcinoma, a lesion with abundant numbers of large pleomorphic cells.

DeMay RM, The Art & Science of Cytopathology.
Parakeratosis, atypical parakeratosis, p. 220.

28. **D** GMS staining for confirmation of *Pneumocystis carinii*

Pneumocystis carinii, once considered an opportunistic protozoan but now thought to be a fungus, often infects patients with acquired immunodeficiency syndrome. Immunocompromised patients and premature infants are considered suitable hosts for infection. Cytological identification is based on the presence of foamy-to-frothy casts/mats of eosinophilic material with interspersed "contact lens"–shaped refractile structures containing intranuclear trophozoites (Pap stain). GMS will stain the cell wall of the cyst black with central black dots. In Wright-Giemsa or other Romanovsky-based stains, the alveolar casts of *P. carinii* stain as basophilic masses with the trophozoites appearing as eosinophilic specks within the mass.

DeMay RM, The Art & Science of Cytopathology.
Fungi, p. 57, and Specific infections (miscellaneous infections), p. 223.

29. **D** bronchial metaplastic cells

The replacement of normal bronchial epithelium with a squamous protective epithelium in the lung is consistent with squamous metaplasia. This process may occur in response to a reparative/reactive process secondary to toxic agents such as cigarette smoke, bronchiectasis, tuberculosis, and pneumonia. The cytologic identification is based on the finding of monolayer sheets or single cells with cobblestone pavement configuration and well-defined borders, predictable round to oval nuclei, and cyanophilic staining cytoplasm. Differential diagnoses include those of atypical nature.

DeMay RM, The Art & Science of Cytopathology.
Squamous metaplasia, p. 220.

30. **C** normal lymphocytes

Lymphocytes are small, round, single cells without cohesive cytoplasmic features. The presence of lymphogranular bodies distributed throughout the background (best visualized with air-dried preparations, see FNA chapter) may also help in confirming the lymphoid origin of these cells.

DeMay RM, The Art & Science of Cytopathology.
Inflammatory cells, p. 217.

31. **D** atypical squamous metaplasia

Atypical squamous metaplasia or squamous dysplasia is an antecedent for squamous cell carcinoma of the lung. The finding of small cells in sheets and as single cells with slight pleomorphism, hyperchromatic nuclei, moderate N/C ratios, finely granular regularly distributed chromatin staining cyanophilic to orangeophilic is diagnostic of this process.

DeMay RM, The Art & Science of Cytopathology.
Squamous dysplasia, carcinoma in situ, and occult cancers, pp. 227–228.

32. **C** Curschmann spirals

Curschmann spirals are casts of inspissated mucus created by occluded or stenotic bronchi. The association of these structures with hypersensitivity reactions such as asthma as well as other mucus-producing pulmonary disorders is common.

DeMay RM, The Art & Science of Cytopathology.
Curschmann spirals, p. 217.

33. **B** nonkeratinizing stratified squamous

The presence of nonkeratinizing epithelium in respiratory specimens may represent cells from the oral cavity, epiglottis, vocal cords, oropharynx, and the pharynx.

DeMay RM, The Art & Science of Cytopathology.
Introduction and squamous cells, p. 213.

34. **A** lipoid pneumonia

The finding of lipid-laden histiocytes or lipophages may be seen in patients who chronically abuse lipid solvent nose inhalants, in patients who have aspirated food material, or in lipoid pneumonia. Cytologic changes associated with pneumonia are common. These macrophages contain abundant intracytoplasmic clear to granular vacuoles. Confirmation with oil red O or Sudan black is helpful in establishing the presence of lipid due to the fact that the alcoholic Papanicolaou stain dissolves these products.

DeMay RM, The Art & Science of Cytopathology.
Lipophages, p. 216.

35. **D** inflammatory pseudotumor

The finding of eosinophils is more likely to be associated with parasitic infections and hypersensitivity reactions.

DeMay RM, The Art & Science of Cytopathology.
Charcot-Leyden crystals, p. 219.

36. **D** reserve cell hyperplasia

Subcolumnar cells with uniform features, scanty cytoplasm, and dark nuclei, found in sheets, as single cells, or attached to mature bronchial cells, are consistent with reserve cell hyperplasia (RCH). RCH may be related to an assortment of bronchial disorders including pneumonia, fungal infections, viral infections, or tuberculosis. Caution must be exercised to differentiate these benign entities from small cell carcinoma.

DeMay RM, The Art & Science of Cytopathology.
Reserve cell hyperplasia, p. 219.

37. C ciliocytophthoria

Viral infections such as adenovirus, measles, and parainfluenza, often with less specific cytomorphologic criteria, may have associated ciliocytophthoria (CCP). The cytology shows degenerative nuclear changes (karyorrhexis) and pinched off ciliated tufts with eosinophilic nonspecific intracytoplasmic inclusions. Other causes of CCP include nonspecific injury, air pollution, and hot or dry air.

DeMay RM, The Art & Science of Cytopathology.
Ciliocytophthoria, p. 215.

38. C plant cells

Cells with double cell walls, squared-off cytoplasm containing smudgy nuclei, and intracytoplasmic granules are diagnostic of vegetable contaminant. Care should be taken not to diagnose these as metaplasia or squamous carcinoma.

DeMay RM, The Art & Science of Cytopathology.
Contaminants (plant cells/food), p. 219.

39. A asthma

Bronchial hyperplasia is often found in patients with asthma. The presence of papillary three-dimensional clusters of cells with well-defined cytoplasmic interior borders, along with the presence of terminal bars and/or cilia, is diagnostic of "creola" bodies. These groupings may easily be differentiated from well-differentiated bronchogenic adenocarcinoma due to the presence of cilia and/or terminal bars. Curschmann spirals are casts of inspissated mucus created by occluded or stenotic bronchi. The association of these structures with hypersensitivity reactions such as asthma as well as other mucus-producing pulmonary disorders is common. Small crystalline structures with sharp, pointed ends represent Charcot-Leyden crystals, often associated with asthma. These structures, in addition to creola bodies, Curschmann spirals, and eosinophils, are nonspecific findings of this hypersensitivity reaction.

DeMay RM, The Art & Science of Cytopathology.
Asthma, p. 224.

40. B lipid pneumonia

Aspiration pneumonia (milk) can be confirmed with oil red O staining by the presence of lipid-laden macrophages.

DeMay RM, The Art & Science of Cytopathology.
Lipophages, p. 216.

41. A ferruginous bodies

Ferruginous bodies are hemosiderin-coated fibers and may be detected in the respiratory samples of patients who have inhaled any one of a variety of mineral fibers, most notably asbestos. They may be identified by the presence of rod- or dumbbell-shaped golden brown structures with an iron protein matrix. Their association with mesothelioma has been established, and a role in the carcinogenesis of the lung has been suggested.

DeMay RM, The Art & Science of Cytopathology.
Ferruginous (asbestos) bodies, p. 218.

42. A reactive bronchial epithelial cells

Multinucleated bronchial cells are associated with a variety of pulmonary conditions, including viral pneumonitis, previous bronchoscopy, bronchiectasis, or fume inhalation. Their presence indicates a reactive process. Cells with typical reactive criteria reveal enlarged hypochromatic nuclei with finely granular, evenly distributed chromatin, prominent nucleoli, and well-preserved cytoplasmic borders (often with terminal bars and/or cilia).

DeMay RM, The Art & Science of Cytopathology.
Benign, reactive atypia, p. 214.

43. B creola bodies

Bronchial hyperplasia is often found in patients with asthma. The presence of papillary three-dimensional clusters of cells with well-defined cytoplasmic interior borders, along with the presence of terminal bars and/or cilia, is diagnostic of these "creola" bodies. These groupings may easily be differentiated from well-differentiated bronchogenic adenocarcinoma due to the presence of cilia and/or terminal bars.

DeMay RM, The Art & Science of Cytopathology.
Bronchial hyperplasia and creola bodies, p. 220.

44. A carbon histiocyte

The presence of abundant carbon-laden histiocytes is commonly associated with anthracosis, a pneumoconiosis (dust disease) related to carbon inhalation.

DeMay RM, The Art & Science of Cytopathology.
Pneumoconiosis and miscellaneous diseases, p. 224.

45. **D** psammoma bodies

Psammoma bodies (calcospherites) are composed of calcifying concentric rings of phosphate, iron, and magnesium. These eosinophilic structures may be associated with bronchioloalveolar adenocarcinomas, metastatic papillary carcinoma, tuberculosis, and less common conditions such as pulmonary Lithia sis.

DeMay RM, The Art & Science of Cytopathology.
Calcospherites and psammoma bodies, p. 218.

46. **C** atypical squamous metaplasia

Atypical squamous metaplasia or squamous dysplasia is an antecedent for squamous cell carcinoma of the lung. The finding of small cells in sheets and as single cells with slight pleomorphism, hyperchromatic nuclei, moderate N/C ratios, finely granular, regularly distributed chromatin, and cytoplasm staining cyanophilic to orangeophilic is diagnostic of this process.

DeMay RM, The Art & Science of Cytopathology.
Squamous dysplasia, carcinoma in situ, and occult cancers, pp. 227–228.

47. **B** corpora amylacea

Corpora amylacea are condensed glycoproteins associated with heart failure, pulmonary infarction, or bronchitis. The cytologic finding of these round masses may be differentiated from psammoma bodies by their lack of calcification; however, they are birefringent.

DeMay RM, The Art & Science of Cytopathology.
Corpora amylacea, p. 218.

48. **B** oat cell carcinoma

Small cell carcinoma is a highly malignant neuroendocrine neoplasm that is ultrastructurally part of amine precursor uptake and decarboxylation (APUD) tumors. These cells contain hyperchromatic stippled chromatin, coarse clumping, nuclear molding, scanty cytoplasm, and micronucleoli. They characteristically have vertebral column formation, microbiopsy aggregates, cords, nests, or ribbons. The oat cell type, which may represent a degenerated form of the tumor, typically is found in streams of mucin when evaluating the cells using the pick-and-smear or crush technique. The Saccomanno technique may not preserve the molding patterns. The intermediate cell small cell carcinoma represents both fusiform and polygonal variants, which are typically better preserved cells with open coarse chromatin patterns and enlarged cell areas. Immunocytochemical staining with chromogranin is helpful in establishing the neurosecretory nature of this tumor.

DeMay RM, The Art & Science of Cytopathology.
Small cell carcinoma, oat cell type, p. 231.

49. **B** squamous cell carcinoma

Cells from poorly differentiated squamous lesions present as single cells and monolayer tissue fragments. Anisocytosis, dense basophilic, hard or waxy cytoplasm often with characteristic cytoplasmic ringing and coarse, irregular chromatin and macronucleoli may be present.

DeMay RM, The Art & Science of Cytopathology.
Nonkeratinizing "poorly differentiated" squamous cell carcinoma, pp. 226–227.

50. **D** *Aspergillus* sp.

The cytologic presentation of thick-walled hyphae with dichotomous acute angled branching is characteristic of *Aspergillus* sp.

DeMay RM, The Art & Science of Cytopathology.
Fungi, p. 56.

51. **B** asthma

Bronchial hyperplasia is often found in patients with asthma. The presence of papillary three-dimensional clusters of cells with well-defined cytoplasmic interior borders, along with the presence of terminal bars and/or cilia, is diagnostic of "creola" bodies. These groupings may easily be differentiated from well-differentiated bronchogenic adenocarcinoma due to the presence of cilia and/or terminal bars.

DeMay RM, The Art & Science of Cytopathology.
Bronchial hyperplasia and creola bodies, p. 220.

52. **B** neuroendocrine tumor

Small cell carcinoma is a highly malignant neuroendocrine neoplasm that is ultrastructurally part of the amine precursor uptake and decarboxylation (APUD) tumors. These cells contain hyperchromatic stippled chromatin, coarse clumping, nuclear molding, scanty cytoplasm, and micronucleoli. They characteristically have vertebral column formation and microbiopsy aggregates, and are grouped as cords, nests, or ribbons. The oat cell type, which may represent a degenerated form of the tumor, typically is found in streams of mucin when evaluating the cells using the pick-and-smear or crush technique. The Saccomanno technique may not preserve the molding patterns as often. The intermediate cell small cell carcinoma represents both fusiform and polygonal variants, which are typically better preserved with open coarse chromatin patterns and enlarged cell areas. Immunocytochemical staining with chromogranin is helpful in establishing the neurosecretory nature of this tumor.

DeMay RM, The Art & Science of Cytopathology.
Small cell carcinoma, pp. 231–233.

53. **C** pharynx

Small regular elliptical eosinophilic or orangeophilic single cells with degenerated nuclei and parakeratotic features may represent non-pulmonary cells such as those from the pharynx or upper respiratory tract ("Pap cells").

DeMay RM, The Art & Science of Cytopathology.
Pap cells, p. 220.

54. **C** small cell carcinoma

These cells contain hyperchromatic stippled chromatin, coarse clumping, nuclear molding, scanty cytoplasm, and micronucleoli. They characteristically have vertebral column formation, microbiopsy aggregates, cords, nests, or ribbons. The oat cell type, which may represent a degenerated form of the tumor, typically is found in streams of mucin when evaluating the cells using the pick-and-smear or crush technique. The Saccomanno technique may not preserve the molding patterns as often. The intermediate cell small cell carcinoma represents both fusiform and polygonal variants, which are typically better preserved with open coarse chromatin patterns and enlarged cell areas. Immunocytochemical staining with chromogranin is helpful in establishing the neurosecretory nature of this tumor.

DeMay RM, The Art & Science of Cytopathology.
Small cell carcinoma, intermediate type, p. 232.

55. **C** acid-fast bacilli, *Mycobacterium avium-intracellulare*

Mycobacterium avium-intracellulare may be seen within macrophages using Kinyoun or Ziehl-Neelsen stain, where it appears as rod-shaped bacilli.

DeMay RM, The Art & Science of Cytopathology.
Bacteria, p. 55.

56. **C** *Alternaria* sp.

Alternaria sp. are cytologically identified as dark brown conidia in chains often resembling "snow shoes."

DeMay RM, The Art & Science of Cytopathology.
Fungi, p. 56.

57. **D** non-Hodgkin lymphoma

Large cell cleaved lymphomas typically present with a predominant population (80%) of large cleaved lymphomas with coarse irregular chromatin and prominent nucleoli. A smaller population of small round or cleaved lymphocytes completes the cytologic picture.

DeMay RM, The Art & Science of Cytopathology.
Malignant lymphoma, pp. 234–235.

58. **C** epithelioid histiocytes

Elongated, round, or oval cells presenting singly or in syncytial aggregates with oval/reniform nuclei containing finely granular, evenly distributed chromatin and micronucleoli are diagnostic of epithelioid histiocytes. These cells are part of the spectrum of granulomatous inflammation. Other cells associated with granulomatous inflammation include multinucleated histiocytes, fibroblasts, and assorted white blood cells.

DeMay RM, The Art & Science of Cytopathology.
Granulomatous inflammation, pp. 222–223.

59. **C** arise from type II pneumocytes

Bronchioloalveolar adenocarcinomas present cytologically in large tissue fragments, flower or petal-like acinar clusters with great depth of focus, and mucinous or non-mucinous cytoplasm. The cells are typically uniform in size and shape and contain round-to-oval nuclei. These malignant cells are often accompanied by alveolar macrophages or rare psammoma bodies.

DeMay RM, The Art & Science of Cytopathology.
Bronchioloalveolar carcinoma, pp. 229–230.

60. **A** *Blastomyces dermatitidis*

Blastomyces dermatitidis is a yeast-like organism that cytologically presents as single organisms with thick-walled refractile cytoplasm. The organism reproduces by single broad-based budding, which characteristically differentiates it from *Cryptococcus neoformans.*

DeMay RM, The Art & Science of Cytopathology.
Fungi, p. 56.

61. **B** carcinoid tumor; chromogranin (+)

Carcinoid tumors are slow-growing neuroendocrine tumors that have association with small cell carcinoma etiology. The polyploid tumors cytologically present as small cells with high N/C ratios and hypochromatic, finely granular, evenly distributed chromatin patterns, with typical oat cell grouping of cords, nests, ribbons, and vertebral column formations. Reactive/reparative cells can be discriminated from these lesions based on the absence of terminal bars and/or cilia with carcinoid tumors. A radiographically detectable lesion and physiological changes are essential elements in diagnosing carcinoid lesions. Immunocytochemical staining with chromogranin will confirm neuroendocrine origin. Atypical carcinoid, usually associated with the physiological carcinoid syndrome of right-sided fibrosis of the heart, cyanotic flushing of the skin, and liver metastasis, generally has classical neuroendocrine malignant features that may be difficult to distinguish from small cell carcinomas.

DeMay RM, The Art & Science of Cytopathology.
Carcinoids, pp. 233–234.

62. **C** **common leukocytic antigen**

The image represents a hypercellular population of polymorphic cells diagnostic of normal/reactive lymphocytes. Lymphocytes present as small, round, single cells without cohesive cytoplasmic features. The presence of lymphogranular bodies distributed throughout the background (best visualized with air-dried preparations, see FNA chapter) may also help in confirming the lymphoid origin of these cells.

DeMay RM, The Art & Science of Cytopathology.
Inflammatory cells (lymphocytes), p. 217.

63. **B** **glycoproteins (and do not calcify)**

Corpora amylacea are condensed glycoproteins associated with heart failure, pulmonary infarction, or bronchitis. The cytologic finding of these round masses may be differentiated from psammoma bodies by their lack of calcification; however, they are birefringent.

DeMay RM, The Art & Science of Cytopathology.
Corpora amylacea, p. 218.

64. **A** **cytomegalovirus**

Large cells with intranuclear basophilic inclusions surrounded by halos resembling an "owl's eye" are diagnostic of cytomegalovirus.

DeMay RM, The Art & Science of Cytopathology.
Viruses, p.54.

65. **A** ***Candida* sp.**

The presence of thin pseudohyphae with interrupted cell walls ("sticks") or spore formations ("stones") represents *Candida albicans.* Oral cavity contamination must be ruled out.

DeMay RM, The Art & Science of Cytopathology.
Fungi, p. 56.

66. **B** ***Histoplasma capsulatum***

Histoplasma capsulatum is a reticuloendothelial organism cytologically presenting as small, thick refractile spherules with endospores that invariably must be identified as intracytoplasmic inclusions within histiocytes. Confirmation with GMS is imperative.

DeMay RM, The Art & Science of Cytopathology.
Fungi, p. 56.

67. **C** ***Coccidioides immitis***

Coccidioides immitis is associated with mild respiratory tract infections. The organisms are cytologically identified as spherical structures containing multiple endospores and revealing a pomegranate appearance.

DeMay RM, The Art & Science of Cytopathology.
Fungi, p. 56.

68. **C** **reactive bronchial epithelial cells**

Reactive/reparative bronchial cells may be secondary to granulomatous disease, pneumonitis, or bronchitis. Cells with typical reactive criteria including enlarged hypochromatic nuclei with finely granular, evenly distributed chromatin, prominent nucleoli, and well-preserved cytoplasmic borders are characteristic of these benign cellular changes.

DeMay RM, The Art & Science of Cytopathology.
Regenerative/reparative bronchial cells, p. 214.

69. **B** ***Actinomyces* sp.**

Actinomyces sp., branching diphtheroid saprophytic organisms, produce sulfur granules that contain radiating bacillary fragments. Care must be taken to rule out possible contamination from the oral cavity or tonsils.

DeMay RM, The Art & Science of Cytopathology.
Bacteria, p. 55.

70. **D** **bronchogenic adenocarcinoma**

Bronchogenic adenocarcinomas cytologically present in three-dimensional acinar clusters and single cells, have hypochromatic/bland chromatin, or, if less well-differentiated, hyperchromasia. The presence of central macronucleoli is helpful in establishing this disease process. These true tissue fragments possess frothy cytoplasm, high N/C ratios, and uniform or lobulated nuclei.

DeMay RM, The Art & Science of Cytopathology.
Bronchogenic adenocarcinoma, pp. 228–229.

71. **D** **reserve cell hyperplasia**

Subcolumnar cells with uniform features, scanty cytoplasm and dark nuclei, found in sheets, as single cells, or attached to mature bronchial cells, are consistent with reserve cell hyperplasia (RCH). RCH may be related to an assortment of bronchial disorders including pneumonia, fungal infections, viral infections, or tuberculosis. Caution must be exercised to differentiate these benign entities from small cell carcinoma.

DeMay RM, The Art & Science of Cytopathology.
Reserve cell hyperplasia, p. 219.

72. **B** reactive/reparative changes

Reactive/reparative bronchial cells may be secondary to granulomatous disease, pneumonitis, or bronchitis. Cells with typical reactive criteria including enlarged hypochromatic nuclei with finely granular, evenly distributed chromatin, prominent nucleoli, and well preserved cytoplasmic borders are characteristic of these benign cellular changes.

DeMay RM, The Art & Science of Cytopathology.
Regenerative/reparative bronchial cells, p. 214.

73. **C** multinucleated bronchial cells

Multinucleated bronchial cells are associated with a variety of pulmonary conditions, including viral pneumonitis, previous bronchoscopy, bronchiectasis, or fume inhalation. Their presence indicates a reactive process.

DeMay RM, The Art & Science of Cytopathology.
Multinucleation, p. 214.

74. **C** siderophages

The presence of hemosiderin-laden (iron positive) macrophages or siderophages is associated with blood within the alveolar septum. These cells may be secondary to hemorrhage, heart failure, necrosis, or pulmonary hemosiderosis.

DeMay RM, The Art & Science of Cytopathology.
Alveolar macrophages (siderophages), p. 216.

75. **B** normal metaplastic cells

The replacement of normal bronchial epithelium with a squamous protective epithelium in the lung is consistent with squamous metaplasia. This process may occur in response to a reparative/reactive process secondary to toxic agents such as cigarette smoke, bronchiectasis, tuberculosis, and pneumonia. The cytologic identification is based on the finding of monolayer sheets or single cells with cobblestone pavement configuration and well-defined borders, predictable round to oval nuclei, and cyanophilic-staining cytoplasm. Differential diagnoses include those of atypical nature.

DeMay RM, The Art & Science of Cytopathology.
Squamous metaplasia, p. 220.

76. **A** mucicarmine

The presence of single yeast-like structures with mucinous capsules is diagnostic of *Cryptococcus neoformans*. These organisms reproduce by tear-drop budding. Special staining with mucicarmine will help elucidate the distinctive mucoid capsule.

DeMay RM, The Art & Science of Cytopathology.
Specific infections (miscellaneous infections), p. 223.

77. D asthma

Small crystalline structures with sharp, pointed ends represent Charcot-Leyden crystals, often associated with asthma. These structures, in addition to creola bodies, Curschmann spirals, and eosinophils, are nonspecific findings of this hypersensitivity reaction.

DeMay RM, The Art & Science of Cytopathology.
Charcot-Leyden crystals, p. 218.

78. **B** bone marrow

The pulmonary macrophage is a bone marrow-derived cell that has an eccentrically located round, oval or reniform-shaped nucleus with or without nucleoli.

DeMay RM, The Art & Science of Cytopathology.
Alveolar macrophages, pp. 215–216.

79. **D** *Pneumocystis carinii*

Pneumocystis carinii, once considered an opportunistic protozoan but now thought to be a fungus, often infects patients with acquired immunodeficiency syndrome. Immunocompromised patients and premature infants are considered suitable hosts for infection. Cytological identification is based on the presence of foamy-to-frothy casts/mats of eosinophilic material with interspersed "contact lens"-shaped refractile structures containing intranuclear trophozoites (Pap stain). GMS will stain the cell wall of the cyst black with central black dots. In Wright-Giemsa or other Romanovsky-based stains, the alveolar casts of *P. carinii* stain as basophilic masses with the trophozoites appearing as eosinophilic specks within the mass.

DeMay RM, The Art & Science of Cytopathology.
Fungi, p. 57, and Specific infections (miscellaneous infections), p. 223.

80. **D** nose inhalant abuse

The finding of lipid-laden histiocytes or lipophages may be seen in patients who chronically abuse lipid solvent nose inhalants, in patients who have aspirated food material, or in lipoid pneumonia. These macrophages contain abundant intracytoplasmic clear to granular vacuoles. Confirmation with oil red O or Sudan black is helpful in establishing the presence of lipid due to the fact that the alcoholic Papanicolaou stain dissolves these products.

DeMay RM, The Art & Science of Cytopathology.
Lipophages, p. 216.

81. **B** hypersensitivity reaction

Curschmann spirals are casts of inspissated mucus created by occluded or stenotic bronchi. The association of these structures with hypersensitivity reactions such as asthma as well as other mucus-producing pulmonary disorders is common.

DeMay RM, The Art & Science of Cytopathology.
Curschmann spirals, p. 217.

82. B carbon histiocytes

The pulmonary macrophage is a bone marrow-derived cell that has an eccentrically located round, oval or reniform-shaped nucleus with or without nucleoli. Pulmonary macrophages with engulfed intracytoplasmic carbonaceous inclusions are referred to as "dust cells." The presence of dust cells is essential in establishing the adequacy of a satisfactory deep sputum specimen.

DeMay RM, The Art & Science of Cytopathology.
Alveolar macrophages (carbon histiocytes), p. 215.

Adequacy of Sputum Sample

83. **C** herpesvirus

Herpesvirus infections may be seen in immunocompromised hosts, including patients affected with concomitant HIV infections, patients receiving therapy for malignant disease, or those with other chronic debilitating disorders. Cytologic identification is based on the findings of cells containing ground-glass nuclei, karyolytic chromatin, nuclear molding, and eosinophilic Cowdry Type A inclusions. Possible contamination from the oral cavity must be considered in the absence of clinically apparent pulmonary infections.

DeMay RM, The Art & Science of Cytopathology.
Viruses, p. 54, and Specific infections (viral pneumonia), p. 223.

84. **A** viral infection

Viral infections such as adenovirus, measles, and parainfluenza, often with less specific cytomorphologic criteria, may have associated ciliocytophthoria (CCP). The cytology shows degenerative nuclear changes (karyorrhexis) and pinched off ciliated tufts with eosinophilic nonspecific intracytoplasmic inclusions. Other causes of CCP include nonspecific injury, air pollution, and hot or dry air.

DeMay RM, The Art & Science of Cytopathology.
Ciliocytophthoria, p. 215.

85. **A** starch granulomatosis

The structures with characteristic Maltese cross formations are associated with starch contamination. Their presence may be associated with a granulomatous response.

DeMay RM, The Art & Science of Cytopathology.
Contaminants (talc/starch), p. 219.

86. **D** striated muscle (meat) contamination, repeat sputum

The finding of striated muscle within sputum cytology most often represents meat contamination associated with masticated food.

DeMay RM, The Art & Science of Cytopathology.
Contaminants (plant cells/food), p. 219.

87. **B** mesothelioma

Ferruginous bodies are hemosiderin-coated fibers that may be detected in the respiratory samples of patients who have inhaled any one of a variety of mineral fibers, most notably asbestos. These structures are identified by the presence of a rod- or dumbbell-shaped golden brown structure with an iron protein matrix. Their association with mesothelioma has been established, and a role in the carcinogenesis of the lung has been suggested.

DeMay RM, The Art & Science of Cytopathology.
Ferruginous (asbestos) bodies, p. 218

88. **C** normal bronchial epithelial cells

The presence of columnar to prismatic-shaped cells with centrally to basally located nuclei and finely granular, regularly distributed chromatin, often containing micronucleoli, is diagnostic of normal bronchial mucosa. Terminal bars and/or cilia also help confirm the normality of these cells.

DeMay RM, The Art & Science of Cytopathology.
Glandular cells, pp. 213–214.

89. **B** vegetable cells

Cells with double cell walls, squared-off cytoplasm containing smudgy nuclei, and intracytoplasmic granules are diagnostic of vegetable contaminant. Caution should be given not to overdiagnose these cells as true indigenous processes such as metaplasia or squamous carcinoma.

DeMay RM, The Art & Science of Cytopathology.
Contaminants (plant cells/food), p. 219.

90. **C** pollen contamination

Small symmetrical structures with centrally located pores and spiky surfaces are indicative of pollen contamination. These structures should be differentiated from fungal infections such as *Blastomyces dermatitidis* or *Cryptococcus neoformans*.

DeMay RM, The Art & Science of Cytopathology.
Arthropods and contaminants, p. 58, and Contaminants (pollen), p. 219.

91. **C reactive bronchial cells**

Reactive/reparative bronchial cells may be secondary to granulomatous disease, pneumonitis, or bronchitis. Cells, arranged singly or in clusters, with typical reactive criteria including enlarged hypochromatic nuclei with finely granular, evenly distributed chromatin, prominent nucleoli, and well-preserved cytoplasmic borders are characteristic of these benign cellular changes. Cells secondary to pulmonary infarct may exhibit "atypical features," but on close examination terminal bars or cilia are often found.

DeMay RM, The Art & Science of Cytopathology.
Regenerative/reparative bronchial cells, p. 214.

92. **C** ***Pneumocystis carinii***

Pneumocystis carinii, once considered an opportunistic protozoan but now thought to be a fungus, often infects patients with acquired immunodeficiency syndrome. Immunocompromised patients and premature infants are considered suitable hosts for infection. Cytological identification is based on the presence of foamy-to-frothy casts/mats of eosinophilic material with interspersed "contact lens"-shaped refractile structures containing intranuclear trophozoites (Pap stain). GMS will stain the cell wall of the cyst black with central black dots. In Wright-Giemsa or other Romanovsky-based stains, the alveolar casts of *P. carinii* stain as basophilic masses with the trophozoites appearing as eosinophilic specks within the mass.

DeMay RM, The Art & Science of Cytopathology.
Fungi, p. 57 and Specific infections (miscellaneous infections), p. 223.

Chapter 4

Body Fluids

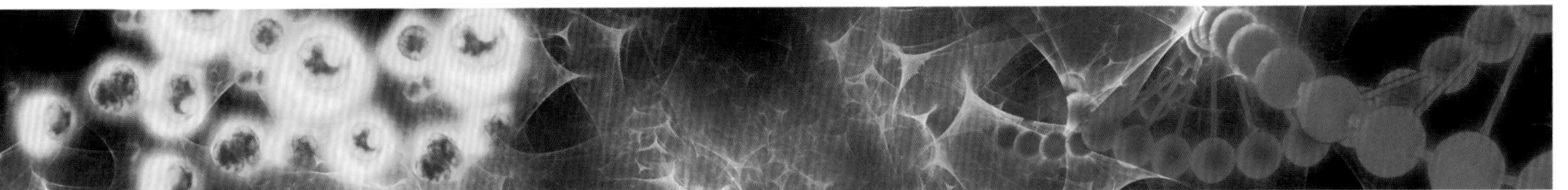

1. **In gouty arthritis, which type of crystal may be visualized under polarized microscopy?**

   A. calcium phosphate
   B. monosodium urate
   C. triple phosphate
   D. calcium carbonate

2. **A synovial disease often found in elderly women that manifests cytologically as multiple fragments of chondrocytes, osteoclasts, lymphocytes, and reactive synovial lining cells is:**

   A. rheumatoid arthritis
   B. septic arthritis
   C. osteoarthritis
   D. osteocalcinosis

3. **The most common metastatic tumor diagnosed by cerebrospinal fluid cytology is:**

   A. lung
   B. liver
   C. stomach
   D. colon

4. **Which of the following tumors has the greatest predisposition for brain metastasis?**

   A. choriocarcinoma
   B. clear cell carcinoma
   C. cholangiocarcinoma
   D. adenoid cystic carcinoma

5. **Polymorphonuclear neutrophils, trapezoidal histiocytes, cholesterol crystals, cells with intracytoplasmic inclusions, and a dense eosinophilic granular background in synovial fluid are diagnostic of:**

   A. osteoarthritis
   B. rheumatoid arthritis
   C. Reiter syndrome
   D. gout

6. **The presence of siderophages (hemosiderin-laden macrophages) in CSF could be related to:**

   A. post-oil myelogram
   B. subdural hematoma
   C. tuberculosis
   D. bacterial meningitis

7. **A tumor often involving the long bones and found in children in their second decade cytologically presents in synovial fluid as small, mononuclear cells scattered among blood vessels and fibrous stroma. The diagnosis is:**

   A. villonodular synovitis
   B. giant cell tumor
   C. Ewing sarcoma
   D. gout

8. **A synonym for pseudogout is:**

   A. osteochondritis
   B. acidosis
   C. sodium biuratosis
   D. chondrocalcinosis

9. **A plasma cell infiltrate seen in a CSF specimen may be related to:**

A. acute bacterial meningitis
B. epileptic seizure
C. hemorrhage
D. multiple sclerosis

10. **The cytologic/histologic pattern of cells from an intraventricular mass in the choroid plexus reveals which architecture pattern?**

A. papillary
B. acinar
C. sheets
D. signet ring

11. **A pea-sized lesion composed of anaplastic cells located posterior to the third ventricle over the brain stem is diagnostic of:**

A. medulloblastoma
B. retinoblastoma
C. meningioma
D. pineoblastoma

12. **In cerebrospinal fluid, round-to-cuboidal neuronal elements with vacuolated and pigmented cytoplasm exhibiting small, eccentric, vesicular nuclei are identified as:**

A. ependymal cells
B. nucleus pulposus cells
C. chondrocytes
D. leptomeningeal cells

13. **A CSF specimen shows numerous blood cells, neutrophils, lymphocytes, and a few single cells exhibiting giant cell features and multinucleation. These cells are diagnostic of:**

A. peripheral blood contamination
B. chronic lymphocytic leukemia
C. metastatic sarcoma
D. metastatic giant cell carcinoma

14. **A 41-year-old woman presents with a meningeal tumor contained within the cerebral hemispheres. Cytology shows cells in a whorl-like formation and cigar-shaped cells with delicate chromatin, micronucleoli, and intranuclear inclusions. The diagnosis is:**

A. meningioma
B. schwannoma
C. pituitary adenoma
D. Rathke pouch cyst

15. **What infectious agent in cerebrospinal fluid stains positively with mucicarmine?**

A. *Blastomyces dermatitidis*
B. *Cryptococcus neoformans*
C. *Candida albicans*
D. cytomegalovirus

16. **Which tumor is neural crest in origin?**

A. oligodendroglioma
B. astrocytoma
C. meningioma
D. medulloblastoma

17. **A circumscribed tumor found in adolescents, which may arise in the fourth ventricle of the posterior fossa, comprises elongated cells and rosettes with round, eccentric nuclei and micronucleoli. These cells are diagnostic of:**

A. medulloblastoma
B. neuroblastoma
C. astrocytoma
D. ependymoma

18. **A cerebellar neoplasm identified in a 5-year-old boy sheds cells into the CSF. Lumbar puncture reveals small spindle cells with fibrillar, fine, and lacy cytoplasm. The nuclei have a bland appearance. These cells are representative of:**

A. ependymoma
B. medulloblastoma
C. astrocytoma
D. glioblastoma multiforme

19. **A patient receiving intrathecal therapy for acute lymphocytic leukemia has a lumbar puncture two weeks after treatment. Cytology reveals a heterogeneous population of lymphocytes, many of which have nucleoli. The diagnosis is:**

A. reactive pleocytosis
B. recurrent leukemia
C. atypical changes suggestive of recurrent leukemia
D. peripheral blood contamination

20. **Lipid-laden histiocytes found in a CSF specimen may be related to:**

A. post-oil myelogram
B. melanoma
C. neurosyphilis
D. viral meningitis

21. **A disease of young adults that may involve the knee is cytologically diagnosed as a highly cellular anaplastic tumor. Histologically, slit-like spaces are found within the tissue. The cellular findings suggest:**

A. Ewing sarcoma
B. villonodular synovitis
C. giant cell tumor of tendon sheath
D. synovial sarcoma

22. **A primary tumor of the cerebellum, usually found in children, that sheds small cells with hyperchromatic nuclei forming pseudorosettes is characteristic of:**

A. medulloblastoma
B. oligodendroglioma
C. glioblastoma multiforme
D. pituitary adenoma

23. **A benign tumor of neural sheath arising predominantly in adults is termed:**

A. meningioma
B. schwannoma
C. pituitary adenoma
D. craniopharyngioma

24. **A periorbital mass infiltrating the optic tract and shedding cells into CSF is:**

A. medulloblastoma
B. retinoblastoma
C. neuroblastoma
D. pinealoma

25. **A 3-year-old girl presents with evaluated catecholamines in the urine and abdominal enlargement. CSF cytology reveals anaplastic cells forming rosettes. Electron microscopy reveals secretory granules. The diagnosis is:**

A. nephroblastoma
B. medulloblastoma
C. neuroblastoma
D. schwannoma

26. **A 68-year-old man presents with diplopia. CSF analysis reveals a population of pleomorphic cells with large, eccentrically located, hyperchromatic nuclei with irregular chromatin and dense, hard, refractile cytoplasm. A previous pleural fluid was malignant. The most likely diagnosis/primary site of this malignancy is:**

A. metastatic carcinoma, lung
B. metastatic carcinoma, pancreas
C. metastatic carcinoma, colon
D. metastatic carcinoma, prostate

27. **An elderly woman with a previously diagnosed extra-CNS malignancy currently presents with hemiparesis and disorientation. A lumbar puncture is performed. The CSF reveals cells in three-dimensional groupings and loose clusters with fine chromatin, macronucleoli, and granular cytoplasm. Which of the following most likely represents the primary site?**

A. muscle
B. skin
C. breast
D. liver

28. **A joint-related disease that is related to chlamydial infection is referred to as:**

A. rheumatoid arthritis
B. Reiter syndrome
C. gout
D. chondrocalcinosis

29. **Which of the following may present as neutrophilia in a cerebrospinal fluid specimen?**

A. viral encephalitis
B. acute bacterial meningitis
C. neurosyphilis
D. metastatic carcinoma

30. **A small group of cohesive cells with macronucleoli is seen in synovial fluid from an elderly man. Elevated acid phosphatase is noted. The diagnosis/origin is :**

A. squamous carcinoma/lung (parathormone +)
B. adenocarcinoma/kidney (lipid +)
C. adenocarcinoma/prostate (PSA +)
D. osteogenic sarcoma/bone (vimentin –)

31. **A 32-year-old man presents with frequent headaches and a recent onset of seizures. Nuclear magnetic resonance reveals a 3-cm mass located in the left cerebral hemisphere. A ventricular tap reveals a pleomorphic sample with stellate bipolar cells exhibiting hyperchromatic nuclei, anisocytosis, and multinucleated giant cells scattered in a granular background. Many single cells as well as aggregates are seen. Based on the cytologic findings, the diagnosis is:**

A. astrocytoma
B. glioblastoma multiforme
C. oligodendroglioma
D. ependymoma

32. **What special stain might prove useful in distinguishing oligodendrogliomas from other primary brain tumors?**

A. PAS
B. oil red O
C. mucicarmine
D. Giemsa

33. **A benign congenital nest intracranial cystic tumor shedding keratin pearls and anucleate squames into the CSF is diagnostic of:**

A. meningioma
B. craniopharyngioma
C. pinealoma
D. ependymoma

34. **A 22-year-old HIV-positive patient with meningoencephalitis and myocarditis submits for a lumbar puncture because of a spiking fever. Cytology reveals mononuclear pleocytosis. Giemsa staining reveals many crescent-shaped cystic structures within the cytoplasm of histiocytes. The diagnosis is:**

A. *Cryptosporidium*
B. *Toxoplasma gondii*
C. *Entamoeba histolytica*
D. Kaposi sarcoma

35. **A 44-year-old man with a previously diagnosed extra-CNS malignancy presents for CSF analysis. Cytology reveals large cells containing large, eccentrically located hyperchromatic nuclei and double mirror image nuclei with macronucleoli. Intranuclear cytoplasmic invaginations are present in many of the cells. Which of the following is the most likely diagnosis?**

A. adenocarcinoma, bronchogenic
B. adenocarcinoma, stomach
C. malignant melanoma
D. histiocytic lymphoma

36. **A patient with pleurisy secondary to pneumonia presents with a 500-mL pleural effusion. A large population of cells are present in the cytology analysis of a filter preparation. Cells have frothy cytoplasm and eccentrically located vesicular/reniform nuclei. These cells are:**

A. macrophages
B. mesothelial cells
C. associated with Hodgkin disease
D. atypical mesothelial cells

37. **The most commonly identified fungus found in cerebrospinal fluid specimens is:**

A. *Blastomyces dermatitidis*
B. *Cryptococcus neoformans*
C. *Histoplasma capsulatum*
D. *Candida albicans*

38. **The presence of mitotic figures in effusion cytology:**

A. is of little significance
B. most likely represents malignancy
C. suggests an infectious process
D. should recommend a biopsy

39. **In differentiating metastatic adenocarcinoma from malignant mesothelioma in a pleural fluid, which special stains would confirm metastatic adenocarcinoma?**

A. PAS-D (+)
B. PAS-D (–)
C. hyaluronic acid (+)
D. alcian blue-hyaluronidase (–)

40. **Which of these cytologic findings favors a metastatic effusion over a benign condition?**

A. "knobby" cytoplasmic borders
B. community borders
C. prominent nucleoli
D. monolayer sheets

41. **A 69-year-old man with a two-pack-per-day history of cigarette smoking presents with a pleural effusion. A thoracentesis reveals cells in vertebral column formation with molding and coarse irregular chromatin. Which of the following is the most likely diagnosis?**

A. squamous carcinoma, nonkeratinizing
B. sclerosing hemangioma
C. small cell carcinoma
D. bronchioloalveolar adenocarcinoma

42. **Cells presenting with increased nuclear sizes, micronucleoli, round and uniform nuclear contours, and "knobby" cytoplasmic borders in an ascitic fluid specimen are diagnostic of:**

A. lymphocytic lymphoma
B. reactive mesothelial cells
C. small cell carcinoma
D. Hodgkin disease

43. **A young child with a history of embryonal rhabdomyosarcoma presents with a peritoneal effusion. Which stain may confirm a metastatic neoplasm?**

A. PAS
B. melanin
C. lipid
D. amyloid

44. **A 44-year-old woman presents with a butterfly rash on her face and a pleural effusion. Cytology reveals severe acute inflammation. Many cells contain eosinophilic intracytoplasmic inclusions. The diagnosis is:**

A. rheumatoid pleuritis
B. systemic lupus erythematosus
C. tuberculous effusion
D. eosinophilic pleural effusion

45. **The organism most commonly associated with elephantiasis of the genitalia or extremities is:**

A. *Echinococcus granulosus*
B. *Paragonimus westermani*
C. *Mycobacterium tuberculosis*
D. *Nocardia asteroides*

46. **When discriminating adenocarcinoma from mesothelioma, which of the following is true?**

A. mesothelioma is positive for vimentin
B. adenocarcinoma is positive for vimentin
C. mesothelioma is positive for Leu-M1 and secretory component
D. adenocarcinoma is positive for beta human chorionic gonadotropin

47. A pleural effusion from a 51-year-old woman reveals a foreign population of multiple three-dimensional round, cohesive tissue fragments resembling "cannonballs," blastulas, or proliferation spheres with community borders. Multiple Barr bodies are identified. The likely diagnosis/origin of these cells is:

A. poorly differentiated adenocarcinoma/lung
B. adenocarcinoma/breast
C. adenocarcinoma/colon
D. adenocarcinoma/ovary

48. Effusions that are composed predominantly of eosinophils are:

A. most often related to Wegener granulomatosis
B. specific for tuberculosis
C. idiopathic
D. diagnostic of sarcoidosis

49. Which of the following organisms is highly antigenic, often resulting in anaphylaxis when aspirated?

A. *Mycobacterium tuberculosis*
B. *Wuchereria bancrofti*
C. *Echinococcus granulosus*
D. *Nocardia asteroides*

50. Cells staining positive for PAS-D and mucicarmine in an effusion could be diagnostic of:

A. mesothelioma
B. adenocarcinoma
C. lymphoma
D. squamous carcinoma

51. A 65-year-old shipyard worker with a history of asbestos exposure and persistent pleural effusions currently presents with shortness of breath. Sputum and bronchoscopic analyses show no evidence of malignancy. Pleural fluid cytology reveals abundant single cells with nuclear enlargement, multiple macronucleoli, hyperchromasia, and coarse irregular chromatin. The cytoplasm has a dense nature with an ectoplasm/endoplasm two-toned staining. Which special stain would have a negative reaction with these cells?

A. alcian blue
B. alcian blue-hyaluronidase
C. PAS
D. cytokeratin

52. In the evaluation of malignant processes involving the serous cavities, what factor is essential before rendering a diagnosis?

A. identification of a blood cell component
B. patient history
C. special stains for mucin
D. cytochemical staining

53. A malignant teratoid renal tumor found in children is:

A. Grawitz tumor
B. Wilms tumor
C. neuroblastoma
D. embryonal rhabdomyosarcoma

54. One of the most helpful criteria in determining malignancy in effusion cytology is:

A. a single cell population of abnormal cells
B. a discrete population of foreign cells and normal cells
C. identification of nucleoli
D. presence of mitotic figures

55. A pleural fluid reveals many large elongated "snake" cells exhibiting basophilia, well-defined cell borders, finely granular regularly distributed chromatin, and round to oval well-preserved nuclei. Another population of multinucleated cells with cytoplasmic inclusions were found. The background exhibits an eosinophilic granular debris. The cytologic findings suggest:

A. metastatic squamous cell carcinoma
B. synovial sarcoma
C. systemic lupus erythematosus
D. rheumatoid pleuritis

56. A malignant population of cohesive cells staining mucicarmine negative may represent:

A. a poorly differentiated adenocarcinoma, not otherwise specified
B. ductal carcinoma of the breast
C. well-differentiated adenocarcinoma of the lung
D. colonic adenocarcinoma

57. A 41-year-old woman presents with abdominal ascites. Cytologic analysis of the effusion reveals large clusters of transparent, elongated cells with distended vacuoles and community borders staining positive with mucicarmine. The origin of these cells is most likely:

A. liver
B. colon
C. ovary
D. kidney

58. A 62-year-old woman with a history of radiation exposure to the head and neck presents with a 300-mL pleural effusion. Cytologic analysis reveals clusters of malignant cells and many eosinophilic, calcifying structures with concentric rings. What may be the site of origin?

A. thyroid
B. trachea
C. salivary glands
D. esophagus

59. A peritoneal effusion from a 72-year-old man is represented by a heterogeneous population of cells possessing central granular and clear peripheral cytoplasm and large, hyperchromatic nuclei with macronucleoli. Clinical symptoms include hypercalcemia, hypertension, and polycythemia. Prostatic acid phosphatase and mucicarmine stains were negative. Special staining with oil red O was strongly positive. The most likely diagnosis/origin is:

A. adenocarcinoma/colon
B. renal cell carcinoma/kidney
C. hepatocellular carcinoma/liver
D. melanoma/skin

60. An abdominal centesis from a 56-year-old man yields an abundant population of cohesive cells in papillary clusters with tall, columnar morphology, irregular chromatin, and nucleoli. The most likely diagnosis/origin of these cells is:

A. adenocarcinoma/pancreas
B. cholangiocarcinoma/bile duct
C. mesothelioma/parietal peritoneal
D. adenocarcinoma/colon

61. A chylous effusion may be associated with:

A. scleroderma
B. rheumatoid arthritis
C. cirrhosis
D. systemic lupus erythematosus

62. Septic arthritis in a synovial fluid is related to:

A. a generalized body infection
B. an autoimmune disease
C. *Chlamydia*
D. trauma

63. What type of cell found in an ascitic fluid might suggest extramedullary hematopoiesis associated with myeloid metaplasia?

A. plasma cell
B. megakaryocyte
C. immunoblasts
D. reticulocyte

64. Which of the following diagnoses has an associated hyaluronic acid background and does not stain positive with alcian-blue hyaluronidase?

A. adenocarcinoma, pancreas
B. carcinoid tumor, lung
C. hepatocellular carcinoma
D. mesothelioma, carcinomatous

65. A 44-year-old man with a known primary malignancy presents with a 400-mL pleural effusion. The cells are predominantly single in nature with large, eccentrically located nuclei and intranuclear cytoplasmic invaginations. Many cells have multiple nuclei as well as macronucleoli. Which of the following is most likely represented?

A. melanoma
B. poorly differentiated adenocarcinoma
C. squamous cell carcinoma
D. pancreatic adenocarcinoma

66. **A 4-year-old girl presents with an abdominal mass and a peritoneal effusion. Analysis of the serous fluid reveals small, immature cells with high N/C ratios. The cells are found in small aggregates with a central lumen, resembling rosettes. Special stains for chromogranin are positive. The most likely diagnosis/ origin is:**

A. Wilms tumor/kidney
B. Ewing sarcoma/bone
C. embryonal rhabdomyosarcoma/vagina
D. neuroblastoma/adrenals

67. **Which of the following is associated with septic arthritis in a synovial fluid?**

A. decrease in fibrin
B. sarcoid
C. rheumatoid factor
D. tuberculosis

68. Normal mesothelial cells are:

A. positive for neutral mucin
B. positive for DPAS
C. negative for neutral mucin
D. always positive with Leu-M5

69. **Single cells with "windows" and dense endoplasm/ pale ectoplasm features seen in serous fluids are characteristic of:**

A. macrophages
B. mesothelial cells
C. lymphocytes
D. oat cell carcinoma

70. **The diagnosis of traumatic arthritis in a synovial fluid specimen is associated with the cytologic identification of:**

A. immunoblasts
B. lymphocytic effusion
C. hemosiderin-laden macrophages
D. chlamydial inclusions

71. **These cells, identified in a pleural effusion from a 53-year-old man with a history of a gastrointestinal disorder, represent:**

A. metastatic squamous cell carcinoma
B. pleuro-esophageal fistula
C. skin contaminant
D. collagen balls

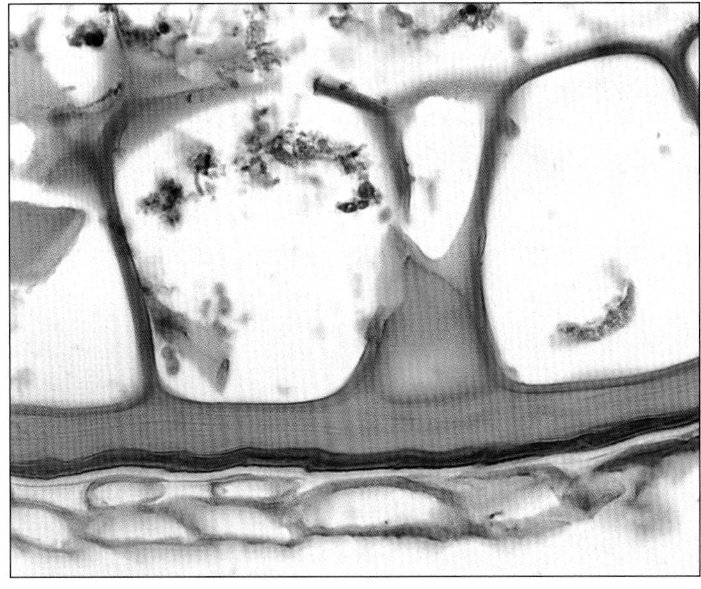

72. **A 44-year-old man, after intrathecal therapy for chronic myelogenous leukemia, presents for follow-up analysis via the ventricular shunt. These cells are diagnostic of:**

A. reactive lymphocytosis
B. recurrent CML
C. viral meningitis
D. acute bacterial meningitis

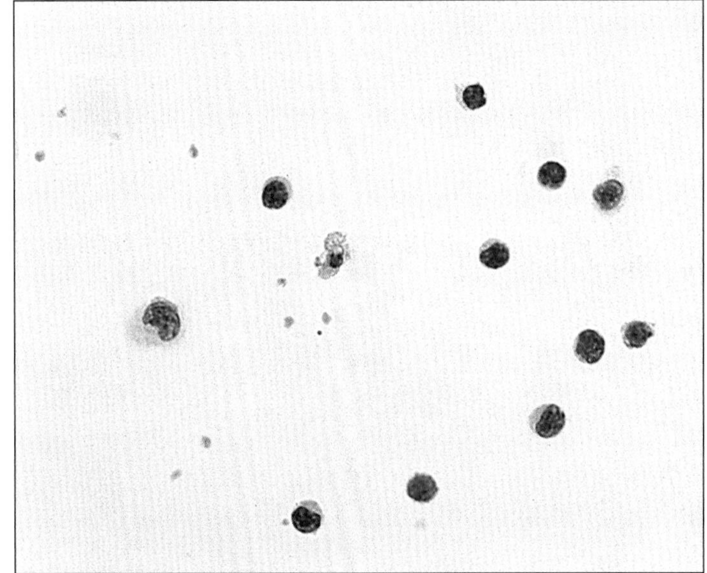

73. **The cellular process as demonstrated in this lumbar puncture specimen (stained with mucicarmine) represents:**

A. starch
B. *Cryptococcus neoformans*
C. *Taenia solium*
D. coxsackievirus infection

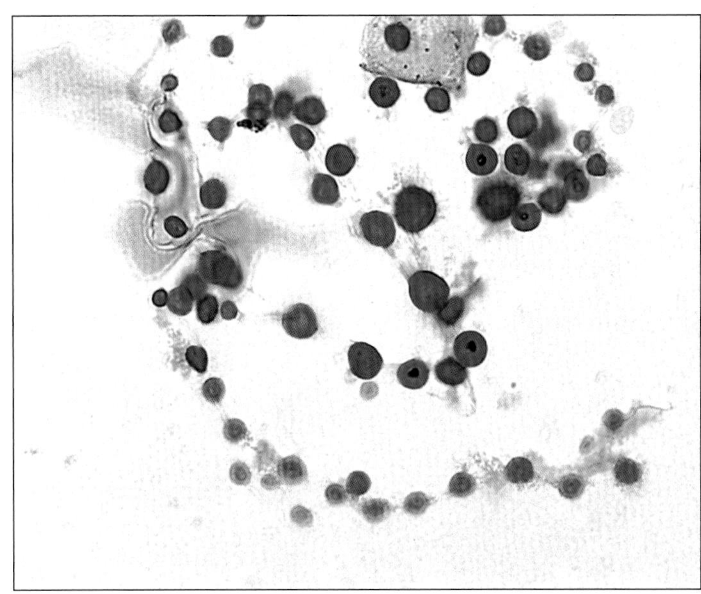

74. These cells are from a 63-year-old alcoholic man with a left-sided pleural effusion. Clinical findings include a low hematocrit value and high amylase levels. 800 mL of a dark brown fluid was obtained for evaluation. Cytology reveals:

A. normal/reactive mesothelial cells
B. normal/reactive hepatocytes
C. mesothelioma
D. pancreatic adenocarcinoma

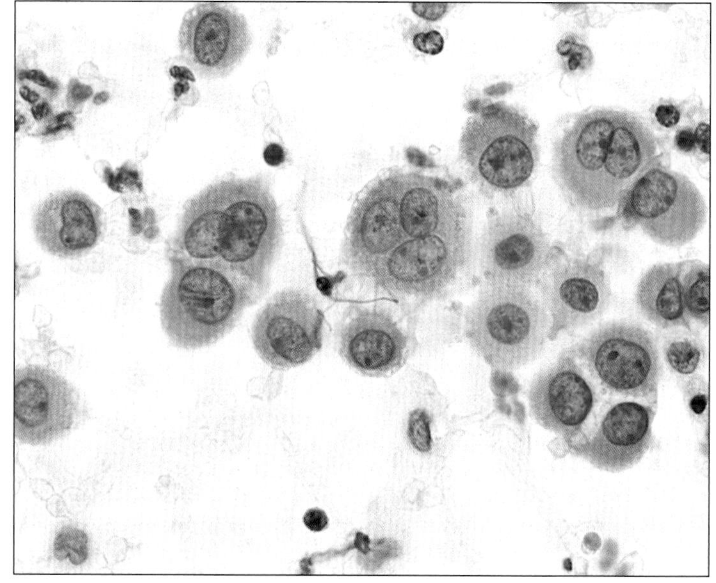

75. These cells are from the CSF specimen of a 5-year-old child previously diagnosed with acute lymphoblastic leukemia and now presenting with a spiking fever and malaise. What special stain would aid in establishing the possibility of recurrence?

A. tumor marker: terminal deoxytransferase
B. S-100
C. alpha-fetoprotein
D. chromogranin

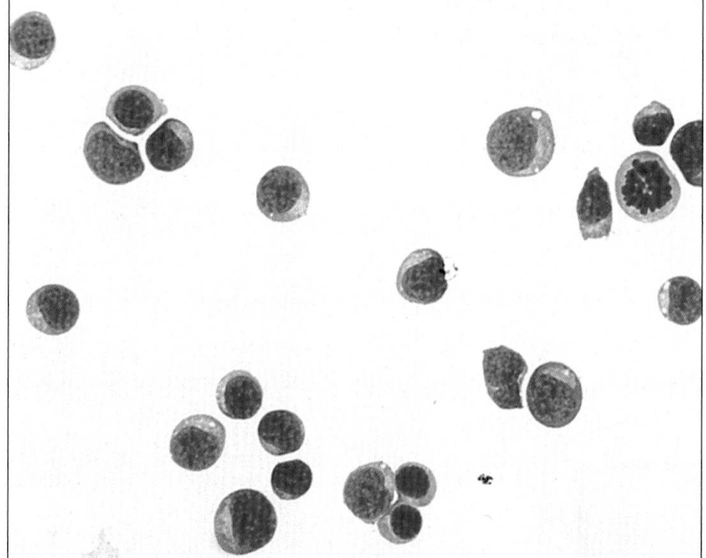

76. A 44-year-old man with recent fainting spells presents with a large cerebral mass. No history of cancer is noted. A ventricular aspiration is performed. Based on the cytological findings, the diagnosis is:

A. astrocytoma, grade I
B. glioblastoma multiforme
C. ependymoma
D. oligodendroglioma

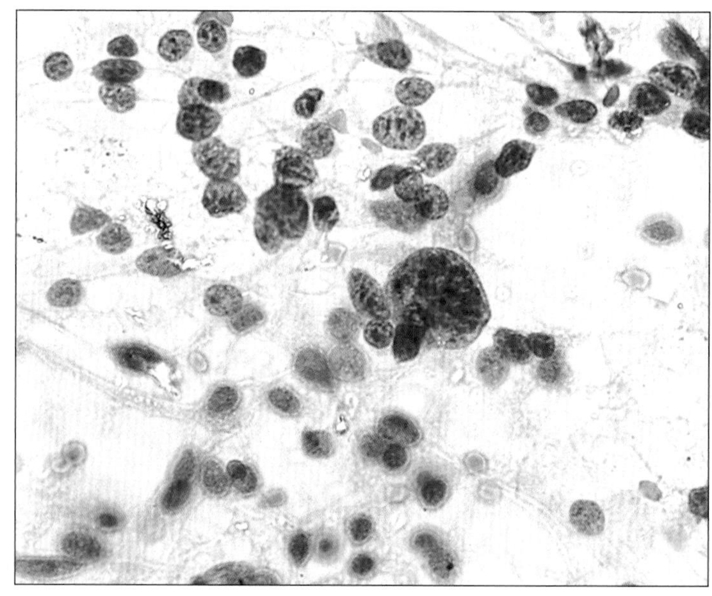

77. **A 44-year-old woman with joint inflammation, multiple tophi deposits, and a history of an inborn uric acid metabolism disorder undergoes synovial fluid analysis. These structures were found with polarized light. Cytology reveals:**

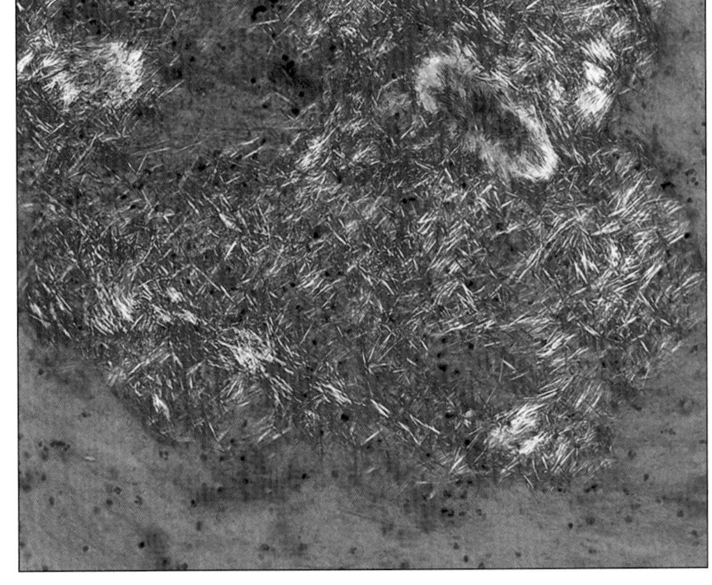

A. chondrocalcinosis/monosodium urate monohydrate
B. gout/monosodium urate monohydrate
C. chondrocalcinosis/bisodium urate monohydrate
D. gout/bisodium urate bihydrate

78. **A lumbar puncture was performed on a 44-year-old AIDS patient. The cytologic pattern represents:**

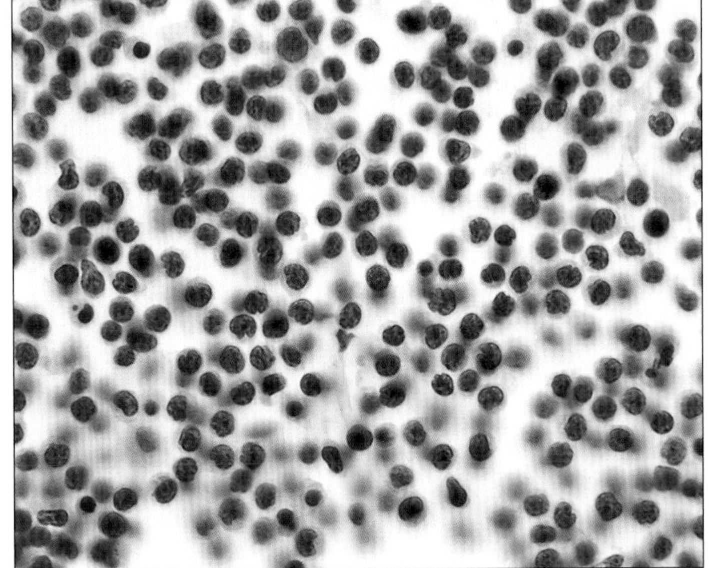

A. bacterial meningitis
B. viral meningitis
C. lymphocytic lymphoma
D. neuroblastoma

79. **A ventricular tap from a 10-year-old child with a history of acute lymphocytic leukemia status post-intrathecal therapy (via ventricular peritoneal shunt catheter) yields a 1-mL specimen for analysis. The findings are consistent with:**

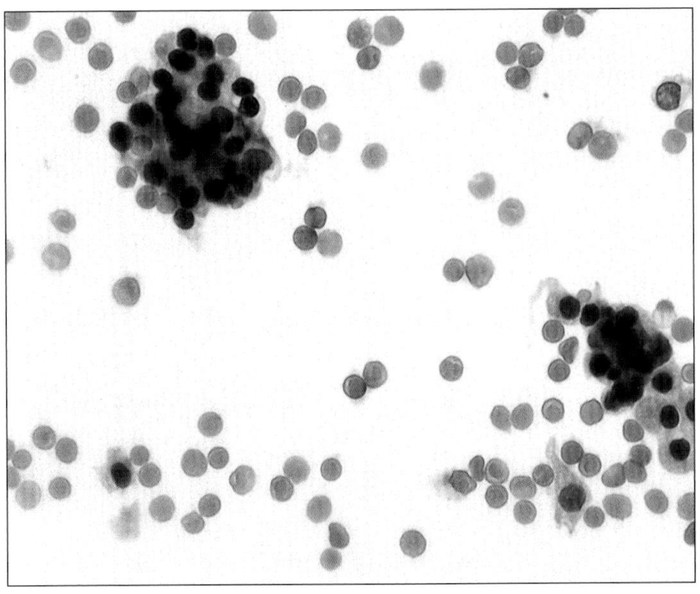

A. recurrent leukemia
B. acute inflammation, secondary to bacterial meningitis
C. neural elements
D. chronic inflammation, secondary to viral meningitis

80. A lumbar puncture is performed on a 44-year-old man with a history of severe headaches. Cytology reveals:

A. normal cellular findings
B. hypocellular sample, suggest repeat
C. viral meningitis
D. leptomeningeal cells

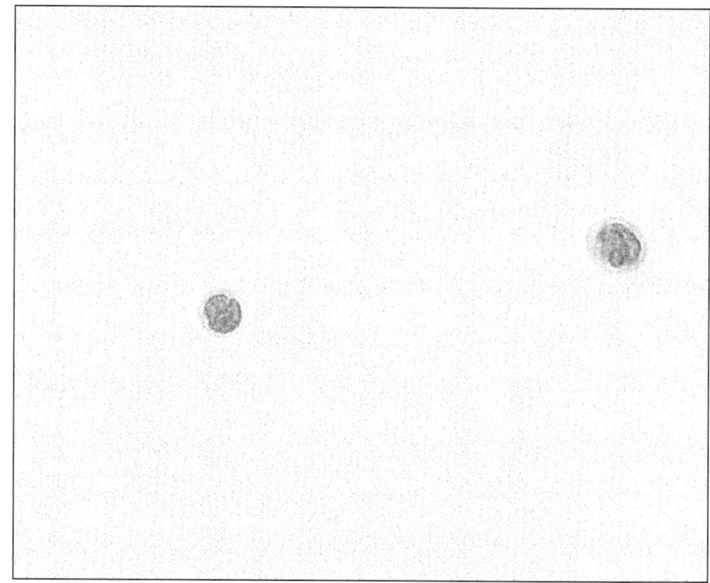

81. An 8-year-old girl presents with a 2-cm midline cerebellar lesion. These cells are found on ventricular tap. They are diagnostic of:

A. neuroblastoma
B. lymphoma
C. astrocytoma
D. medulloblastoma

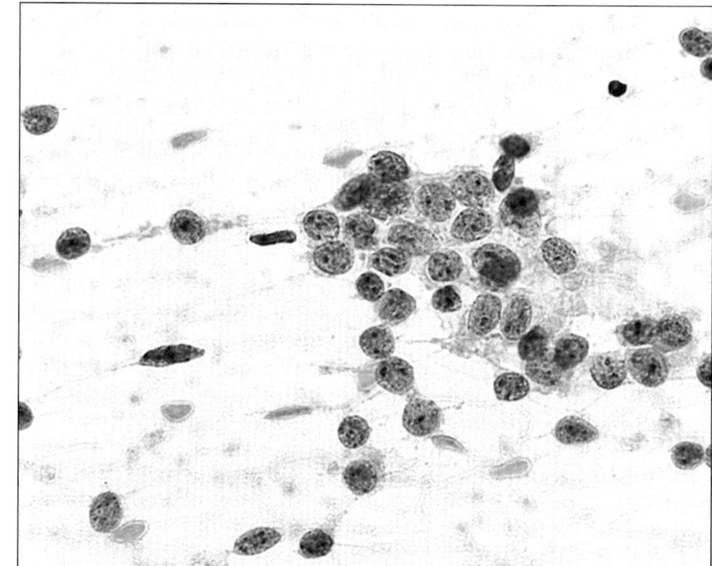

82. These cells were identified in a pleural effusion from a 55-year-old woman with a bilateral 300-mL pulmonary effusion and a history of congestive heart failure. The diagnosis is:

A. mesothelioma
B. metastatic adenocarcinoma, breast
C. metastatic large cell carcinoma, lung
D. reactive mesothelial cells

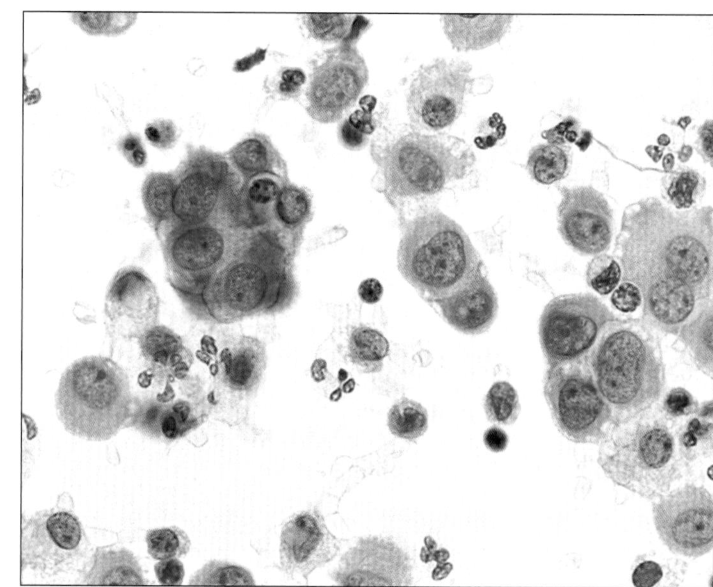

83. A 40-year-old woman with no history of malignancy presents with a midline tumor of the left cerebral hemisphere. These cells are detected in a lumbar puncture specimen. They are consistent with a diagnosis of:

A. meningioma
B. squamous cell carcinoma
C. pinealoma
D. pituitary adenoma

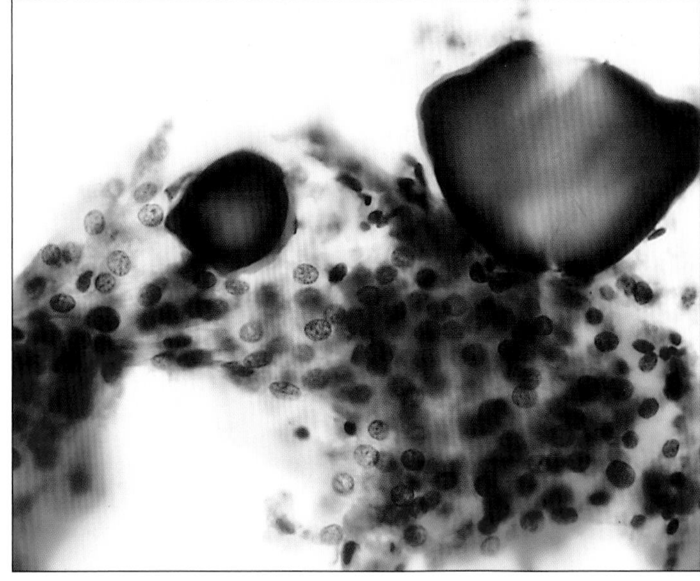

84. A 56-year-old woman with a history of lung carcinoma presents with diplopia and vomiting. A lumbar puncture specimen reveals these cells. A suspicion of metastasis can be confirmed by positive immunocytochemical staining with:

A. high-molecular-weight keratin
B. chromogranin
C. alpha-fetoprotein
D. common leukocyte antigen

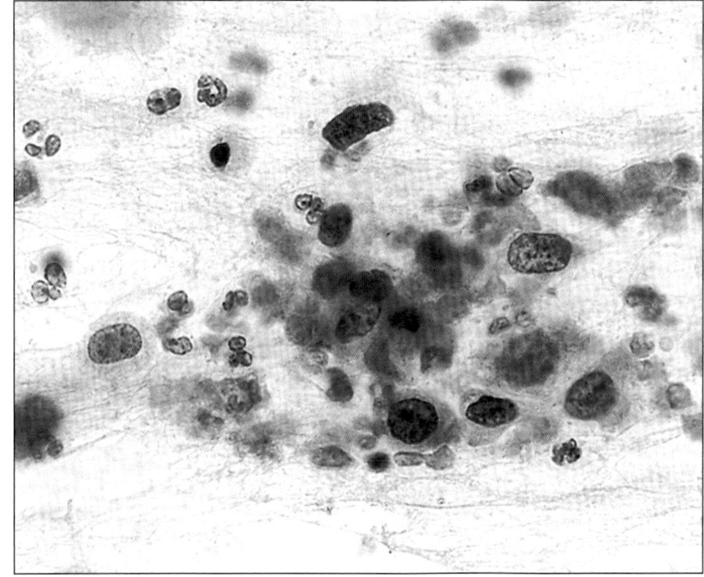

85. The depicted cells represent a pelvic washing specimen from a 48-year-old woman who had undergone surgery for a 3 × 5-cm ovarian mass. The depicted cells represent:

A. liver parenchyma
B. mucinous cystadenocarcinoma of ovary
C. normal mesothelial cells
D. squamous cells, contaminant from the skin

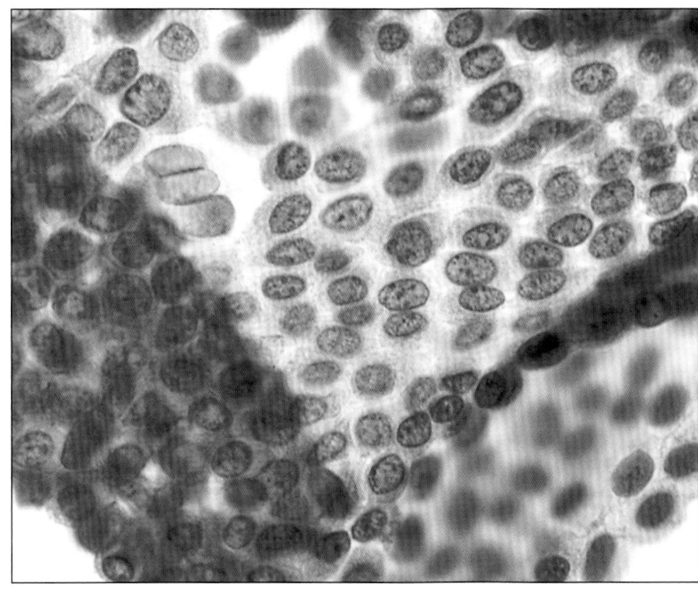

86. A 67-year-old man with a history of cancer presents with meningeal carcinomatosis. Based on the cellular morphology, the most likely primary site is:

A. colon
B. lung
C. pancreas
D. bladder

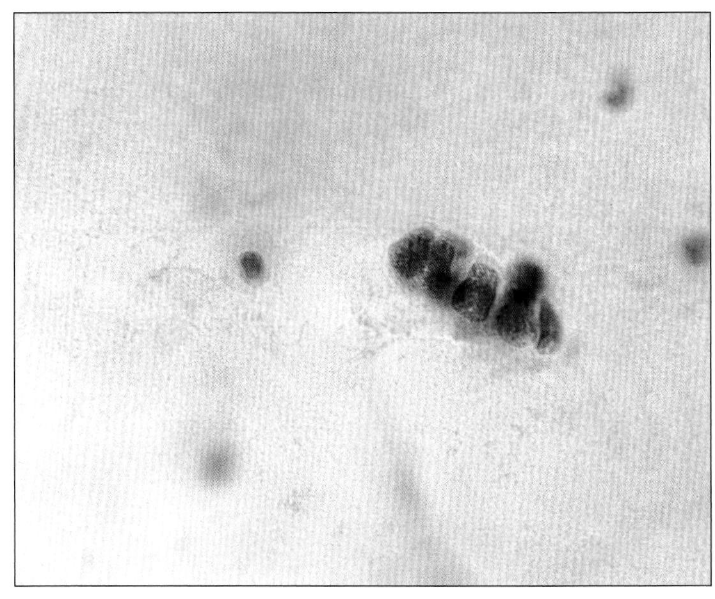

87. These cells, when detected in a pleural effusion, are:

A. idiopathic
B. suggestive of a parasitic effusion
C. suggestive of a hypersensitivity reaction
D. suggestive of asthma

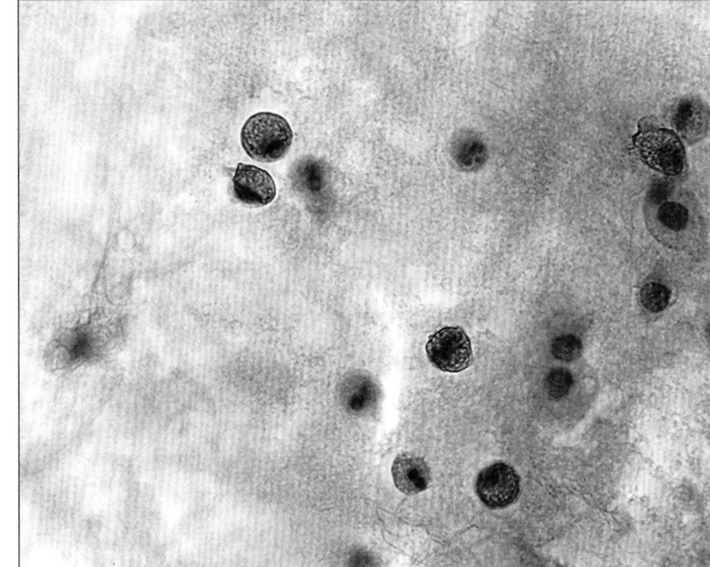

88. A 55-year-old man with a history of tuberculosis presents with dizziness and diplopia. Cytology reveals:

A. viral meningitis
B. acute bacterial meningitis
C. intracranial hemorrhage
D. lymphoma

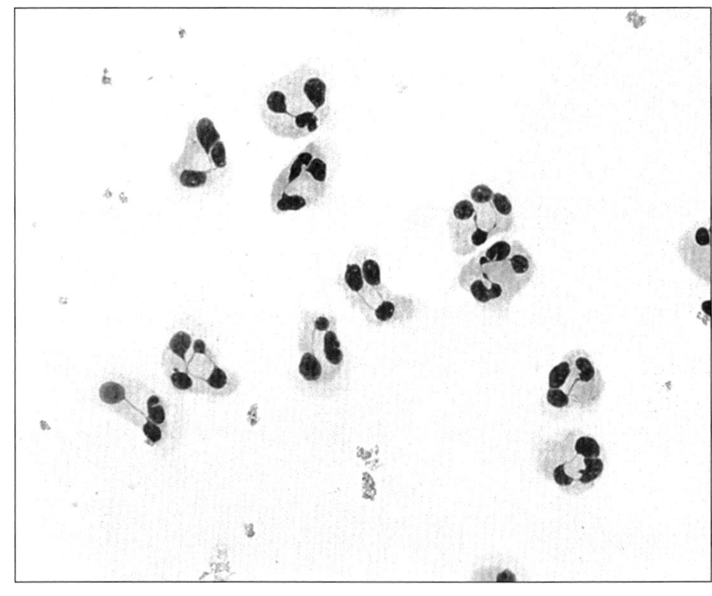

89. A 66-year-old man presents with unilateral chest pain and shortness of breath. 300 mL of bloody pleural fluid underwent cytologic analysis. These cells represent a Papanicolaou-stained smear. The findings are consistent with:

A. large cell carcinoma
B. mesothelioma
C. reactive mesothelial cells
D. poorly differentiated adenocarcinoma

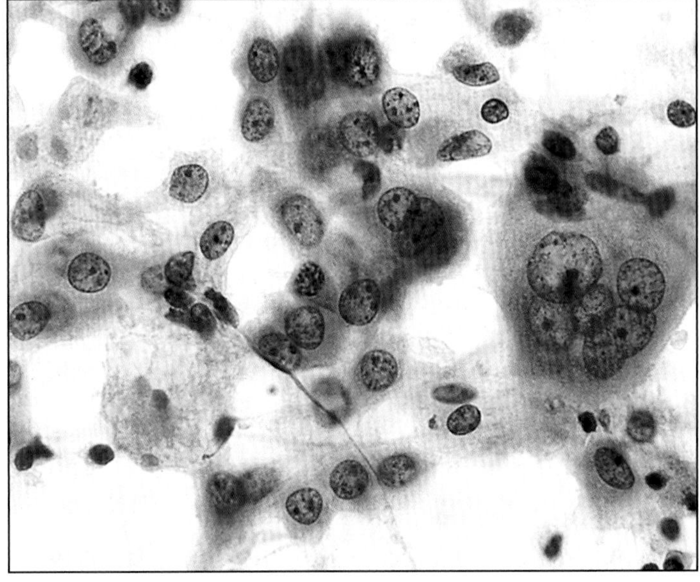

90. This cellular sample is from a 67-year-old man with a pulmonary disorder and a bilateral pleural effusion. Which of the following is supported by the cellular findings?

A. adenosquamous carcinoma
B. adenocarcinoma, bronchogenic type
C. large cell undifferentiated carcinoma
D. carcinosarcoma

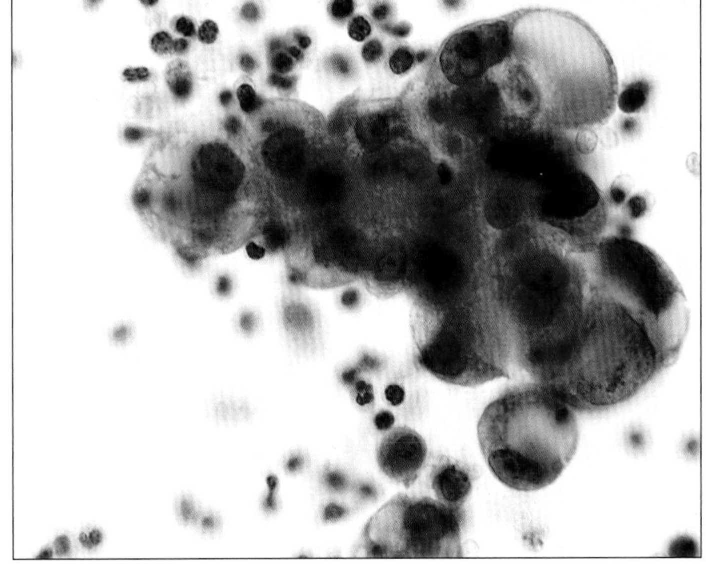

91. The presence of these cells from synovial fluid with PAS-D (+) granules is often diagnostic of a (an):

A. LE cell
B. macrophage
C. metastatic carcinoma, breast
D. Mott cell

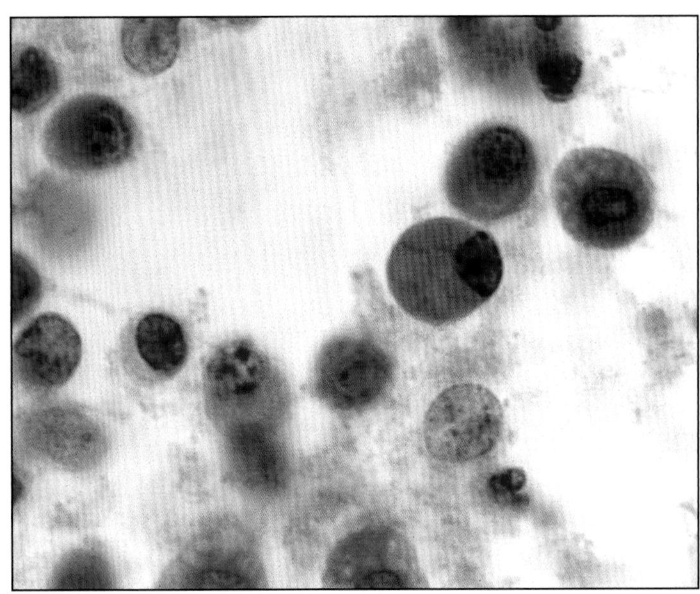

92. What would be the best stain to confirm a diagnosis of this pleural effusion from a 44-year-old man?

A. chromogranin
B. S-100
C. common leukocyte antigen
D. alpha-fetoprotein

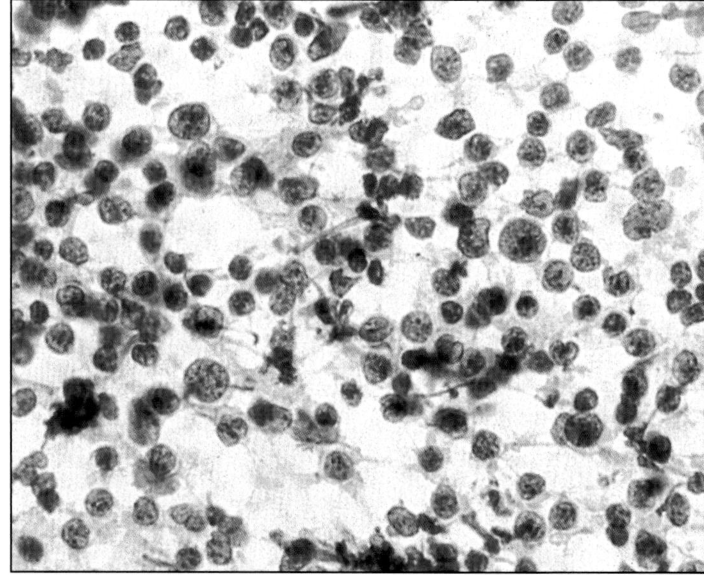

93. A 36-year-old woman with swollen joints, subcutaneous nodules, and pain has 3 mL of synovial fluid submitted for evaluation. The cells suggest:

A. systemic lupus erythematosus
B. Reiter syndrome
C. gouty arthritis
D. rheumatoid arthritis

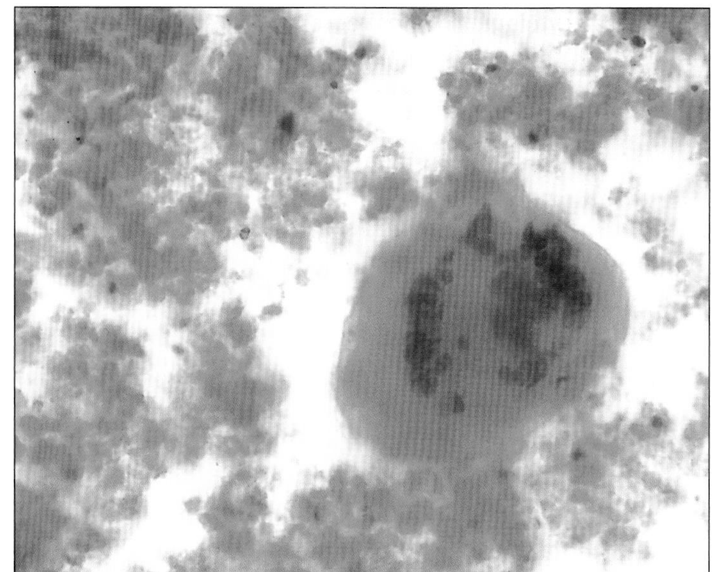

94. These cells were found in a 62-year-old woman with an increasing abdominal girth. Ultrasonography revealed a 3×4-cm mass near the common bile duct. Paracentesis yielded 500 mL of proteinaceous fluid. The cytologic pattern represents:

A. pancreaticobiliary carcinoma
B. epithelioid histiocytes
C. mesothelioma
D. reactive mesothelial cells

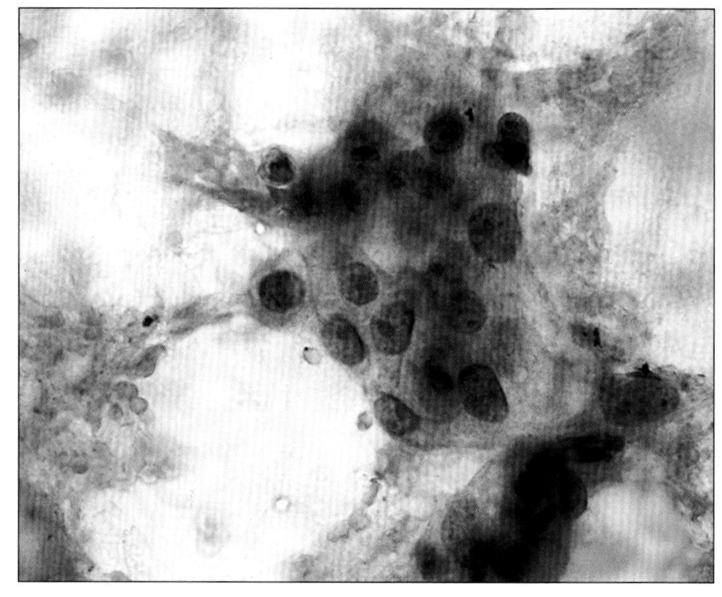

95. **These cells were observed in a pericardial effusion from a 44-year-old woman suffering from an autoimmune disease. A serum specimen was positive for antinuclear antibodies. These findings are diagnostic of:**

A. acute inflammation with "tart cells"
B. a Mallory body
C. systemic lupus erythematosus
D. rheumatoid arthritis

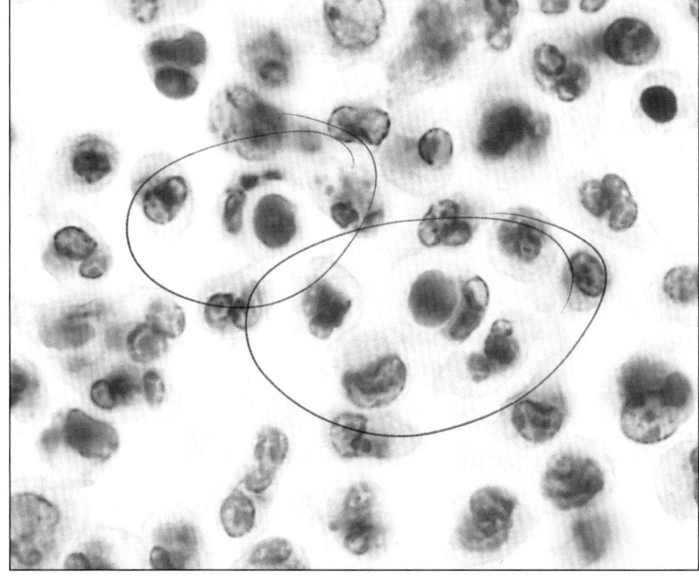

96. **These cytologic findings represent a pleural effusion from a 57-year-old man suffering from a collagen disease. The cellular pattern represents:**

A. systemic lupus erythematosus
B. rheumatoid pleuritis
C. scleroderma
D. tuberculosis

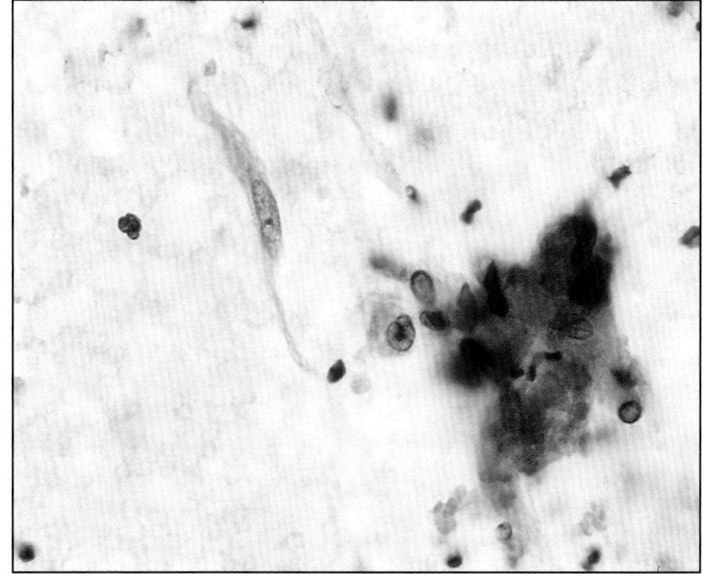

97. **These cells were found in a pericardial effusion from a 60-year-old man. The cytologic pattern shows:**

A. small cell carcinoma
B. large cleaved lymphoma
C. lobular carcinoma, breast
D. reactive lymphoid process

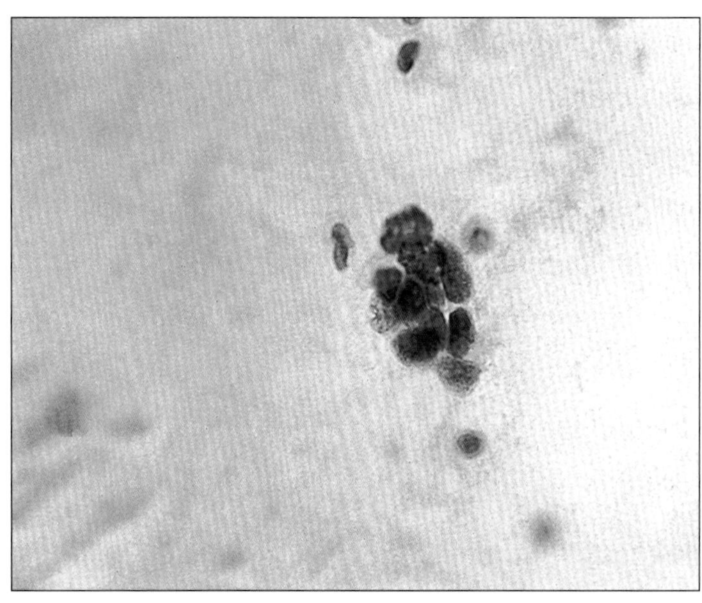

98. These cells, found in an ascitic fluid specimen from a 50-year-old woman, are often associated with:

A. rheumatoid peritonitis
B. mucicarmine (–)
C. an ovarian mass
D. an increase in ACTH

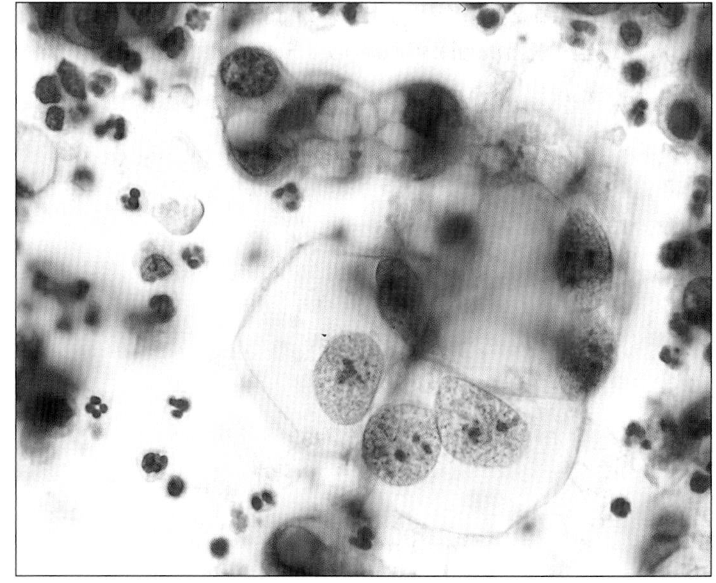

99. Represented is cerebrospinal fluid (CSF) (lumbar puncture) from a 42-year-old man with AIDS. The patient presents to the clinician with weakness, malaise, a spiking fever, and cervical adenopathy. The diagnosis is:

A. metastatic small cell carcinoma (pulmonary origin)
B. small noncleaved lymphoma
C. reactive lymphocytes secondary to viral meningitis
D. bacterial meningitis

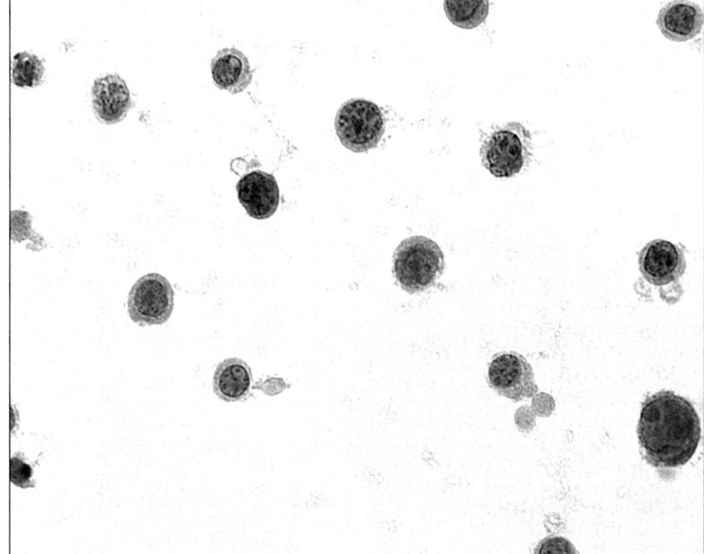

100. These cells were present in a peritoneal effusion from a 2-year-old girl with a retroperitoneal tumor and increased levels of urine catecholamine and vanillylmandelic acid. The cytologic pattern represents:

A. angiomyolipoma
B. retroperitoneal sarcoma
C. neuroblastoma
D. Wilms tumor

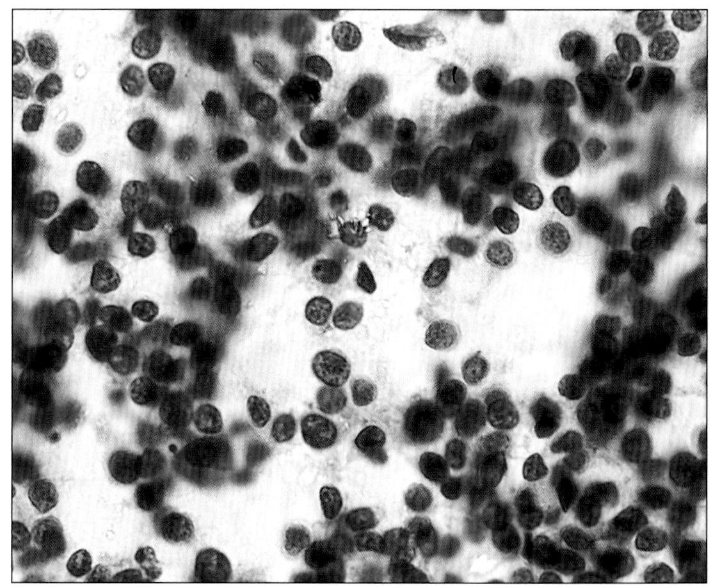

101. What stain would help identify these cells obtained from a peritoneal effusion in a 50-year-old man?

A. chromagranin
B. alpha-fetoprotein
C. neuron-specific enolase
D. S-100

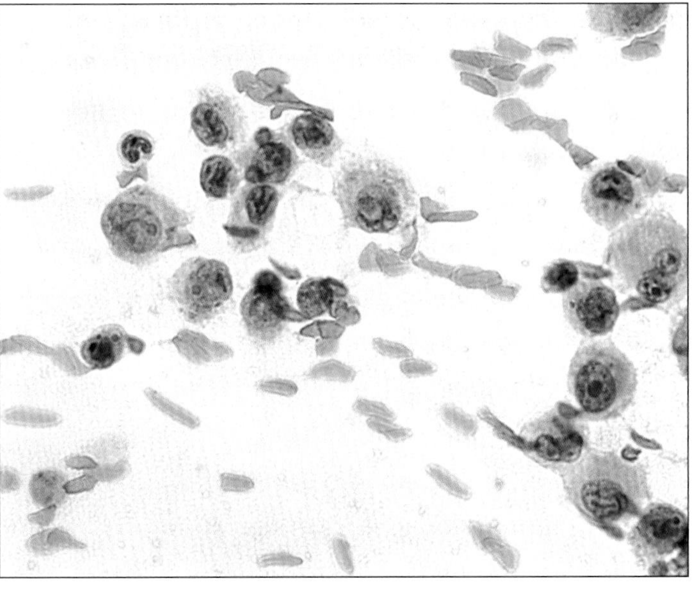

102. These cells were identified in a synovial fluid specimen from a 42-year-old athlete with joint pain. The findings are consistent with:

A. reactive synovial lining cells
B. histiocytes
C. cartilaginous material
D. synovial sarcoma

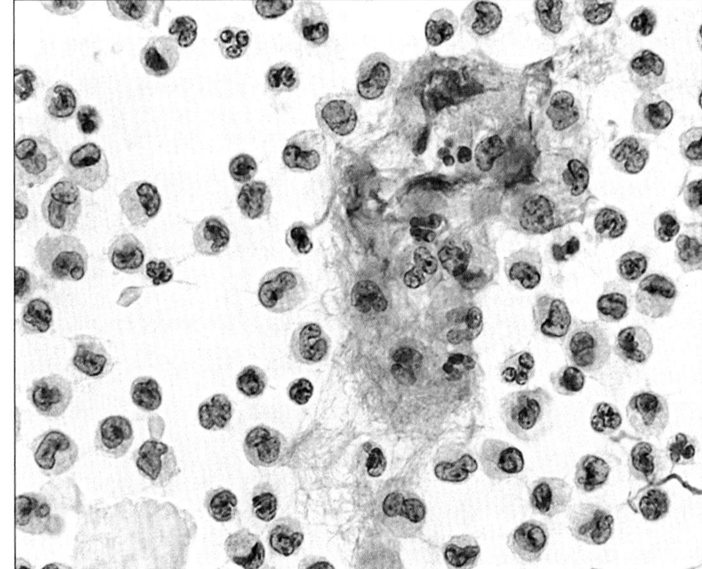

103. A peritoneal effusion from a 40-year-old woman with an abdominal mass reveals these cells. They are diagnostic of:

A. adenocarcinoma, pancreatic
B. mucinous cystadenocarcinoma, ovarian
C. adenocarcinoma, endometrial
D. serous cystadenocarcinoma, ovarian

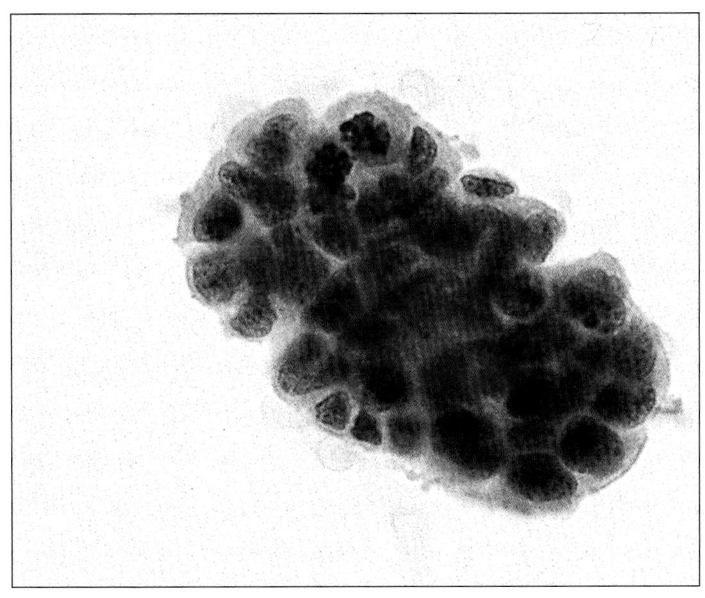

104. A 72-year-old man presents with a peritoneal effusion and a history of a genitourinary tract primary neoplasm. These cells:

A. are reactive mesothelial in origin
B. could be verified as renal cell carcinoma by using a Giemsa stain
C. could be verified as prostatic adenocarcinoma by using a prostate-specific antigen (PSA) immunohistochemical stain
D. represent a chronic infectious process

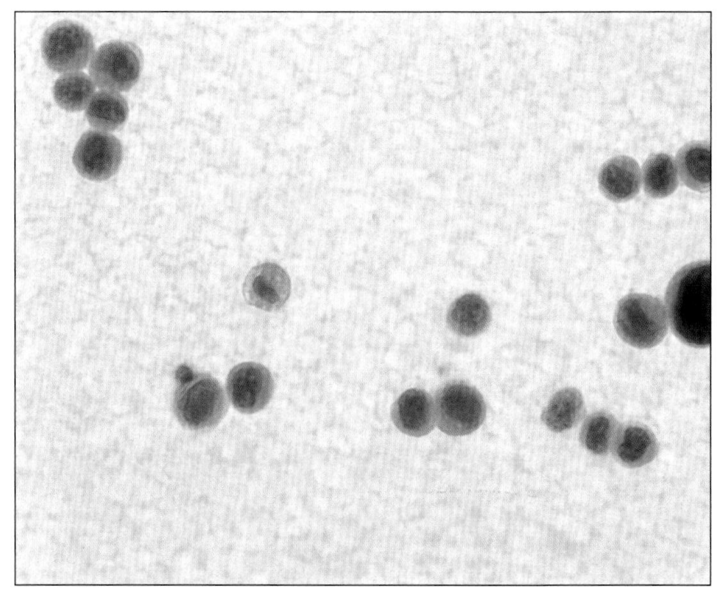

105. These cells were found in an ascitic effusion specimen from a 3-year-old boy with a flank mass. Immunocytochemical staining for chromogranin is negative. The cellular findings are representative of:

A. neuroblastoma
B. Ewing sarcoma
C. pheochromocytoma
D. Wilms tumor

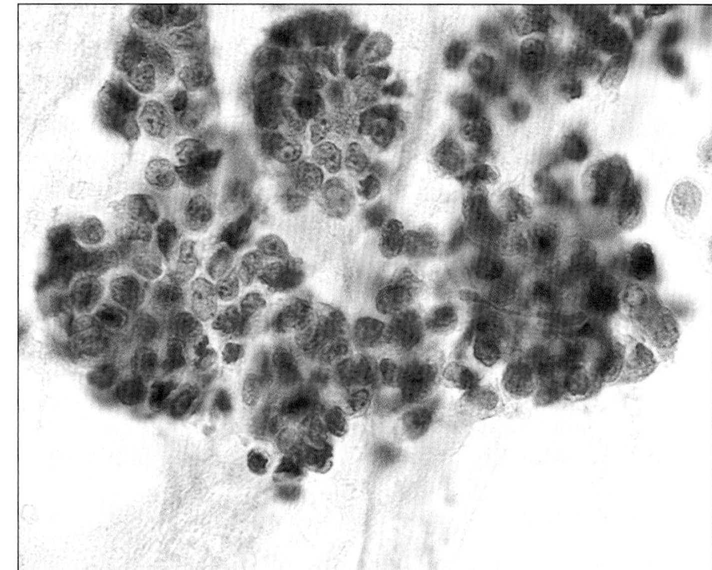

106. These cells were taken from a 52-year-old woman presenting with a 300-mL pleural effusion. The cellular findings represent:

A. mesothelial hyperplasia
B. changes secondary to pulmonary infarct
C. collagen balls
D. metastatic breast carcinoma

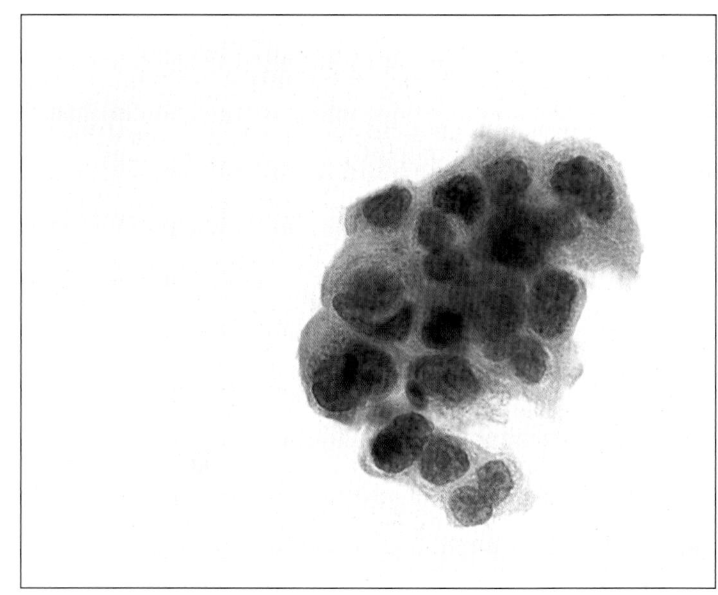

Body Fluids *Answer Key*

1. **B** monosodium urate

Monosodium urate crystals (strongly negative birefringence with pointed ends) polarize and help confirm the presence of gouty arthritis. The differential diagnosis includes pseudogout/chondrocalcinosis, which is marked by calcium phosphate crystals that are not enhanced by polarized light.

DeMay RM, The Art & Science of Cytopathology.
Gout, p. 292.

2. **C** osteoarthritis

A degenerative joint disease, osteoarthritis usually occurs in the weight-bearing joints due to repeated trauma to the articular cartilage.

DeMay RM, The Art & Science of Cytopathology.
Degenerative arthritis (osteoarthritis), p. 291.

3. **A** lung

The most common metastatic carcinoma to the brain is lung cancer. Of these lesions, adenocarcinoma is the most frequently diagnosed tumor, followed by small cell and squamous carcinomas, respectively. In addition to lung cancer, other common metastatic lesions include carcinoma of the breast, malignant melanoma, and adenocarcinoma of the stomach.

DeMay RM, The Art & Science of Cytopathology.
Metastatic malignancy, pp. 449–450.

4. **A** choriocarcinoma

Choriocarcinomas are placental lesions that metastasize to the brain. Cytologic findings consist of mononuclear and multinucleated cells with high nuclear-to-cytoplasmic ratios, granular chromatin, anisonucleosis, and prominent nucleoli. Clinical history is important as well as positive staining with beta-human chorionic gonadotropin.

DeMay RM, The Art & Science of Cytopathology.
Metastatic malignancy, p. 449.

5. **B** rheumatoid arthritis

This collagen disease may be identified by the presence of multinucleated histiocytes and epithelioid histiocytes ("snake cells") among a granular, "sandy" or "fluffy" eosinophilic necrotic background. Large numbers of ragocytes, which represent mono- or multilobulated neutrophils with dark blue cytoplasmic inclusions (immunoglobulin) are specific for this disease. These findings are consistent with a necrotizing granuloma. Clinical symptoms include joint pain and/or synovitis and a positive serum test for rheumatoid factor. Rheumatoid arthritis usually affects women; nevertheless, effusion-related disease is seen more often in men.

DeMay RM, The Art & Science of Cytopathology.
Rheumatoid arthritis, p. 291.

6. **B** subdural hematoma

Intracranial hemorrhaging will often result in cytological presence of hemosiderin-laden macrophages or siderophages, which are macrophages with a refractile, gold intracytoplasmic pigment. The differential diagnosis of siderophages may include metastatic melanoma, which can be excluded based on their negative reaction with S-100, HMB-45, Melan A or positivity with an iron stain.

DeMay RM, The Art & Science of Cytopathology.
The cells (siderophages), p. 433.

7. **C** Ewing sarcoma

Ewing sarcoma cytologically presents as small, round cells with granular cytoplasm found in clusters or rosette formations. The nuclei contain coarsely granular, irregularly distributed chromatin with nucleoli. Tumor diathesis is a reliable cytomorphologic feature of these lesions. Differentiation of synovial sarcoma, osteogenic sarcoma, and other neuroendocrine lesions is permitted by the positive staining of intracytoplasmic glycogen, as demonstrated with periodic acid-Schiff. Ewing sarcoma lesions are found in serous or synovial effusions.

DeMay RM, The Art & Science of Cytopathology.
Ewing sarcoma, p. 278.

8. **D** chondrocalcinosis

Pseudogout/chondrocalcinosis is marked by calcium phosphate crystals that are not enhanced by polarized light.

DeMay RM, The Art & Science of Cytopathology.
Pseudo-gout/chrondrocalcinosis, p. 292.

9. **D** multiple sclerosis

The mere presence of plasma cells in CSF specimens represents a pathologic process. Some of the disease processes include neurosyphilis, multiple sclerosis, viral infections, sarcoidosis, or sclerosing panencephalitis. Answers A, B, and C are conditions associated with neutrophilic infiltrates.

DeMay RM, The Art & Science of Cytopathology.
Plasma cells, p. 433.

10. **A** papillary

Cells derived from choroid plexus papillomas appear in papillary cohesive clusters with irregular nuclear membranes. The cytoplasm is generous and basophilic. These cells are often difficult to distinguish from normal choroid plexus cells, ependymomas, and pineocytomas; therefore, the clinical history of an intraventricular mass is imperative.

DeMay RM, The Art & Science of Cytopathology.
Choroid plexus tumors, p. 442.

11. **D** pineoblastoma

Pineoblastomas present cytologically with "small blue cell" tumor morphology. The cells may be either pleomorphic or monomorphic, with scanty, ill-defined cytoplasm and hyperchromasia. The differential diagnosis includes pineocytoma, its benign counterpart (which lacks malignant criteria), and medulloblastoma (differentiated by location).

DeMay RM, The Art & Science of Cytopathology.
Pineal gland tumors (pineoblastomas), p. 444.

12. **D** leptomeningeal cells

These cells resemble mesothelial cells or monocytes and are derived from the pia-arachnoid layers of the brain covering.

DeMay RM, The Art & Science of Cytopathology.
CNS cells (pia-arachnoid cells), p. 435.

13. **A** peripheral blood contamination

Peripheral blood contamination in a CSF specimen renders it unsatisfactory. The presence of megakaryocytes may at first seem alarming based on their giant cell size, multinucleation, and coarse appearing chromatin patterns. However, these sparse cells found in conjunction with other peripheral blood cells should suggest their blood-derived origin.

DeMay RM, The Art & Science of Cytopathology.
Miscellaneous cells (giant cells), p. 435.

14. **A** meningioma

Cells with fibroblastic appearance found in whorls and sheets with benign nuclear features represent meningioma. These meningeal tumors are generally found in adolescents. These benign lesions need to be discriminated from their malignant counterpart, meningiosarcoma, a tumor which presents with classic sarcomatous features.

DeMay RM, The Art & Science of Cytopathology.
Miscellaneous primary tumors, pp. 448–449.

15. **B** ***Cryptococcus neoformans***

The presence of single, yeast-like structures (5–15 μm) with mucinous capsules is diagnostic of *Cryptococcus neoformans.* These organisms reproduce by tear-drop budding. Special staining with mucicarmine will help elucidate the distinctive capsule. Differentiation includes starch crystals, which possess a Maltese cross birefringence.

DeMay RM, The Art & Science of Cytopathology.
Fungal infections, p. 437.

16. **D** medulloblastoma

The finding of small, anaplastic cells ("small blue cell tumors") in the CSF of children may indicate the presence of medulloblastoma, neuroblastoma, or retinoblastoma. Special attention should focus on possible clinical history. Medulloblastomas are neural crest tumors that arise from the cerebellum and are found in children or adolescents. Neuroblastomas (rare in the brain) typically arise within the cerebral hemisphere. Retinoblastomas involve the orbit and optic tract.

DeMay RM, The Art & Science of Cytopathology.
Medulloblastoma, p. 443.

17. **D** ependymoma

Ependymoma, a benign common spinal cord lesion that generally occurs in children and adolescents, presents readily in CSF specimens due to its ventricular origin. Cytologically, the cells demonstrate columnar morphology and possess finely granular, evenly distributed chromatin patterns with occasional nucleoli. Small cluster or rosettes may be seen; furthermore, the presence of blepharoplasts (basal bodies), which are positive with phosphotungstic acid hematoxylin, is a confirmatory finding. Differential diagnosis must exclude neural crest tumors, the cells of which stain positive for chromogranin.

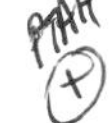

DeMay RM, The Art & Science of Cytopathology.
Ependymoma, p. 441.

18. C astrocytoma

Astrocytomas are the most common primary brain neoplasm found in children. Uniform cells with oval nuclei and hypochromasia mimic their normal benign counterpart. Because the cytology may be difficult to distinguish from normal astrocytes, the history of a radiographically identified cerebellar lesion is extremely important.

DeMay RM, The Art & Science of Cytopathology.
Astrocytoma, p. 440.

19. A reactive pleocytosis

Severe inflammation/reactive lymphocytosis is often difficult to distinguish from recurrent leukemia, with the exception that reactive changes consist of a polytypic population of small mature lymphocytes and immunoblasts (often containing prominent nucleoli), as well as plasma cells. The absence of malignant blasts with irregular, notched, or cleaved nuclear membranes and hyperchromatic, coarse, irregular chromatin with prominent nucleoli is important when differentiating reactive processes secondary to intrathecal therapy or infection from recurrent leukemic involvement. A negative reaction with tumor marker terminal deoxytransferase is useful in ruling out recurrent leukemia.

20. A post-oil myelogram

When lipophages are observed, a differential diagnosis may include metastatic adenocarcinoma. Confirmation with oil red O and clinical history of a recent oil myelogram or pneumoencephalogram are key in corroborating the benign nature of these cells.

DeMay RM, The Art & Science of Cytopathology.
The cells (lipophages), p. 433.

21. D synovial sarcoma

Malignant synovioma or synovial sarcoma is an extremely aggressive neoplasm that presents as a very cellular monotonous population of anaplastic cells. Differential staining will differentiate it from metastatic neuroendocrine tumors (latter stains positive for chromogranin). Although these lesions represent indigenous neoplasms, they rarely arise in the joints.

DeMay RM, The Art & Science of Cytopathology.
Tumors, p. 293

22. A medulloblastoma

The finding of small, anaplastic cells ("small blue cell tumors") in the CSF of children may indicate the presence of medulloblastoma, neuroblastoma, or retinoblastoma. Special attention should focus on possible clinical history. Medulloblastomas are neural crest tumors that arise from the cerebellum and are found in children or adolescents. Neuroblastomas (rare in the brain) typically arise within the cerebral hemisphere. Retinoblastomas involve the orbit and optic tract.

DeMay RM, The Art & Science of Cytopathology.
Medulloblastoma, p. 443.

23. B schwannoma

Schwannomas cytologically present as hypocellular, monotonous clusters of spindle-appearing cells. The presence of Verocay bodies, clusters of cells with peripherally palisading nuclei, central fibrillar cores, and "flame-like" cytoplasm, is an essential component in diagnosing a primary schwannoma.

DeMay RM, The Art & Science of Cytopathology.
Nerve sheath tumors (schwannoma and neurofibroma), pp. 585–587.

24. B retinoblastoma

The finding of small, anaplastic cells ("small blue cell tumors") in the CSF of children may indicate the presence of medulloblastoma, neuroblastoma, or retinoblastoma. Special attention should focus on possible clinical history. Medulloblastomas are neural crest tumors that arise from the cerebellum and are found in children or adolescents. Neuroblastomas (rare in the brain) typically arise within the cerebral hemisphere. Retinoblastomas involve the orbit and optic tract.

DeMay RM, The Art & Science of Cytopathology.
Retinoblastoma, p. 443.

25. C neuroblastoma

Should small, anaplastic cells be identified in serous effusions from children, the diagnostic focus should be differentiating between neuroblastoma of adrenal origin and Wilms tumor (nephroblastoma). The former is a neuroendocrine lesion that will immunologically stain positive for chromogranin. Wilms tumors are negative for chromogranin.

DeMay RM, The Art & Science of Cytopathology.
Neuroblastoma, p. 443.

26. **A** metastatic carcinoma, lung

Cytology reveals pleomorphic cells with hyperchromatic, eccentrically located nuclei, irregular nuclear membranes, macronucleoli, and dense, hard cytoplasm. Positive staining with high molecular weight keratin would indicate a squamous cell carcinoma (the most common lung neoplasm).

DeMay RM, The Art & Science of Cytopathology.
Metastatic malignancy (lung), p. 450.

27. **C** breast

Metastatic carcinoma of the breast is the most common malignancy of the CNS. The most common morphologic variant, ductal adenocarcinoma, may be cytologically identified as "cannon balls," three-dimensional proliferation spheres, or morula formations. However, metastatic adenocarcinoma of the breast in the CSF can also present as single cells with cohesive features with plasmacytoid morphology. In this case, the presence of these true tissue fragments with community cell borders is strongly suggestive of breast metastasis.

DeMay RM, The Art & Science of Cytopathology.
Metastatic malignancy (breast), p. 450.

28. **B** Reiter syndrome

Reiter syndrome is associated with polyarthritis and is diagnosed cytologically by the finding of intracytoplasmic eosinophilic inclusions within synovial cells. Mononucleated leukocytes and fibrinous protein are found within the background. A clinical history of conjunctivitis or nongonococcal urethritis is important in correlating the disease process.

DeMay RM, The Art & Science of Cytopathology.
Reiter syndrome, p. 292.

29. **B** acute bacterial meningitis

A hypercellular population of neutrophilic leukocytes are commonly associated with acute bacterial infections. Culture analysis should be performed to specify the etiology of the infection. Differential diagnosis includes a tuberculous effusion. Clinical history is imperative in discriminating these two diagnoses.

DeMay RM, The Art & Science of Cytopathology.
The cells (neutrophils), p. 432.

30. **C** adenocarcinoma/prostate (PSA +)

Prostatic adenocarcinomas present in serous effusions as small cells in microacinar clusters containing hyperchromatic nuclei and macronucleoli. A history of prostate cancer is helpful in conjunction with immunohistochemical staining with prostatic-specific antigen or acid phosphatase.

DeMay RM, The Art & Science of Cytopathology.
Prostate-specific antigen, p. 18.

31. **B** glioblastoma multiforme

Glioblastomas (grade IV astrocytomas) represent the most common primary brain neoplasm (often contained within the frontal lobes) detected in adults. The cytomorphologic criteria associated with this lesion are the finding of pleomorphic, bizarre, frankly malignant cells with opaque or lacy cytoplasm and wispy cytoplasmic appendages, either singularly or in cell balls. These cells are easily recognized as malignant; however, the differential diagnosis may include a pleomorphic carcinoma or sarcoma. Immunocytochemical staining with glial fibrillary acidic protein will confirm CNS origin.

DeMay RM, The Art & Science of Cytopathology.
Glioblastoma multiforme, p. 441.

32. **A** PAS

Oligodendrogliomas appear benign by cytomorphologic criteria, possessing round, uniform shapes, and are found in sheets or syncytial aggregates with predictable patterns and finely granular, evenly distributed chromatin. Special staining with PAS is positive for intracytoplasmic glycogen and may be a key differential feature in discriminating these lesions from other adult glial tumors.

DeMay RM, The Art & Science of Cytopathology.
Oligodendroglioma, p. 441.

33. **B** craniopharyngioma

These supracellular cystic tumors, which arise within the Rathke pouch, are cytologically diagnosed only after rupture of the cyst into the meninges. Cells lining the cyst are composed of columnar cells, anucleate squames, and/or keratin pearls. Occasionally, degenerative components and cholesterol crystals may be seen.

DeMay RM, The Art & Science of Cytopathology.
Craniopharyngioma, p. 444.

34. **B** *Toxoplasma gondii*

Toxoplasma gondii is an intracellular parasite acquired by exposure to uncooked meats or blood transfusions. 20%–70% of Americans have antibody titers but are asymptomatic, unless there is a reactivation of a dormant disease secondary to failed cell-mediated immunity. Cerebrospinal fluid infections may be seen in patients with AIDS. The cysts are readily demonstrated by staining with PAS, Giemsa, Romanovsky (Diff-Quik), or immunocytochemistry.

DeMay RM, The Art & Science of Cytopathology.
Meningitis (toxoplasma), p. 438.

35. **C malignant melanoma**

Melanoma typically presents in single cells, aggregates, or as spindle cells with bizarre malignant nuclear features, macronucleoli, intranuclear cytoplasmic inclusions, and possibly intracytoplasmic golden brown pigment. Due to the fact that these diseases may be amelanotic, it may be helpful to confirm this disease process with S-100, HMB-45, Melan A or MITF (microphthalmia-associated transcription factor)—all which preferentially react with melanoma cells.

Wang JF, Sarma DP, Ulmer P. Diagnostic dilemma: HMB-45 and Melan-A negative tumor, can it be still a melanoma?: MITF (Microphthalmia-associated transcription factor) stain may confirm the diagnosis. The Internet Journal of Dermatology. 2007. Volume 5 Number 1.

DeMay RM, The Art & Science of Cytopathology.
Metastatic malignancy (melanoma), p. 450.

36. **A macrophages**

Macrophages are commonly identified elements in serous effusions. These cells are roughly the same size as mesothelial cells but possess frothy, indistinct cytoplasm with eccentric, bean-shaped, reniform, boomerang, or round nuclei. The chromatin is fine and regular in Papanicolaou-stained specimens while resembling "raked sand" in air dried material. These phagocytes may have intracytoplasmic inclusions often containing the phagosome, such as hemosiderin-laden macrophages or siderophages. Histiocytes stain positive for neutral red and Janus green (supravital stains), whereas mesothelial cells are negative.

DeMay RM, The Art & Science of Cytopathology.
Histiocytes, p. 264.

37. **B** *Cryptococcus neoformans*

The presence of single, yeast-like structures (5–15 µm in diameter) with mucinous capsules is diagnostic of *Cryptococcus neoformans*. These organisms reproduce by tear-drop budding. Special staining with mucicarmine will help elucidate the distinctive capsule. Differentiation includes starch crystals, which possess a Maltese cross birefringence.

DeMay RM, The Art & Science of Cytopathology.
Fungal infections, p. 437.

38. **A is of little significance**

Mitotic figures are common findings in effusion cytology. Their presence is related to hyperplastic and/or reactive as well as malignant conditions. Mesothelial cells have the ability to proliferate within the fluid matrix.

DeMay RM, The Art & Science of Cytopathology.
The cells (mesothelial), p. 262.

39. **A PAS-D (+)**

Identifying the cells as mesothelial cell lineage is the first step in establishing the diagnosis of carcinomatous mesothelioma. Cytology reveals many cells possessing homogeneous cytoplasm with "skirts" or "blebs," multinucleation, single cells and clusters, and coarse, irregular chromatin with multiple macronucleoli. Irregular papillae and knobby three-dimensional clusters with cytoplasmic vacuolation are found among a metachromatic precipitous background (demonstrated with Diff-Quik staining). The differential diagnosis is metastatic adenocarcinoma; however, special staining with alcian blue-hyaluronidase and PAS-D is negative for carcinomatous mesothelioma, but positive for adenocarcinoma. Immunocytochemical staining with CEA and B72.3 is also negative for mesothelioma but positive for adenocarcinoma.

DeMay RM, The Art & Science of Cytopathology.
Special studies in diagnosis of mesothelioma, p. 283.

40. **B community borders**

Benign reactive mesothelial cells may present with pseudoacinar or papillae structures; however, the cytoplasmic borders are described as "knobby" or flower-like. In contrast, the most common metastatic malignancies to the serous cavities are adenocarcinomas, which present as three-dimensional true acinar, papillary, or morula groupings with smooth community borders.

DeMay RM, The Art & Science of Cytopathology.
General features of a malignant effusion (group contours), p. 270, and General patterns of adenocarcinoma, p. 272.

41. **C** small cell carcinoma

Metastatic small cell carcinoma presents with hyperchromatic, stippled chromatin, coarse clumping, nuclear molding, scanty cytoplasm, and micronucleoli. The cells are arranged characteristically in vertebral column formation ("stack of dishes"), microbiopsy aggregates, and as cords, nests, or ribbons.

DeMay RM, The Art & Science of Cytopathology.
Small cell carcinoma, p. 274.

42. **B** reactive mesothelial cells

Reactive mesothelial cells (reactive hyperplasia) show papillae and pseudoacini with knobby borders instead of true community borders, and single cells with "windows" between adjacent cells—a result of centrifugation and maintenance of the cytoplasmic brush border. The finding of a brush border infers benignity, and is often described as indistinct or fuzzy in appearance. The nuclei of these cells are round and centrally located with well-defined, regular nuclear membranes and finely granular, regularly distributed chromatin with nucleoli. The cytoplasmic morphology is homogeneous and dense with peripheral fading, often demonstrating an endo-ectoplasmic demarcation. The density of the cytoplasm may give a false "atypical" impression of hyperchromatic nuclei; however, when the nuclear intensity is compared with that of the cytoplasm, there is little divergence. The presence of psammoma bodies may also be seen in reactive conditions such as mesothelial hyperplasia and endosalpingiosis. Psammoma bodies are more commonly seen in benign effusions than in malignant effusions (eg, ovarian cancer).

DeMay RM, The Art & Science of Cytopathology.
Reactive changes in mesothelial cells, p. 263.

43. **A** PAS

Embryonal rhabdomyosarcoma is considered an uncommon vaginal lesion affecting young girls generally less than 5 years of age. The cytological identification of small single cells, clusters, and cells with elongated tadpole-like morphology with broad bands ("strap cells") is helpful in identifying this lesion. Special staining for PAS and myoglobulin may help confirm these lesions.

DeMay RM, The Art & Science of Cytopathology.
Malignant effusions in children (rhabdomyosarcoma, embryonal type), p. 278.

44. **B** systemic lupus erythematosus

Systemic lupus erythematosus may be cytologically confirmed by finding characteristic LE cells, a neutrophil containing a large hematoxylin inclusion consisting of antinuclear antibody-coated, degenerative nuclear material. This disease, generally affecting women in childbearing years, presents with idiopathic pleural effusions. It must be confirmed with antinuclear antibodies and clinical manifestations such as a butterfly facial rash and joint pain. In the absence of a previously established clinical and serological diagnosis, the diagnosis may be difficult and suggestive only. The differential diagnosis includes the more commonly found tart cell, however, this cell does not have discernible chromatin within the hematoxylin body.

DeMay RM, The Art & Science of Cytopathology.
Miscellaneous findings, p. 266, and Systemic lupus erythematosus, p. 268.

45. **B** *Paragonimus westermani*

This unusual parasite has been described in effusion cytology as yellowish ova with a flat, thick operculum at one end and a rounded, thickened shell on the opposite end. It should be differentiated from *Echinococcus granulosus,* a cestode which often presents with hydatid sand consisting of associated scoleces and hooks.

DeMay RM, The Art & Science of Cytopathology.
Parasites, p. 57.

46. **A** mesothelioma is positive for vimentin

Vimentin is an intermediate filament that immunocytochemically will stain positive in mesenchymal cells (mesothelial) but negative in epithelial cells.

DeMay RM, The Art & Science of Cytopathology.
Other special studies (immunocytochemistry), p. 285.

47. **B** adenocarcinoma/breast

Metastatic carcinoma of the breast is the most common malignancy involving the pleural cavity in women. The most common morphologic variant, ductal adenocarcinoma, may be cytologically identified as "cannon balls," three-dimensional proliferation spheres, or morula formations. The presence of these true tissue fragments with community cell borders is strongly suggestive of breast metastasis in light of the clinical history.

DeMay RM, The Art & Science of Cytopathology.
"Specific" patterns of adenocarcinoma (breast cancer), p. 272.

48. C idiopathic

The presence of a vast majority of eosinophils in serous fluids may be idiopathic in the absence of a specific clinical history such as trauma, hypersensitivity, pneumothorax, or pulmonary infarct. Idiopathic eosinophilia is self-limiting and tends to spontaneously resolve.

DeMay RM, The Art & Science of Cytopathology.
Other blood cells (eosinophils), p. 264.

49. C *Echinococcus granulosus*

Echinococcus granulosus is a cestode that often presents with hydatid sand consisting of associated scoleces and hooks. Aspiration of *Echinococcus granulosus* is a contraindication due to the possibility of creating anaphylactic shock.

DeMay RM, The Art & Science of Cytopathology.
Parasites, p. 57.

50. B adenocarcinoma

Mesothelial cells do not contain neutral mucin but rather mesenchymal mucin or hyaluronic acid; therefore, neutral mucin positivity as identified by special staining with mucicarmine or alcian blue would indicate an adenocarcinoma. Mesothelial cells may be peripherally positive with PAS, but after digestion with diastase the cells are negative, whereas adenocarcinomas will remain positive.

DeMay RM, The Art & Science of Cytopathology.
Special studies in diagnosis of mesothelioma, pp. 283–284.

51. B alcian blue-hyaluronidase

Mesotheliomas stain negative with alcian blue-hyaluronidase, whereas adenocarcinomas are positive. Both mesotheliomas and adenocarcinomas may be positive for alcian blue (without hyaluronidase), PAS (mesotheliomas peripherally positive), and immunostaining with cytokeratin. Therefore, the latter stains will be of little value in differentiating the two tumor types.

DeMay RM, The Art & Science of Cytopathology.
Special studies in diagnosis of mesothelioma, pp. 283–285.

52. B patient history

It is imperative to have appropriate clinical history to correctly identify the origin of a metastatic neoplasm. Correlation with the original primary tissue is also of great utility in establishing metastasis. In the absence of clinical history, special stains and immunocytochemical marking may be useful, but oftentimes are not reliable.

DeMay RM, The Art & Science of Cytopathology.
Malignant effusions, pp. 269–270.

53. B Wilms tumor

Wilms tumors cytologically present as small cells with anaplastic features and infrequent spindle cells, often mimicking neuroblastoma of the adrenal gland. The clinical history is important, as well as the use of adjunctive immunocytochemistry.

DeMay RM, The Art & Science of Cytopathology.
Malignant effusions in children (Wilms tumor), p. 278

54. B a discrete population of foreign cells and normal cells

A foreign population of cells with foreign features may suggest a metastatic malignant process when found in association with a benign population of mesothelial cells and histiocytes.

DeMay RM, The Art & Science of Cytopathology.
General features of a malignant effusion, p. 270.

55. D rheumatoid pleuritis

This collagen disease may be identified by the presence of multinucleated histiocytes and epithelioid histiocytes ("snake cells") in a granular, "sandy" or "fluffy" eosinophilic necrotic background. These findings are consistent with a necrotizing granuloma. Occasional cholesterol crystals and multinucleated or trapezoidal histiocytes are seen in rheumatoid pleuritis. Large numbers of ragocytes, which represent mono- or multilobulated neutrophils with dark blue cytoplasmic inclusions (immunoglobulin), are specific for this disease. Serum confirmation of rheumatoid factor is necessary to establish this disease process.

DeMay RM, The Art & Science of Cytopathology.
Rheumatoid effusion, p. 268.

56. A a poorly differentiated adenocarcinoma, not otherwise specified

Poorly differentiated adenocarcinomas (PDA) may not actively produce mucin. Therefore, the possibility of PDA cannot be ruled out when the cells are negative for mucicarmine staining. Immunocytochemical staining with CEA and B72.3 is positive for adenocarcinoma.

DeMay RM, The Art & Science of Cytopathology.
Special studies in diagnosis of mesothelioma, pp. 283–284.

57. **C** ovary

These cells represent metastatic mucinous cystadenocarcinoma of the ovary. The presence of irregular, transparent clusters with large distended, degenerated cytoplasmic vacuoles, "signet ring" morphology, and classic malignant nuclear features often suggests this metastatic neoplasm. Although ovarian tumors often produce peritoneal effusions, pleural effusions may be seen without ascites. Staining with alcian blue-hyaluronidase will be positive for most mucinous adenocarcinomas.

DeMay RM, The Art & Science of Cytopathology.
"Specific" patterns of adenocarcinoma (ovarian cancer), p. 273

58. **A** thyroid

Psammoma bodies are common findings associated with papillary carcinomas of the thyroid; however, the presence of psammoma bodies per se is neither sensitive nor specific in the differentiation of benign and malignant disease.

DeMay RM, The Art & Science of Cytopathology.
Adenocarcinomas, p. 538.

59. **B** renal cell carcinoma/kidney

Renal cell carcinomas contain intracytoplasmic lipids that stain positive with oil red O or Sudan black. Colonic adenocarcinoma, hepatocellular carcinoma, and melanoma will all be negative for lipid.

DeMay RM, The Art & Science of Cytopathology.
Kidney cancer, p. 273, and Renal cell carcinoma, p. 1088.

60. **D** adenocarcinoma/colon

Tall columnar cells in clusters with granular cytoplasm and hyperchromatic nuclei containing finely granular, irregularly distributed chromatin with macronucleoli are suggestive of metastatic colonic adenocarcinoma. Special emphasis should be placed on the columnar or cigar-shaped cellular morphology when differentiating these lesions from other possible metastatic sites.

DeMay RM, The Art & Science of Cytopathology.
"Specific" patterns of adenocarcinoma (colorectal cancer), p. 273.

61. **A** scleroderma

Chylous effusions, those containing emulsified neutral lipids, are milky in nature and often associated with diseases such as scleroderma, tuberculosis, or cancer (most commonly lymphoreticular malignancies).

DeMay RM, The Art & Science of Cytopathology.
Special types of effusions (chylous effusion), p. 261.

62. **A** a generalized body infection

The diagnosis of septic arthritis in synovial fluid specimens is grounded upon the finding of an admixture of neutrophils, fibrin, and sheets of synovial cells. The etiology is usually related to bacteria (often mycobacteria or pyogenic), a virus, or fungus; however, the exact etiology of the disorder must be ascertained.

DeMay RM, The Art & Science of Cytopathology.
Infectious arthritis, p. 292.

63. **B** megakaryocyte

The presence of numerous megakaryocytes might raise suspicion of a possible myeloid metaplasia, a condition considered a precursor for myelocytic leukemia. Care must be taken not to overestimate the importance of these findings, especially if peripheral blood contamination is present.

DeMay RM, The Art & Science of Cytopathology.
Miscellaneous findings, p. 266.

64. **D** mesothelioma, carcinomatous

Identifying the cells as mesothelial cell lineage is the first step in establishing the diagnosis of carcinomatous mesothelioma. Cytology reveals many cells possessing homogeneous cytoplasm with "skirts" or "blebs," multinucleation, single cells and clusters, and coarse, irregular chromatin with multiple macronucleoli. Irregular papillae and knobby three-dimensional clusters with cytoplasmic vacuolation are found among a metachromatic precipitous background (demonstrated with Diff-Quik staining). The differential diagnosis is metastatic adenocarcinoma; however, special staining with alcian blue-hyaluronidase and PAS-D is negative for carcinomatous mesothelioma, but positive for adenocarcinoma. Immunocytochemical staining with CEA and B72.3 is also negative for mesothelioma, but positive for adenocarcinoma.

DeMay RM, The Art & Science of Cytopathology.
Background, p. 282.

65. **A** melanoma

Melanoma typically presents in single cells, aggregates, or as spindle cells with bizarre malignant nuclear features, macronucleoli, intranuclear cytoplasmic inclusions, and possibly intracytoplasmic golden brown pigment. Due to the fact that these diseases may be amelanotic, it may be helpful to confirm this disease process with S-100, HMB-45, Melan A or MITF (microphthalmia-associated transcription factor)—all which preferentially react with melanoma cells.

Wang JF, Sarma DP, Ulmer P. Diagnostic dilemma: HMB-45 and Melan-A negative tumor, can it be still a melanoma?: MITF (Microphthalmia-associated transcription factor) stain may confirm the diagnosis. The Internet Journal of Dermatology. 2007. Volume 5 Number 1.

66. **D** neuroblastoma/adrenals

Should the presence of small anaplastic cells be identified in serous effusions from children, the diagnostic focus should be discriminating between neuroblastoma of adrenal origin and Wilms tumor (nephroblastoma) of kidney origin. The former is a neuroendocrine lesion that will immunologically stain positive for chromogranin. Wilms tumors are negative for chromogranin.

DeMay RM, The Art & Science of Cytopathology.
Malignant effusions in children, p. 278.

67. **D** tuberculosis

The diagnosis of septic arthritis in synovial fluid specimens is grounded upon the finding of an admixture of neutrophils, fibrin, and sheets of synovial cells. The etiology is usually related to bacteria (often mycobacteria or pyogenic), a virus, or fungus; however, the exact etiology of the disorder must be ascertained.

DeMay RM, The Art & Science of Cytopathology.
Infectious arthritis, p. 292.

68. **C** negative for neutral mucin

Mesothelial cells do not contain neutral mucin but rather mesenchymal mucin or hyaluronic acid; therefore, neutral mucin positivity as identified by special staining with mucicarmine or alcian blue would indicate an adenocarcinoma. Mesothelial cells may be peripherally positive with PAS, but after digestion with diastase, the cells are negative, whereas adenocarcinomas will remain positive.

DeMay RM, The Art & Science of Cytopathology.
Mesothelial cells, pp. 262–264.

69. **B** mesothelial cells

Mesothelial cells show papillae and pseudoacini with knobby borders instead of true community borders, and single cells with "windows" between adjacent cells—a result of centrifugation and maintenance of the cytoplasmic brush border. The finding of a brush border infers benignity, and is often described as indistinct or fuzzy in appearance. The nuclei of these cells are round and centrally located with well-defined, regular nuclear membranes and finely granular, regularly distributed chromatin with nucleoli. The cytoplasmic morphology is homogeneous and dense with peripheral fading, often demonstrating an endo-ectoplasmic demarcation. The density of the cytoplasm may give a false "atypical" impression of hyperchromatic nuclei; however, when the nuclear intensity is compared with that of the cytoplasm, there is little divergence. The presence of psammoma bodies may also be seen in reactive conditions such as mesothelial hyperplasia and endosalpingiosis. Psammoma bodies are more commonly seen in benign effusions than in malignant effusions (eg, ovarian cancer).

DeMay RM, The Art & Science of Cytopathology.
Mesothelial cells, pp. 262–264.

70. **C** hemosiderin-laden macrophages

Hemosiderin macrophages (siderophages), neutrophils, cartilaginous elements, sheets of synovial lining cells, and multinucleated histiocytes, in a plethora of proteinaceous debris, are descriptive of traumatic arthritis.

DeMay RM, The Art & Science of Cytopathology.
Traumatic arthritis, p. 292.

71. **B** pleuro-esophageal fistula

The depicted cells represent vegetable material from a pleuro-esophageal fistula. A fistula may be suspected should the cytology contain benign glandular cells (perirectal), squamous cells (periesophageal), bacteria, or detritus. Cells with double cell walls, squared-off cytoplasm containing smudgy nuclei and intracytoplasmic granules are diagnostic of vegetable contaminant.

DeMay RM, The Art & Science of Cytopathology.
Nonreactive mesothelial cells, p. 287.

72. **A** reactive lymphocytosis

Severe inflammation/reactive lymphocytosis is often difficult to distinguish from recurrent leukemia, with the exception that reactive changes consist of a polytypic population of small mature lymphocytes and immunoblasts (often containing prominent nucleoli) as well as plasma cells. The absence of malignant blasts with irregular, notched, or cleaved nuclear membranes and hyperchromatic, coarse, irregular chromatin with prominent nucleoli is important when differentiating reactive processes secondary to intrathecal therapy or infection from recurrent leukemic involvement. A negative reaction with tumor marker terminal deoxytransferase is useful in ruling out recurrent leukemia.

DeMay RM, The Art & Science of Cytopathology.
Lymphocytes, p. 432, and Reactive conditions: hemorrhage, inflammation, infection. p. 436.

73. **B** *Cryptococcus neoformans*

The presence of single, yeast-like structures (5–15 microns) with mucinous capsules is diagnostic of *Cryptococcus neoformans.* These organisms reproduce by tear-drop budding. Special staining with mucicarmine will help elucidate the distinctive capsule. Differentiation includes starch crystals, which have a Maltese cross birefringence.

DeMay RM, The Art & Science of Cytopathology.
Fungal infections, p. 437.

74. **A** normal/reactive mesothelial cells

Pancreatitis may often be associated with a hemorrhagic effusion. In such cases, a bloody or dark "chocolate" effusion, representative of old blood, may be withdrawn along with a population of normal mesothelial cells and inflammatory cells. The depicted mesothelial cells possess distinct cell windows between adjacent cells that are representative of the microvillus borders. An endo-ectoplasmic demarcation is seen and the cytoplasm is homogeneous. The nuclei are variable, round to oval, and possess well-defined smooth nuclear membranes. The chromatin is finely granular, evenly distributed, with variable nucleoli. An occasional multinucleated or "atypical" mesothelial cell with aberrant nuclear features may be seen. However, in benign processes, a one-cell population is seen instead of the typical two-cell population associated with metastatic carcinomatosis (normal mesothelial cells and a second population of "foreign" cells).

DeMay RM, The Art & Science of Cytopathology.
Bloody or dark brown ("chocolate") effusions, p. 261

75. **A** tumor marker: terminal deoxytransferase

The cellular findings are consistent with recurrent acute lymphoblastic leukemia (ALL). Recurrent leukemia may often be difficult to separate from benign/reactive processes. Terminal deoxytransferase is a DNA polymerase leukemic marker that is absent in normal or reactive lymphocytes; therefore, a positive reaction may help confirm the emergence of recurrent ALL.

DeMay RM, The Art & Science of Cytopathology.
Lymphoma/leukemia (acute lymphoblastic leukemia), pp. 444–446.

76. **B** glioblastoma multiforme

Glioblastomas (grade IV astrocytomas) represent the most common primary brain neoplasm (often contained within the frontal lobes) detected in adults. The cytomorphologic criteria associated with this lesion are the finding of pleomorphic, bizarre, frankly malignant cells with opaque or lacy cytoplasm and wispy cytoplasmic appendages, either singularly or in cell balls. These cells are easily recognized as malignant; however, the differential diagnosis may include a pleomorphic carcinoma or sarcoma. Immunocytochemical staining with glial fibrillary acidic protein will confirm CNS origin.

DeMay RM, The Art & Science of Cytopathology.
Glioblastoma multiforme, p. 441.

77. **B** gout/monosodium urate monohydrate

Monosodium urate crystals (strongly negative birefringence with pointed ends) polarize and help confirm the presence of gouty arthritis. The differential diagnosis includes pseudo-gout/chondrocalcinosis, a condition that features calcium phosphate crystals that are not enhanced by polarized light.

DeMay RM, The Art & Science of Cytopathology.
Gout, p. 292.

78. **B** viral meningitis

A hypercellular population of polytypic reactive lymphocytes in this patient suggests a possible viral meningitis. Care should be taken to discriminate these cells from those of a primary leukemia/lymphoma, which are usually monomorphic. It may be difficult if not impossible to discriminate these cells as benign if a lymphopoietic malignancy had been diagnosed in the past.

DeMay RM, The Art & Science of Cytopathology.
Viral meningitis, p. 437.

79. **C** neural elements

Choroid/ependymal cells may be seen following intrathecal therapy. The cells present as single cells and in microacinar or papillary clusters. They have moderate lacy cytoplasm (often containing a yellow pigment) and uniform nuclear sizes with fine, even chromatin. Although cilia are generally absent, club-shaped microvilli may be present.

DeMay RM, The Art & Science of Cytopathology.
Choroid plexus cells, p. 434.

80. **A** normal cellular findings

Normal cerebrospinal fluid taken from lumbar taps reveals a hypocellular population of small round mature lymphocytes or monocytes (0–5 cells per μL, or 20–70 if cytocentrifuged). Rarely, the presence of leptomeningeal, ependymal, or neuronal elements are identified in lumbar taps, but appear more frequently in ventricular taps.

DeMay RM, The Art & Science of Cytopathology.
Blood cells, p. 432.

81. **D** medulloblastoma

The finding of small anaplastic cells ("small blue cell tumors") in the CSF of children may indicate the presence of medulloblastoma, neuroblastoma, or retinoblastoma. Special attention should focus on possible clinical history. Medulloblastomas are neural crest tumors that arise from the cerebellum and are found in children or adolescents. Neuroblastomas (rare in the brain) typically arise within the cerebral hemisphere. Retinoblastomas involve the orbit and optic tract.

DeMay RM, The Art & Science of Cytopathology.
Medulloblastoma, p. 443.

82. D reactive mesothelial cells

Reactive mesothelial cells (reactive hyperplasia) occur as papillae and pseudoacini with knobby borders (instead of true community borders) and as single cells with "windows" between adjacent cells—a result of centrifugation and maintenance of the cytoplasmic brush border. The finding of a brush border infers benignity, and is often described as indistinct or fuzzy in appearance. The nuclei of these cells are round and centrally located with well-defined, regular nuclear membranes and finely granular, regularly distributed chromatin with nucleoli. The cytoplasmic morphology is homogeneous and dense with peripheral fading, often demonstrating an endo-ectoplasmic demarcation. The density of the cytoplasm may give a false "atypical" impression of hyperchromatic nuclei; however, when the nuclear intensity is compared to that of the cytoplasm, there is little divergence. The presence of psammoma bodies may also be seen in reactive conditions such as mesothelial hyperplasia and endosalpingiosis. Psammoma bodies are more commonly seen in benign effusions than in malignant effusions (eg, ovarian cancer).

DeMay RM, The Art & Science of Cytopathology.
Reactive mesothelial cells, pp. 263–264.

83. A meningioma

Small cells found in whorls and sheets with benign nuclear features (often accompanied by psammoma bodies) indicate meningioma. These meningeal tumors are generally found in adolescents. These benign lesions need to be discriminated from their malignant counterpart, meningiosarcoma, a tumor that presents with classic sarcomatous features.

DeMay RM, The Art & Science of Cytopathology.
Miscellaneous primary tumors, pp. 448–449.

84. A high-molecular-weight keratin

Cytology reveals pleomorphic cells with hyperchromatic, eccentrically located nuclei, irregular nuclear membranes, macronucleoli, and dense, hard cytoplasm. Positive staining with high-molecular-weight keratin would indicate a squamous cell carcinoma (the most common lung neoplasm).

DeMay RM, The Art & Science of Cytopathology.
Metastatic malignancy (lung), p. 450.

85. C normal mesothelial cells

The depicted cells are representative of normal or nonreactive mesothelial cells from body cavity washings. The cells are usually seen in flat sheets with polygonal cytoplasm and polygonal borders (stripped away by the saline jet). The nuclei are usually single and often paracentrically located with fine, regular chromatin. "Daisy cells," benign cells with lobulated nuclei that may be seen in women at midcycle, may also be found in body cavity washings. In addition to the normal mesothelial cells, body cavity washings may have associated white and red blood cells, starch granules (from gloves), and debris. In contrast to body cavity washings, serous effusions often contain mesothelial cells with reactive features.

DeMay RM, The Art & Science of Cytopathology.
Nonreactive mesothelial cells, p. 287.

86. B lung

These cells are consistent with small cell carcinoma of the lung. Cytology reveals the typical presentation of anaplastic cells with nuclear molding and vertebral column formation arranged in cords, nests, or ribbons. The nuclei exhibit coarse, irregular chromatin and hyperchromasia. Extreme importance should be given to correlative studies with the original tissue section, or a previous history. Differential diagnoses include undifferentiated gliomas, large cell lymphomas, lobular carcinoma of the breast in women, and Merkel cell tumor of the skin.

DeMay RM, The Art & Science of Cytopathology.
Metastatic malignancy (lung), p. 450.

87. A idiopathic

The presence of a very large number of eosinophils in serous fluids may be idiopathic in the absence of a specific clinical history such as trauma, hypersensitivity, pneumothorax, or pulmonary infarct. Idiopathic eosinophilia is self-limiting and tends to spontaneously resolve.

DeMay RM, The Art & Science of Cytopathology.
Other blood cells (eosinophils), p. 264.

88. B acute bacterial meningitis

A hypercellular population of neutrophilic leukocytes are commonly associated with acute bacterial infections. Culture analysis should be performed to specify the etiology of the infection.

DeMay RM, The Art & Science of Cytopathology.
Meningitis (bacterial), pp. 436–437.

89. **B** mesothelioma

Identifying the cells as mesothelial cell lineage is the first step in establishing the diagnosis of carcinomatous mesothelioma. Cytology reveals many cells possessing homogeneous cytoplasm with "skirts" or "blebs," multinucleation, single cells and clusters, and coarse, irregular chromatin with multiple macronucleoli. Irregular papillae and knobby three-dimensional clusters with cytoplasmic vacuolation are found among a metachromatic precipitous background (demonstrated with Diff-Quik staining). The differential diagnosis is metastatic adenocarcinoma; however, special staining with alcian blue-hyaluronidase and PAS-D is negative for carcinomatous mesothelioma, but positive for adenocarcinoma. Immunocytochemical staining with CEA and B72.3 are also negative for mesothelioma but positive for adenocarcinoma.

DeMay RM, The Art & Science of Cytopathology.
Mesothelioma, pp. 278–285.

90. **B** adenocarcinoma, bronchogenic type

Metastatic bronchogenic adenocarcinoma cytologically presents in clusters and as single cells with vacuolated cytoplasm positive for mucin, hyperchromatic nuclei with irregular nuclear membranes, fine to coarse chromatin with irregular distribution, and macronucleoli. Clinical history and tissue comparison with the original primary site is important in confirming this metastatic process.

DeMay RM, The Art & Science of Cytopathology.
"Specific" patterns of adenocarcinoma, p. 273.

91. **D** Mott cell

Mott cells are of plasma cell lineage with PAS (+) intracytoplasmic granules (Russell bodies).

DeMay RM, The Art & Science of Cytopathology.
Synovial fluid (the cells, etc.), p. 291.

92. **C** common leukocyte antigen

Immunocytochemical confirmation with common leukocyte antigen separates a lymphopoietic malignancy (lymphoma) from a metastatic carcinoma such as small cell carcinoma or other neuroendocrine metastases.

DeMay RM, The Art & Science of Cytopathology.
Lymphoma/leukemia, pp. 275–276.

93. **D** rheumatoid arthritis

A predominance of neutrophilic inflammatory cells among a fibrinous, granular or "sandy" necrotic background (which stain from blue to pink to orange) with occasional cholesterol crystals and multinucleated or trapezoidal histiocytes is suggestive of rheumatoid arthritis. Serum confirmation of rheumatoid factor is necessary to establish this disease process.

DeMay RM, The Art & Science of Cytopathology.
Rheumatoid arthritis, p. 291.

94. **A** pancreaticobiliary carcinoma

Cells in vertebral column formations or three-dimensional clusters containing pleomorphic cytoplasm, classic malignant nuclear features, prominent nucleoli, and evidence of mucus secretion or papillary formation are helpful features in establishing the diagnosis of metastatic pancreatic and biliary adenocarcinoma. The morphologic differentiation between pancreatic and biliary duct carcinoma is difficult; however, pancreatic lesions are generally less differentiated. The diagnosis, however, must be correlated with a previously established malignancy or related clinical history as indicated by this question.

DeMay RM, The Art & Science of Cytopathology.
"Specific" patterns of adenocarcinoma, p. 273.

95. **C** systemic lupus erythematosus

Systemic lupus erythematosus may be cytologically confirmed by finding the characteristic LE cell, a neutrophil containing a large hematoxylin inclusion consisting of antinuclear antibody-coated, degenerated nuclear material. This disease, generally affecting women in childbearing years, presents with idiopathic pleural effusions, and must be clinically diagnosed with antinuclear antibodies and clinical manifestations such as a butterfly facial rash and joint pain. In the absence of a previously established clinical and serological diagnosis, the diagnosis may be difficult.

DeMay RM, The Art & Science of Cytopathology.
Miscellaneous findings, p. 266,
and Systemic lupus erythematosus, p. 268.

96. B rheumatoid pleuritis

This collagen disease may be identified by the presence of multinucleated histiocytes and epithelioid histiocytes ("snake cells") amongst a granular, "sandy" or "fluffy" eosinophilic necrotic background. Large numbers of ragocytes, which represent mono- or multilobulated neutrophils with dark blue cytoplasmic inclusions (immunoglobulin), are specific for this disease. These findings are consistent with a necrotizing granuloma. Clinical symptoms include joint pain and/or synovitis and a positive serum test for rheumatoid factor. Rheumatoid pleuritis usually affects women; nevertheless, effusion-related disease is seen more often in men.

DeMay RM, The Art & Science of Cytopathology.
Rheumatoid effusion, p. 268.

97. A small cell carcinoma

Metastatic small cell carcinoma presents with hyperchromatic, stippled chromatin, coarse clumping, nuclear molding, scanty cytoplasm, and micronucleoli. The cells are arranged characteristically in vertebral column formation ("stack of dishes"), microbiopsy aggregates, and in cords, nests, or ribbons.

DeMay RM, The Art & Science of Cytopathology.
Small cell carcinoma, pp. 274–275.

98. C mucicarmine (–)

These cells represent metastatic mucinous cystadenocarcinoma of the ovary. The presence of irregular transparent clusters with large distended, degenerated cytoplasmic vacuoles, "signet ring" morphology and classic malignant nuclear features, in combination with the clinical history, suggests this metastatic neoplasm. Although ovarian tumors suggest peritoneal effusions, pleural effusions may often be seen without ascites. Staining with alcian blue-hyaluronidase will be positive for most mucinous adenocarcinomas.

99. B small noncleaved lymphoma

Small noncleaved lymphomas may be secondary to AIDS, or more commonly, seen in children (Burkitt and non-Burkitt lymphoma). The cytology reveals a small-to-medium size population of immature lymphocytes with a monomorphic cellular pattern. The cells have round nuclei, moderately clumped chromatin, macronucleoli, and abundant cytoplasm.

DeMay RM, The Art & Science of Cytopathology.
Lymphoma, p. 447.

100. C neuroblastoma

The clinical findings suggest the adrenal neoplasm neuroblastoma. Small cells appear in clusters with rosette formations and anaplastic nuclear features. Immunocytochemical positivity for chromogranin and PAS-D negativity would help confirm the malignancy.

DeMay RM, The Art & Science of Cytopathology.
Malignant effusions in children, p. 278.

101. D S-100

Amelanotic melanoma typically presents in single cells, aggregates, or as spindle cells with bizarre malignant nuclear features, macronucleoli, intranuclear cytoplasmic inclusions. Due to the fact that these cells do not contain the melanin typically associated with metastatic melanoma, it becomes essential to attempt to confirm this disease process with immunocytochemistry markers such as S-100, HMB-45, Melan A or MITF (microphthalmia-associated transcription factor)—all which preferentially react with melanoma cells.

Wang JF, Sarma DP, Ulmer P. Diagnostic dilemma: HMB-45 and Melan-A negative tumor, can it be still a melanoma?: MITF (Microphthalmia-associated transcription factor) stain may confirm the diagnosis. The Internet Journal of Dermatology. 2007. Volume 5 Number 1.

102. A reactive synovial lining cells

Synovial cells resemble mesothelial cells, possessing round to oval, often eccentrically placed nuclei containing finely granular, regularly distributed chromatin and abundant basophilic cytoplasm. They are seen in sheets or in single cells, which resemble macrophages.

DeMay RM, The Art & Science of Cytopathology.
Synovial fluid, p. 290.

103. D serous cystadenocarcinoma, ovarian

The diagnosis of serous cystadenocarcinoma of the ovary cytologically presents as three-dimensional aggregates with hyperchromatic nuclei and finely granular, irregularly distributed chromatin. The presence of psammoma bodies may help in identifying these lesions as ovarian primary. These cells recapitulate fallopian tube cells and may be difficult to distinguish from reactive or malignant mesothelial cells.

DeMay RM, The Art & Science of Cytopathology.
Ovarian cancer, p. 273.

104. **C** could be verified as prostatic adenocarcinoma by using a prostate-specific antigen (PSA) immunohistochemical stain

Prostatic carcinomas metastatic to the serous cavities are generally poorly differentiated lesions, presenting in small, microacinar groups and as single cells with hyperchromatic, irregular nuclei, and prominent nucleoli. Clinical history and special staining with prostatic specific antigen is important in confirming this disease process.

DeMay RM, The Art & Science of Cytopathology.
Adenocarcinoma, p. 1142.

105. **D** Wilms tumor

When small anaplastic cells are identified in serous effusions from children, the diagnostic focus should be discriminating between neuroblastoma of adrenal origin and Wilms tumor of kidney origin (nephroblastoma). The former is a neuroendocrine lesion which will immunologically stain positive for chromogranin. Wilms tumors are negative for chromogranin. Wilms tumors represent small blue cell tumors that present cytologically as anaplastic cells in clusters and balls. A spindle cell component may be identified (not seen in this photograph).

DeMay RM, The Art & Science of Cytopathology.
Malignant effusions in children, p. 278.

106. **D** metastatic breast carcinoma

Metastatic carcinoma of the breast is the most common malignancy involving the pleural cavity in women. The most common morphologic variant, ductal adenocarcinoma, may be cytologically identified as "cannon balls," three-dimensional proliferation spheres, or morula formations. The presence of these true tissue fragments with community cell borders is strongly suggestive of breast metastasis in light of provided clinical history.

DeMay RM, The Art & Science of Cytopathology.
"Specific" patterns of adenocarcinoma (breast cancer), p. 272.

Chapter 5

Gastrointestinal Tract

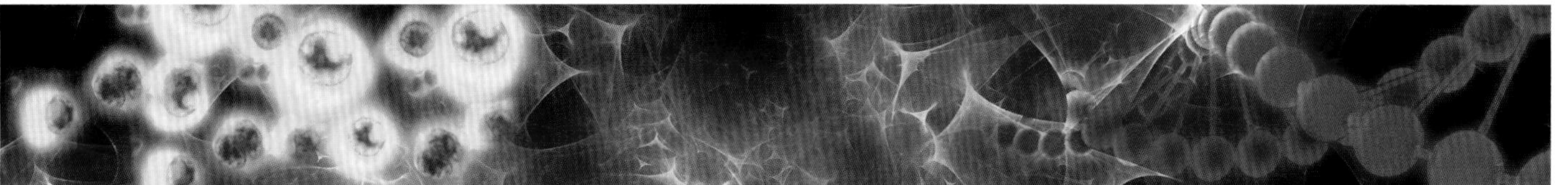

1. **A hereditary condition that manifests itself by the existence of melanotic pigmentation on the lips of infants is often concomitant with intestinal adenomatosis. The disease is:**

   A. Peutz-Jeghers syndrome
   B. Crohn disease
   C. melanoma
   D. melanosis cerebri

2. **A gastric tumor that frequently metastasizes to the ovaries is:**

   A. well differentiated
   B. non-signet ring adenocarcinoma
   C. Krukenberg tumor
   D. lymphoma

3. **What places a patient at an increased risk for the development of colonic carcinoma?**

   A. ulcerative colitis
   B. *Giardia lamblia*
   C. intestinal metaplasia
   D. chronic follicular colitis

4. **Leiomyosarcoma is often differentiated histologically from its benign counterpart by:**

   A. counting >10 mitotic figures per high-power field
   B. enlarged nuclear features as determined cytologically
   C. presence of single cells
   D. fusiform appearance

5. **A 44-year-old woman presents with a polypoid mass in the rectum. Cytology reveals cells in sheets, elongated "trumpet"-shaped cells with granular cytoplasm and basally located nuclei, and hypochromatic nuclei without nucleoli. The diagnosis is:**

   A. villous adenoma
   B. adenocarcinoma
   C. ulcerative colitis
   D. reparative/regenerative changes

6. **Which special stain would prove useful in the diagnosis of intestinal metaplasia as seen in gastric brushings?**

   A. PAS
   B. oil red O
   C. GMS
   D. Congo red

7. **A colonic brushing consists of abundant cells in cohesive, orderly sheets with hypochromatic nuclei and macronucleoli. Single cells are not identified. The diagnosis is:**

   A. adenocarcinoma, well differentiated
   B. reparative/regenerative changes
   C. leiomyoma
   D. villous adenoma

8. **A radioimmunoassay for carcinoembryonic antigen may be a false-positive predictor of colonic adenocarcinoma if the patient has:**

   A. cervical carcinoma
   B. mesothelioma
   C. cystitis
   D. alcoholic cirrhosis

9. **Clusters of columnar cells with multiple distinct vacuoles, varying nuclear locations, hypochromatic nuclei, mild anisocytosis, naked nuclei, and the absence of single cells as found in duodenal specimens are diagnostic of:**

   A. leiomyosarcoma
   B. adenocarcinoma, well differentiated
   C. hemangioma
   D. reactive/reparative changes

10. **A 44-year-old woman presents with chronic diarrhea, cyanotic flushing of the skin, and 5 hydroxyindoleacetic acid urinary changes. CAT scan reveals a 2-cm nodule located in the ileum. Brush cytology shows a population of monomorphic plasmacytoid-appearing cells in loose aggregates. The diagnosis is:**

   A. adenocarcinoma, well differentiated
   B. metastatic ovarian adenocarcinoma
   C. carcinoid tumor
   D. adenoma, Brunner gland

11. **In comparison with other gastrointestinal neoplasms, cancer of the small bowel is:**

   A. common
   B. rare
   C. most often sarcomatous
   D. most often lymphopoietic

12. **A mixed population of lymphoid elements including small and large lymphocytes, tingible body macrophages, and plasma cells is diagnostic of:**

   A. large cell lymphoma
   B. multiple myeloma
   C. Hodgkin disease
   D. chronic follicular gastritis

13. **Bipolar spindle cells in aggregates and overlapping single cells associated with ulcerative gastric specimens are:**

   A. reparative/regenerative changes
   B. smooth muscle in origin
   C. adenocarcinoma, poorly differentiated
   D. carcinoid

14. **Which of the following is associated with gastric and peptic ulcer disease?**

   A. *Entamoeba histolytica*
   B. *Helicobacter pylori*
   C. *Mycobacterium* sp.
   D. human papillomavirus

15. **The most common primary neoplasm of the small intestine cytologically resembles:**

   A. colorectal adenocarcinoma
   B. gastric-type adenocarcinoma
   C. signet ring adenocarcinoma
   D. leiomyosarcoma

16. **Clusters of cells with cyanophilic granular cytoplasm, enlarged hyperchromatic nuclei, macronucleoli, and tall columnar single cells with irregular chromatin and eccentrically located nuclei identified in colonic brushings represent:**

   A. carcinoid tumor
   B. villous adenoma
   C. reparative/regenerative changes
   D. adenocarcinoma

17. **What special stain is helpful in the diagnosis of carcinoid tumors of the intestinal tract?**

   A. mucicarmine
   B. Fontana
   C. PAS
   D. alcian blue

18. **A 42-year-old man presents with abdominal distention, nausea, and hemiparesis. A 2 × 3-cm periampullar lesion is identified in the small intestine. An intestinal brushing reveals many clusters of hyperchromatic cells with nuclear compression, irregular chromatin, macronucleoli, and cells with large distended vacuoles. A large population of single cells with abnormal features are present. The diagnosis is most consistent with:**

   A. adenocarcinoma
   B. reactive/reparative cellular changes
   C. carcinoid
   D. adenoma

19. **A patient with a dull right-sided pain is evaluated for anemia. An ulcerative lesion is identified on endoscopic examination. Cytology reveals many single cells and epithelial aggregates with a high N/C ratio, granular and vacuolated cytoplasm, hyperchromasia, macronucleoli, and many cells with signet ring morphology. The diagnosis is:**

   A. adenocarcinoma, well differentiated
   B. adenocarcinoma, poorly differentiated
   C. reparative/regenerative changes
   D. primary lymphoma

20. **Which of the following is associated with steatorrhea and malnutrition?**

   A. *Allescheria boydii*
   B. *Schistosoma haematobium*
   C. *Toxoplasma gondii*
   D. *Giardia lamblia*

21. **A gastric brushing reveals normal cells with goblet cell features and windows between adjacent cells. The diagnosis is:**

   A. respiratory contaminants
   B. normal gastric mucosa
   C. intestinal metaplasia
   D. chronic atrophic gastritis

22. **An esophageal scraping reveals squamous cells with abundant cytoplasm, normal nuclear-to-cytoplasm ratios, degenerative nuclear features, and chromatic membranes. These cells are representative of:**

   A. reparative/regenerative changes
   B. nonkeratinizing squamous cell carcinoma
   C. pernicious anemia
   D. granulomatous reaction

23. **An esophageal brushing specimen from the distal third reveals squamous cells as well as nongoblet glandular cells. The presence of the glandular cells suggests:**

   A. Barrett esophagitis
   B. normal representative findings
   C. reparative/regenerative cellular changes
   D. respiratory contaminants

24. **The most common esophageal malignancy is:**

   A. squamous carcinoma, nonkeratinizing
   B. adenocarcinoma, poorly differentiated
   C. adenocarcinoma, signet ring
   D. squamous carcinoma, keratinizing

25. **Sheets of cells with abundant cytoplasm exhibiting hypochromasia, enlarged nuclei, well-defined cellular borders, and cytoplasmic streaming and containing fine, regular chromatin patterns in esophageal specimens are diagnostic of:**

   A. adenocarcinoma, well differentiated
   B. squamous carcinoma
   C. reparative/regenerative changes
   D. chronic atrophic gastritis

26. **What cell types might be found in a small bowel brushing from a patient suffering from Peutz-Jeghers syndrome?**

   A. granulomatous inflammation
   B. smooth muscle cells
   C. acute inflammation
   D. intestinal metaplasia

27. **What is considered an important feature in the cytologic diagnosis of gastric adenocarcinoma?**

   A. single cells
   B. macronucleoli
   C. bare nuclei
   D. fibropurulent exudate

28. **Poorly differentiated gastric adenocarcinoma of the stomach reveals which cytological criteria?**

   A. 3-D clusters of malignant cells
   B. sheets of anaplastic cells
   C. signet ring cells, single malignant cells
   D. polygonal cells with hyperchromatic opaque nuclei

29. **A 55-year-old man with a history of tobacco smoking and ETOH abuse presents with dysphagia. Esophageal brushing cytology reveals many clusters of cells with granular cytoplasm, fine, irregular chromatin patterns, nuclear compression, and macronucleoli in every cell. The diagnosis is:**

A. squamous carcinoma
B. adenocarcinoma
C. reparative/regenerative changes
D. granulomatous reaction

30. **Eosinophilic staining cells with intracytoplasmic granules and centrally located nuclei found in gastric specimens represent:**

A. surface neck cells
B. chief cells
C. parietal cells
D. respiratory contaminants

31. **The signet ring form of gastric adenocarcinoma is considered:**

A. well differentiated
B. moderately well differentiated
C. moderately differentiated
D. poorly differentiated

32. **Gastric adenomatous polyps have (are):**

A. premalignant predisposition
B. no premalignant predisposition
C. inflammatory in nature
D. hamartomatous

33. **A 44-year-old woman with a history of achlorhydria submits for evaluation. Gastric washings reveal numerous columnar appearing cells with karyolytic bland nuclear features, cytomegaly, karyomegaly, and nuclear folds. The diagnosis is:**

A. pernicious anemia
B. intestinal metaplasia
C. reparative/regenerative changes
D. adenocarcinoma, well differentiated

34. **The presence of small single cells without cohesive features, with scanty cytoplasm and lobulated nuclear features containing macronucleoli is diagnostic of:**

A. metastatic small cell carcinoma
B. primary lymphoma
C. inflammatory changes
D. leiomyoma

35. **Which is etiologically related to esophageal carcinoma?**

A. tuberculosis
B. Plummer-Vinson syndrome
C. ulcerative esophagitis
D. herpetic esophagitis diverticula

36. **The histologic representation most commonly associated with esophageal carcinoma is:**

A. fungating
B. ulcerative
C. flat
D. inverted

37. **A 55-year-old patient presents with GI bleeding and anemia. Gastric cytology reveals cells in well-defined clusters, altered polarity, anisonucleosis, slight nuclear compression, hyperchromasia, and frequent macronucleoli. Few single cells are present. The diagnosis is:**

A. reactive/reparative cellular changes
B. a malignant glandular tumor arising from intestinal metaplasia
C. a malignant glandular tumor that does not arise from intestinal metaplasia
D. leiomyosarcoma

38. **The most common lymphoma involving the stomach is:**

A. small cell cleaved
B. small cell non-cleaved
C. large cell type
D. Burkitt lymphoma

39. Cells with well-defined borders exhibiting good polarity, enlarged nuclei, and macronucleoli in an esophageal specimen are suggestive of:

A. pernicious anemia
B. squamous carcinoma, nonkeratinizing
C. herpetic esophagitis
D. reparative/regenerative cellular changes

40. Cells in sheets, single cells, and hyperchromatic syncytia with irregular chromatin, nucleoli, cellular cannibalism, and cytoplasmic ringing in esophageal brushings are representative of:

A. adenocarcinoma, poorly differentiated
B. squamous carcinoma, nonkeratinizing
C. squamous carcinoma, keratinizing
D. adenocarcinoma, well differentiated

41. **These cells from a gastric brushing were most likely collected from a patient with a history of:**

A. intestinal metaplasia
B. chronic follicular gastritis
C. pernicious anemia
D. hyperplastic polyps

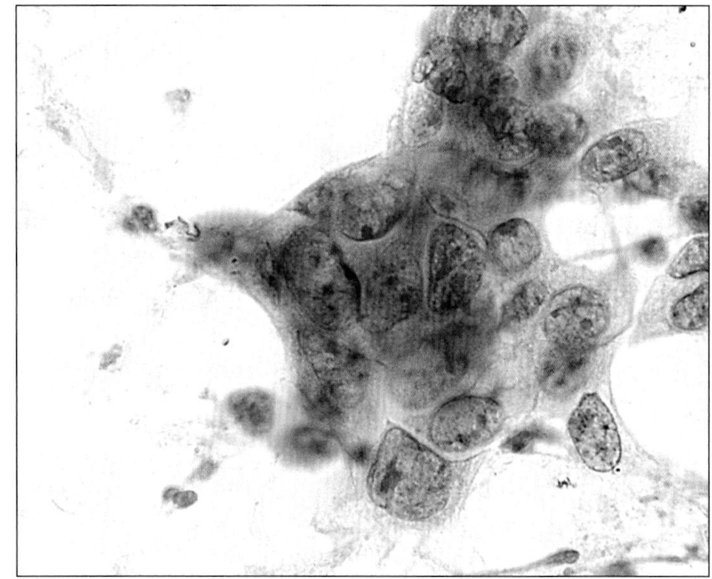

42. **These cells were identified in a gastric washing specimen. They are diagnostic of:**

A. adenocarcinoma, well differentiated
B. adenocarcinoma, poorly differentiated signet ring
C. reactive/reparative process
D. Crohn disease

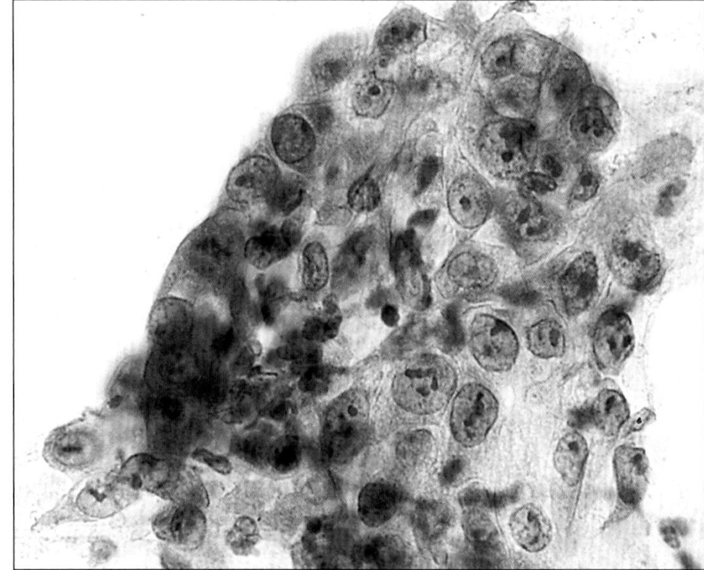

43. **A 60-year-old man presents with unexplained nausea and vomiting. A barium swallow identified a 3-cm lesion in the ileum of the small intestine. Brushings revealed these cells, which represent :**

A. adenomatosis
B. hemangioma
C. adenocarcinoma
D. reactive/reparative process

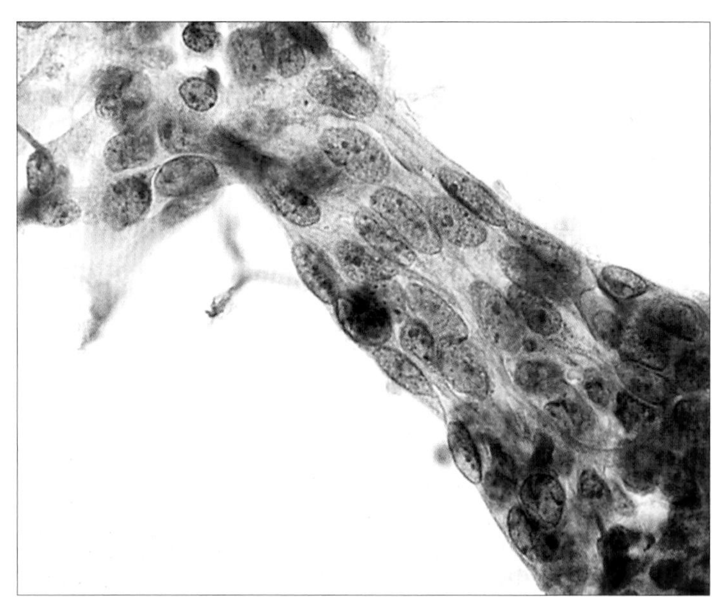

44. **A 67-year-old man with dysphagia, iron deficiency anemia, and positive guaiac testing results presents for a gastric brushing. Which of the following may give rise to the depicted cells?**

A. intestinal metaplasia
B. native gastric epithelium
C. Peutz-Jeghers syndrome
D. aspirin gastritis

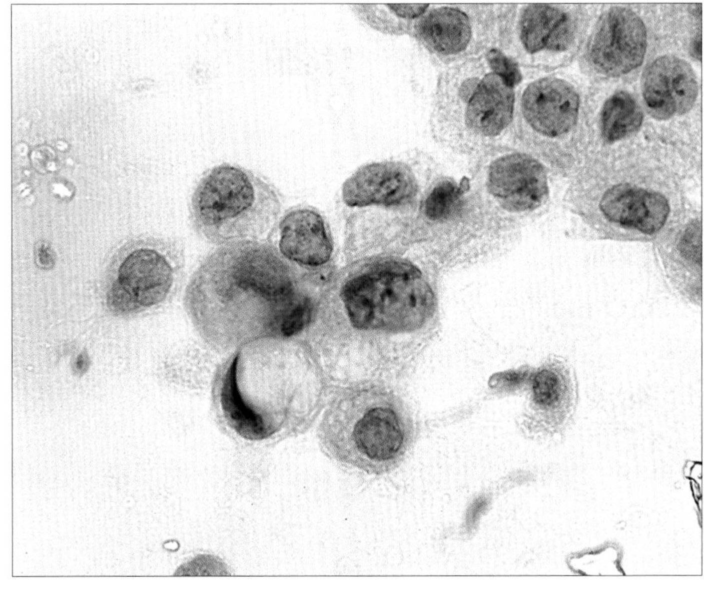

45. **These cells were taken from a 45-year-old man with multiple ulcerative lesions of the rectum. A colonic brushing specimen reveals these cells. They are diagnostic of:**

A. reactive/reparative changes
B. adenocarcinoma, well differentiated
C. carcinoid tumor
D. villous adenoma

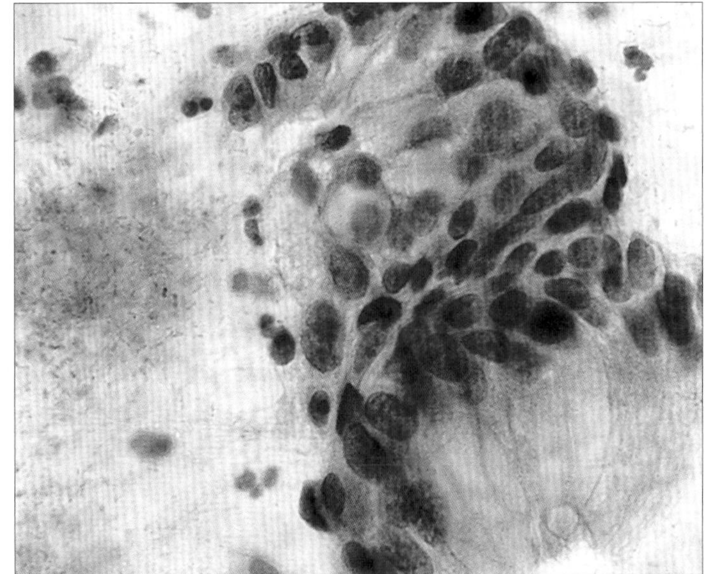

46. **A 66-year-old woman with a history of ulcerative colitis presents with a polypoid mass in the rectum. A colonic brushing specimen reveals:**

A. adenocarcinoma, well differentiated
B. villous adenoma
C. hamartomatous polyp
D. reactive/reparative changes

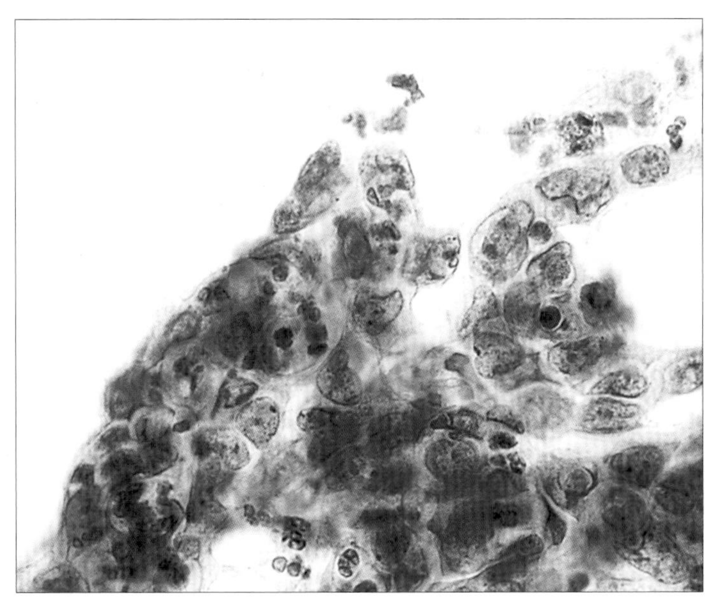

47. **These cells were found in a gastric brushing specimen taken from a 55-year-old man with a history of celiac disease. They are diagnostic of:**

A. poorly differentiated adenocarcinoma
B. pseudolymphoma
C. small cell cleaved lymphoma
D. large cell lymphoma

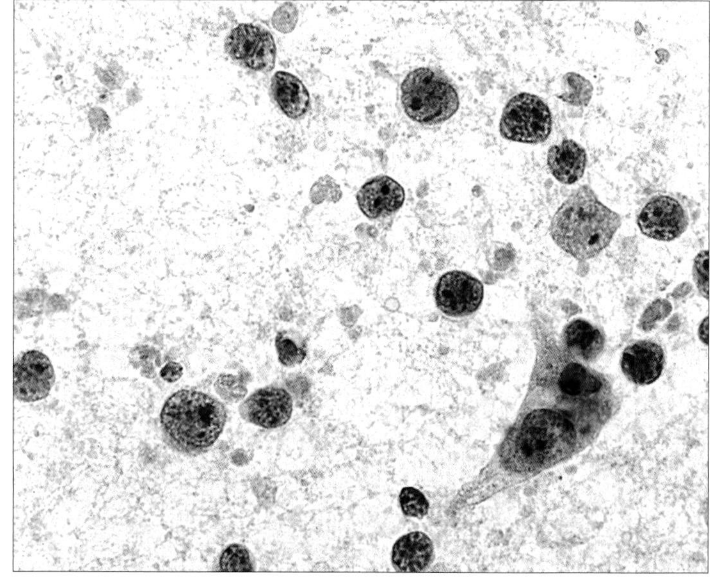

48. **This structure was found in a duodenal brushing specimen from a 44-year-old woman who had recently traveled abroad. The clinical finding/diagnosis is:**

A. vomiting/*Helicobacter pylori* infection
B. nonspecific clinical findings/*Entamoeba histolytica* infection
C. steatorrhea/*Giardia lamblia* infection
D. bloody stool/*Strongyloides stercoralis* infection

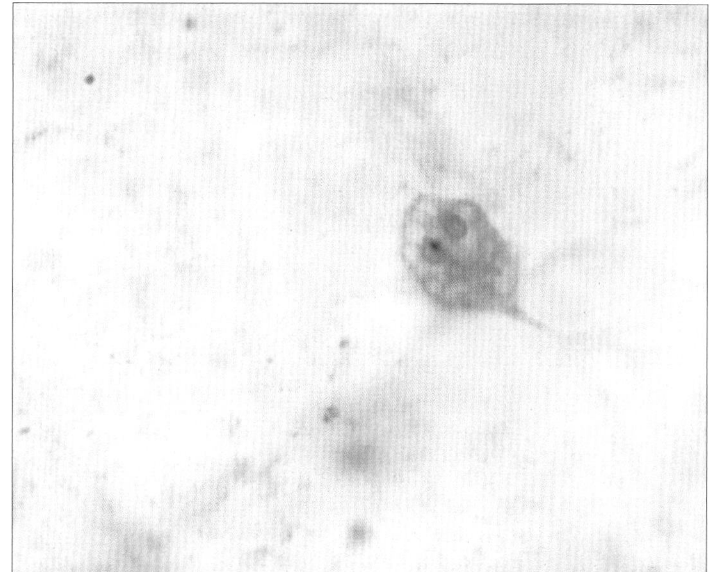

49. **A 56-year-old man with a history of colonic adenocarcinoma presents with a 300-mL peritoneal effusion. Which of the following might aid in confirmation of a metastatic colonic adenocarcinoma?**

A. S-100 (+)
B. vimentin (+)
C. serotonin (+)
D. carcinoembryonic antigen (+)

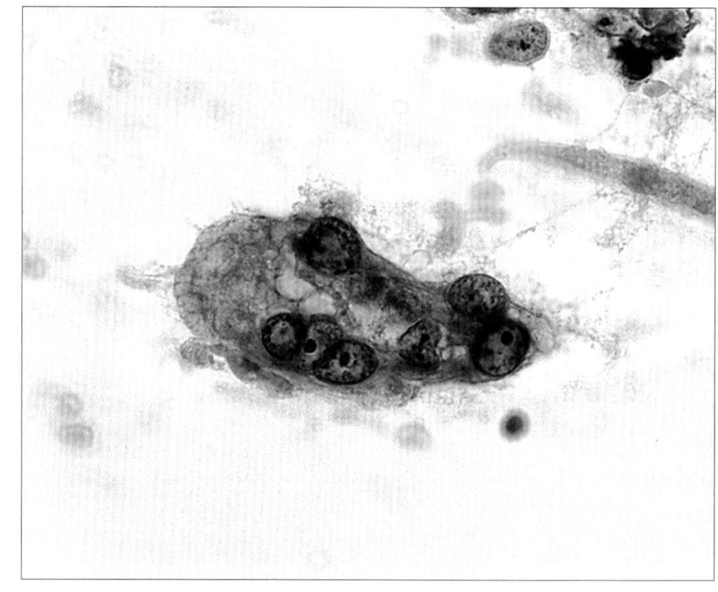

50. The finding of these cells in an esophageal brushing specimen from the middle third of the esophagus is diagnostic of:

A. villous adenoma
B. reactive/reparative changes
C. Barrett esophagus
D. adenocarcinoma, well differentiated

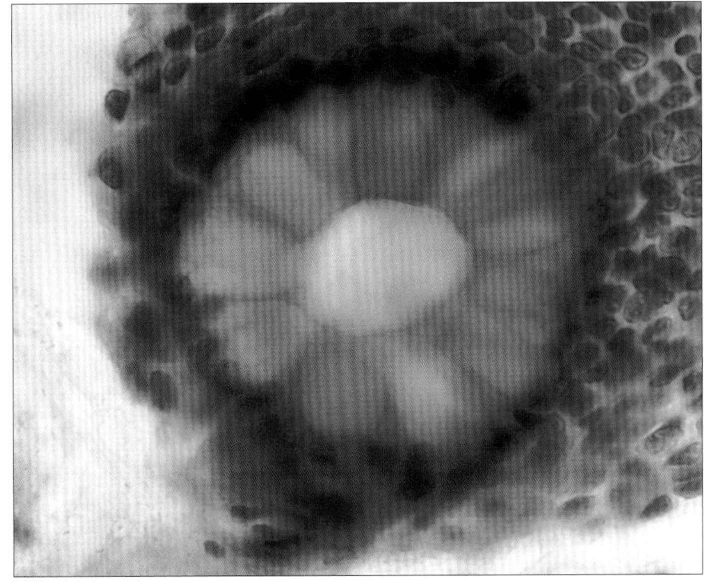

51. A 43-year-old woman with unexplained gastritis undergoes gastric lavage. These cells represent:

A. large cell lymphoma
B. pseudolymphoma
C. small cell lymphoma
D. signet ring adenocarcinoma

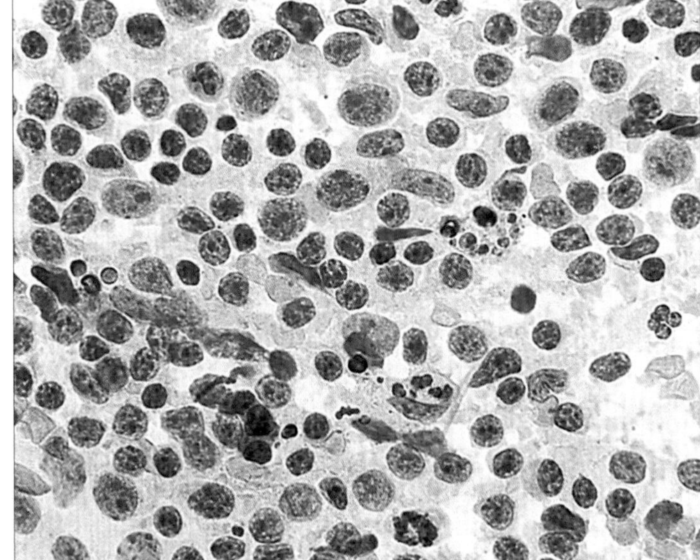

52. A 55-year-old Japanese farmer presents with vomiting of long duration. Results of a gastric lavage are diagnostic of:

A. adenocarcinoma, well-differentiated intestinal type
B. adenocarcinoma, signet ring type
C. intestinal metaplasia
D. reactive/reparative process

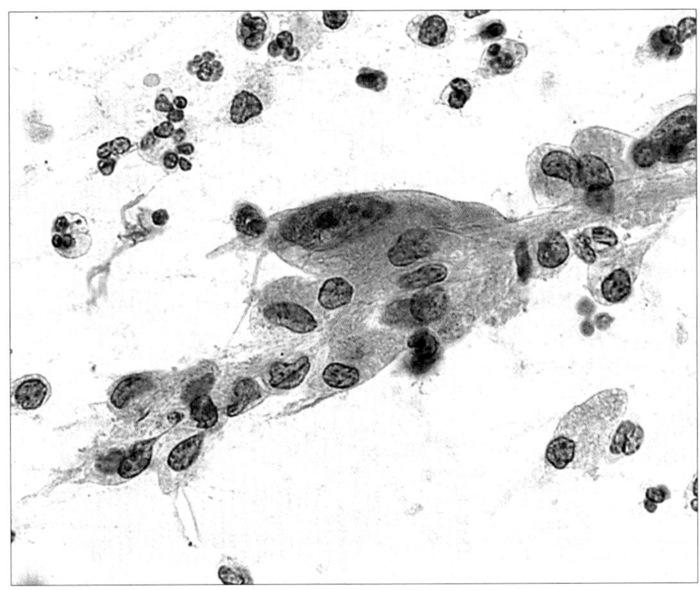

53. A 55-year-old man with a dull pain located on the right side of his abdomen presents for evaluation. The physician notes anorexia and anemia. Guaiac is positive for occult blood. Colonic brushings reveal these cells. The diagnosis is most consistent with:

A. villous adenoma
B. large cell lymphoma
C. adenocarcinoma, poorly differentiated
D. melanoma

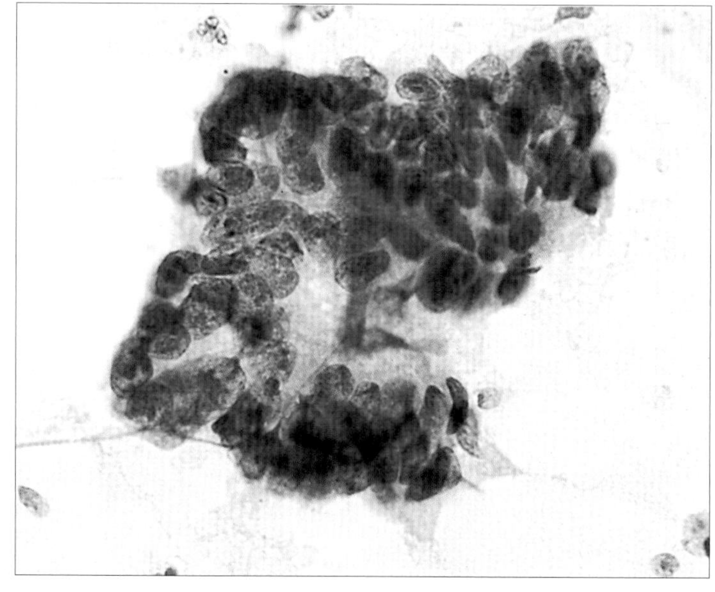

54. A 34-year-old AIDS patient presents with rectal adhesions. These cells, identified upon rectal swabbing, are diagnostic of:

A. cytomegalovirus
B. herpesvirus
C. reactive/reparative changes
D. adenocarcinoma

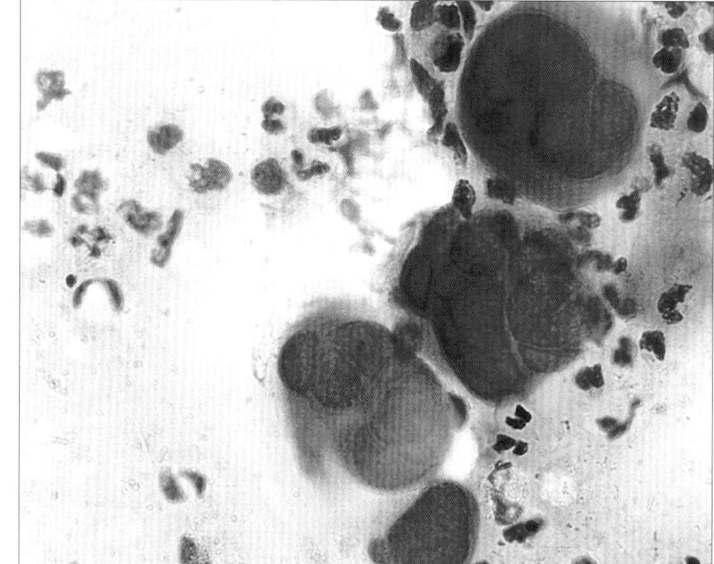

55. A 44-year-old man complaining of rectal bleeding presents with a 2-cm lesion of the sigmoid region of the colon. These cells, identified in a colonic brushing, are diagnostic of:

A. adenocarcinoma, well differentiated
B. normal colonic mucosa
C. ulcerative colitis
D. villous adenoma

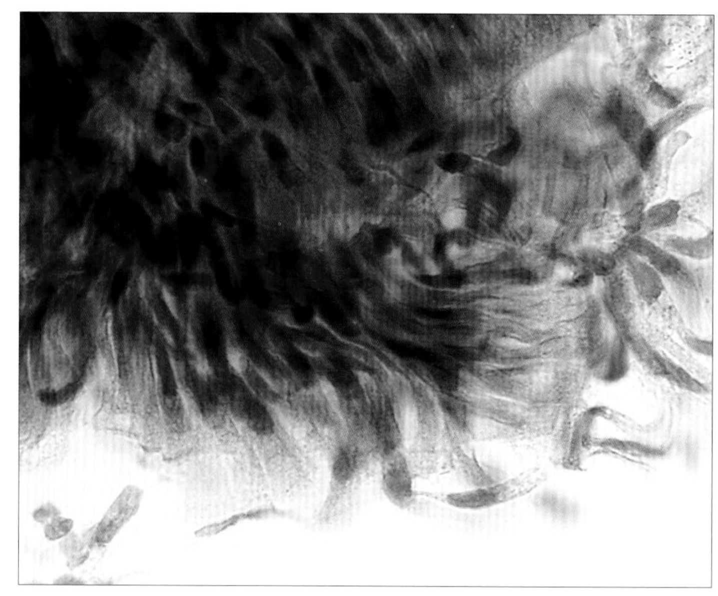

56. This photomicrograph is from a cell block of an alimentary tract neoplasm. A clinical symptom of this patient would be:

A. long-standing dysphagia
B. aspirin gastritis
C. steatorrhea
D. bloody stool

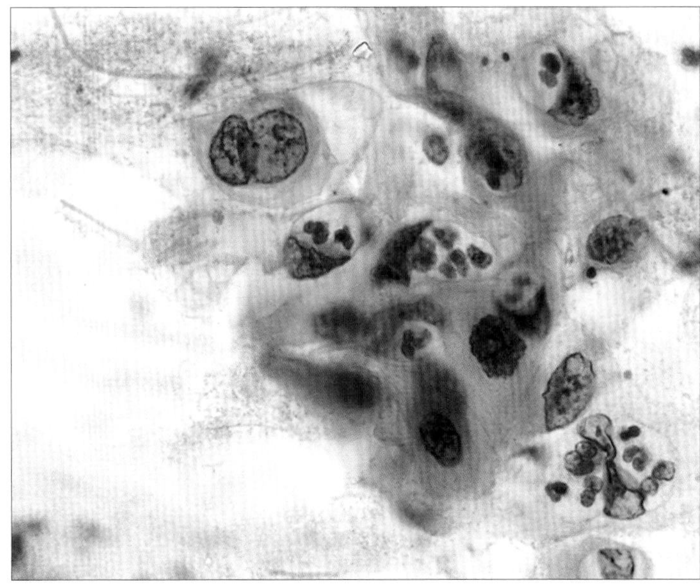

57. A 50-year-old woman underwent an esophageal brushing. Which clinical condition best explains these cellular findings?

A. chronic esophageal reflux
B. herpetic esophagitis
C. granulomatous esophagitis
D. syphilitic esophagitis

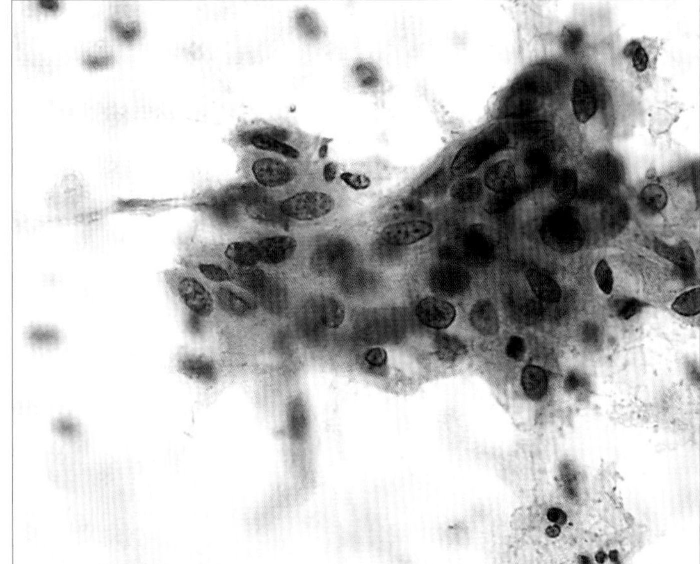

58. This is a histologic section of gastric mucosa stained with periodic acid–Schiff. The findings are consistent with:

A. adenocarcinoma, well differentiated
B. adenocarcinoma, poorly differentiated
C. intestinal metaplasia
D. normal mucus neck cells

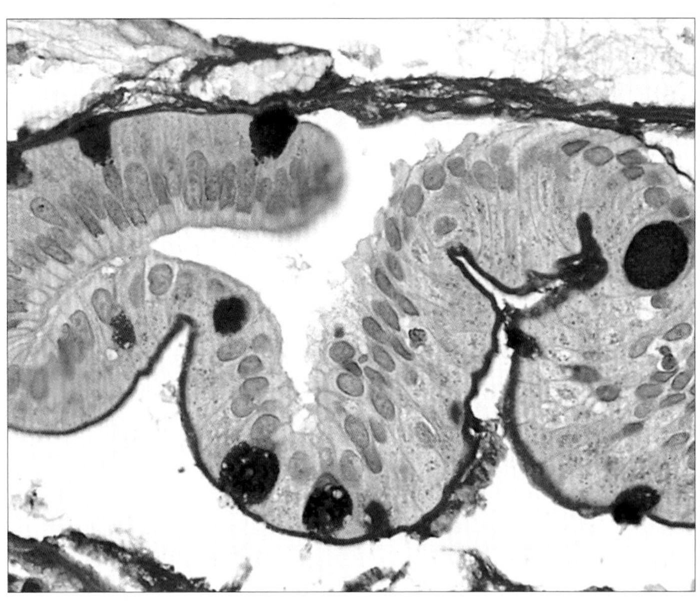

59. **Represented is a gastric wash specimen taken from a 55-year-old man. The cellular finding is:**

A. primary adenocarcinoma
B. reparative/regenerative changes
C. respiratory tract contaminants
D. pernicious anemia

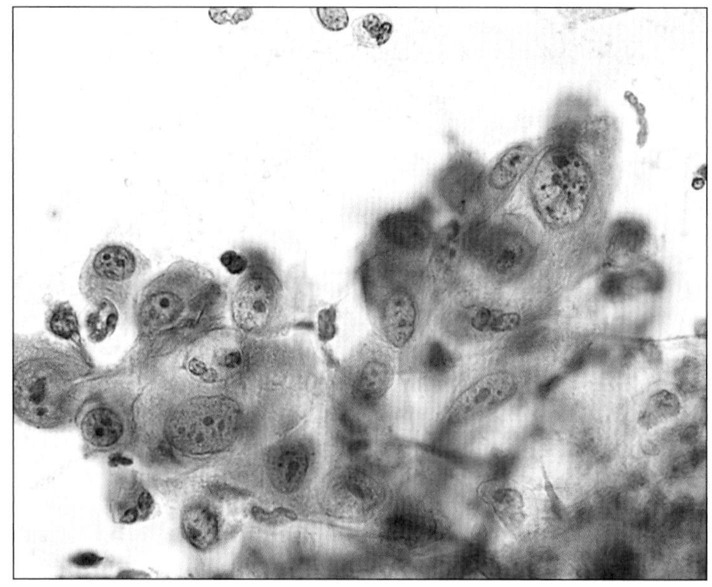

60. **These elements identified in an esophageal brushing from a 50-year-old man with dysphagia suggest:**

A. leiomyosarcoma
B. food contamination
C. leiomyoma
D. metastatic sarcoma, not otherwise specified

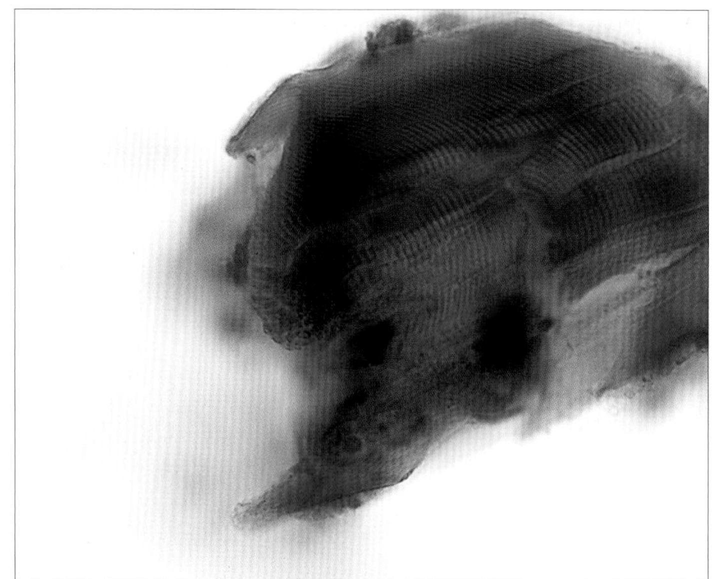

61. **A 60-year-old man with a 20-year history of excessive alcohol intake as well as smoking presents with a 2-cm mucosal lesion. An esophageal brushing reveals:**

A. squamous cell carcinoma, nonkeratinizing
B. atypical laryngeal cells, "Pap" cells
C. moderate keratinizing squamous dysplasia
D. squamous cell carcinoma, keratinizing

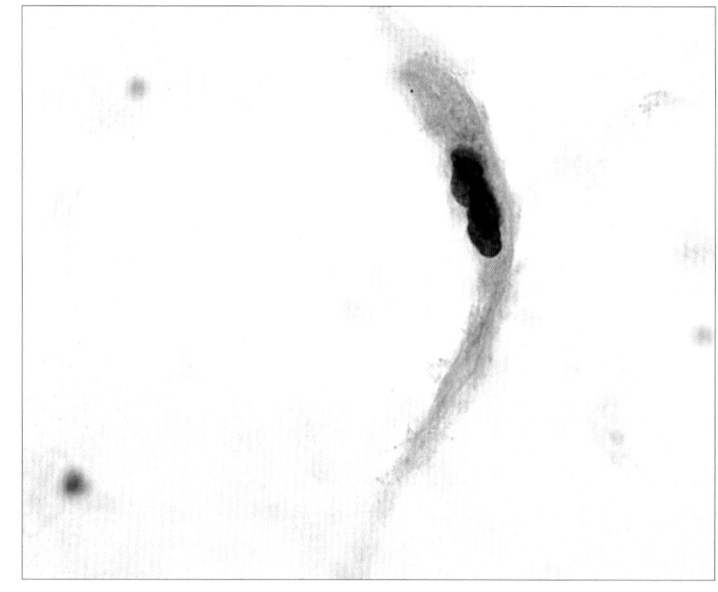

62. **A 62-year-old woman previously diagnosed with reflux esophagitis presents with dysphagia. Esophageal brushings reveal these cells, which are compatible with:**

A. reactive/reparative changes
B. squamous cell carcinoma
C. atypical squamous cells
D. squamous dysplasia

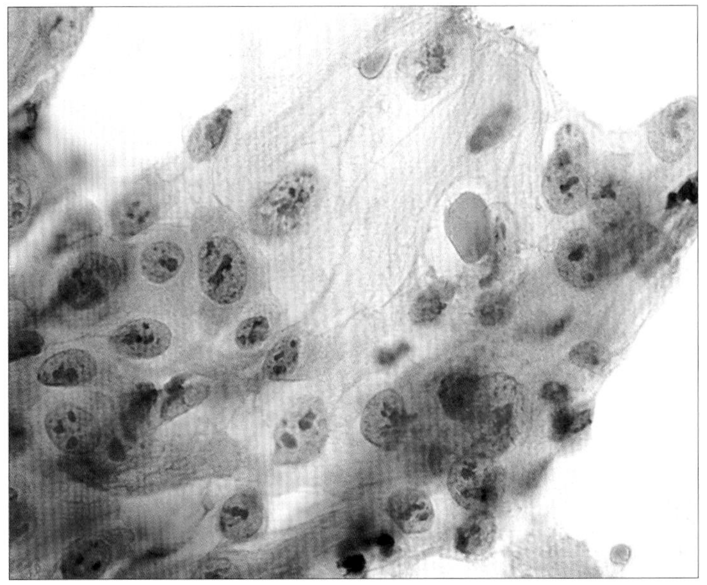

63. **These cells represent a gastric brushing from a 65-year-old man with a history of chronic atrophic gastritis secondary to pernicious anemia. The cellular pattern represents:**

A. parietal cells
B. intestinal metaplasia
C. Crohn disease
D. a gastric ulcer

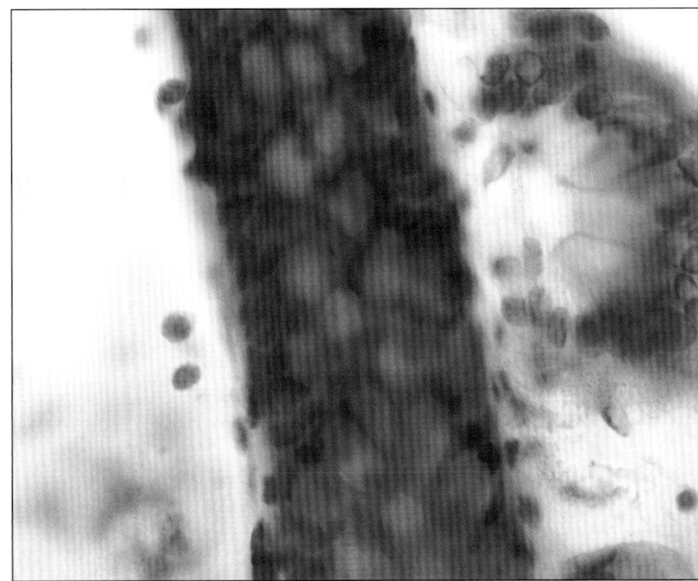

64. **A 55-year-old man with Crohn disease presents for an esophageal brushing. The cytologic pattern depicted is:**

A. squamous cell carcinoma, nonkeratinizing
B. granulomatous esophagitis
C. pemphigus vulgaris
D. Barrett metaplasia

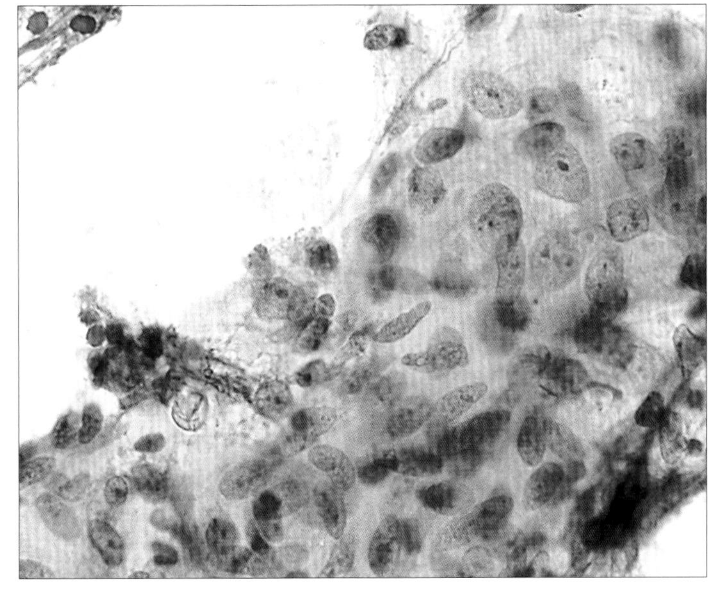

65. **These cells were identified in a gastric washing specimen from a patient with hematemesis. The findings are consistent with:**

A. normal gastric mucosa
B. intestinal metaplasia
C. parasitic infection
D. vegetable contaminant

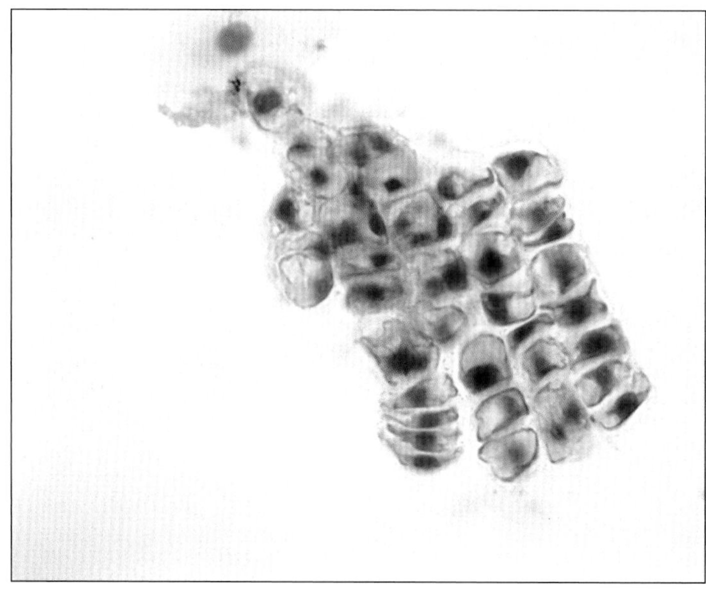

66. **These cells were collected from a gastric brush specimen in a patient complaining of GI pain and weight loss. GI bleeding was clinically confirmed. Cytology reveals:**

A. adenocarcinoma, well-differentiated intestinal type
B. reactive/reparative
C. granulation tissue
D. adenocarcinoma, poorly differentiated gastric type

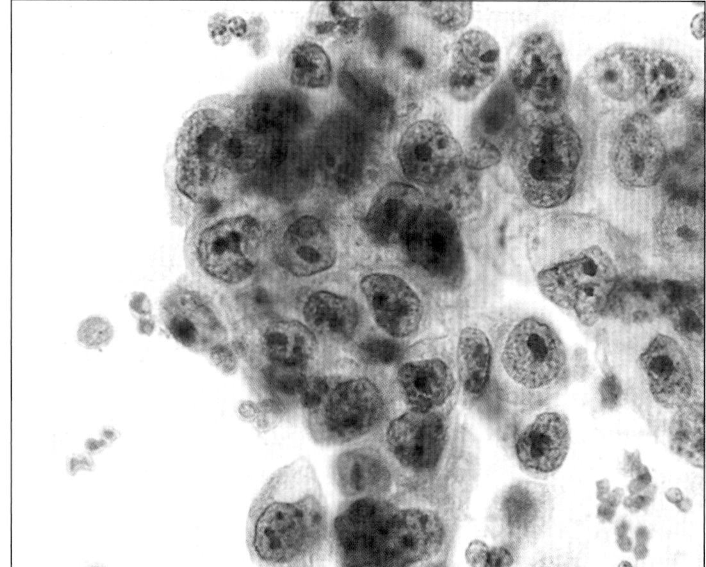

67. **A patient receiving corticosteroid therapy for advanced rheumatoid arthritis underwent esophageal brushing. This process reveals:**

A. rheumatoid granuloma
B. *Candida albicans*
C. *Geotrichum candidum*
D. *Aspergillus* sp.

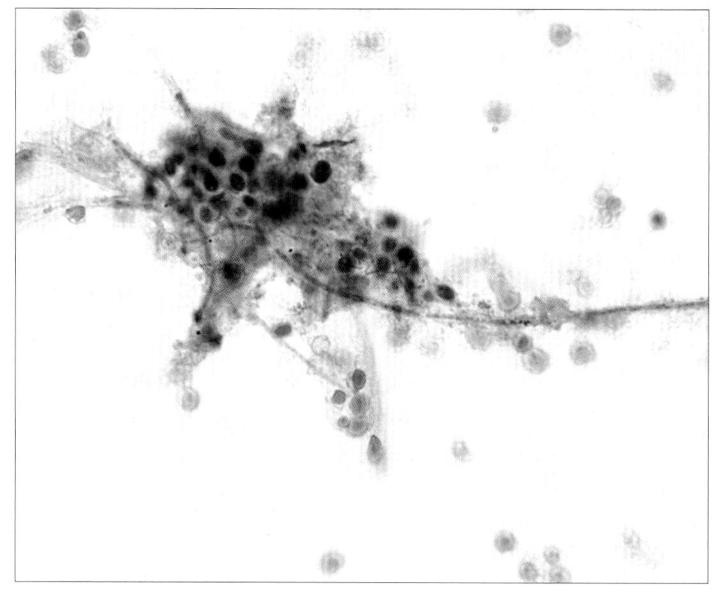

68. **These cells were collected from a 66-year-old man with a history of hyperplastic gastric polyps. The cytologic pattern represents:**

A. intestinal metaplasia
B. normal gastric mucosa
C. pernicious anemia/B_{12} deficiency
D. granulation tissue associated with ulceration

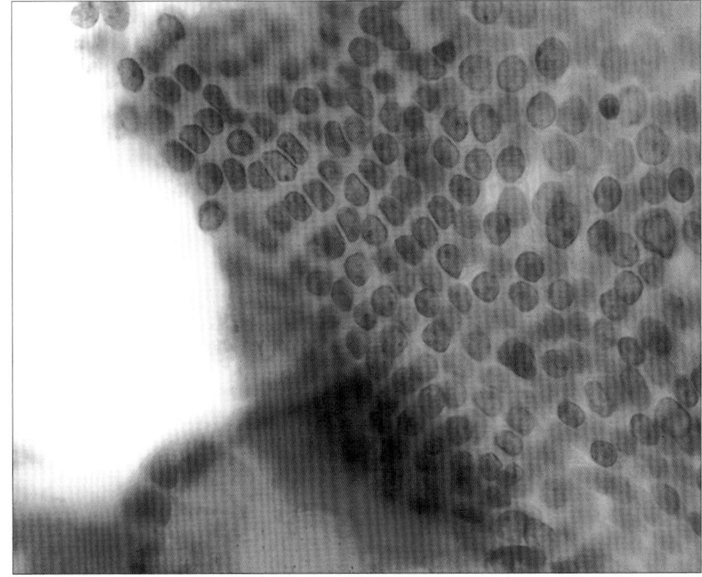

69. **A 55-year-old man with a history of giardiasis presents for a colonoscopy. Colonic brushings reveal these cells. These cells are associated with:**

A. adenocarcinoma, well differentiated
B. villous adenoma
C. fibroma
D. reactive/reparative changes secondary to ulcerative colitis

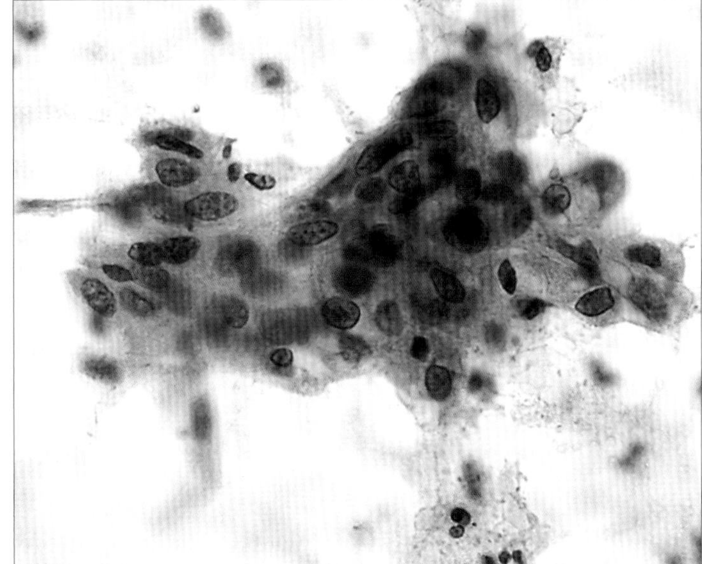

70. **A 44-year-old transplant recipient develops multiple sores within the esophagus. An esophageal brushing is performed. The cellular finding is most compatible with:**

A. pernicious anemia
B. Plummer-Vinson syndrome
C. herpes
D. pemphigus vulgaris

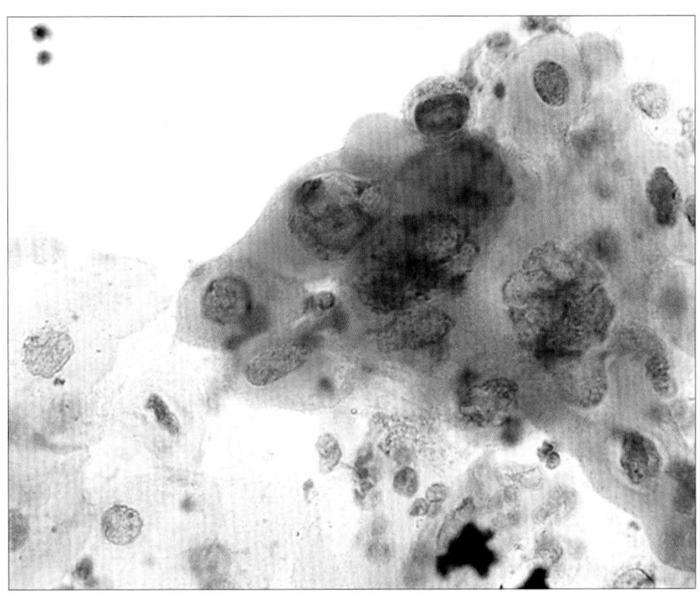

Gastrointestinal Tract ***Answer Key***

1. **A Peutz-Jeghers syndrome**

These lesions are hamartomatous polyps composed of benign glandular elements and smooth muscle.

DeMay RM, The Art & Science of Cytopathology.
Benign tumors, p. 352.

2. **C Krukenberg tumor**

Poorly differentiated adenocarcinomas may metastasize bilaterally to the ovaries. These metastases are renamed Krukenberg tumors.

DeMay RM, The Art & Science of Cytopathology.
Photomicrograph 18.54, p. 304.

3. **A ulcerative colitis**

These patients have an increased risk for development of malignant neoplasia. Lesions arising from ulcerative colitis are generally poorly differentiated with multiple foci.

DeMay RM, The Art & Science of Cytopathology.
Ulcerative colitis, p. 354.

4. **A counting >10 mitotic figures per high-power field**

It may be quite difficult to distinguish leiomyomas from leiomyosarcomas using conventional cytological morphology. Generally, leiomyosarcomas are more cellular, contain irregular chromatin, and are impressively pleomorphic. However, it is important to count the number of mitotic figures per high-power field (HPF) with histopathology to accurately evaluate the aggressiveness of this lesion or determine its malignant nature. Lesions containing less than 5 mitotic figures per HPF are usually considered benign, between 5 and 10 is borderline, while those possessing over 10 mitoses per HPF are considered malignant.

DeMay RM, The Art & Science of Cytopathology.
Smooth muscle tumors, p. 350.

5. **A villous adenoma**

Villous adenomas are considered premalignant lesions found within the gastrointestinal tract. The sensitivity of cytologic morphology may be inadequate in distinguishing these lesions from well-differentiated adenocarcinomas. It is estimated that 25–75% of villous adenomatous polyps will undergo malignant transformation if surgical resection is not performed. These papillary lesions are also diagnostic within the colon.

DeMay RM, The Art & Science of Cytopathology.
Adenoma, p. 354.

6. **A PAS**

Periodic acid-Schiff (PAS) will stain mucoproteins, mucolipids, and glycoproteins. Cells associated with intestinal metaplasia contain mucin-containing "windows." Oil red O stains lipids/fat (answer B), GMS stains fungi (answer C), and Congo red stains amyloid (answer D).

DeMay RM, The Art & Science of Cytopathology.
Intestinal metaplasia, pp. 343–344.

7. **B reparative/regenerative changes**

Reactive/reparative changes seen within the colon are associated with ulcerative colitis, chronic irritation, or trauma. It is imperative to differentiate these conditions from well-differentiated adenocarcinomas. Cellular predictability, preserved polarity, hypochromasia, and the absence of nuclear compression are found with repair. Single malignant cells, true tissue fragments, and tall columnar cell morphology containing hyperchromatic nuclei with irregular chromatin are critical for establishing a diagnosis of colonic adenocarcinoma.

DeMay RM, The Art & Science of Cytopathology.
Reactive cells: repair/regeneration, p. 353.

8. **D alcoholic cirrhosis**

Carcinoembryonic antigen (CEA) is associated with colonic adenocarcinoma and may prove to be a useful indicator of metastatic carcinoma. There are several conditions, however, which may be falsely positive for CEA, including alcoholic cirrhosis, inflammatory bowel disease, and pancreatitis.

DeMay RM, The Art & Science of Cytopathology.
Oncofetal antigens (carcinoembryonic antigen [CEA]), p. 18.

9. **D reactive/reparative changes**

Reactive/reparative changes seen within the colon are associated with ulcerative colitis, chronic irritation, or trauma. It is imperative to differentiate these conditions from well-differentiated adenocarcinomas. Cellular predictability, preserved polarity, hypochromasia, and the absence of nuclear compression are found with repair. Single malignant cells, true tissue fragments, and tall columnar cell morphology containing hyperchromatic nuclei with irregular chromatin are critical for establishing a diagnosis of colonic adenocarcinoma.

DeMay RM, The Art & Science of Cytopathology.
Reactive and degenerative changes, p. 351.

10. **C** carcinoid tumor

Carcinoid tumors are the second most common tumor of the duodenum. These argentaffin tumors are neural ectodermal in origin and represent an amine precursor uptake and decarboxylase (APUD) lesion. Their stem cell is the Kulchitsky cell. The diagnosis of carcinoid tumors relies on two-dimensional aggregates of cells with finely granular, regularly distributed chromatin, inconspicuous nucleoli, and abundant granular cytoplasm. Immunocytochemical staining for chromogranin will help elucidate these lesions.

DeMay RM, The Art & Science of Cytopathology.
Carcinoid tumors, p. 352.

11. **B** rare

Although most carcinomas of the small bowel are metastatic, primary lesions can include adenocarcinomas, large cell lymphocytic lymphomas, and carcinoid tumors. MC

DeMay RM, The Art & Science of Cytopathology.
Malignant tumors, p. 352, and Small intestine, p. 351.

12. **D** chronic follicular gastritis

A polymorphic population of small mature lymphocytes, larger immunoblasts, plasma cells, and tingible body macrophages is pathognomonic of pseudolymphoma, chronic follicular gastritis, or benign lymphoreticular hyperplasia. Most cases of chronic follicular gastritis are associated with gastric ulcers and may be concomitantly associated with highly reactive epithelial fragments.

DeMay RM, The Art & Science of Cytopathology.
Lymphocytes, p. 342.

13. **B** smooth muscle in origin

The presence of smooth muscle cells may be associated with leiomyoma and leiomyosarcoma. It may be quite difficult to distinguish leiomyomas from leiomyosarcomas using conventional cytological morphology. Generally, leiomyosarcomas are more cellular, contain irregular chromatin, and are impressively pleomorphic. However, it is important to count the number of mitotic figures per high power field (HPF) with histopathology to accurately evaluate the aggressiveness of this lesion or determine its malignant nature. Lesions containing less than 5 mitotic figures per HPF are usually considered benign, between 5 and 10 is borderline, while those possessing over 10 mitoses per HPF are considered malignant.

DeMay RM, The Art & Science of Cytopathology.
Leiomyoma, p. 345.

14. **B** *Helicobacter pylori*

These gram-negative, spiral-shaped flagellated, bacteria stain positive with Warthin-Starry, Giemsa, or Dieterle stains. Papanicolaou staining may reveal these bacteria, although often poorly (oil immersion may be required).

DeMay RM, The Art & Science of Cytopathology.
Organisms (Helicobacter [campylobacter] pylori), p. 344.

15. **A** colorectal adenocarcinoma

Adenocarcinomas arising within the small bowel cytologically recapitulate intestinal-type adenocarcinoma. The differential diagnoses include adenocarcinomas of the pancreas, bile duct, and ampulla of Vater.

DeMay RM, The Art & Science of Cytopathology.
Malignant tumors, p. 352.

16. **D** adenocarcinoma

Colonic adenocarcinomas may be related to benign conditions such as ulcerative colitis, villous adenomas, or familial polyposis. Most adenocarcinomas occur within the rectosigmoid region, are polypoid or ulcerative, and are generally moderately well differentiated at the time of detection.

DeMay RM, The Art & Science of Cytopathology.
Adenocarcinoma, p. 355.

17. **B** Fontana

Carcinoid tumors contain argentaffin granules (serotonin) which stain positively with the Fontana stain.

DeMay RM, The Art & Science of Cytopathology.
Carcinoid tumors, p. 352.

18. **A** adenocarcinoma

Duodenal adenocarcinomas mimic colonic adenocarcinoma, possessing polypoid growth patterns, and often create stenosis. These lesions are extremely uncommon.

DeMay RM, The Art & Science of Cytopathology.
Adenocarcinoma, p. 352.

19. **B** adenocarcinoma, poorly differentiated

Poorly differentiated adenocarcinomas are generally not difficult to establish as malignant due to myriad abnormal features as well as signet ring cells.

DeMay RM, The Art & Science of Cytopathology.
Adenocarcinoma, p. 355.

20. **D** *Giardia lamblia*

These protozoa are associated with fatty stools, or steatorrhea, and may be diagnosed cytologically as blue to gray organisms with four pairs of flagella. Trophozoites closely resemble those of *Trichomonas* with the exception that *Giardia* are binucleated and have a ventral sucking disk. In addition, they lack an undulating membrane.

DeMay RM, The Art & Science of Cytopathology.
Giardia lamblia, p. 351.

21. **C intestinal metaplasia**

Intestinal metaplasia is a premalignant gastric condition related to chronic atrophic gastritis in which normal columnar epithelial cells are replaced with cells of intestinal type. Cytology reveals sheets of normal glandular epithelium with interspersed goblet cells. Periodic acid-Schiff will stain mucoproteins, mucolipids, and glycoproteins. Cells associated with intestinal metaplasia possess mucin-containing "windows." Cytology represents cohesive sheets of mucus neck cells with scattered goblet cells with large signet ring vacuoles.

DeMay RM, The Art & Science of Cytopathology.
Intestinal metaplasia, p. 343.

22. **C pernicious anemia**

Pernicious anemia (PA) occurs as a result of impaired absorption of vitamin B_{12} due to the absence of intrinsic factor. This condition gives rise to atrophic gastritis due to the loss of gastric parietal cells. Cytologically, cells possess enlarged nuclei with karyolytic features and bland nuclear folds. An increase in gastric carcinoma has been associated with PA.

DeMay RM, The Art & Science of Cytopathology.
Vitamin deficiency, pp. 333–334.

23. **B normal representative findings**

Squamous mucosa and nongoblet glandular mucosa (a contaminant from the cardiac region of the stomach) represent normal cytologic findings when brushing the distal third of the esophagus. The absence of goblet cell morphology mitigates against a possible diagnosis of Barrett esophagitis.

DeMay RM, The Art & Science of Cytopathology.
The cells, p. 333.

24. **D squamous carcinoma, keratinizing**

Ninety percent of primary esophageal tumors are keratinizing squamous cell carcinomas. Generally, these lesions occur in the middle to distal third of the esophagus. Most lesions are polypoid in nature, but may be endophytic or ulcerative. However, the incidence of signet ring adenocarcinomas (answer C) arising from Barrett esophagus is increasing.

DeMay RM, The Art & Science of Cytopathology.
Squamous cell carcinoma, p. 338.

25. **C reparative/regenerative changes**

The differential diagnosis between reactive/reparative conditions is imperative in gastrointestinal tract specimens. Reparative/regenerative changes that occur in squamous mucosa of the esophagus resemble those found in the female genital tract. Sheets of cells with well-defined cytoplasmic borders, preserved nuclear polarity, predictable nuclear features, fine regular chromatin patterns, micro- to macronucleoli, and characteristic cytoplasmic streaming (squamous) or honeycombing polarity (glandular) are pathognomonic of repair. This process is often associated with ulcerative esophagitis, trauma, reflux, and inflammatory etiology.

DeMay RM, The Art & Science of Cytopathology.
Esophagitis, p. 334.

26. **B smooth muscle cells**

The presence of hamartomatous polyps containing normal gastric mucosa with concomitant smooth muscle proliferation is associated with Peutz-Jeghers syndrome.

DeMay RM, The Art & Science of Cytopathology.
Benign tumors, p. 352.

27. **A single cells**

Single or isolated malignant cells are extremely important in establishing the diagnosis of gastric adenocarcinoma. These cells possess irregular chromatin, macronucleoli, and hyperchromasia. Should single cells be found from changes secondary to reactive/reparative conditions, they would possess normal chromatin features and be next to or associated with the coexisting reparative sheets.

DeMay RM, The Art & Science of Cytopathology.
Adenocarcinoma, pp. 346–347.

28. **C** signet ring cells, single malignant cells

Poorly differentiated adenocarcinoma of the stomach arises from native gastric epithelium—not from intestinal metaplasia. Poorly differentiated adenocarcinomas present as syncytial aggregates or single signet ring cells with nuclear overlapping and compression, increased N/C ratios, pleomorphism, irregular chromatin distribution, and macronucleoli. Malignancies arising from intestinal metaplasia are generally well differentiated.

DeMay RM, The Art & Science of Cytopathology.
Gastric-type adenocarcinoma, p. 347.

29. **B** adenocarcinoma

Predisposition to Barrett metaplasia is often considered an important premalignant change for the subsequent development of adenocarcinoma. Adenocarcinomas of the esophagus must be differentiated from reactive/reparative changes, which generally occur in sheets, not in two- or three-dimensional clusters with malignant nuclear features as described in this explanation. Reparative/regenerative changes that occur in squamous mucosa of the esophagus resemble those found in the female genital tract. Sheets of cells with well-defined cytoplasmic borders, preserved nuclear polarity, predictable nuclear features, fine regular chromatin patterns, micro- to macronucleoli, and characteristic cytoplasmic streaming (squamous) or honeycombing polarity (glandular) are pathognomonic of repair. This process is often associated with ulcerative esophagitis, trauma, reflux, and inflammatory etiology.

DeMay RM, The Art & Science of Cytopathology.
Adenocarcinoma, p. 339.

30. **C** parietal cells

Parietal cells are responsible for the production of hydrochloric acid as well as intrinsic factor. The finding of these cells and chief cells (pepsinogen, rennin, gelatinase) in gastric brush specimens is somewhat rare.

DeMay RM, The Art & Science of Cytopathology.
Parietal cells, p. 342.

31. **D** poorly differentiated

Poorly differentiated adenocarcinoma of the stomach arises from native gastric epithelium—not from intestinal metaplasia. Poorly differentiated adenocarcinomas present as syncytial aggregates or single signet ring cells with nuclear overlapping and compression, increased N/C ratios, pleomorphism, irregular chromatin distribution, and macronucleoli. Malignancies arising from intestinal metaplasia are generally well differentiated. Well-differentiated gastric adenocarcinomas (WDGA) arise from areas of intestinal metaplasia but lack the so-called signet ring cells.

DeMay RM, The Art & Science of Cytopathology.
Gastric-type adenocarcinoma, p. 347.

32. **A** premalignant predisposition

Villous adenomas are considered premalignant lesions found within the gastrointestinal tract. It is estimated that 25–75% of villous adenomatous polyps will undergo malignant transformation if surgical resection is not performed. These papillary lesions are also diagnostic within the colon. The sensitivity of cytologic morphology may be inadequate in distinguishing these lesions from well-differentiated adenocarcinomas.

DeMay RM, The Art & Science of Cytopathology.
Adenomatous polyps, p. 345.

33. **A** pernicious anemia

Pernicious anemia (PA) occurs as a result of impaired absorption of vitamin B_{12} due to the absence of intrinsic factor. This condition gives rise to atrophic gastritis due to the loss of gastric parietal cells. Cytologically, cells possess enlarged nuclei with karyolytic features and bland nuclear folds. An increase in gastric carcinoma has been associated with PA.

DeMay RM, The Art & Science of Cytopathology.
Pernicious anemia, p. 344.

34. **B** primary lymphoma

The absence of cohesive features, scattered bimorphic single cells without vacuolated cytoplasm, and an absence of true tissue fragments is helpful in discriminating this lesion from one of epithelial nature.

DeMay RM, The Art & Science of Cytopathology.
Malignant lymphoma, pp. 349–350.

35. **B** Plummer-Vinson syndrome

Tobacco smoking, increased ethanol intake, achalasia, hiatal hernia, and Plummer-Vinson syndrome may be predisposing conditions for the subsequent development of esophageal cancer.

DeMay RM, The Art & Science of Cytopathology.
Malignant neoplasms, pp. 337–338.

36. **A** fungating

Ninety percent of primary esophageal tumors are keratinizing squamous cell carcinomas. Generally, these lesions occur in the middle to distal third of the esophagus. Most lesions are polypoid in nature, but may be endophytic or ulcerative.

DeMay RM, The Art & Science of Cytopathology.
Squamous cell carcinoma, p. 338.

37. **B** a malignant glandular tumor arising from intestinal metaplasia

Well-differentiated gastric adenocarcinomas (WDGA) arise from areas of intestinal metaplasia but lack the so-called signet ring cells associated with poorly differentiated adenocarcinomas.

DeMay RM, The Art & Science of Cytopathology.
Intestinal-type adenocarcinoma, pp. 346–347.

38. **C** large cell type MC type of lymphoma in GI Tract

Histiocytic or large cell lymphoma is the most common lymphopoietic lesion involving the gastrointestinal tract, including the stomach. These lesions often produce crater-like ulcerations of the gastric mucosa; therefore, a pronounced diathesis may be associated with these malignancies.

DeMay RM, The Art & Science of Cytopathology.
Malignant lymphoma, pp. 349–350.

39. **D** reparative/regenerative cellular changes

Reparative/regenerative changes that occur in the squamous mucosa of the esophagus resemble those found in the female genital tract. Sheets of cells with well-defined cytoplasmic borders, preserved nuclear polarity, predictable nuclear features, fine regular chromatin patterns, micro- to macronucleoli, and characteristic cytoplasmic streaming (squamous) or honeycombing polarity (glandular) are pathognomonic of repair. This process is often associated with ulcerative esophagitis, trauma, reflux, and inflammatory etiology.

DeMay RM, The Art & Science of Cytopathology.
Esophagitis, p. 334.

40. **B** squamous carcinoma, nonkeratinizing

Cell-in-cell arrangement or cannibalism as seen in single, noncohesive cells with the described criteria are suggestive of a poorly differentiated nonkeratinizing squamous carcinoma. These lesions cytologically resemble those poorly differentiated squamous malignancies found elsewhere in the body, often making it difficult to distinguish from adenocarcinoma. Special stains may be needed for confirmation; however, cells negative for mucin do not rule out the possibility of a poorly differentiated adenocarcinoma.

DeMay RM, The Art & Science of Cytopathology.
Squamous cell carcinoma, p. 338.

41. **A** intestinal metaplasia

Intestinal-type adenocarcinoma is derived from long-standing intestinal metaplasia, a benign condition related to chronic atrophic gastritis. These non-signet ring cancers may be well to poorly differentiated. Cytology reveals disorderly thick groups in sheets or microacinar structures with columnar or cuboidal shapes. The nucleus has irregular nuclear membranes, pleomorphic shapes, and is hyperchromatic with coarse irregular chromatin and multiple nucleoli. The presence of abnormal single cells is a key diagnostic feature of gastric adenocarcinoma.

DeMay RM, The Art & Science of Cytopathology.
Adenocarcinoma (intestinal-type adenocarcinoma), pp. 346–347.

42. **C** reactive/reparative process

Reparative/reactive conditions, as found in gastrointestinal specimens, are commonly associated with chronic duodenitis, colitis, giardiasis, benign ulcers, and polyposis. It is imperative to differentiate these conditions from well-differentiated adenocarcinomas. Cellular predictability, preserved polarity, hypochromasia, and the absence of nuclear compression are found with repair. Single malignant cells, true tissue fragments, and tall columnar cell morphology containing hyperchromatic nuclei with irregular chromatin are critical for establishing a diagnosis of colonic adenocarcinoma.

DeMay RM, The Art & Science of Cytopathology.
Reactive/reparative cells and degeneration, p. 342.

43. **C** adenocarcinoma

Duodenal adenocarcinomas mimic colonic adenocarcinoma, possessing polypoid growth patterns, and often create stenosis. These lesions are extremely uncommon.

DeMay RM, The Art & Science of Cytopathology.
Adenocarcinoma, p. 352.

44. **B** native gastric epithelium

Poorly differentiated adenocarcinoma of the stomach arises from native gastric epithelium—not from intestinal metaplasia. Poorly differentiated adenocarcinomas present as syncytial aggregates or single signet ring cells with nuclear overlapping and compression, increased N/C ratios, pleomorphism, irregular chromatin distribution, and macronucleoli. Malignancies arising from intestinal metaplasia are generally well differentiated.

DeMay RM, The Art & Science of Cytopathology.
Gastric-type adenocarcinoma, p. 347.

45. A reactive/reparative changes

Sheets of cells with well-defined cytoplasmic borders, preserved nuclear polarity, predictable nuclear features, fine regular chromatin patterns, micro- to macronucleoli, and honeycombing polarity (glandular) are pathognomonic of repair.

DeMay RM, The Art & Science of Cytopathology.
Reactive cells: repair/regeneration, p. 353.

46. A adenocarcinoma, well differentiated

Colonic adenocarcinomas may be related to benign conditions such as ulcerative colitis, villous adenomas, or familial polyposis. Most adenocarcinomas occur within the recto/sigmoid region, are polypoid or ulcerative, and are generally moderately well differentiated at the time of detection.

DeMay RM, The Art & Science of Cytopathology.
Adenocarcinoma, p. 355.

47. D large cell lymphoma

Histiocytic or large cell lymphoma is the most common lymphopoietic lesion involving the gastrointestinal tract, including the stomach. These lesions often produce crater-like ulcerations of the gastric mucosa; therefore, a pronounced diathesis may be associated with these malignancies.

DeMay RM, The Art & Science of Cytopathology.
Malignant lymphoma, pp. 349–350.

48. C steatorrhea/*Giardia lamblia* infection

This protozoan is associated with fatty stools, or steatorrhea, and may be diagnosed cytologically as blue to gray organisms with four pairs of flagella (some of which will not be visible in a single plane). Trophozoites closely resemble those of *Trichomonas* with the exception that *Giardia* are binucleated and have a ventral sucking disk. In addition, they lack an undulating membrane.

DeMay RM, The Art & Science of Cytopathology.
Giardia lamblia, p. 351.

49. D carcinoembryonic antigen (+)

Carcinoembryonic antigen levels may be monitored by radioimmunoassay analysis. Increased serum levels are associated with recurrent or metastatic colonic adenocarcinoma.

DeMay RM, The Art & Science of Cytopathology.
Oncofetal antigens (carcinoembryonic antigen), p. 18.

50. C Barrett esophagus

Barrett esophagitis/metaplasia is a result of chronic esophageal reflux. The cells must be of goblet cell (signet ring) morphology if the diagnosis is to be established within the distal third of the esophagus because of possible contamination of the esophageal brush from the cardiac region of the stomach. The presence of "cell windows" is helpful in establishing the diagnosis of Barrett esophagus. It is possible to diagnose the condition should intestinal type (goblet) or non-intestinal type gastric epithelium be found in the mid to upper regions of the esophagus. The lesion has been associated with chronic atrophic gastritis and achlorhydria (decreased parietal cells).

DeMay RM, The Art & Science of Cytopathology.
Barrett esophagus, pp. 334–336.

51. B pseudolymphoma

A polymorphic population of small mature lymphocytes, larger immunoblasts, plasma cells, and tingible body macrophages is pathognomonic of pseudolymphoma, chronic follicular gastritis, or benign lymphoreticular hyperplasia. Most cases of chronic follicular gastritis are associated with gastric ulcers and may be concomitantly associated with highly reactive epithelial fragments.

DeMay RM, The Art & Science of Cytopathology.
Miscellaneous cells (lymphocytes), p. 342.

52. A adenocarcinoma, well-differentiated intestinal type

Intestinal-type adenocarcinoma is derived from intestinal metaplasia, a benign condition related to chronic atrophic gastritis. These non-signet ring cancers may be well to poorly differentiated. Cytology reveals disorderly thick groups in sheets or microacinar structures with columnar or cuboidal shapes. The nucleus has irregular nuclear membranes, pleomorphic shapes, and is hyperchromatic with coarse irregular chromatin and multiple nucleoli. The presence of abnormal single cells is a key diagnostic feature of gastric adenocarcinoma.

DeMay RM, The Art & Science of Cytopathology.
Adenocarcinoma (intestinal-type adenocarcinoma), pp. 346–347.

53. C adenocarcinoma, poorly differentiated

True tissue fragments and columnar cell morphology containing hyperchromatic nuclei with irregular chromatin are anticipated findings in colonic adenocarcinoma.

DeMay RM, The Art & Science of Cytopathology.
Adenocarcinoma, p. 355.

54. **B** herpesvirus

Infection with herpesvirus is generally associated with immunocompromised hosts, including patients affected with concomitant HIV infections, patients receiving therapy for malignant disease, or those with other chronic debilitating disorders. Cytologic identification is based on the finding of multinucleated cells containing ground glass nuclei, karyolytic chromatin, nuclear molding, and eosinophilic Cowdry Type A inclusions. Possible contamination from the oral cavity must be considered in the absence of clinically indicated infections.

DeMay RM, The Art & Science of Cytopathology.
Herpes, p. 337.

55. **D** villous adenoma

Villous adenomas are considered premalignant lesions found within the gastrointestinal tract. The sensitivity of cytologic morphology may be inadequate in distinguishing these lesions from well-differentiated adenocarcinomas.

DeMay RM, The Art & Science of Cytopathology.
Adenoma, p. 354.

56. **A** long-standing dysphagia

Ninety percent of primary esophageal tumors are keratinizing squamous cell carcinomas. Generally, these lesions occur in the middle to distal third of the organ. Most lesions are polypoid in nature, but may be endophytic or ulcerative.

DeMay RM, The Art & Science of Cytopathology.
Squamous cell carcinoma, pp. 338–339.

57. **A** chronic esophageal reflux

Reparative/regenerative changes which occur in squamous mucosa of the esophagus resemble those found in the female genital tract. Sheets of cells with well-defined cytoplasmic borders, preserved nuclear polarity, predictable nuclear features, fine regular chromatin patterns, micro- to macronucleoli, and characteristic cytoplasmic streaming (squamous) or honeycombing polarity (glandular) are pathognomonic of repair. This process is often associated with ulcerative esophagitis, trauma, reflux, and inflammatory etiology.

DeMay RM, The Art & Science of Cytopathology.
Esophagitis, p. 334.

58. **C** intestinal metaplasia

Periodic acid-Schiff will stain mucoproteins, mucolipids, and glycoproteins. Cells associated with intestinal metaplasia possess mucin-containing "windows." Cytology represents cohesive sheets of mucus neck cells with scattered goblet cells with large signet ring vacuoles.

DeMay RM, The Art & Science of Cytopathology.
Intestinal metaplasia, pp. 343–344.

59. **B** reparative/regenerative changes

Reparative/reactive conditions, as found in gastrointestinal specimens, are commonly associated with chronic duodenitis, colitis, giardiasis, benign ulcers, and polyposis.

DeMay RM, The Art & Science of Cytopathology.
Reactive/regenerative cells and degeneration, p. 342.

60. **B** food contamination

The finding of striated muscle most often represents meat contamination associated with masticated food.

DeMay RM, The Art & Science of Cytopathology.
Miscellaneous cells (contaminants), p. 343,
and Contaminants (plant cells/food), p. 219.

61. **D** squamous cell carcinoma, keratinizing

Ninety percent of primary esophageal tumors are keratinizing squamous cell carcinomas. Generally, these lesions occur in the middle to distal third of the organ. Most lesions are polypoid in nature, but may be endophytic or ulcerative.

DeMay RM, The Art & Science of Cytopathology.
Squamous cell carcinoma, p. 338.

62. **A** reactive/reparative changes

Reparative/regenerative changes that occur in squamous mucosa of the esophagus resemble those found in the female genital tract. Sheets of cells with well-defined cytoplasmic borders, preserved nuclear polarity, predictable nuclear features, fine regular chromatin patterns, micro- to macronucleoli, and characteristic cytoplasmic streaming (squamous) or honeycombing polarity (glandular) are pathognomonic of repair. This process is often associated with ulcerative esophagitis, trauma, reflux, and inflammatory etiology.

DeMay RM, The Art & Science of Cytopathology.
Esophagitis, p. 334.

63. **B** intestinal metaplasia

Periodic acid-Schiff will stain mucoproteins, mucolipids, and glycoproteins. Cells associated with intestinal metaplasia possess mucin-containing "windows." Cytology represents cohesive sheets of mucus neck cells with scattered goblet cells with large signet ring vacuoles.

DeMay RM, The Art & Science of Cytopathology.
Intestinal metaplasia, pp. 343–344.

64. **B** granulomatous esophagitis

Granulomatous esophagitis resembles granulomatous disease elsewhere in the body—characteristic epithelioid histiocytes and foreign body giant cells are detected cytologically. Acid-fast stains would confirm a tuberculosis etiology; however, other diseases such as sarcoid, syphilis, or Crohn disease may also be related.

DeMay RM, The Art & Science of Cytopathology.
Granulomatous esophagitis, p. 334.

65. **D** vegetable contaminant

Cells with translucent, refractile, squared-off cytoplasm containing smudgy nuclei and intracytoplasmic granules indicate vegetable contamination. Caution should be taken not to confuse these cells with indigenous elements such as metaplasia or squamous carcinoma.

DeMay RM, The Art & Science of Cytopathology.
Miscellaneous cells (contaminants), p. 343,
and Contaminants (plant cells/food), p. 219.

66. **A** adenocarcinoma, well-differentiated intestinal type

Well-differentiated gastric adenocarcinomas (WDGA) arise from areas of intestinal metaplasia but lack the so-called signet ring cells. WDGA must be differentiated from poorly differentiated adenocarcinomas (signet ring type).

DeMay RM, The Art & Science of Cytopathology.
Malignant disease (adenocarcinoma), pp. 346–347.

67. **B** *Candida albicans*

The presence of thin pseudohyphae with interrupted cell walls or spore formations represents *Candida albicans.* The presence of this yeast should be clinically correlated due to its possible representation of oral cavity contamination.

DeMay RM, The Art & Science of Cytopathology.
Candida, p. 336.

68. **B** normal gastric mucosa

Hyperplastic polyps are composed of normal to reactive glandular cells. The cytologic presence of sheets of glandular cells with honeycombing features or cells with enlarged nuclei and well-preserved polarity is characteristic. These lesions have no premalignant association and are often linked to benign inflammatory processes.

DeMay RM, The Art & Science of Cytopathology.
The cells (mucous cells), pp. 341–342.

69. **D** reactive/reparative changes secondary to ulcerative colitis

Reactive/reparative changes seen within the colon are associated with ulcerative colitis, chronic irritation, or trauma. It is imperative to differentiate these conditions from well-differentiated adenocarcinomas. Cellular predictability, preserved polarity, hypochromasia, and the absence of nuclear compression are found with repair. Single malignant cells, true tissue fragments, and tall columnar cell morphology containing hyperchromatic nuclei with irregular chromatin are critical for establishing a diagnosis of colonic adenocarcinoma.

DeMay RM, The Art & Science of Cytopathology.
Ulcerative colitis, p. 354.

70. **C** herpes

Infection with herpesvirus is generally associated with immunocompromised hosts, including patients affected with concomitant HIV infections, patients receiving therapy for malignant disease, or those with other chronic debilitating disorders. Cytologic identification is based on the finding of multinucleated cells containing ground glass nuclei, karyolytic chromatin, nuclear molding, and eosinophilic Cowdry Type A inclusions. Possible contamination from the oral cavity must be considered in the absence of clinically indicated infections.

DeMay RM, The Art & Science of Cytopathology.
Herpes, p. 336.

Chapter 6

Urinary Tract

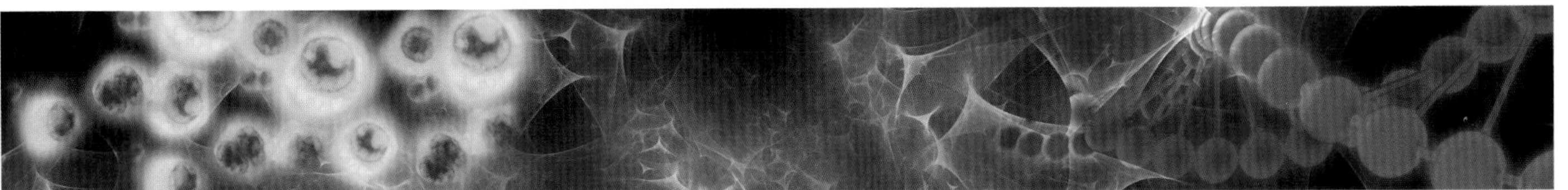

1. When evaluating papillary clusters in a urine specimen, what is imperative?

   A. knowledge of specimen color/texture
   B. knowledge of specimen collection method
   C. knowledge of a history of prostatic carcinoma
   D. knowledge of a history of prostatic hyperplasia

2. A voided urine specimen from a 68-year-old woman reveals a large population of cells with cohesive features, tall columnar morphology, and palisading hyperchromatic nuclei with irregular nuclear membranes and irregular chromatin. A bloody, granular, "dirty" background is noted. What clinical finding would explain these cells?

   A. cystitis
   B. calculi
   C. rectovesical fistula shedding colonic adenocarcinoma
   D. nonpapillary transitional cell carcinoma

3. A 60-year-old man, status post-radical prostatectomy two years, presents with microhematuria and dysuria. Cytologic examination reveals abundant polymorphonuclear leukocytes, red blood cells, and a granular "dirty" background. Scattered degenerated and few well-preserved single and clustered epithelial cells presenting with enlarged smudgy nuclei, irregular nuclear membranes, and macronucleoli are present. The cytoplasm, usually absent, is poorly preserved and vacuolated when present. The cytoplasm is often invaded with neutrophils. The cytologic findings are consistent with:

   A. cystitis-related changes
   B. malacoplakia
   C. heavy metal-related poisoning
   D. transitional cell carcinoma, grade III

4. Cells presenting in loose clusters or papilla, with increased N/C ratios, enlarged hyperchromatic nuclear features, micronucleoli, and irregular chromatin from a voided urine are diagnostic of:

   A. renal cell carcinoma, grade I
   B. reactive urothelial cells
   C. papilloma
   D. transitional cell carcinoma, low grade

5. A 66-year-old man presents with microhematuria and dysuria. Cystoscopy reveals red velvety focal patches on the bladder wall. A voided urine reveals papillary structures with irregular borders, crowded nuclei, and nuclear atypia. The chromatin is coarse and demonstrates clearing. The diagnosis is: 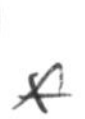

   A. transitional cell carcinoma in situ
   B. papilloma
   C. papillary transitional cell carcinoma, grade I
   D. normal urothelial cells

6. A voided urine specimen from a 42-year-old woman reveals an abundance of squamous cells among a mild inflammatory background. Your interpretation is:

   A. bilharzia
   B. squamous cell carcinoma, well differentiated
   C. unsatisfactory: contamination
   D. pathognomonic of bladder diverticula

7. **A malignancy that may be derived from Brunn nests or cystitis glandularis is:**

A. squamous carcinoma
B. adenocarcinoma
C. renal cell carcinoma
D. transitional cell carcinoma

8. **Bilharzia is associated with an increased risk of developing:**

A. squamous carcinoma of the bladder
B. adenocarcinoma of the bladder
C. transitional cell carcinoma
D. renal cell carcinoma

9. **A bladder washing from a 55-year-old woman showed many flat sheets of polyhedral cells with increased cellular and nuclear size. Cystoscopy was normal. The findings indicate:**

A. transitional cell carcinoma, grade I
B. benign papilloma
C. normal cellular findings
D. atypical hyperplasia

10. **Adenocarcinomas arising within the urinary bladder cytologically resemble:**

A. reactive urothelial cells
B. renal cell carcinoma
C. colonic adenocarcinoma
D. pancreatic adenocarcinoma

11. **In the United States, bladder cancer is more common in ____.**

A. Caucasian women
B. Caucasian men
C. African American women
D. African American men

12. **A post-prostatic massage urine specimen reveals round, concentric, non-calcifying structures in a population of columnar cells. These structures are identified as:**

A. psammoma bodies
B. corpora amylacea
C. cytomegalovirus
D. nonspecific degeneration

13. **Carcinoma of the bladder is ____ common than carcinoma of the renal pelvis?**

A. more
B. less
C. bladder and renal cancer are similar in incidence
D. the incidence of bladder and renal cancer are exactly the same

14. **A catheterized urine specimen contains a sparse population of cells presenting in clusters with scalloping knobby borders and enlarged nuclei with central micronucleoli. A large population of normal transitional cells is also present. The diagnosis is:**

A. reactive transitional cells associated with catheterization
B. transitional cell carcinoma, grade I
C. papilloma
D. adenocarcinoma of the kidney

15. **Cells from a voided urine specimen have abundant vacuolated cytoplasm and large nuclei with macronucleoli. Oil red O stains are positive. The diagnosis is:**

A. renal cell carcinoma
B. melanoma
C. metastatic colonic carcinoma
D. hepatocellular carcinoma

16. **A catheterized urine reveals single cells with coarse, irregular chromatin, and irregular nuclear membranes in a bloody, necrotic background. The diagnosis is:**

A. transitional cell carcinoma, grade III
B. transitional cell carcinoma, grade I
C. squamous cell carcinoma
D. adenocarcinoma

17. **A 55-year-old woman with dysuria undergoes a negative cystoscopy. Cytology of a voided urine specimen reveals many single cells with high N/C ratios, hyperchromasia, and macronucleoli. The diagnosis is:**

A. transitional cell carcinoma, grade III
B. papillary transitional cell carcinoma
C. reactive urothelial cells
D. transitional cell carcinoma in situ

18. **A voided urine specimen contains papillary structures with fibrovascular cores and well-preserved vesicular nuclear features. The best cytologic diagnosis is:**

A. benign papilloma
B. papillary neoplasm, transitional cell carcinoma cannot be excluded
C. transitional cell carcinoma, grade II
D. renal cell carcinoma

19. **A 4-year-old boy presents with hematuria and flank pain. Cytology of a voided urine specimen reveals a mixed population of small, round cells with scanty cytoplasm and hyperchromasia as well as a rare population of spindle cells. The diagnosis is consistent with:**

A. Ewing sarcoma
B. neuroblastoma
C. Wilms tumor
D. embryonal rhabdomyosarcoma

20. **A mucosal neoplasm measuring 2-cm in diameter is found in the urinary bladder of a 61-year-old woman. Cytology of a voided urine specimen reveals a population of small cells occurring singly and clustered with nuclear molding. Nuclear chromatin is coarse and irregular, and micronucleoli are identified. The patient has no previous history of malignancy. Which of the following may represent the findings?**

A. transitional cell carcinoma, low grade
B. Wilms tumor
C. primary lymphoma
D. small cell carcinoma, rule out bladder primary

21. **A 57-year-old woman presents to the clinician with flank pain, microhematuria, longstanding fatigue, and mental confusion. Serum analysis reveals hypercalcemia and abnormal liver function. Cytologic examination of a voided urine specimen reveals abundant degenerated cells found singly or in small groups with large, round, eccentrically located hyperchromatic nuclei and prominent macronucleoli. The cytoplasm, although sparse, is wispy or frothy. Special stains with oil red O, using fresh unfixed urine, reveal rare positive cells. The diagnosis is most suggestive of:**

A. prostatic adenocarcinoma
B. renal cell carcinoma
C. melanoma
D. transitional cell carcinoma

22. **Keratinizing pearls were found along with a population of malignant transitional cells in a voided urine specimen taken from a 51-year-old woman. A hemorrhagic lesion is identified on the anterior wall of the bladder. Your diagnosis is:**

A. metastatic squamous carcinoma
B. normal constituents of the trigone
C. trigone hyperplasia
D. squamous differentiated transitional carcinoma

23. **Which of the following is associated with transitional cell carcinoma of the urinary bladder?**

A. aniline dye exposure
B. asbestos
C. neuroendocrine conditions
D. radium

24. **The observation of isolated cells displaying variation in size and shape; cyanophilic cytoplasm; some cells with intracytoplasmic eosinophilic granules; fine, regular chromatin patterns; micronucleoli; and some multinucleated cells is diagnostic of:**

A. transitional epithelial cells
B. squamous cell contaminant
C. navicular cells
D. renal tubule cells

25. A urine sample containing abundant degenerated columnar cells in a highly cellular inflammatory exudate is most often derived from which of the following collection types?

A. catheterized urine
B. voided "clean catch" urine
C. ileal conduit urine
D. bladder washing

26. Michaelis-Gutmann bodies are associated with:

A. malacoplakia
B. polyomavirus
C. sulfonamides
D. cholesterol plaques

27. A cystic condition involving the Brunn nests is termed:

A. cystitis
B. urethritis
C. barbotage
D. cystitis glandularis

28. Cystoscopy reveals glistening yellow plaques on the bladder mucosa. A voided urine specimen contains a few cyanophilic macrophages with laminated, calcified, intracytoplasmic, PAS-positive structures.
The diagnosis is:

A. *Schistosoma* infection
B. lithiasis
C. transitional hyperplasia
D. malacoplakia

29. Large numbers of cells in groups and clusters, numerous multinucleated cells, vesicular and degenerative nuclear features, and slight anisonucleosis are characteristic of which collection method?

A. voided
B. catheterized
C. post-prostatic massage
D. ileal conduit

30. A patient receiving estrogen therapy for prostatic cancer submits a voided urine speciment for evaluation. Many cells with elongated cytoplasm, low N/C ratios, round to oval nuclei, and finely granular chromatin represent:

A. squamous metaplasia
B. renal tubule cells
C. seminal vesicle cells
D. prostatic adenocarcinoma

31. An HIV-positive patient with complaints of fever and petechiae submits a voided urine specimen for cytologic analysis. Cells with large nuclei and basophilic intranuclear inclusions that demonstrate a clear zone between the inclusions and the nuclear rim are identified. These cells are associated with:

A. cytomegalovirus
B. transitional cell carcinoma
C. polyomavirus
D. lithiasis

32. Colorless flat plate-like structures with cut-out corners in 9 "stairsteps" configuration found in a voided urine are diagnostic of:

A. bilirubin
B. sulfa
C. ammonium urate
D. cholesterol

33. Nuclear degeneration, necrosis, large numbers of erythrocytes, lymphocytes, and neutrophils among a scattered population of renal tubular cells are associated with:

A. chemotherapy-associated changes
B. renal parenchymal disease
C. malacoplakia
D. transitional cell carcinoma

34. What organism possesses a midlateral spine and is often associated with gastrointestinal disease?

A. *Schistosoma haematobium*
B. *Schistosoma mansoni*
C. *Schistosoma japonicum*
D. *Schistosoma egyptii*

35. **A 60-year-old man presents with ureteral obstruction, hematuria, and flank pain. Cytology reveals rare cells with large nuclei, large multiple nucleoli, and abundant clear/vacuolated cytoplasm. Which stain might aid in the diagnosis?**

A. alcian blue-hyaluronidase
B. Gomori methenamine silver
C. Wright-Giemsa
D. Sudan black

36. **A 44-year-old man on corticosteroid therapy presents with urinary stasis. A catheterized urine reveals small cells with elongated/stretched cytoplasm and degenerative smudged nuclei. These cells may represent:**

A. transitional cell carcinoma, grade III
B. hypernephroma
C. polyomavirus infection
D. cytomegalovirus infection

37. **A 50-year-old man being evaluated for prostatic hyperplasia submits a urine specimen for evaluation. Seen are cuboidal to bizarre cells with large, irregular, hyperchromatic nuclei and micronucleoli in single forms and clusters. Cyanophilic cytoplasm with golden-orange granules are found. These cells represent:**

A. transitional cell carcinoma, grade III
B. seminal vesicle cells
C. prostatic adenocarcinoma
D. renal cell carcinoma

38. **The presence of intracytoplasmic eosinophilic inclusions composed of mucopolysaccharide is diagnostic of:**

A. degeneration
B. lithiasis
C. polyomavirus infection
D. herpesvirus infection

39. **A 44-year-old airline flight attendant presents with spiking fever. Urine cytology reveals abundant binucleated single cells with eosinophilic refractile intracytoplasmic granules. Also found were multiple large oval structures with a terminal spine-like structure. Cytology is consistent with a diagnosis of:**

A. idiopathic eosinophilia
B. *Schistosoma haematobium*
C. calculus
D. malacoplakia

40. **The major cause of death related to cervical cancer is:**

A. uremia
B. brain metastasis
C. cervical stenosis
D. meningitis

41. **A 42-year-old man with a history of transitional cell carcinoma is treated intravesicularly with triethylenethiophosphoramide (thiotepa). Cytology reveals many large cells with abundant cytoplasm and proportionately enlarged nuclei. Many cells demonstrate normochromasia and others reveal smudgy nuclear features. Multinucleation is common. Based on the following, these cells are:**

A. recurrent transitional cell carcinoma
B. renal cell carcinoma
C. chemotherapy-associated changes
D. transitional cell carcinoma in situ

42. **Crystalline structures that are described as fine silky needles in sheaves or rosettes are:**

A. cystine
B. calcium carbonate
C. calcium oxalate
D. tyrosine

43. **Areas of mucus-secreting glandular epithelium may represent:**

A. heavy metal exposure
B. cystitis cystica
C. fecal contaminant
D. pyelogram effect

44. **Acid-fast intranuclear inclusions staining eosinophilic with the Papanicolaou stain are found within the cytoplasm of cells of a voided urine specimen. The specimen was taken from a 4-year-old child with abdominal pain. The diagnosis is:**

A. polyomavirus infection
B. degenerative changes
C. infectious mononucleosis
D. lead poisoning

45. **A voided urine specimen from an immunosuppressed patient reveals cells with large basophilic intranuclear inclusions obliterating the nucleus. Electron microscopy indicates many non-encapsulated virions arranged in a crystalline fashion. The diagnosis is:**

A. herpesvirus
B. cytomegalovirus
C. human polyomavirus
D. human papillomavirus

46. **The cytologic findings represent a voided urine specimen from a 55-year-old Egyptian immigrant. These cells represent:**

A. squamous cell carcinoma, bladder primary
B. metastatic squamous cell carcinoma
C. squamous dysplasia
D. normal contaminant from the uterine corpus

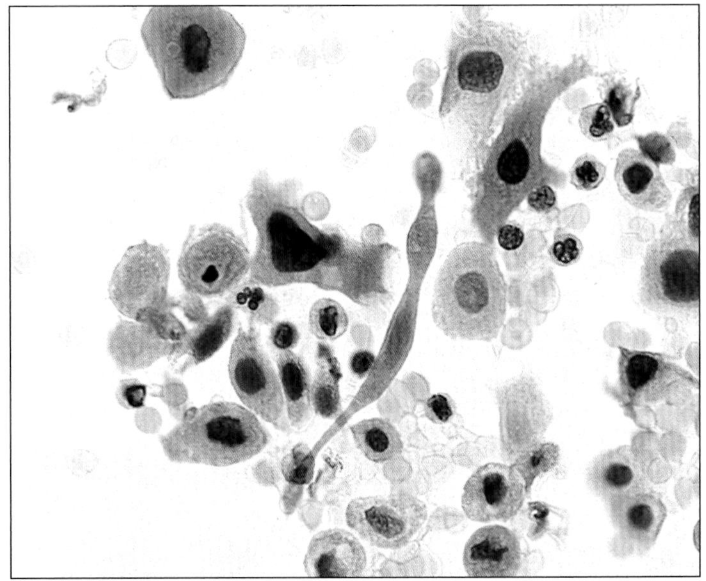

47. **A 66-year-old woman with a history of urinary stones presents with these structures in a voided urine specimen. They represent:**

A. uric acid crystals
B. triple phosphate crystals
C. calcium phosphate crystals
D. calcium carbonate crystals

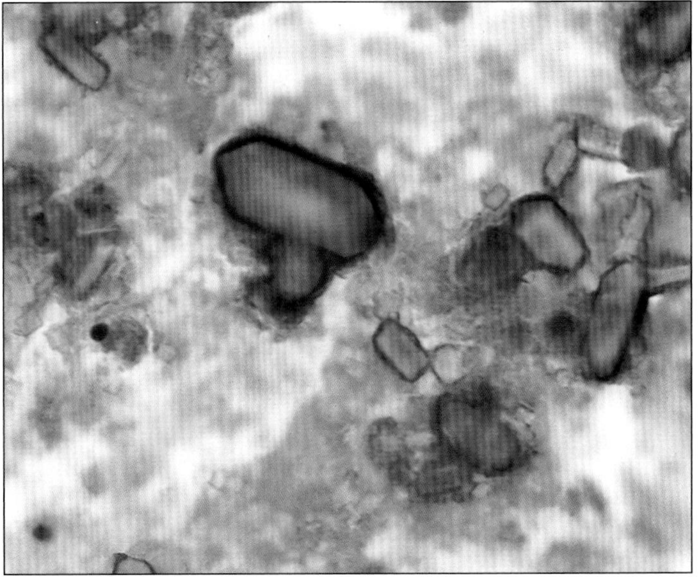

48. **A 26-year-old woman being treated for a gynecologic infection with broad-spectrum antibiotics presents with cystitis and microhematuria. The cytologic findings suggest an infection by:**

A. *Blastomyces* sp.
B. *Aspergillus* sp.
C. *Candida* sp.
D. *Nocardia* sp.

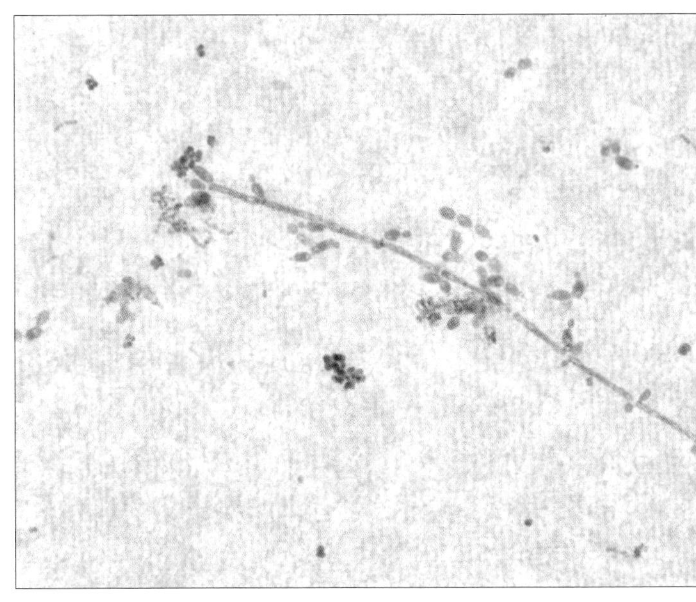

49. **A catheterized urine specimen is collected from a 44-year-old woman with urinary obstruction. The findings suggest:**

A. lithiasis, cholesterol crystals
B. lithiasis, calcium phosphate crystals
C. lithiasis, calcium oxalate crystals
D. lithiasis, calcium carbonate crystals

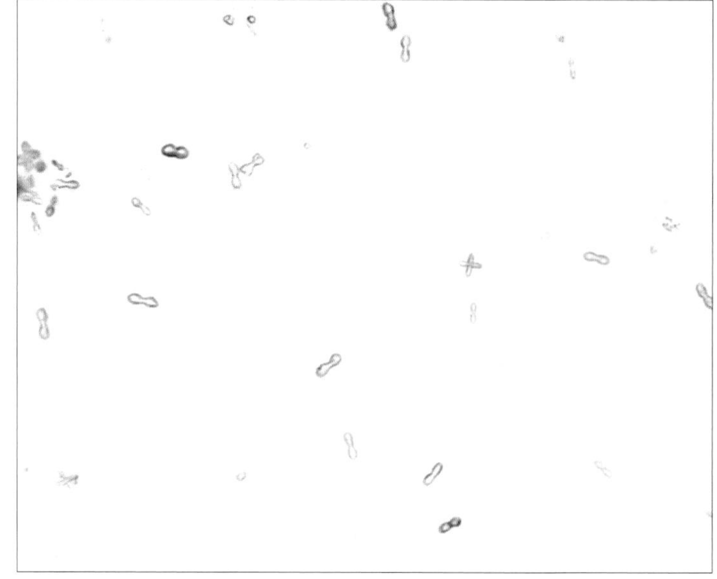

50. **A voided urine specimen from a patient with a negative cystoscopic test result yields these cells for analysis. Their presence suggests:**

A. transitional cell carcinoma, grade III
B. transitional cell carcinoma in situ
C. papillary transitional cell carcinoma, grade I
D. degenerating transitional epithelial cells

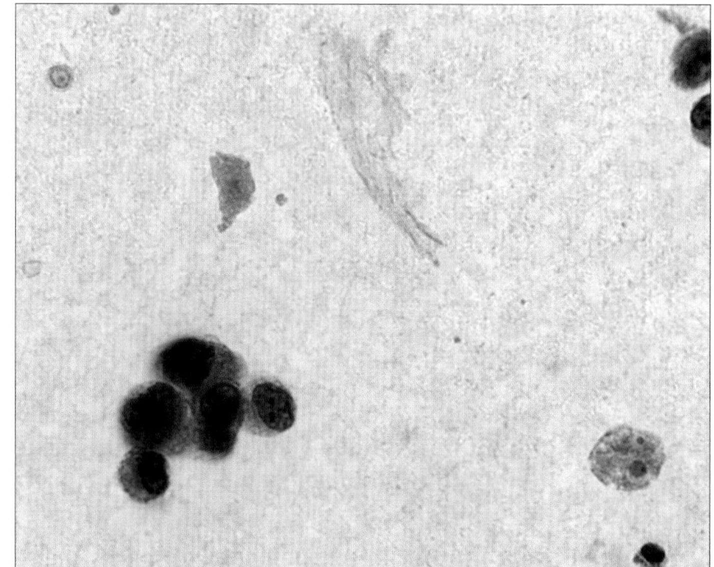

51. **A voided urine specimen from a 55-year-old man yields these cells. The best diagnosis is:**

A. benign papilloma
B. papillary neoplasm, rule out transitional cell carcinoma
C. transitional cell carcinoma in situ
D. reactive/reparative cellular changes

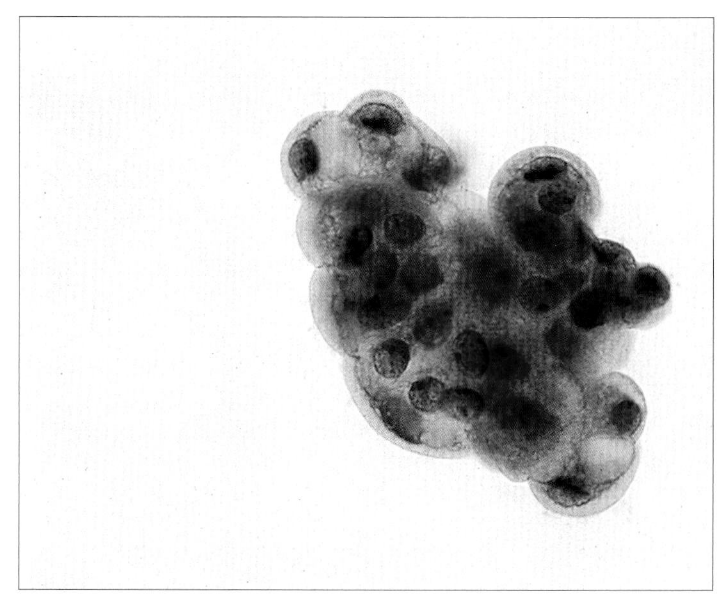

52. A 67-year-old man with urethral obstruction and elevated alkaline phosphatase levels yields a catheterized urine specimen. The cytologic pattern represents:

A. transitional cell carcinoma
B. renal cell carcinoma
C. squamous cell carcinoma
D. prostate adenocarcinoma

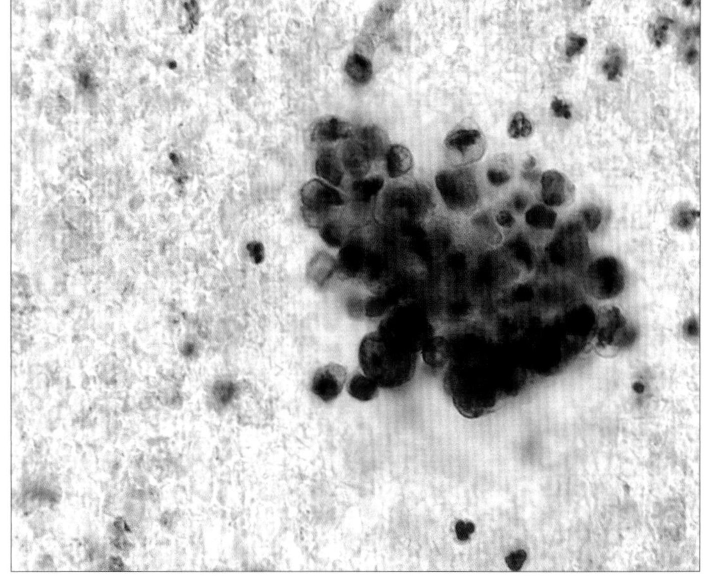

53. These cells are identified in a voided urine specimen in a 45-year-old woman with flank pain and microhematuria. A 3-cm lesion is identified within the renal calyces. What stain will help confirm the diagnosis?

A. mucicarmine
B. oil red O
C. alcian blue
D. Warthin-Starry

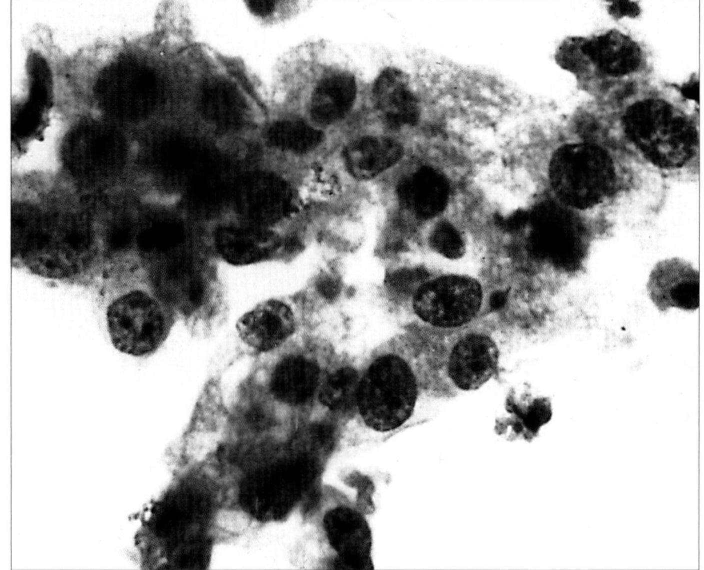

54. These cells were identified in a catheterized urine specimen from a 69-year-old man with an ulcerative lesion and microhematuria. The diagnosis is consistent with:

A. transitional cell carcinoma, grade I
B. renal cell carcinoma
C. transitional cell carcinoma, grade III
D. adenocarcinoma arising from cystitis glandularis

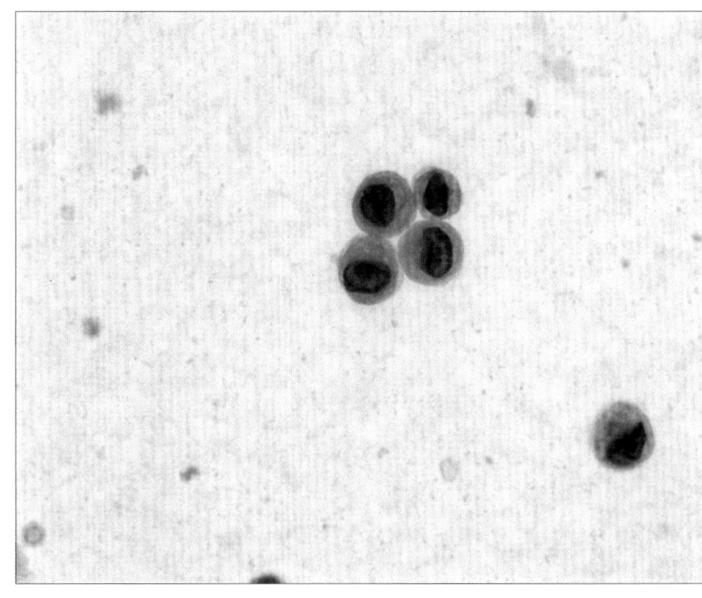

55. These cells in a voided urine specimen are from a 44-year-old woman with hematuria. Their presence is most likely related to:

A. well-differentiated squamous carcinoma
B. vaginal contamination
C. lead poisoning
D. lithiasis

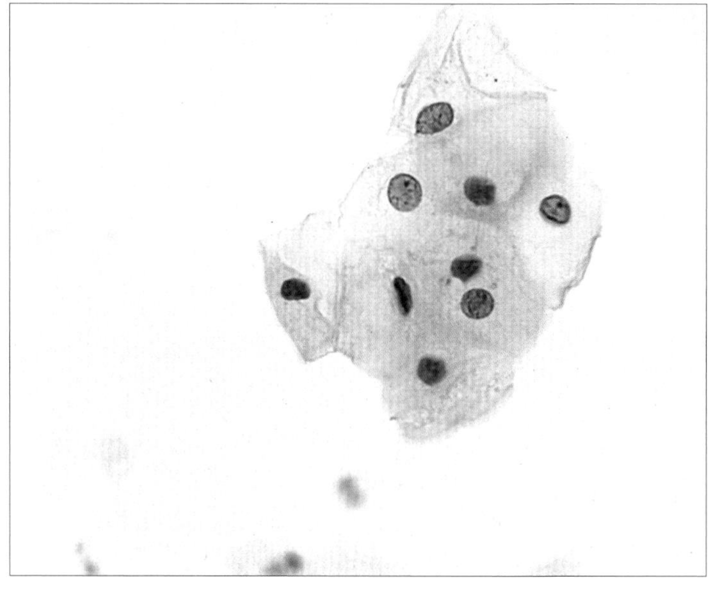

56. This catheterized urine specimen from a 44-year-old woman with cystitis shows:

A. normal catheterized urothelial changes
B. *Escherichia coli*
C. human polyomavirus
D. transitional cell carcinoma, grade I

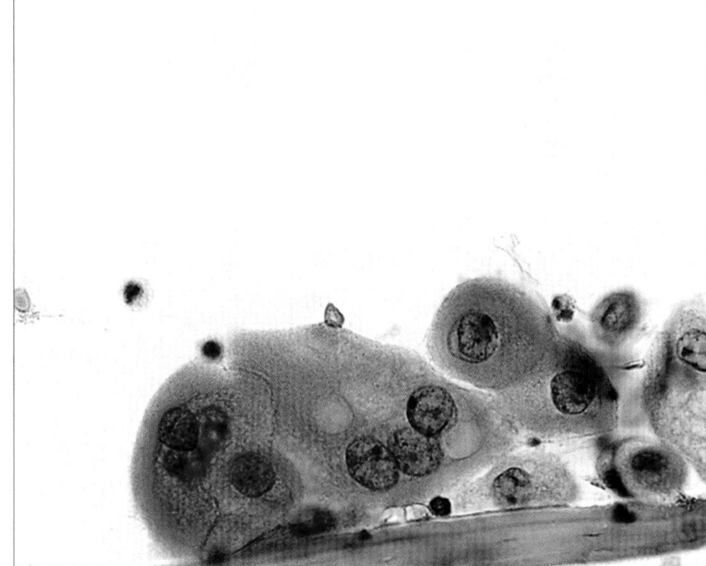

57. These cells in a voided urine specimen may arise from:

A. malacoplakia
B. vulva
C. bladder dome
D. nephron

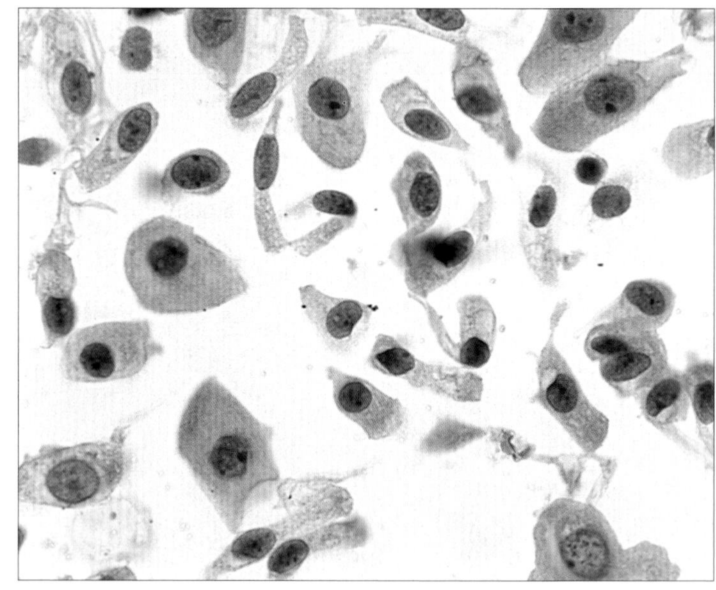

58. **An alkaline urine sample reveals these structures. They are suggestive of:**

A. uric acid crystals
B. triple phosphate crystals
C. calcium phosphate crystals
D. calcium carbonate crystals

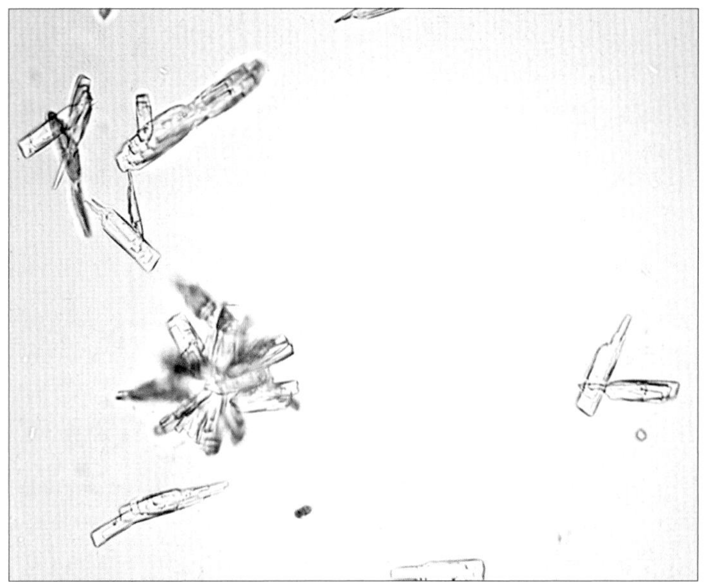

59. **These structures identified in a post-prostate massage specimen are suggestive of:**

A. psammoma body
B. corpora amylacea
C. navicular cell
D. metastatic adenocarcinoma

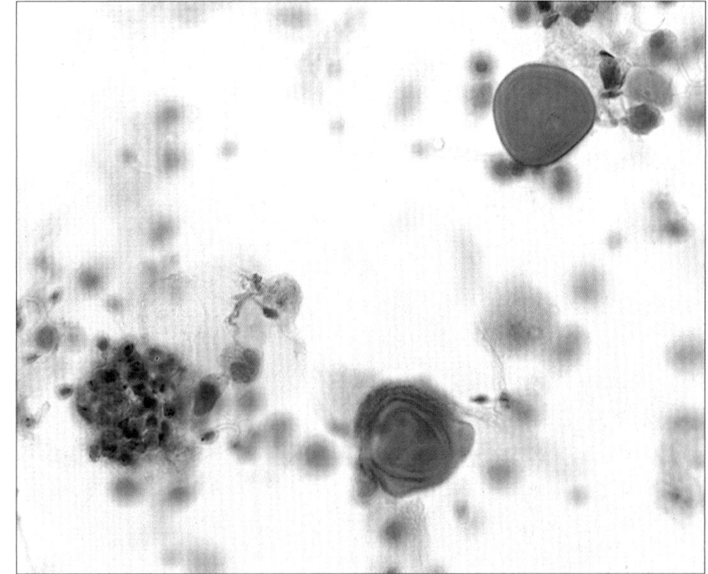

60. **This structure is found in a 55-year-old woman. Which of the following statements is most applicable?**

A. the findings are consistent with malignant renal cell carcinoma
B. the patient has a history of schistosomiasis exposure
C. the patient has a history of malacoplakia
D. this cell is infected with the human polyomavirus

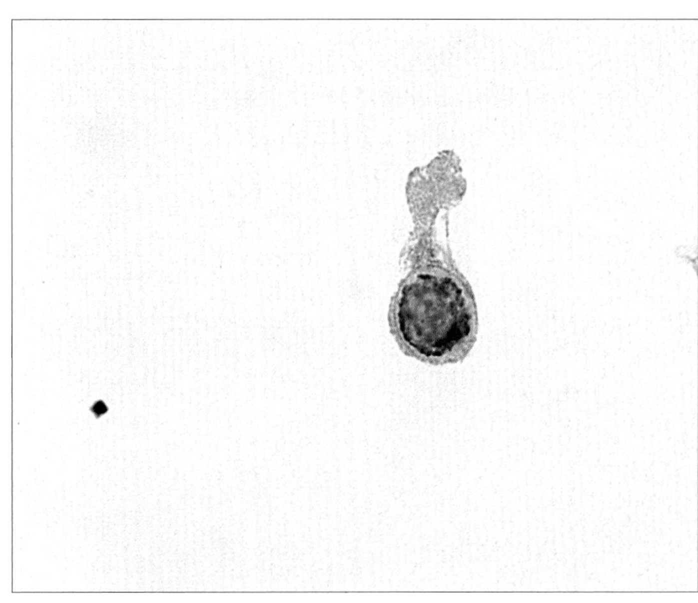

61. **These structures are associated with:**

A. urinary calculi
B. malacoplakia
C. *Escherichia coli* infection
D. carcinoma of the bladder

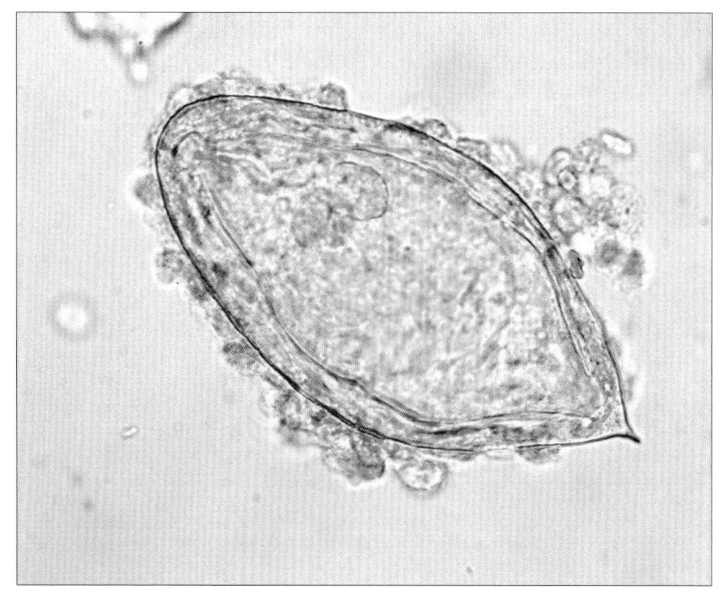

62. **A febrile 2-year-old girl is unable to urinate. A catheterized urine sample reveals these cells. They represent:**

A. herpesvirus
B. cytomegalovirus
C. polyomavirus
D. nonspecific cellular findings

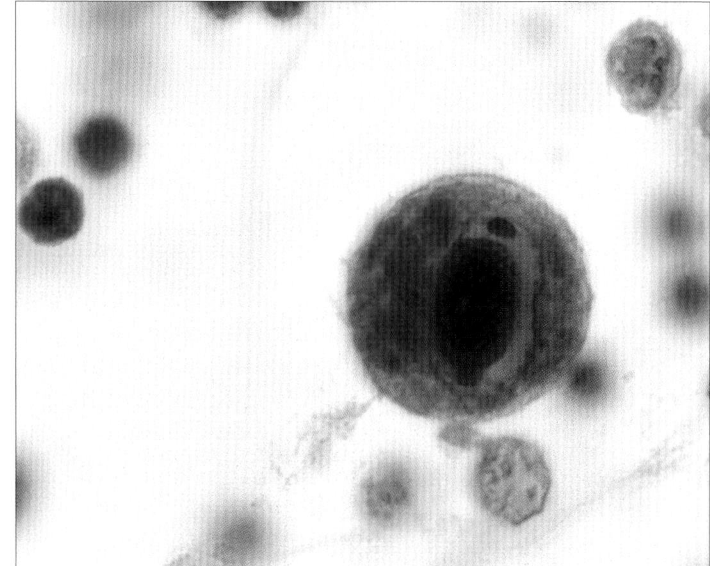

63. **A 55-year-old diabetic man who recently underwent kidney transplantation presents with microhematuria and flank pain. A voided urine specimen reveals these structures. They are:**

A. renal casts
B. columnar transitional cells
C. prostatic cells
D. glomeruli

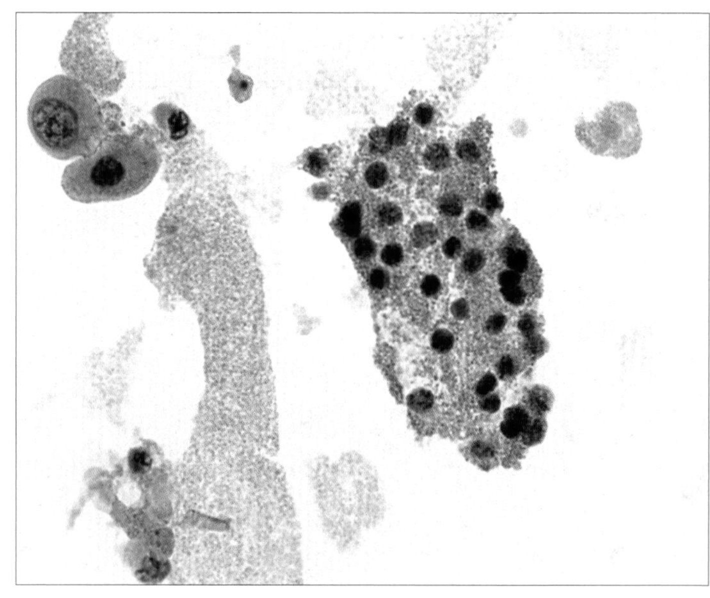

64. **A voided urine specimen from a 55-year-old man with a recent urinary obstruction reveals these cells. The diagnosis is:**

A. prostatic adenocarcinoma
B. benign prostatic hypertrophy
C. normal urothelial cells
D. human polyomavirus infection

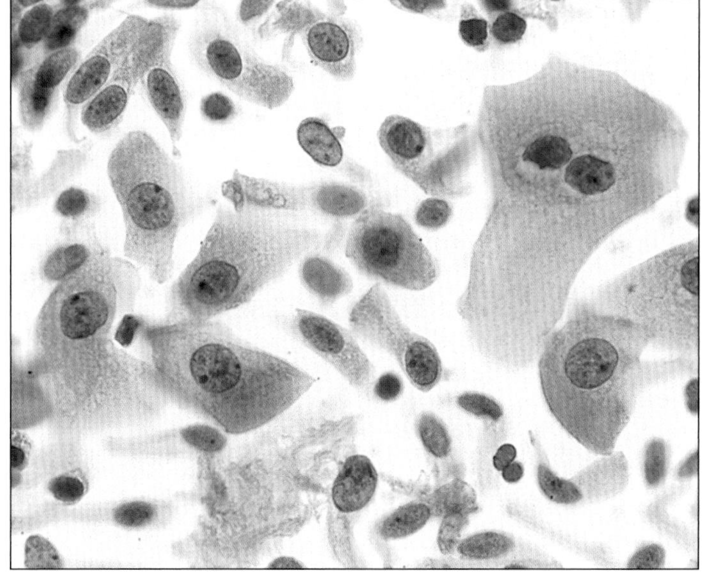

Urinary Tract *Answer Key*

1. **B** knowledge of specimen collection method

Normal catheterized urine specimens contain a hypercellular and heterogeneous population of normal transitional cells that includes dome or superficial cells, sheets of oval intermediate type urothelial cells, squamous cells, and occasional columnar cells, usually from the Brunn nests. The urothelial cells contain round, hypochromatic or degenerative nuclei and granular cytoplasm. Reactive nuclear changes may be detected by the observation of slightly enlarged nuclei and prominent nucleoli; however, normal N/C ratios and benign chromatin patterns detected in well-preserved transitional cells establish their benignity. Careful attention should be given to the differentiation of pseudoclusters (associated with catheterization) from true papillary groupings (such as those found with low-grade papillary neoplasms).

DeMay RM, The Art & Science of Cytopathology.
Catheterization, p. 392, and Papilloma (well differentiated papillary transitional cell neoplasm), p. 401.

2. **C** rectovesical fistula shedding colonic adenocarcinoma

Colonic adenocarcinomas extending into the bladder present with columnar morphology, apical cytoplasmic densities ("terminal bar-like"), and palisading nuclei with classic malignant nuclear criteria. Due to its direct invasion, a granular, necrotic diathesis is also present (most metastatic lesions appear in a clean background unless they have seeded). Clinical history is important in establishing any metastatic lesion.

DeMay RM, The Art & Science of Cytopathology.
Other metastases, p. 409.

3. **A** cystitis-related changes

Cystitis is a common finding in women (due to the short nature of the urethra), often secondary to fecal contamination (infection by *Escherichia coli, Proteus, Klebsiella, Enterobacter, Streptococcus, Pseudomonas*) and in patients who have had genitourinary surgery (such as transurethral resection of the prostate or prostatectomy). Degenerative cells are common, although the preserved transitional cells will often have alarming features, including hyperchromatic nuclei and coarse chromatin with clearing. Malignancy, however, is generally associated with increased necrosis and less inflammation (unless ulcerative), and is usually composed of well-preserved cells with crisp, distinct nuclei and typical malignant features (coarsely granular, irregularly distributed chromatin). Other infectious agents which may be cytologically detected in urinary specimens include trichomonads, amebae, and schistosomes. Cellular changes secondary to tuberculosis may also create mild to severe reactive epithelial atypia.

DeMay RM, The Art & Science of Cytopathology.
Cystitis, pp. 393–395.

4. **D** transitional cell carcinoma, low grade

Loosely cohesive groups and papillae with frankly malignant criteria are diagnostic of transitional cell carcinoma, grade II (low grade). The presence of abnormal nuclear features, including enlarged nuclei and irregular chromatin distribution represent key features of urothelial cell malignancies. Suspicion should be raised if the background contains a population of small pyknotic urothelial cells.

DeMay RM, The Art & Science of Cytopathology.
Low grade TCC, p. 402.

5. **C** papillary transitional cell carcinoma, grade I

The presence of true papillary clusters identified in urinary specimens is suggestive of a low-grade papillary neoplasm. These lesions cannot be excluded from grade I transitional cell carcinoma. In the absence of classic malignant nuclear morphology, the diagnosis of carcinoma remains. These cells present with uniform cell borders, micronucleoli and finely granular, regularly distributed chromatin (when visible). Differentiating these low-grade neoplasms in catheterized specimens may prove difficult; however, the presence of true cohesive smooth borders will help confirm a neoplastic process.

DeMay RM, The Art & Science of Cytopathology.
Significance of papillary clusters, pp. 389–390, and Papilloma (well-differentiated papillary transitional cell neoplasm), pp. 401–402.

6. **C** unsatisfactory: contamination

Vaginal contamination may preclude the possibility of a satisfactory diagnosis in voided urine specimens. Voided urine specimens normally contain a hypocellular population of transitional cells. Squamous contamination may easily obscure urothelial cells or be the sole representative population in unsatisfactory urine specimens.

DeMay RM, The Art & Science of Cytopathology.
Squamous cells and squamous metaplasia, p. 390.

7. **B** adenocarcinoma

Two varieties of adenocarcinoma may arise within the bladder. The first type resembles colonic adenocarcinoma (mucin-positive), while the second variety is a signet ring carcinoma (also mucin-positive).

DeMay RM, The Art & Science of Cytopathology.
Adenocarcinoma, pp. 407–408.

8. **A** **squamous carcinoma of the bladder**

Schistosoma haematobium is a parasitic fluke found in Africa and the Middle East that embeds within the bladder mucosa, eventually creating squamous metaplasia and squamous cell carcinoma. The cytology reveals transparent ova with a terminal spine. Schistosomiasis is also referred to as bilharzia. Differential diagnosis is the lemon drop form of uric acid crystals.

DeMay RM, The Art & Science of Cytopathology.
Transitional cell carcinoma (risk factors), p. 400, and Parasites, p. 394.

9. **C** **normal cellular findings**

Bladder washings or barbotage yield hypercellular specimens consisting of sheets of transitional cells, pseudopapillary fragments, and single cells. Cells from the deeper regions of the transitional epithelium are small, hypochromatic, and exhibit macronucleoli. Reactive nuclear changes may necessitate the differential diagnosis of neoplasia.

DeMay RM, The Art & Science of Cytopathology.
Bladder washes, p. 392.

10. **C** **colonic adenocarcinoma**

Two varieties of adenocarcinoma may arise within the bladder. The first type resembles colonic adenocarcinoma (mucin-positive), while the second variety is a signet ring carcinoma (also mucin positive).

DeMay RM, The Art & Science of Cytopathology.
Adenocarcinoma, pp. 407–408.

11. **B** **Caucasian men**

Bladder cancer is three times more common in men than women, and twice as common in Caucasians than African-Americans.

DeMay RM, The Art & Science of Cytopathology.
Urinary tract cancer, p. 399.

12. **B** **corpora amylacea**

Corpora amylacea are basophilic, condensed, concentrically laminated, glycogenated, noncalcifying structures originating from the prostate.

DeMay RM, The Art & Science of Cytopathology.
Corpora amylacea, p. 391.

13. **A** **more**

In the United States, there are 50,000 new cases of bladder cancer annually and 11,000 deaths, representing about 2% of all cancer-related mortalities. Bladder cancer is 10 to 20 times more common than carcinoma of the renal pelvis and ureter and is increasing in incidence. The average age of patients is between 65 and 70 years (rare before age 40).

DeMay RM, The Art & Science of Cytopathology.
Urinary tract cancer, p. 399.

14. **A** **reactive transitional cells associated with catheterization**

Normal catheterized urine specimens contain a hypercellular and heterogeneous population of normal transitional cells that includes dome or superficial cells, sheets of oval intermediate type urothelial cells, squamous cells, and occasional columnar cells, usually from the Brunn nests. The urothelial cells contain round, hypochromatic or degenerative nuclei and granular cytoplasm. Reactive nuclear changes may be detected by the observation of slightly enlarged nuclei and prominent nucleoli; however, normal N/C ratios and benign chromatin patterns detected in well-preserved transitional cells establish their benignity. Careful attention should be given to the differentiation of pseudoclusters (associated with catheterization) from true papillary groupings (found with low-grade papillary neoplasms).

DeMay RM, The Art & Science of Cytopathology.
Significance of papillary clusters, pp. 389–390,
Catheterization, p. 392.

15. **A** **renal cell carcinoma**

Renal cell adenocarcinomas cytologically present with large nuclei, prominent nucleoli, and abundant vacuolated neutral lipid-laden cytoplasm. Special staining with oil red O or Sudan black must be performed with air-dried preparations due to the dissolution of fat in the alcoholic Papanicolaou stain. Primary adenocarcinoma of the bladder generally arises within the Brunn nest as a result of cystitis cystica and presents cytologically with classic malignant mucinous glandular morphology, often resembling colonic adenocarcinoma.

DeMay RM, The Art & Science of Cytopathology.
Renal cell carcinoma, pp. 408–409.

16. **A** transitional cell carcinoma, grade III

Grade III transitional cell carcinomas yield a hypercellular population of single cells with few clusters, anisokaryosis and pleomorphism, coarsely granular, irregularly distributed chromatin, and macronucleoli.

An adverse host response and necrotic diathesis are found within the background. These cells are easily recognized as malignant; however, in the absence of a necrotic background (a "clean" background), the diagnosis of carcinoma in situ might be entertained due to its frequency of exfoliation and mimicking cytomorphology.

DeMay RM, The Art & Science of Cytopathology.
High-grade TCC, pp. 402–403.

17. **D** transitional cell carcinoma in situ

Carcinoma in situ recapitulates grade III non-papillary transitional cell carcinoma, with the exception that these preinvasive lesions present with a clean background and a negative or "cystitis-mimicking" red transitional mucosa. The cytologic diagnosis may be of great importance in high-risk groups (industrial or aniline dye workers and patients with previously resected carcinoma).

DeMay RM, The Art & Science of Cytopathology.
Dysplasia and carcinoma in situ, pp. 404–405.

18. **B** papillary neoplasm, transitional cell carcinoma cannot be excluded

The presence of true papillary clusters identified in urinary specimens is suggestive of a low-grade papillary neoplasm. These lesions cannot be excluded from grade I transitional cell carcinoma. In the absence of classic malignant nuclear morphology, the diagnosis of carcinoma remains. These cells present with uniform cell borders, micronucleoli and finely granular, regularly distributed chromatin (when visible). Differentiating these low-grade neoplasms in catheterized specimens may prove difficult; however, the presence of true cohesive smooth borders is helpful.

DeMay RM, The Art & Science of Cytopathology.
Significance of papillary clusters, pp. 404–405, and Papilloma (well-differentiated papillary transitional cell neoplasm), pp. 401–402.

19. **C** Wilms tumor

Wilms tumors cytologically present as small cells with anaplastic features and infrequent spindle cells, often mimicking neuroblastoma of the adrenal gland as well as other "small blue cell tumors." Clinical history is extremely important in establishing this disease process.

DeMay RM, The Art & Science of Cytopathology.
Wilms tumor, p. 409.

20. **D** small cell carcinoma, rule out bladder primary

Although rare, small cell carcinomas resemble their diagnostic counterparts in the lung. The cells contain hyperchromatic stippled chromatin, coarse clumping, nuclear molding, scanty cytoplasm, and micronucleoli. They characteristically have vertebral column formation, microbiopsy aggregates, and cords, nests, or ribbons. The oat cell type, which may represent a degenerated form of the tumor, typically is found in streams of mucin.

DeMay RM, The Art & Science of Cytopathology.
Small cell carcinoma, p. 408.

21. **B** renal cell carcinoma

Renal cell carcinoma may be diagnosed in urine specimens, however, the cells are generally not shed until the latter stages of the disease; therefore, the early detection of this disease by cytologic examination has limited practical utility. Degenerated cells may accompany the cytologic findings detailed in the question. The identification of neutral lipid by special stains may aid in the confirmation of a kidney primary, however, a negative reaction does not mitigate against the diagnosis of a less well-differentiated lesion. Conversely, false-positive lipid reactions may be associated with lithiasis, transplant rejection, bladder outlet obstruction, and metastatic carcinoma.

DeMay RM, The Art & Science of Cytopathology.
Renal cell carcinoma, pp. 408, and 1087–1091.

22. **D** squamous differentiated transitional carcinoma

The concomitant finding of squamous cell carcinoma and transitional cell carcinoma (TCC) indicates a squamous differentiation of TCC. These coexisting findings, which are quite common, suggest a high grade neoplasm.

DeMay RM, The Art & Science of Cytopathology.
Squamous cell carcinoma, p. 407.

23. **A** aniline dye exposure

Other "high-risk" groups include textile workers, painters, and occupations that involve work with metal and rubber. Exposure to naphthylamine derivatives (aniline dye) has been shown to have a carcinogenic effect. By far, cigarette smoking is the greatest risk factor for the subsequent development of urothelial cancer—accounting for greater than 40% of all lesions.

DeMay RM, The Art & Science of Cytopathology.
Transitional cell carcinoma (risk factors), pp. 399–400.

24. **A** **transitional epithelial cells**

Normal voided urine specimens are hypocellular, containing predominantly superficial/dome/umbrella/cap-like transitional cells. Transitional cells contain dense granular cytoplasm with homogeneous texture. Urothelial nuclei may be round and slightly enlarged and possess finely granular, evenly distributed chromatin patterns and micronucleoli. The N/C ratios of urothelial cells are low. Scattered squamous cells, either indigenous or contamination from the vaginal mucosa, and rare columnar cells from the renal tubules, Brunn nests, or glands of Littre may be observed. Inflammatory exudate is typically mild unless an inflammatory process exists.

DeMay RM, The Art & Science of Cytopathology.
Transitional cells, pp. 388–389.

25. **C** **ileal conduit urine**

Normal urine from ileal conduit bladders will contain abundant degenerative columnar cells, necrotic debris, and a background containing bacteria and mucus.

DeMay RM, The Art & Science of Cytopathology.
Ileal conduit urine, pp. 405–406.

26. **A** **malacoplakia**

This granulomatous disease grossly appears as yellow plaques in place of the bladder mucosa. Cytology reveals rare histiocytes and giant cells (von Hansemann histiocytes) containing granular intracytoplasmic inclusions representing bacteria, as well as macrophages with intracytoplasmic, cyanophilic, spherical, laminated calcospherites, referred to as Michaelis-Gutmann bodies.

DeMay RM, The Art & Science of Cytopathology.
Malacoplakia, p. 395.

27. **D** **cystitis glandularis**

Brunn nests are areas of columnar epithelium in which transitional cells extend into the lamina propria, separate, and form mucus-producing nests (cystitis glandularis). These cystic nests are lined by normal colonic-type mucosal cells.

DeMay RM, The Art & Science of Cytopathology.
Brunn nests, cystitis cystica, and glandularis, p. 394.

28. **D** **malacoplakia**

This granulomatous disease grossly appears as yellow plaques in place of the bladder mucosa. Cytology reveals rare histiocytes and giant cells (von Hansemann histiocytes) containing granular intracytoplasmic inclusions representing bacteria, as well as macrophages with intracytoplasmic, cyanophilic, spherical, laminated calcospherites, referred to as Michaelis-Gutmann bodies.

DeMay RM, The Art & Science of Cytopathology.
Malacoplakia, p. 395.

29. **B** **catheterized**

Normal catheterized urine specimens contain a hypercellular and heterogeneous population of normal transitional cells that includes dome or superficial cells, sheets of oval intermediate type urothelial cells, squamous cells, and occasional columnar cells, usually from the Brunn nests. The urothelial cells contain round, hypochromatic or degenerative nuclei and granular cytoplasm. Reactive nuclear changes may be detected by the observation of slightly enlarged nuclei and prominent nucleoli; however, normal N/C ratios and benign chromatin patterns detected in well-preserved transitional cells establish their benignity. Careful attention should be given to the differentiation of pseudoclusters (associated with catheterization) from true papillary groupings (such as those found with low-grade papillary neoplasms).

DeMay RM, The Art & Science of Cytopathology.
Transitional cells, pp. 388–389.

30. **A** **squamous metaplasia**

Squamous metaplasia resembling "navicular" cells is often identified in urinary specimens from females, representing a progesterone-stimulated epithelium, such as that found within the vaginal mucosa in pregnant patients. In men, their presence may represent squamous metaplastic cells of the prostatic ducts secondary to estrogen therapy for prostatic adenocarcinoma.

DeMay RM, The Art & Science of Cytopathology.
Squamous cells and squamous metaplasia, p. 390.

31. **A** **cytomegalovirus**

Cytomegalovirus may be identified in immunosuppressed patients such as those infected with HIV, patients with cancer, or renal transplant recipients. Large renal tubular cells with intranuclear basophilic inclusions surrounded by halos resembling an "owl's eye" are diagnostic of cytomegalovirus.

DeMay RM, The Art & Science of Cytopathology.
Viruses, p. 394.

32. **D** cholesterol

Cholesterol crystals abnormally appear as colorless structures in urine specimens.

DeMay RM, The Art & Science of Cytopathology
Miscellaneous, p. 392.

33. **B** renal parenchymal disease

Renal tubular cells, oval cells with granular cytoplasm and eccentrically located nuclei, or polygonal cells occurring singly or in clusters are found in patients with renal parenchymal diseases, such as glomerulonephritis or pyelonephritis. Other associated changes include cellular casts, necrosis, and erythrocytes.

DeMay RM, The Art & Science of Cytopathology.
Renal tubular cells, p. 390, and Renal transplant, pp. 396–397.

34. **B** *Schistosoma mansoni*

The location of the spine differentiates this species from *Schistosoma haematobium* (which possesses a terminal spine).

DeMay RM, The Art & Science of Cytopathology.
Parasites, p. 394.

35. **D** Sudan black

Renal cell carcinomas cytologically present with large nuclei, prominent nucleoli, and abundant vacuolated neutral lipid-laden cytoplasm. Special staining with oil red O or Sudan black must be performed with air-dried preparations due to the dissolution of fat in the alcoholic Papanicolaou stain. Primary adenocarcinoma of the bladder generally arises within the Brunn nest as a result of cystitis cystica and presents cytologically with classic malignant mucinous glandular morphology, often resembling colonic adenocarcinoma.

DeMay RM, The Art & Science of Cytopathology.
Renal cell carcinoma, pp. 408–409.

36. **C** polyomavirus infection

Polyomavirus infections present in urine cytology with enlarged, degenerated, karyopyknotic, eccentrically located nuclei with trailing cytoplasmic tails, often described as decoy (mimicking CIS) or "comet cells" (long cytoplasmic tails). Basophilic intranuclear inclusions are necessary to establish this diagnosis. Care should be exercised to differentiate these benign infections from true neoplastic cells.

DeMay RM, The Art & Science of Cytopathology.
Viruses, p. 394.

37. **B** seminal vesicle cells

Cells originating from the seminal vesicles in males cytologically appear as single cuboidal cells with intracytoplasmic yellow lipofusion granules. The nuclei of these cells may appear quite abnormal; however, the cytoplasmic pigment should indicate the benignity of these cells.

DeMay RM, The Art & Science of Cytopathology.
Seminal vesicle cells, p. 390.

38. **A** degeneration

Eosinophilic (or cyanophilic) intracytoplasmic inclusions in transitional cells commonly represent nonspecific mucopolysaccharide degeneration, or giant lysosomes. These cells are not associated with urinary pathology and care should be exercised when interpreting the significance of their presence.

DeMay RM, The Art & Science of Cytopathology.
Globular, or hyaline, inclusion bodies, p. 391.

39. **B** *Schistosoma haematobium*

Schistosoma haematobium is a parasitic fluke found in Africa and the Middle East that embeds within the bladder mucosa, eventually creating squamous metaplasia and squamous cell carcinoma. The cytology reveals transparent ova with a terminal spine. Schistosomiasis is also referred to as bilharzia. Differential diagnosis is the lemon drop form of uric acid crystals.

DeMay RM, The Art & Science of Cytopathology.
Parasites, p. 394.

40. **A** uremia

Metastasis of cervical carcinomas to the ureters accounts for the most common cause of death in patients with cervical carcinoma. Urinary specimens may yield diagnostic malignant cells in patients with late-stage disease.

DeMay RM, The Art & Science of Cytopathology.
Other metastases, p. 409.

41. **C** **chemotherapy-associated changes**

The presence of large cells with elevated N/C ratios, degenerated nuclear features, and chromatic margination (associated with degeneration) in single cells is related to therapeutic changes secondary to treatment of malignant disease. More "atypical" cytologic changes may be seen with Cytoxan or busulfan therapy, whereas the administration of thiotepa usually creates more reactive urothelial changes. The differential diagnosis of chemotherapy-associated changes includes high-grade transitional cell carcinoma, carcinoma in situ, and polyomavirus infection; however, the absence of single cells with well-preserved, classic malignant nuclear morphology should mitigate against the possibility of a neoplastic process.

DeMay RM, The Art & Science of Cytopathology.
Chemotherapy (thiotepa, mitomycin c, and others), pp. 397–398.

42. **D** **tyrosine**

Tyrosine crystals are typically found in urine from patients with hepatitis, cirrhosis, or trauma to the liver.

DeMay RM, The Art & Science of Cytopathology.
Miscellaneous, p. 392.

Keebler CM, Somrak TM, The Manual of Cytotechnology.
Genitourinary tract samples, pp. 422–423.

43. B **cystitis cystica**

Columnar cells identified in urinary specimens are most commonly derived from the bladder dome or Brunn nests, areas in which columnar mucosa extends into the lamina propria. Other sources include cystitis glandularis, gland os, lacunae of Morgagni, female genital system, prostate or renal tubules.

DeMay RM, The Art & Science of Cytopathology.
Columnar cells, p. 389.

44. **D** **lead poisoning**

Cellular changes secondary to lead poisoning are often found in children who consume paint or water high in lead content.

DeMay RM, The Art & Science of Cytopathology.
Other inclusions, p. 391.

45. **C** **human polyomavirus**

Polyomavirus infections present in urine cytology with enlarged, degenerated, karyopyknotic, eccentric nuclei with trailing cytoplasmic tails, often described as decoy (mimicking CIS) or "comet cells" (long cytoplasmic tails). Basophilic intranuclear inclusions are necessary to establish this diagnosis. Care should be exercised to differentiate these benign infections from true neoplastic cells.

DeMay RM, The Art & Science of Cytopathology.
Viruses, p. 394.

46. **A** **squamous cell carcinoma, bladder primary**

Schistosoma haematobium is a parasitic fluke found in Africa and the Middle East that embeds within the bladder mucosa, eventually creating squamous metaplasia and squamous cell carcinoma. Squamous cell carcinoma of the bladder (secondary to bilharzia) presents with typical pleomorphic keratinizing morphology identical to that found in other primary sites. These lesions may be very well differentiated; therefore, extreme caution should be exercised when discriminating these lesions from normal squamous cells.

DeMay RM, The Art & Science of Cytopathology.
Squamous cell carcinoma, p. 407.

47. **B** **triple phosphate crystals**

Triple phosphate crystals generally present with "coffin lid" or prism morphology in urinary tract specimens.

DeMay RM, The Art & Science of Cytopathology.
Miscellaneous, p. 392.

Keebler CM, Somrak TM, The Manual of Cytotechnology.
Genitourinary tract samples, pp. 422–423.

48. **C** *Candida* **sp.**

Immunocompetent individuals taking broad spectrum antibiotics are at an increased risk for isolated fungal infections, however, immunocompromised patients (such as diabetics) are more commonly at risk. The photomicrograph illustrates an infection by *Candida* sp., demonstrated by the presence of pseudohyphae or elongated yeast with attached buds (resembling "balloon dogs") as well as scattered budding yeast (often collectively referred to as "sticks and stones"). Other fungal infections, such as *Blastomyces* sp., *Cryptococcus* sp., and *Aspergillus* sp., may also be seen in urine specimens as a part of a local or systemic infection.

DeMay RM, The Art & Science of Cytopathology.
Fungus infections, p. 394, and Fungi, p. 56.

49. D lithiasis, calcium carbonate crystals

Calcium carbonate crystals are easily identified in urinary specimens as dumbbell and granule structures. Their presence may be associated with the over consumption of vegetables.

DeMay RM, The Art & Science of Cytopathology.
Miscellaneous, p. 392.

50. B transitional cell carcinoma in situ

Carcinoma in situ recapitulates grade III non-papillary transitional cell carcinoma, with the exception that these preinvasive lesions present with a clean background and a negative or "cystitis-mimicking" red transitional mucosa. The cytologic diagnosis may be of great importance in high-risk groups (industrial or aniline dye workers and patients with previously resected carcinoma).

DeMay RM, The Art & Science of Cytopathology.
Dysplasia and carcinoma in situ, pp. 404–405.

51. B papillary neoplasm, rule out transitional cell carcinoma

The presence of true papillary clusters identified in urinary specimens is suggestive of a low-grade papillary neoplasm. These lesions cannot be excluded from grade I transitional cell carcinoma. In the absence of classic malignant nuclear morphology, the diagnosis of carcinoma remains. These cells present with uniform cell borders, micronucleoli and finely granular, regularly distributed chromatin (when visible). Differentiating these low-grade neoplasms in catheterized specimens may prove difficult; however, the presence of true cohesive smooth borders will help confirm a neoplastic process.

DeMay RM, The Art & Science of Cytopathology.
Significance of papillary clusters, pp. 389–390, and Papilloma (well-differentiated papillary transitional cell neoplasm), pp. 401–402.

52. D prostate adenocarcinoma

Prostatic adenocarcinomas cytologically appear in repeating microacinar structures and syncytial groupings with anisonucleosis, crowding nuclear features, finely granular chromatin, and irregular macronucleoli within every cell. The positivity with immunocytochemistry for prostate-specific antigen is helpful in distinguishing these lesions from those from bladder or renal primary sites.

DeMay RM, The Art & Science of Cytopathology.
Prostatic adenocarcinoma, p. 409.

53. B oil red O

Renal cell adenocarcinomas cytologically present with large nuclei, prominent nucleoli, and abundant, faintly vacuolated, lipid-laden cytoplasm. Special staining with oil red O or Sudan black must be performed with air-dried preparations due to the dissolution of fat in the alcoholic Papanicolaou stain. Primary adenocarcinoma of the bladder generally arises within the Brunn nest as a result of cystitis cystica and presents cytologically with classic malignant mucinous glandular morphology, often resembling colonic adenocarcinoma.

DeMay RM, The Art & Science of Cytopathology.
Renal cell carcinoma, pp. 408–409.

54. C transitional cell carcinoma, grade III

Grade III transitional cell carcinomas yield a hypercellular population of single cells with few clusters, anisokaryosis and pleomorphism, coarsely granular, irregularly distributed chromatin, and macronucleoli. An adverse host response and necrotic diathesis are found within the background. These cells are easily recognized as malignant; however, in the absence of a necrotic background (a "clean" background), the diagnosis of carcinoma in situ might be entertained due to its frequency of exfoliation and mimicking cytomorphology.

DeMay RM, The Art & Science of Cytopathology.
High-grade TCC, pp. 402–403.

55. B vaginal contamination

The most common source of squamous cells in urine specimens is vaginal contamination. The urethra and the bladder trigone are also possible sources of squamous mucosa.

DeMay RM, The Art & Science of Cytopathology.
Squamous cells and squamous metaplasia, p. 390.

56. A normal catheterized urothelial changes

Normal catheterized urine specimens contain a hypercellular and heterogeneous population of normal transitional cells, including dome or superficial cells, sheets of oval intermediate type urothelial cells, squamous cells, and occasional columnar cells, usually from the Brunn nests. The urothelial cells contain round, hypochromatic or degenerative nuclei and granular cytoplasm. Reactive nuclear changes may be detected by the observation of slightly enlarged nuclei and prominent nucleoli; however, normal N/C ratios and benign chromatin patterns detected in well-preserved transitional cells establish their benignity. Careful attention should be given to the differentiation of pseudoclusters (associated with catheterization) from true papillary groupings (found with low-grade papillary neoplasms).

DeMay RM, The Art & Science of Cytopathology.
Catheterization, p. 392, and Significance of papillary clusters, pp. 389–390.

57. **C bladder dome**

Columnar cells identified in urinary specimens are most commonly derived from the bladder dome or Brunn nests, areas in which the columnar mucosa extends into the lamina propria. Other sources include cystitis glandularis, gland of Littre, lacunae of Morgagni, female genital system, prostate, and renal tubules.

DeMay RM, The Art & Science of Cytopathology.
Columnar cells, p. 389.

58. **C calcium phosphate crystals**

These transparent crystals cytologically present as wedge-shaped prisms or irregular plate-like structures.

DeMay RM, The Art & Science of Cytopathology.
Miscellaneous, p. 392;

PO4 = prisms plates

Keebler CM, Somrak TM, The Manual of Cytotechnology.
Genitourinary tract samples, pp. 422–423.

59. **B corpora amylacea**

Corpora amylacea are basophilic, condensed, concentrically laminated, glycogenated, noncalcifying structures, originating from the prostate.

DeMay RM, The Art & Science of Cytopathology.
Corpora amylacea, p. 391.

Keebler CM, Somrak TM, The Manual of Cytotechnology.
Genitourinary tract samples, pp. 422–423.

60. **D This cell is infected with the human polyomavirus**

Polyomavirus infections present in urine cytology with enlarged, degenerated, karyopyknotic, eccentrically located nuclei with trailing cytoplasmic tails, often described as decoy (mimicking CIS) or "comet cells" (long cytoplasmic tails). Basophilic intranuclear inclusions are necessary to establish this diagnosis. Care should be exercised to differentiate these benign infections from true neoplastic cells.

DeMay RM, The Art & Science of Cytopathology.
Viruses (human polyomavirus), p. 395.

61. **D carcinoma of the bladder**

Schistosoma haematobium is a parasitic fluke found in Africa and the Middle East that embeds within the bladder mucosa, eventually creating squamous metaplasia and squamous cell carcinoma. The cytology reveals transparent ova with a terminal spine. Schistosomiasis is also referred to as bilharzia. Differential diagnosis is the lemon drop form of uric acid crystals.

DeMay RM, The Art & Science of Cytopathology.
Parasites, p. 394.

62. **B cytomegalovirus**

Cytomegalovirus may be identified in immunosuppressed patients, such as those infected with HIV, patients with cancer, or renal transplant recipients. Large renal tubular cells with intranuclear basophilic inclusions surrounded by halos resembling an "owl's eye" are diagnostic of cytomegalovirus.

DeMay RM, The Art & Science of Cytopathology.
Viruses, p. 54, and Viruses, p. 394.

63. **A renal casts**

The presence of renal casts may be associated with kidney rejection or other renal pathology, although their presence may not indicate pathology (depending upon the type of cast).

DeMay RM, The Art & Science of Cytopathology.
Miscellaneous, p. 409.

64. **C normal urothelial cells**

Normal voided urine specimens are hypocellular, containing predominantly superficial/dome/ umbrella/cap-like transitional cells. Transitional cells contain dense granular cytoplasm with homogeneous texture. Urothelial nuclei may be round and slightly enlarged, and possess finely granular, evenly distributed chromatin patterns and micronucleoli. The N/C ratios of urothelial cells are low. Scattered squamous cells, either indigenous or contamination from the vaginal mucosa, and rare columnar cells from the renal tubules, Brunn nests, or glands of Littre may be observed. Inflammatory exudate is typically mild unless a pathologic process exists.

DeMay RM, The Art & Science of Cytopathology.
Transitional cells, pp. 388–389.

Chapter 7

Breast Secretions/Aspirations

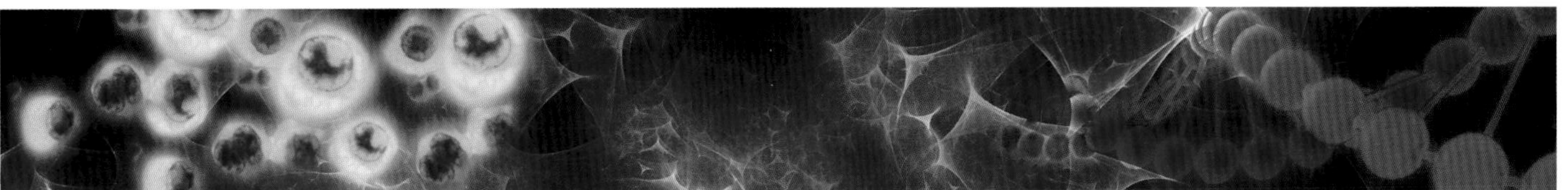

1. A well-demarcated lesion presents cytologically as a large population of cells predominantly in syncytia, few glandular formations, and abundant single cells all possessing large nuclei with coarse, irregular chromatin and macronucleoli. The background contains numerous lymphocytes and plasma cells. The diagnosis is:

   A. poorly differentiated ductal carcinoma
   B. colloid carcinoma
   C. medullary carcinoma
   D. lobular carcinoma

2. FNA reveals apocrine cells with cellular crowding, slightly enlarged nuclei, fine chromatin, smooth nuclear borders, and prominent nucleoli, as well as naked bipolar nuclei. Based on these findings, the cells most likely represent:

   A. fibroadenoma
   B. comedocarcinoma
   C. reactive apocrine cells
   D. apocrine carcinoma

3. Which of the following lesions are more likely to be estrogen receptor-positive by immunocytochemistry?

   A. colloid carcinoma
   B. medullary carcinoma
   C. ductal comedocarcinoma
   D. anaplastic carcinoma

4. Malignant breast tumors that clinically present as red, edematous lesions and have dermal lymphatic involvement are termed:

   A. sclerosing adenosis
   B. comedocarcinoma
   C. inflammatory carcinoma
   D. scirrhous carcinoma

5. Which of the following diagnoses may possibly be clinically managed using ductal lavage cytology?

   A. apocrine metaplasia
   B. fibrocystic disease
   C. ductal carcinoma in situ
   D. atypical ductal hyperplasia

6. A 68-year-old woman presents with a bilateral breast tumor. FNA reveals a hypocellular sample of small cells attached to fibrocollagenous tissue with scanty cytoplasm and little pleomorphism. Single cells with intracytoplasmic lumens are also seen. The diagnosis is:

   A. lobular carcinoma
   B. tubular carcinoma
   C. carcinoid tumor
   D. adenoid cystic carcinoma of the breast

7. A 2-cm circumscribed mass was identified in the right upper outer quadrant of the breast of a 17-year-old girl. FNA cytology reveals a clear fluid containing cells with central nuclei and eosinophilic granular cytoplasm in papillary groups, cells with foamy cytoplasm, a marked population of cells in sheets with uniform polarity, and naked bipolar nuclei. The diagnosis is:

   A. poorly differentiated ductal adenocarcinoma
   B. fibrocystic disease
   C. juvenile papillomatosis
   D. well-differentiated ductal adenocarcinoma

8. The FNA of a breast mass yields a hypercellular population of monotonous, bland cells obtained from an elderly woman. Based on this, these findings are:

   A. consistent with a benign neoplasm
   B. diagnostic of ductal hyperplasia
   C. suggestive of an in situ carcinoma
   D. suspicious for malignancy

9. A 64-year-old woman presented with a 3-cm mass in the right breast. FNA reveals a hypercellular smear containing large fragments of cells in a papillary grouping with dense fibrous cores, elongated pleomorphic nuclei with hyperchromasia and irregular nuclear membranes, and a background of necrosis. The diagnosis suggests:

   A. metastatic melanoma
   B. papillary neoplasm, rule out carcinoma
   C. spindle cell sarcoma
   D. Paget disease

10. The structures that are formed by the terminal ducts and ductules in the non-lactating breast are known as:

   A. myoepithelial layers
   B. fibroadipose tissue
   C. nipples
   D. lobules

11. FNA of nonpalpable mammographically detected microcalcifications in a 52-year-old patient reveals obvious malignant cells. Lymph node biopsies are negative. Which of the following may represent the cellular findings?

   A. ductal carcinoma in situ
   B. apocrine carcinoma
   C. mucinous carcinoma
   D. Paget disease

12. A bulky tumor of the breast that cytologically presents as monomorphic cells appearing singly or in clusters floating in islands of mucin as well as transverse branching capillaries is diagnostic of:

   A. adenoid cystic carcinoma
   B. papillary carcinoma
   C. Paget disease
   D. colloid carcinoma

13. FNA of a 3-cm breast mass yields a hypercellular population of small, uniform, basaloid cells arranged around balls of pink homogeneous globules. A mucinous background is identified as metachromatic with the Romanowsky stain. The diagnosis is:

   A. adenoid cystic carcinoma
   B. comedocarcinoma
   C. medullary carcinoma
   D. ductal carcinoma

14. A 50-year-old woman with a firm, gritty mass in the left breast is evaluated with FNA. Cytology reveals a highly cellular population of disorganized and overlapping cell clusters, microacini, and single cells. Pleomorphic nuclei, prominent nucleoli, irregular nuclear membranes, and chromatin clumping are noted. The diagnosis is:

   A. ductal adenocarcinoma
   B. mucinous adenocarcinoma
   C. lobular carcinoma
   D. comedocarcinoma

15. **An infiltrating ductal carcinoma that invades the epidermis of the breast is termed:**

A. Paget disease
B. adenoid cystic carcinoma
C. papillary carcinoma
D. scirrhous carcinoma

16. **A 55-year-old man with a history of estrogen treatment for prostate cancer presents with bilateral breast enlargement. FNA cytology reveals a large population of cells in sheets, some forming papillary fragments, surrounded by loose connective tissue. The diagnosis is:**

A. ductal adenocarcinoma
B. metastatic prostatic adenocarcinoma
C. gynecomastia
D. idiopathic

17. **When identifying a primary neuroendocrine lesion of the breast, what immunocytochemical stain would help establish its differentiation?**

A. Leu-M5
B. epithelial membrane antigen
C. B72.3
D. serotonin

18. **A 67-year-old woman presents to the clinician with multiple bilateral breast masses. FNA reveals an abundant population of pleomorphic cells with India ink elongated nuclei. Orangeophilic pearls were scattered across the slide. The most likely diagnosis is:**

A. squamous carcinoma, breast primary
B. metastatic carcinoma, lung primary
C. fibromatosis
D. metastatic spindle cell melanoma

19. **Benign mononucleated and multinucleated cells possessing frothy cytoplasm in nipple discharges are diagnostic of:**

A. apocrine cells
B. foam cells
C. ductal cells
D. lipophages

20. **A 52-year-old woman presents with a bloody nipple discharge of three months' duration. Cytology of the breast smear reveals many three-dimensional papillary groupings. The nuclei were oval with irregular nuclear membranes, anisonucleosis, and anisocytosis. Chromatin was finely granular with irregular distribution and macronucleoli were noted in most cells. A necrotic background is identified. These findings suggest:**

A. micropapillomatosis
B. papillary apocrine metaplasia
C. atypical ductal cells
D. adenocarcinoma

21. **A 6-cm breast mass was detected by a 33-year-old woman. Cytology reveals a large population of fibromyxoid stroma and sheets of cells with honeycomb configuration. The lesion was removed. Grossly, the tumor, removed with wide excision, contained slit-like structures across the surface. The diagnosis is:**

A. metaplastic carcinoma
B. primary breast sarcoma
C. fibroadenoma
D. phyllodes tumor

22. **A 45-year-old woman presents with a bloody breast discharge and a subareolar nodule in her right breast. Cytology reveals three-dimensional clusters of cells with smooth or scalloped cohesive borders and containing predictable nuclei that maintain polarity throughout the fragment. The diagnosis is:**

A. ductal adenocarcinoma
B. ductal carcinoma in situ
C. papilloma, neoplasm not excluded
D. apocrine metaplasia

23. **A 32-year-old woman presents with a solid 2×3-cm mass in the upper outer quadrant of the right breast. Cytology reveals a hypercellular sample of cells in sheets with honeycombing characteristics, and cigar-shaped bipolar cells. A fibromyxoid background is present. The diagnosis is:**

A. fibrocystic disease
B. fibroadenoma
C. fat necrosis
D. lipoma

24. **Benign nipple discharges are most often related to:**

A. ductal dilatation
B. granulomatous disease
C. cystosarcoma phyllodes
D. lipoma

25. **A 68-year-old woman presents with thelitis, edematous areola, and nipple discharge. Cytology reveals large cells with abundant cytoplasm containing large nucleoli. Chromatin is fine and irregular in distribution. The diagnosis is:**

A. Paget disease
B. foam cells
C. papillomatosis
D. medullary carcinoma

26. **In the breast, an initial insult of periductal mastitis followed by scarring, stasis of ducts, and ductal dilatation forming macrocysts and fibrosis is considered to be:**

A. tuberculomas
B. fibrocystic disease
C. mammary adenocarcinoma
D. apocrine papillomatosis

27. **A 32-year-old postpartum patient with a painful thick breast discharge reveals abundant neutrophils and round to oval cells with fine regular chromatin, smooth nuclear membranes, and macronucleoli. A necrotic background is noted. The diagnosis is:**

A. cystic disease
B. fibroadenoma
C. lactating adenoma
D. mastitis

28. **A 42-year-old woman presents with a 1-cm firm left breast mass after jogging three days earlier. FNA aspiration shows a yellow, thick substance cytologically containing amorphous debris, hemosiderin-laden macrophages, multinucleated giant cells, as well as a population of cells in honeycomb configuration with enlarged nuclei. The diagnosis is:**

A. fibroadenoma
B. mastitis
C. fat necrosis
D. fibrocystic disease

29. **A 58-year-old woman presents with a nipple discharge. Cytology reveals a monotonous population of cells with intracytoplasmic vacuoles, high N/C ratios, and hyperchromasia. Cellular configuration reveals a slightly cohesive population of cells forming a "stack of coins" or vertebral column. The diagnosis is:**

A. degenerative ductal cells
B. ductal adenocarcinoma
C. carcinoid tumor of the breast
D. lobular carcinoma

30. **Which is not associated with breast disease in pregnancy?**

A. lactating adenoma
B. fibroadenoma
C. fibrocystic disease
D. physiologic nipple discharge without a mass

31. **A 29-year-old pregnant woman in her second trimester presents with a 1.5-cm mass. Cytology presents a dirty background staining positive with PAS. A large population of cells in sheets with good polarity is present, as well as naked oval-shaped cells. The diagnosis is:**

A. lactating adenoma
B. fibrocystic disease
C. ductal adenocarcinoma
D. mucinous adenocarcinoma

32. **A 33-year-old woman presents with a 4-cm mass in the left breast. FNA reveals a colorless material cytologically presenting in an equal population of clusters of enlarged cells with prominent nucleoli and eosinophilic granular cytoplasm, cells with honeycomb appearance, foamy histiocytes, and blood. The diagnosis is:**

A. fibroadenoma
B. ductal adenocarcinoma
C. medullary carcinoma
D. fibrocystic disease

33. What is considered the premalignant disease of the breast?

A. fibrocystic disease
B. fibroadenoma
C. lactating adenoma
D. lipoma

34. Sheets of small epithelial cells with smooth nuclear membranes and prominent cell borders found in nipple secretions are diagnostic of:

A. ductal lining cells
B. apocrine cells
C. foam cells
D. mastitis

35. An FNA specimen of a 2-cm soft nodular mass in the left breast of a woman presents cytologically as cells in sheets, producing a "chicken wire" appearance with criss-crossing capillaries. The diagnosis is:

A. fat necrosis
B. fibrocystic disease
C. fibroadenoma
D. lipoma

36. Cuboidal cells with centrally placed nuclei and eosinophilic granular cytoplasm found in nipple secretions are diagnostic of:

A. intraductal papilloma
B. foam cells
C. apocrine cells
D. lipocytes

37. **FNA of a 2-cm, bulky, gelatinous breast mass yields thick bloody material and malignant cells. What special stain will help confirm the diagnosis?**

A. Congo red/medullary carcinoma
B. oil red O/ductal carcinoma
C. keratin/lobular carcinoma
D. alcian blue/colloid carcinoma

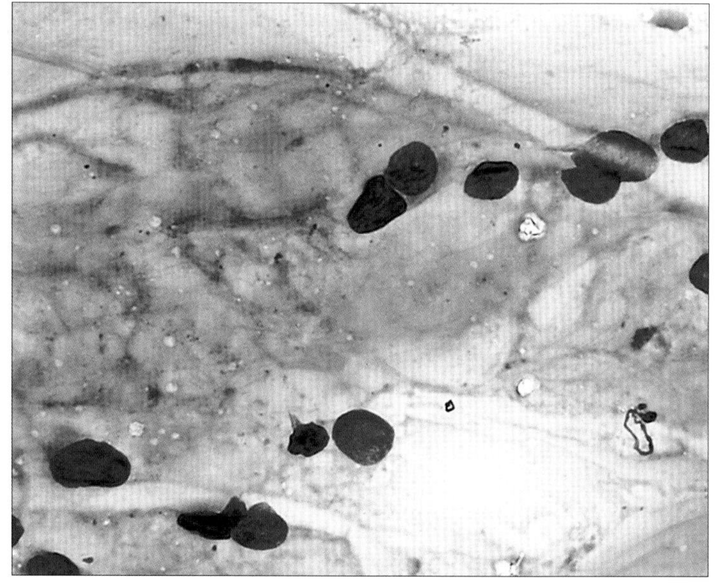

38. **A 0.75-cm nonpalpable mammographically detected breast lesion is found in a 55-year-old woman. FNA performed with a 22-gauge needle yields these cells. The diagnosis is:**

A. mucinous carcinoma
B. tubular carcinoma
C. comedocarcinoma
D. medullary carcinoma

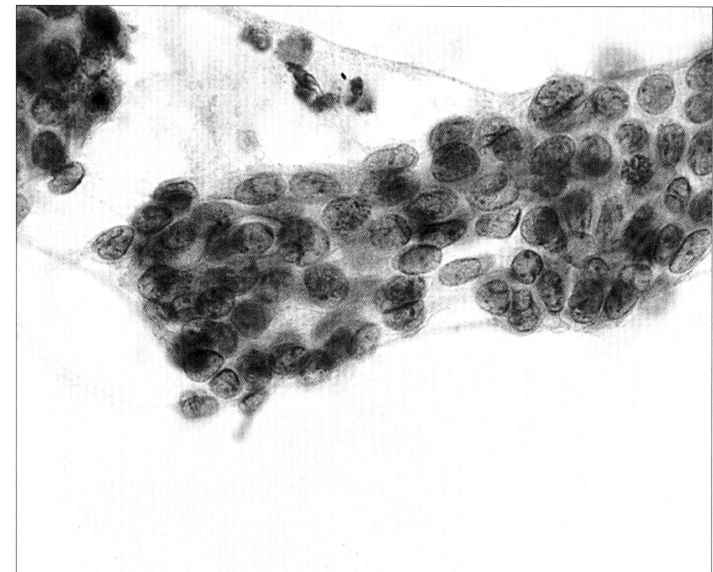

39. **A 77-year-old man with a firm 4-cm lesion of the left breast presents for FNA. Cytology reveals:**

A. ductal adenocarcinoma
B. gynecomastia
C. fat necrosis
D. mastitis

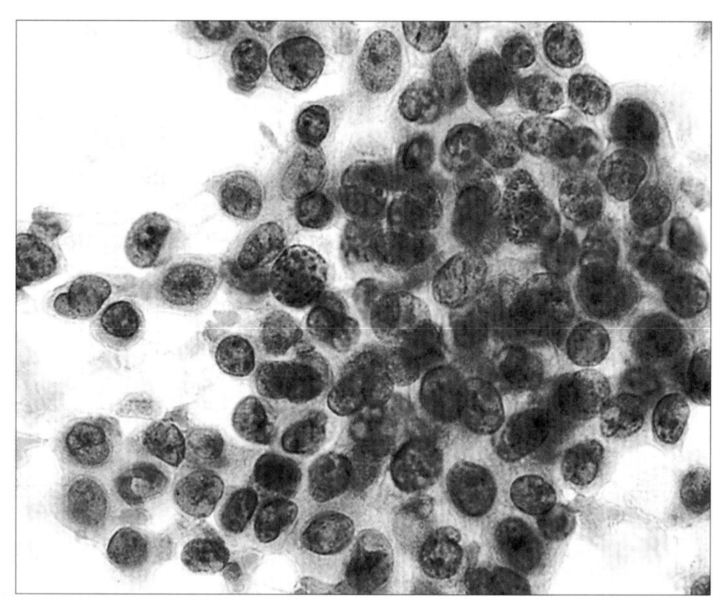

40. A 45-year-old woman with a 4-cm lesion identified on mammography undergoes FNA evaluation. Aspiration of a soft fleshy mass yields copious blood and these cells. The cellular findings are diagnostic of:

A. ductal carcinoma
B. colloid carcinoma
C. medullary carcinoma
D. scirrhous carcinoma

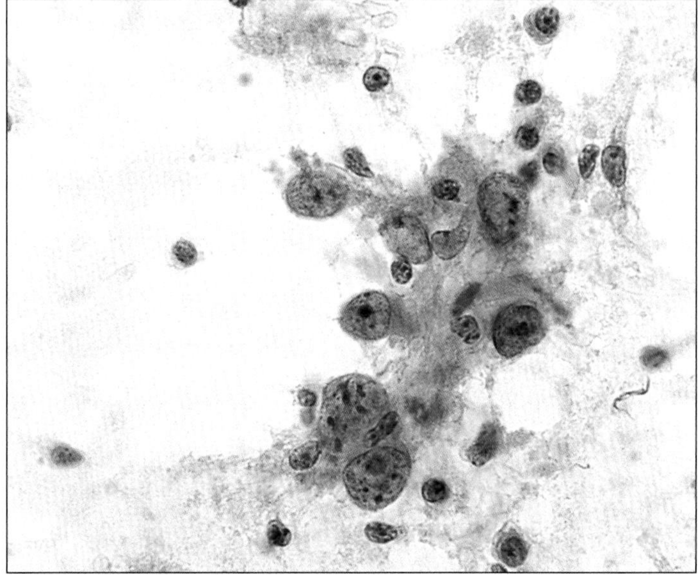

41. A 32-year-old woman in her third trimester presents with a firm 3-cm lesion that had not been present 3 months earlier. The aspirated lesion reveals:

A. lactating adenoma
B. fibrocystic disease
C. ductal adenocarcinoma
D. Paget disease

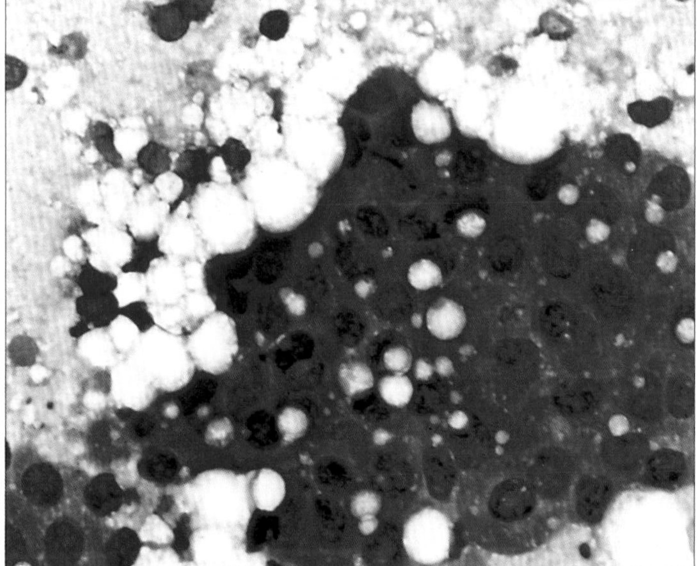

42. A 66-year-old woman presents with an eczematous lesion of the breast and itching. Clinical examination reveals a 1-cm palpable mass. FNA reveals these cells. A positive reaction with which special stain will help confirm the diagnosis?

A. HMB-45/melanoma
B. chromogranin/infiltrating ductal carcinoma
C. S-100/lobular carcinoma
D. mucicarmine/Paget disease

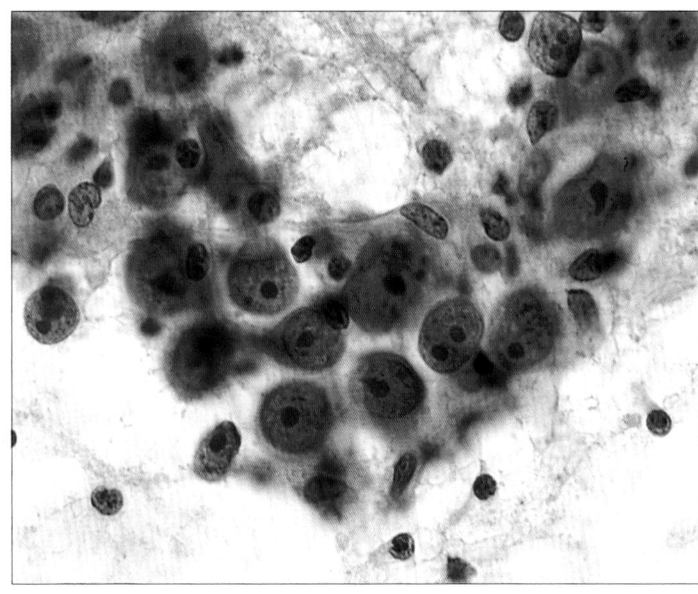

43. **A 32-year-old woman with silicone breast implants presents with a pea-sized lesion located in the left breast. The cellular findings from an FNA specimen with a 22-gauge needle represent:**

A. chronic mastitis
B. inflammatory carcinoma
C. non-Hodgkin lymphoma
D. granulomatous mastitis

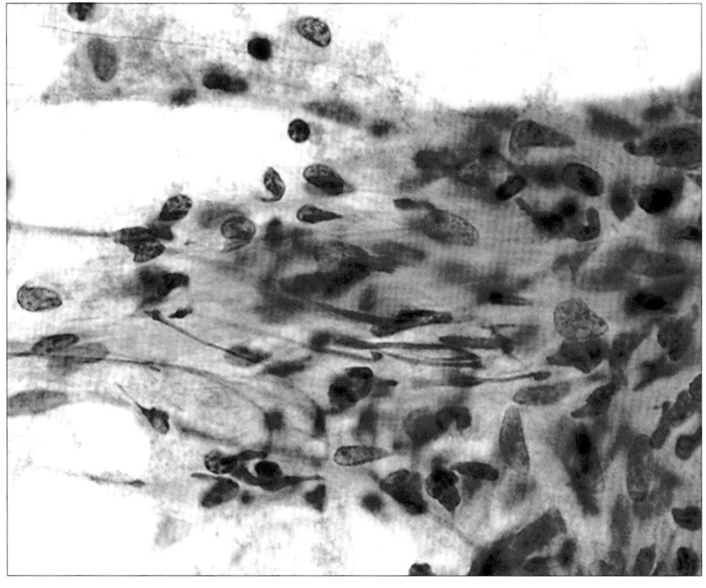

44. **A 62-year-old woman with a 3-cm nonmovable nodule in the upper outer quadrant of the left breast and dimpling of the nipple undergoes FNA. These cells are diagnostic of:**

A. lobular carcinoma
B. fibroadenoma, tubular adenoma variant
C. mucinous adenocarcinoma
D. infiltrating ductal carcinoma

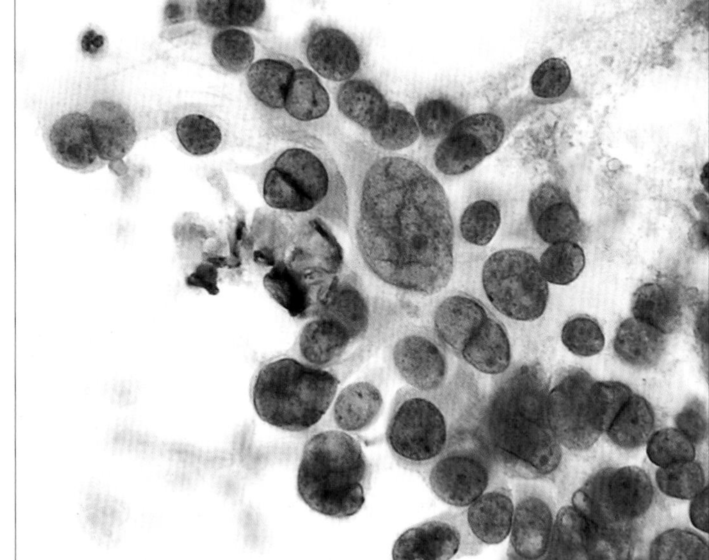

45. **A firm 2-cm lesion of the breast is identified in a 22-year-old female athlete. Retraction of the nipple is evident. FNA of a gritty nodule reveals a yellow pasty material. Cytology reveals:**

A. comedocarcinoma
B. colloid carcinoma
C. fibroadenoma
D. fat necrosis

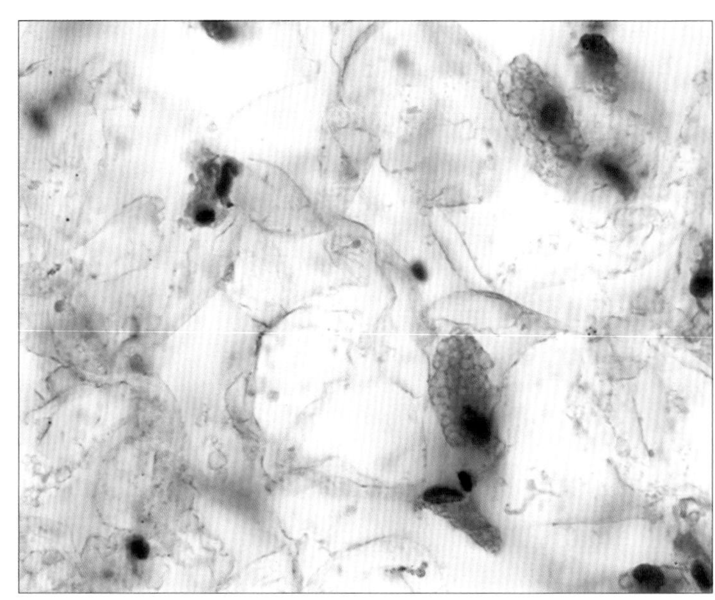

46. A 44-year-old woman with periductal inflammation presents with a cystic mass in the left upper outer quadrant of the breast. Fine-needle aspiration (FNA) reveals a cystic fluid. These cells represent:

A. fibroadenoma, juvenile variant
B. mastitis
C. fat necrosis
D. simple fibrocystic disease

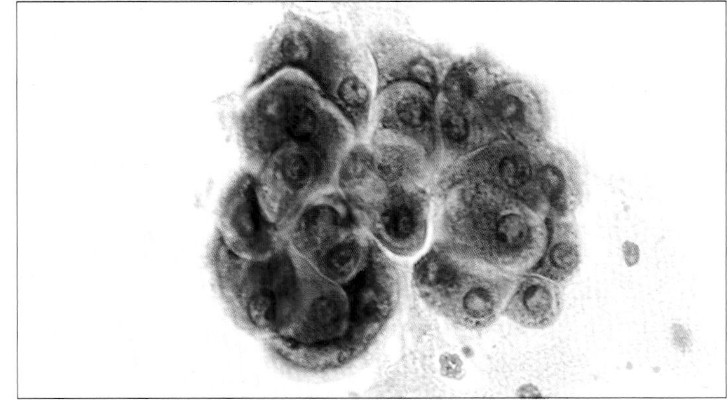

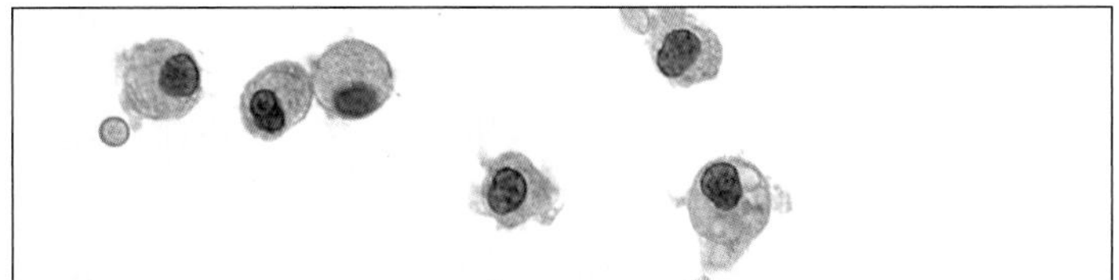

47. This group of cells is observed in a bloody nipple secretion from a 44-year-old woman with no history of malignancy. Cytology reveals:

A. multinucleated foam cells
B. papillary ductal adenocarcinoma
C. papillary apocrine metaplasia
D. papillary clusters, neoplasm not excluded

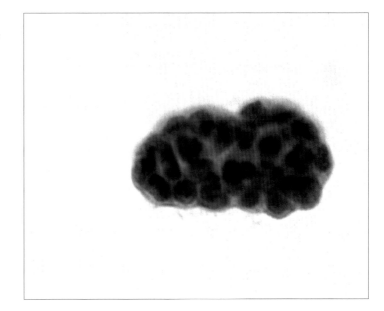

48. When found in nipple discharges, these cells represent holocrine secretion. These findings are consistent with:

A. foam cells
B. apocrine cells
C. ductal lining cells
D. mastitis

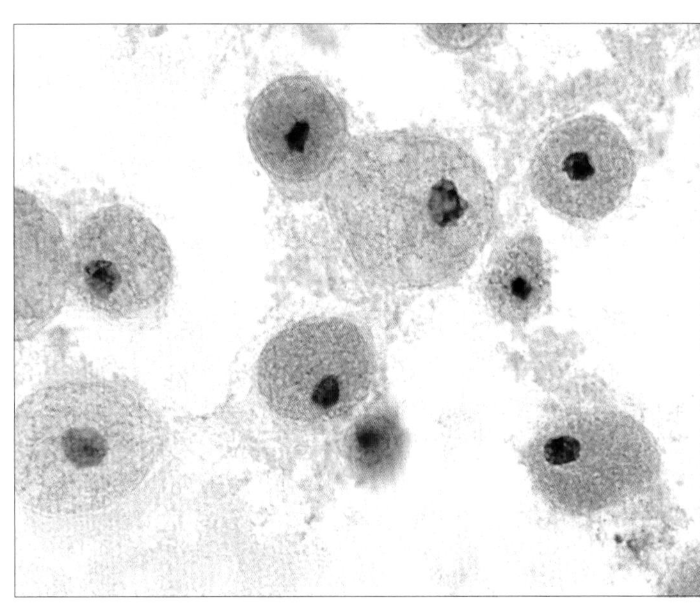

49. A 2-cm, freely mobile mass aspirated from a 28-year-old woman yields these cells upon FNA. The cytologic findings are diagnostic of:

A. fibrocystic disease
B. lipoma
C. ductal carcinoma
D. fibroadenoma

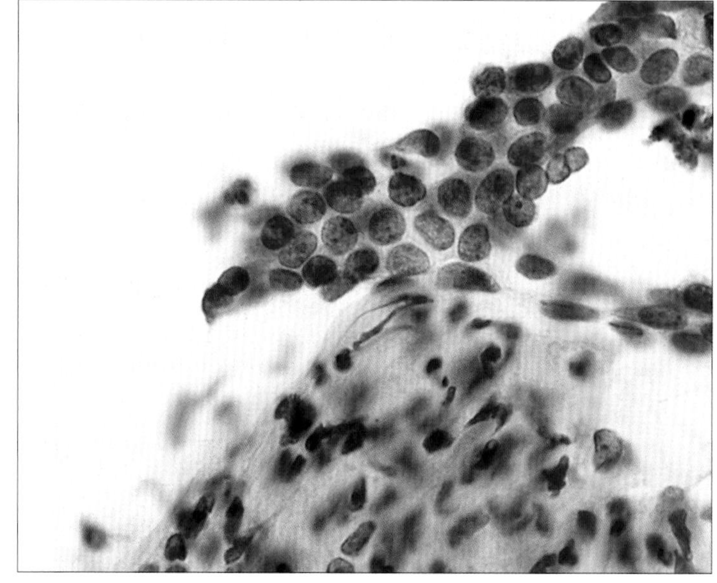

50. An aspiration of a gritty, 2-cm lesion from the left breast of a 50-year-old postmenopausal woman yields little material. These cells, identified upon cytologic evaluation, are diagnostic of:

A. lobular carcinoma
B. ductal carcinoma
C. non-Hodgkin lymphoma
D. colloid carcinoma

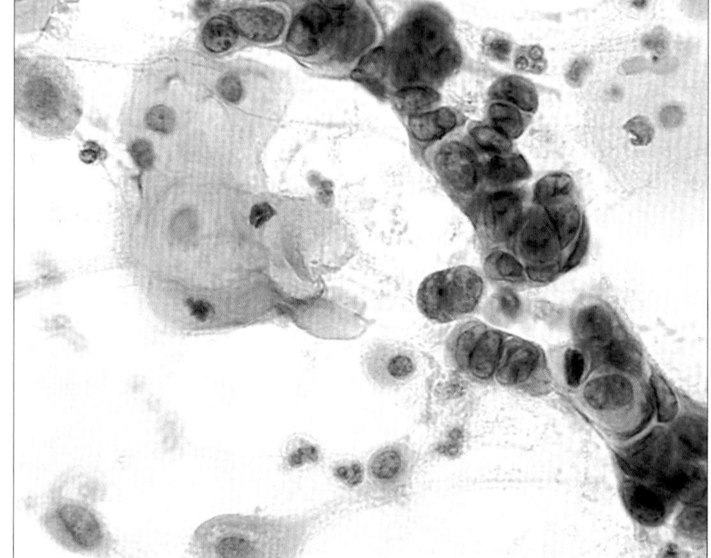

51. A yellowish nipple secretion yields these cells. The cytologic pattern depicted is:

A. papilloma
B. apocrine metaplastic cells
C. ductal lining cells
D. foam cells

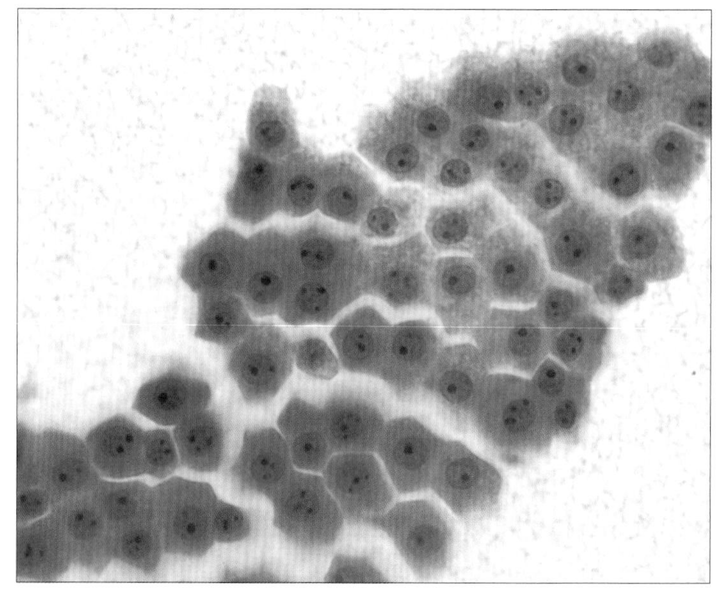

52. **A firm, 5-cm mass is identified in the right breast of a 44-year-old woman. FNA reveals the cells shown. These cells represent:**

A. fibrocystic disease
B. medullary carcinoma
C. tuberculoma
D. phyllodes tumor

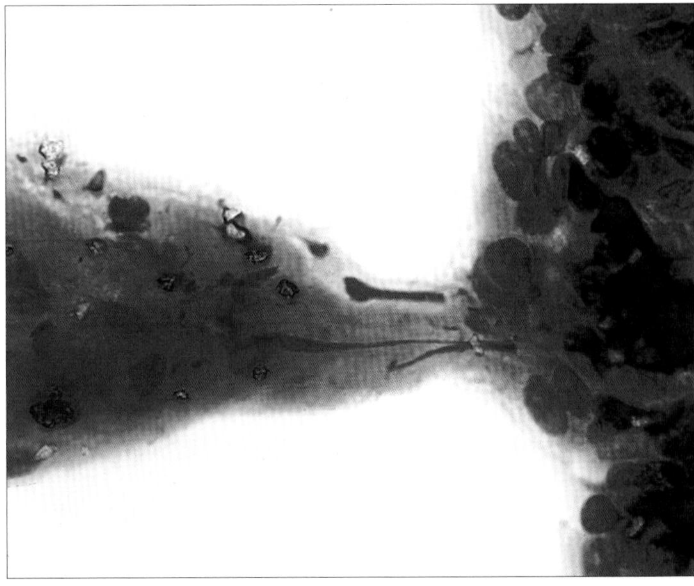

53. **A 55-year-old man with cirrhosis of the liver presents with painful bilateral breast enlargement. FNA yields these cells. The diagnosis is:**

A. ductal carcinoma
B. gynecomastia
C. fat necrosis
D. mastitis

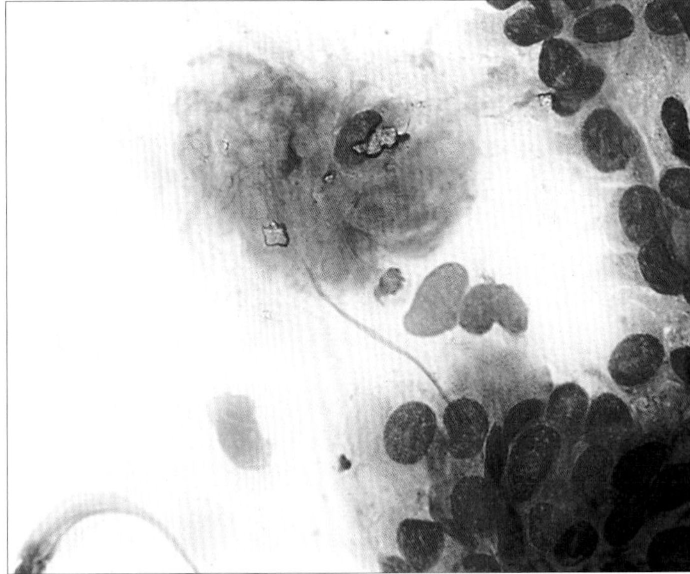

Breast Secretions/Aspirations *Answer Key*

1. **C** medullary carcinoma

These classic malignant features, as well as abnormal mitotic figures in conjunction with a background composed of lymphocytes, plasma cells, and histiocytes, identify this lesion as medullary carcinoma. Care should be exercised to differentiate the benign lymphocytes from lymphoma. Medullary carcinoma is mucin negative.

DeMay RM, The Art & Science of Cytopathology.
Medullary carcinoma, p. 876.

2. **C** reactive apocrine cells

The appearance of "atypical" apocrine morphology is often associated with benign cystic changes. The described morphology suggests a reactive variant; furthermore, the presence of bipolar naked nuclei helps confirm the benign nature of the aspirate. The finding of apocrine cells, regardless of slightly atypical changes, is generally indicative of a benign process. True apocrine carcinoma is rare and often has concomitant ductal carcinoma.

DeMay RM, The Art & Science of Cytopathology.
Atypical apocrine cells, p. 856.

3. **A** colloid carcinoma

Estrogen receptor (ER) status has become an important determinant in the therapeutic evaluation of patients with breast cancer. These steroid receptors may be identified with immunocytochemical techniques using anti-receptor antibodies. Microscopically, ER positivity can be semiquantitated by the number and intensity of the cells staining. ER positive lesions are generally found in older, postmenopausal patients rather than premenopausal females. Small, well-differentiated lesions, such as papillary and colloid carcinoma, are more likely to be ER positive, whereas large, undifferentiated lesions exhibiting aneuploidy are usually ER negative. In addition, tumors that exhibit necrosis or chronic inflammation are typically ER negative.

DeMay RM, The Art & Science of Cytopathology.
Hormone receptors, pp. 870–871.

4. **C** inflammatory carcinoma

Inflammatory carcinomas are underlying carcinomas (usually ductal) which have spread to the dermal lymphatics, thus, the clinical presentation is that of inflammation and mastitis. This diagnosis carries a poor prognosis.

DeMay RM, The Art & Science of Cytopathology.
Inflammatory carcinoma, p. 886.

5. **D** atypical ductal hyperplasia

Women with a cytologic diagnosis of ductal atypia (atypical ductal hyperplasia) from ductal lavage or nipple aspirate fluid specimens are at a 4.9 times greater risk for developing breast cancer compared with women without cellular atypia. Moreover, the risk of breast cancer increases 18-fold in women with confirmed cellular atypia (via ductal lavage) coupled with a family history of breast carcinoma.

O'Shaughnessy JA, Ljung BM, Dooley WC, et al.
Cancer. 2002;94(2):292–298.

6. **A** lobular carcinoma

Lobular carcinomas present as moderate cellular specimens composed of small, monomorphic epithelial cells with minimal nuclear deviation or pleomorphism. The cells possess scanty cytoplasm, often with signet ring morphology or intracytoplasmic lumens. Nuclear overlapping and eccentric nuclei may be noted on high power. Rare vertebral column formation may be noted. Fibrocollagenous tissue may be interspersed amongst the groups of epithelial cells. Mucin positivity is usually noted. Immunopositivity with E-cadherin (a cell-cohesion protein encoded by a gene on chromosome 16q22.1) may help discriminate between lobular and ductal carcinoma of the breast. Lobular carcinomas lack expression while ductal carcinomas typically express cytoplasmic E-cadherin.

DeMay RM, The Art & Science of Cytopathology.
Lobular carcinoma, p. 882.

Yeh I and Mies C. Application of Immunohistochemistry to Breast Lesions Archives of Pathology and Laboratory Medicine: (2007); Vol. 132, No. 3, pp. 349–358.

7. **C** juvenile papillomatosis

The diagnosis of juvenile papillomatosis mirrors the cytologic findings seen with fibroadenoma. The diagnosis is predominately a clinical one; that is, it must be established in adolescent females. In juvenile papillomatosis, both the patient and the mother are at an increased risk for the subsequent development of breast cancer. Fibroadenomas cytologically present as hypercellular specimens containing sheets or clusters of ductal epithelium and abundant fibroconnective tissue (metachromatic with Romanowsky stain). The background contains copious single, naked, oval nuclei (often myoepithelial in origin) that are spindle- or "cigar"-shaped with bipolar features.

DeMay RM, The Art & Science of Cytopathology.
Breast masses in children, adolescents (juvenile papillomatosis), p. 890.

8. **D** suspicious for malignancy

FNA of breast masses from elderly females should be carefully evaluated should the smears reveal a hypercellular population of monomorphic cells. These cells may represent infiltrating ductal carcinoma, mimicking the minimal deviation cytopathy also seen in lobular and colloid carcinoma. Ductal carcinomas found in elderly patients do not resemble their counterparts identified in younger patients. These lesions show little evidence of the classic malignant features detailed in younger females, appearing as monotonous sheets of ductal cells. Despite these cytologic findings, the vast majority of these lesions are histologically malignant; therefore, tissue evaluation must be performed even with the most innocuous-appearing cytomorphology.

DeMay RM, The Art & Science of Cytopathology.
FNA of breast cancer, p. 872.

9. **B** papillary neoplasm, rule out carcinoma

Papillary carcinoma resembles benign papillomas in its architectural patterns, presenting as hypercellular populations of three-dimensional true tissue clusters with smooth borders and central fibrovascular interiors. Overlapping nuclei and nuclear atypia may be observed. Variation in number of cell types is a key in discriminating these malignancies from benign papillomas. Malignant papillary neoplasms are composed of a monotypic population of cells, whereas benign papillomas typically have polytypic populations that include apocrine cells, foam cells, and hemosiderin-laden macrophages in addition to the papillary epithelial fragments. Papillary neoplasms presenting in older females are more likely to be malignant. Together, these minimal deviations may preclude an outright diagnosis of malignancy; therefore, the diagnosis of papillary neoplasm is recommended. Tissue biopsy must be performed to rule out invasion.

DeMay RM, The Art & Science of Cytopathology.
Papillary neoplasms, pp. 884–885.

10. **D** lobules

The breast is composed of 15–25 radially arranged lobes that drain from separate ducts and terminate at the nipple. The ducts are composed of epithelial cells and surrounded by a myoepithelial layer. The lobes are subdivided into lobules that, in the non-lactating breast, result from the terminal ducts and ductules, collectively termed the terminal duct lobular unit.

DeMay RM, The Art & Science of Cytopathology.
Anatomy, embryology, and physiology of the breast, pp. 853–854.

11. **A** ductal carcinoma in situ

Microductal carcinoma in situ (DCIS) may be detected on mammography but is usually nonpalpable. Axillary lymph nodes are disease free. The histologic presentation of these intraductal carcinomas shows a confinement to their basement membrane. The cytologic diagnosis cannot distinguish DCIS from frankly invasive ductal carcinoma. A variant of DCIS, comedo DCIS, presents cytologically as malignant ductal cells among a necrotic background—virtually indistinguishable from its malignant counterpart.

DeMay RM, The Art & Science of Cytopathology.
Ductal carcinoma in situ (DCIS, intraductal carcinoma), p. 875.

12. **D** colloid carcinoma

Colloid or mucinous carcinomas of the breast present as a monomorphic population of cells presenting in balls, acini, sheets, or as single cells scattered amongst a richly mucinous background ("sea of mucin"). The mucin is demonstrated as metachromatic with the Romanowsky stain or pale blue to pink with the Papanicolaou stain. These cells demonstrate few nuclear abnormalities with only slight anisokaryosis. The presence of anatomizing capillaries often accompanies the monotonous epithelial cells. Special stains with alcian blue or PAS will verify the mucinous nature of the background. Differentiation is important to distinguish these neoplasms from benign papillomas and mucocele-like lesions; however, colloid carcinomas generally occur in older patients and cytologically present with more abundant epithelial cells and irregular groupings.

DeMay RM, The Art & Science of Cytopathology.
Colloid carcinoma, p. 877.

13. **A** adenoid cystic carcinoma

Adenoid cystic carcinoma of the breast cytologically presents with metachromatic eosinophilic globules, either free within the background of the smear or contained within central lumens surrounded by acinar cellular formations, resembling "gum balls." The cytologic diagnosis of adenoid cystic carcinoma mimics those lesions arising within the salivary glands.

DeMay RM, The Art & Science of Cytopathology.
Salivary and sweat-gland tumors (adenoid cystic carcinoma), p. 887.

14. A ductal adenocarcinoma

FNA cytomorphology of infiltrating ductal carcinoma of the breast presents as hypercellular epithelial cells arranged in sheets, cords, well-formed microacini, and single cells. Pleomorphic nuclei, nuclear crowding and overlapping, hyperchromasia, irregular nuclear membranes, irregular chromatin and prominent nucleoli make up the malignant nuclear characteristics. Special emphasis should be given to the identification of single cells and intracytoplasmic lumens (often mucin or lipid) with the above-mentioned malignant criteria. Necrosis is exhibited in 60% of the cases.

DeMay RM, The Art & Science of Cytopathology.
Infiltrating ductal carcinoma, pp. 874–875.

15. A Paget disease

Paget disease of the breast is a ductal carcinoma (arising within the lactiferous duct) which has eroded to the surface of the breast, often involving the nipple. Palpable lesions associated with this disease are usually malignant; conversely, nonpalpable lesions may represent an in situ carcinoma. Cytologic criteria mirror a typical ductal carcinoma. Differential diagnosis includes melanoma, a rare disease of the nipple. S-100 and HMB-45 may stain positive for both Paget disease and melanoma, however, the mucin positivity associated with Paget disease excludes melanoma.

DeMay RM, The Art & Science of Cytopathology.
Paget disease of the breast, p. 886.

16. C gynecomastia

Gynecomastia affects 50% of middle-aged men. This disease may be related to an increase in endogenous or exogenous estrogen, illicit drugs, germ cell tumors, cirrhosis, and estrogen therapy for prostate cancer. The cellular findings associated with gynecomastia are similar to those found in fibroadenoma. Fibroadenomas cytologically present as hypercellular specimens containing sheets or clusters of ductal epithelium and abundant fibroconnective tissue (metachromatic with Romanowsky stain). The background contains copious single, naked, oval nuclei (often myoepithelial in origin) that are spindle- or "cigar"-shaped with bipolar features.

DeMay RM, The Art & Science of Cytopathology.
Gynecomastia, p. 890.

17. D serotonin

Carcinoid tumors of the breast have neuroendocrine differentiation, thus they may demonstrate immunocytochemical positivity with serotonin, chromogranin, neuron-specific enolase, or synaptophysin. FNA cytology reveals small monotonous cells with argyrophilic granules in monolayer sheets or singly with minimal nuclear atypia. This positivity, however, does not rule out the possibility of a metastatic neuroendocrine lesion.

DeMay RM, The Art & Science of Cytopathology.
Carcinoid tumors, argyrophilic carcinoma, carcinoma with endocrine differentiation, p. 880.

18. B metastatic carcinoma, lung primary

The described cells represent a keratinizing squamous cell carcinoma, most likely metastatic from the lung. Due to the presence of multiple bilateral masses, a metastatic lesion would be favored over a primary SCC. Primary SCC of the breast is extremely rare and usually has an associated population of malignant ductal cells upon close microscopic examination, thus representing a metaplastic adenosquamous carcinoma. Metastatic malignancies account for less than 5% of all breast tumors. Other metastatic tumors may include melanoma, ovarian carcinoma, lymphoma, and genitourinary malignancies. Prostatic carcinoma should be considered when differentiating malignant breast tumors arising within men. In such cases, special staining with prostate-specific antigen is useful.

DeMay RM, The Art & Science of Cytopathology.
Metastases, pp. 888–889, and Squamous cell carcinoma, p. 882.

19. B foam cells

Foam cells represent histiocytic cells that are often associated with physiologic nipple discharges. Their abundant frothy cytoplasm is easily visualized in cytology, and their nuclei are typically round-to-oval. At times, these cells are multinucleated.

DeMay RM, The Art & Science of Cytopathology.
The cells (foam cells), p. 294.

20. D adenocarcinoma

FNA cytomorphology of infiltrating ductal carcinoma of the breast presents as hypercellular epithelial cells arranged in sheets, cords, well-formed microacini, and single cells. Pleomorphic nuclei, nuclear crowding and overlapping, hyperchromasia, irregular nuclear membranes, irregular chromatin, and prominent nucleoli make up the malignant nuclear characteristics. Special emphasis should be given to the identification of single cells and intracytoplasmic lumens (often mucin or lipid) with the above-mentioned malignant criteria. Necrosis is exhibited in 60% of the cases.

DeMay RM, The Art & Science of Cytopathology.
Infiltrating ductal carcinoma, pp. 874–875.

21. **D** phyllodes tumor

Phyllodes tumors cytologically mimic their counterpart fibroadenoma with the exception that these lesions typically present with greater cellularity. The presence of sheets and clusters (often atypical) of epithelial cells and abundant fibroconnective tissue (generally greater than that of fibroadenoma) with associated capillaries is helpful in establishing the diagnosis. Care should be exercised not to overestimate the atypia within the epithelial sheets. The prominent stroma and the lack of single abnormal cells should help to differentiate this neoplasm from ductal carcinoma of the breast. Conversely, malignant phyllodes tumors show abundant stromal overgrowth in sheets, poorly cohesive clusters, and single cells. The stromal cells exhibit nuclear atypia consisting of irregular nuclear membranes, irregular chromatin, multiple nucleoli, and sometimes, intranuclear cytoplasmic inclusions. In malignant phyllodes tumors, osteosarcoma, chondrosarcoma, liposarcoma, angiosarcoma, or neurofibrosarcoma may represent the sarcomatous neoplasm.

DeMay RM, The Art & Science of Cytopathology.
Phyllodes tumors, pp. 865–866.

22. **C** papilloma, neoplasm not excluded

Three-dimensional glandular fragments with smooth or scalloped cohesive borders and containing predictable nuclei that maintain polarity throughout the fragment are diagnostic of an intraductal papilloma (IP). These fragments may be associated with bloody discharges, thus hemosiderin-laden macrophages may be present. Most papillomas and subareolar ductal lesions are generally of benign origin, often secondary to mastitis. This central breast lesion should not be confused with papillomatosis (also known as epithelial hyperplasia and epitheliosis), a peripheral breast lesion associated with ductal epithelial proliferation and fibrocystic disease. Fibrocystic disease is considered a "dysplasia," which places the patient at an increased risk for subsequent development of carcinoma of the breast. Although IP is a common benign disease, its exclusion from papillary carcinoma cannot be assumed, due to their shared cytomorphology. The diagnosis, "papillary clusters, neoplasm is not possible, excluded" is preferred until tissue biopsy or ductal excision is performed.

DeMay RM, The Art & Science of Cytopathology.
Intraductal papilloma, p. 295.

23. **B** fibroadenoma

Fibroadenomas cytologically present as hypercellular specimens containing sheets or clusters of ductal epithelium and abundant fibroconnective tissue (metachromatic with Romanowsky stain). The background contains copious single, naked, oval nuclei (often myoepithelial in origin) that are spindle-or "cigar"-shaped with bipolar features. Naked oval nuclei are a necessary component in establishing the benign nature of this neoplasm. Care should be taken not to overestimate the importance of rare atypical cells that may sometimes be seen in conjunction with the cellular findings.

DeMay RM, The Art & Science of Cytopathology.
Benign breast neoplasms (fibroadenoma), pp. 862–865.

24. **A** ductal dilatation

Ductal dilatation secondary to fibrocystic disease, papillomas, or mastitis may create unilateral nipple discharges. Bilateral discharges may be subsequent to physiologic or endocrine disturbances.

DeMay RM, The Art & Science of Cytopathology.
Nipple discharge, pp. 293–294.

25. **A** Paget disease

Paget disease represents a ductal carcinoma (arising within the lactiferous duct) that has eroded to the surface of the breast, often involving the nipple and creating a "peau d'orange." Palpable lesions associated with this disease are usually malignant; conversely, nonpalpable lesions may represent an in situ carcinoma. Cytologic criteria mirror a typical ductal carcinoma. Differential diagnosis includes melanoma, a rare disease of the nipple. S-100 and HMB-45 may stain positive for both Paget disease and melanoma, however, the mucin positivity associated with Paget disease excludes melanoma.

DeMay RM, The Art & Science of Cytopathology.
Paget disease of the breast, p. 886.

26. **B** fibrocystic disease

Fibrocystic disease (FCD) is a result of initial periductal mastitis that in time produces scarring, ductal stasis with retrograde dilatation, and macrocystic lesions. FNA cytology reveals mastitis, foam cells, adipose tissue, clusters of normal-appearing ductal epithelium, and apocrine metaplastic cells with their characteristic granular cytoplasm as well as prominent nucleoli. Certain variants of FCD, namely epithelial proliferation predominant, place the patient at an increased risk for subsequent development of carcinoma. FCD is seen as a triad consisting of cysts (fluid), fibrosis (acellular), or epithelial proliferation (papillomas).

DeMay RM, The Art & Science of Cytopathology.
Fibrocystic disease (change) of the breast, pp. 859–861.

27. **D** mastitis

FNA specimens representing acute mastitis reveal acute inflammatory components rich in polymorphonuclear neutrophils and granulomatous tissue (epithelioid histiocytes and/or multinucleated giant cells). Reactive epithelial and mesenchymal cells may complement the cellular findings. Care should be exercised not to overcall these cells—clinical history and the benign nuclear features (smooth nuclear membranes, fine even chromatin) help discriminate these inflammatory lesions from a malignant process.

DeMay RM, The Art & Science of Cytopathology.
Acute mastitis and breast abscess, p. 856.

28. **C** fat necrosis

Smears with rich inflammatory components, including neutrophils, lipid-laden histiocytes, multinucleated giant cells (with normal nuclear features), hemosiderin-laden macrophages, and hypocellular populations of ductal epithelial cells found in association with a bubbly appearing lipid-laden background are characteristic of fat necrosis. Reactive histiocytes and fibroblasts suggest mesenchymal repair. Although atypical nuclear features may be detected in mesenchymal cells, these changes should be treated with skepticism in light of the above benign cytologic findings. Furthermore, a clinical history of trauma and a recently appearing mass help support an acute diagnosis.

DeMay RM, The Art & Science of Cytopathology.
Fat necrosis, p. 858.

29. **D** lobular carcinoma

Lobular carcinomas present as moderate cellular specimens composed of small, monomorphic epithelial cells with minimal nuclear deviation or pleomorphism. The cells possess scanty cytoplasm, often with signet ring morphology or intracytoplasmic lumens. Nuclear overlapping and eccentric nuclei may be noted on high power. Rare vertebral column formation may be noted. Fibrocollagenous tissue may be interspersed amongst the groups of epithelial cells. Mucin positivity is usually noted. Immunopositivity with E-cadherin (a cell-cohesion protein encoded by a gene on chromosome 16q22.1) may help discriminate between lobular and ductal carcinoma of the breast. Lobular carcinomas lack expression while ductal carcinomas typically express cytoplasmic E-cadherin.

DeMay RM, The Art & Science of Cytopathology.
Lobular carcinoma, pp. 882–883.
Yeh I and Mies C. Application of Immunohistochemistry to Breast Lesions Archives of Pathology and Laboratory Medicine: (2007); Vol. 132, No. 3, pp. 349–358.

30. **C** fibrocystic disease

Fibrocystic disease (FCD) is a result of initial periductal mastitis that in time produces scarring, ductal stasis with retrograde dilatation, and macrocystic lesions. FNA cytology reveals mastitis, foam cells, adipose tissue, clusters of normal-appearing ductal epithelium, and apocrine metaplastic cells with their characteristic granular cytoplasm as well as prominent nucleoli. Certain variants of FCD, namely epithelial proliferation predominant, place the patient at an increased risk for subsequent development of carcinoma. FCD is seen as a triad consisting of cysts (fluid), fibrosis (acellular), or epithelial proliferation (papillomas).

DeMay RM, The Art & Science of Cytopathology.
Fibrocystic disease (change) of the breast, pp. 859-861.

31. **A** lactating adenoma

These benign lesions are related to hypersecretory activity of the breast. FNA reveals true acinar cells with foamy cytoplasm that, when smeared, create a proteinaceous background due to the disruption of the intracytoplasmic secretory products. Tight lobules and sheets of ductal epithelium are typically found and may exhibit active nuclear criteria. The presence of bare nuclei that are uniform in size but may contain prominent nucleoli (related to reactivity) may be confused with a true neoplastic process. Slight anisokaryosis may be identified in rare cells. The clinical history of pregnancy should safeguard against the possibility of rendering a malignant diagnosis. Special staining with oil red O or PAS will help elucidate the proteinaceous nature of the background.

DeMay RM, The Art & Science of Cytopathology.
Breast masses and pregnancy (lactating adenoma), pp. 858–859.

32. **D** fibrocystic disease

Fibrocystic disease (FCD) is a result of initial periductal mastitis that in time produces scarring, ductal stasis with retrograde dilatation, and macrocystic lesions. FNA cytology reveals mastitis, foam cells, adipose tissue, clusters of normal-appearing ductal epithelium, and apocrine metaplastic cells with their characteristic granular cytoplasm as well as prominent nucleoli. Certain variants of FCD, namely epithelial proliferation predominant, place the patient at an increased risk for subsequent development of carcinoma. FCD is seen as a triad consisting of cysts (fluid), fibrosis (acellular), or epithelial proliferation (papillomas).

DeMay RM, The Art & Science of Cytopathology.
Fibrocystic disease (change) of the breast, pp. 859–861.

33. **A** fibrocystic disease

Fibrocystic disease (FCD) is a result of initial periductal mastitis that in time produces scarring, ductal stasis with retrograde dilatation, and macrocystic lesions. FNA cytology reveals mastitis, foam cells, adipose tissue, clusters of normal-appearing ductal epithelium, and apocrine metaplastic cells with their characteristic granular cytoplasm as well as prominent nucleoli. Certain variants of FCD, namely epithelial proliferation predominant, places the patient at an increased risk for subsequent development of carcinoma. FCD is seen as a triad consisting of cysts (fluid), fibrosis (acellular), or epithelial proliferation (papillomas).

DeMay RM, The Art & Science of Cytopathology.
Fibrocystic disease (change) of the breast, pp. 859-861.

34. **A** ductal lining cells

Ductal epithelium presents in two-dimensional sheets or clusters with normal polarity or often with honeycombing features, scanty cytoplasm, and round to oval dense-appearing nuclei with micronucleoli. Moderate crowding may be seen (often related to hyperplasia). Should these cells contain secretory mucin, carcinoma should be considered.

DeMay RM, The Art & Science of Cytopathology.
Ductal cells, p. 854.

35. **D** lipoma

Lipomas represent benign neoplasms consisting of soft nodular collections of fat between septa. Capillaries and scanty connective tissue elements may also be seen. Differential diagnoses include fat necrosis or an inadequate sample due to an improperly sampled lesion.

DeMay RM, The Art & Science of Cytopathology.
Miscellaneous, p. 856.

36. **C** apocrine cells

Apocrine cells are metaplastic ductal cells that resemble oncocytes of the salivary gland or thyroid. These cells present in polygonal forms arranged in sheets and clusters, or found as single cells. The cytoplasm is characteristically coarsely granular, containing central nuclei and often prominent nucleoli. DPAS-positive glycolipid deposits may be present (Lendrum granules).

DeMay RM, The Art & Science of Cytopathology.
Apocrine cells, p. 855.

37. **D** alcian blue/colloid carcinoma

Colloid or mucinous carcinomas of the breast present as a monomorphic population of cells presenting in balls, acini, sheets, or as single cells scattered amongst a richly mucinous background ("sea of mucin"). The mucin is demonstrated as metachromatic with the Romanowsky stain or pale blue to pink with the Papanicolaou stain. These cells demonstrate few nuclear abnormalities with only slight anisokaryosis. The presence of anatomizing capillaries often accompanies the monotonous epithelial cells. Special stains with alcian blue or PAS will verify the mucinous nature of the background. Differentiation is important to distinguish these neoplasms from benign papillomas and mucocele-like lesions; however, colloid carcinomas generally occur in older patients and cytologically present with more abundant epithelial cells and irregular groupings.

DeMay RM, The Art & Science of Cytopathology.
Colloid carcinoma, pp. 877–878.

38. **B** tubular carcinoma

Tubular carcinomas may represent a stage in the development of ductal carcinoma, such as carcinoma in situ (DCIS). Cytology reveals cohesive clusters, single cells with intracytoplasmic lumens, tubular "garden hose" structures with central lumens, and glands with arrowhead-like outlines. The nuclei have fine, regular chromatin, and micronucleoli. Irregular nuclear membranes help support a malignant diagnosis. Differential diagnosis includes benign adenosis; however, this condition possesses grapelike glandular morphology.

DeMay RM, The Art & Science of Cytopathology.
Tubular carcinoma, pp. 878–879.

39. **A** ductal adenocarcinoma

Most breast cancers in men represent ductal carcinomas that recapitulate infiltrating ductal carcinoma arising within the female breast. FNA cytomorphology of infiltrating ductal carcinoma of the breast presents as hypercellular epithelial cells arranged in sheets, cords, well-formed microacini, and single cells. Pleomorphic nuclei, nuclear crowding and overlapping, hyperchromasia, irregular nuclear membranes, irregular chromatin, and prominent nucleoli make up the malignant nuclear characteristics. Special emphasis should be given to the identification of single cells and intracytoplasmic lumens (often mucin or lipid) with the above-mentioned malignant criteria. Necrosis is exhibited in 60% of the cases.

DeMay RM, The Art & Science of Cytopathology.
Cancer of the male breast, pp. 890–891.

40. **C** medullary carcinoma

This plate shows large anaplastic cells in sheets, clusters, and as single cells. These classic malignant features, as well as abnormal mitotic figures in conjunction with a background composed of lymphocytes, plasma cells, and histiocytes, identify this lesion as medullary carcinoma. Care should be exercised to differentiate the benign lymphocytes from lymphoma. Medullary carcinoma is mucin negative.

DeMay RM, The Art & Science of Cytopathology.
Medullary carcinoma, pp. 876–877.

41. **A** lactating adenoma

These benign lesions are related to hypersecretory activity of the breast. FNA reveals true acinar cells with foamy cytoplasm that, when smeared, create a proteinaceous background due to the disruption of the intracytoplasmic secretory products. Tight lobules and sheets of ductal epithelium are typical and may exhibit active nuclear criteria. The presence of bare nuclei that are uniform in size but may contain prominent nucleoli (related to reactivity) may be confused with a true neoplastic process. Slight anisokaryosis may be identified in rare cells. The clinical history of pregnancy should safeguard against the possibility of rendering a malignant diagnosis. Special staining with oil red O or PAS will help elucidate the proteinaceous nature of the background.

DeMay RM, The Art & Science of Cytopathology.
Breast masses and pregnancy (lactating adenoma), pp. 858–859.

42. **D** mucicarmine/Paget disease

Paget disease of the breast is a ductal carcinoma (arising within the lactiferous duct) that has eroded to the surface of the breast, often involving the nipple. Palpable lesions associated with this disease are usually malignant; conversely, nonpalpable lesions may represent an in situ carcinoma. Cytologic criteria mirror a typical ductal carcinoma. Differential diagnosis includes melanoma; a rare disease of the nipple. S-100 and HMB-45 may stain positive for both Paget disease and melanoma, however, the mucin positivity associated with Paget disease excludes melanoma.

DeMay RM, The Art & Science of Cytopathology.
Paget disease of the breast, p. 886.

43. **D** granulomatous mastitis

Leaky silicone implants have been associated with granulomatous mastitis, a disease that may clinically mimic infiltrating breast carcinoma. Cytologically, the presence of multinucleated giant cells with asteroid body inclusions, epithelioid histiocytes, and assorted inflammatory cells will be seen amongst a yellow or blue homogeneous, refractile/non-birefringent background; however, silicone may dissolve in the staining process, leaving a background containing clear empty spaces.

DeMay RM, The Art & Science of Cytopathology.
Granulomatous mastitis, pp. 857–858.

44. **D** infiltrating ductal carcinoma

FNA cytomorphology of infiltrating ductal carcinoma of the breast presents as hypercellular epithelial cells arranged in sheets, cords, well-formed microacini, and single cells. Pleomorphic nuclei, nuclear crowding and overlapping, hyperchromasia, irregular nuclear membranes, irregular chromatin, and prominent nucleoli make up the malignant nuclear characteristics. Special emphasis should be given to the identification of single cells and intracytoplasmic lumens (often mucin or lipid) with the above-mentioned malignant criteria. Necrosis is exhibited in 60% of the cases.

DeMay RM, The Art & Science of Cytopathology.
Infiltrating ductal carcinoma, pp. 874–875.

45. **D** fat necrosis

Smears with rich inflammatory components including neutrophils, lipid-laden histiocytes, multinucleated giant cells (with normal nuclear features), hemosiderin-laden macrophages, and hypocellular populations of ductal epithelial cells found in association with a bubbly appearing, lipid-laden background are characteristic of fat necrosis. Reactive histiocytes and fibroblasts suggest mesenchymal repair. Although atypical nuclear features may be detected in mesenchymal cells, these changes should be treated with skepticism in light of the above benign cytologic findings. Furthermore, a clinical history of trauma and a recently appearing mass helps support an acute diagnosis.

DeMay RM, The Art & Science of Cytopathology.
Inflammation (fat necrosis), p. 858.

46. **D** simple fibrocystic disease

Fibrocystic disease (FCD) is a result of initial periductal mastitis, which in time produces scarring, ductal stasis with retrograde dilatation, and macrocystic lesions. FNA cytology reveals mastitis, foam cells, adipose tissue, clusters of normal-appearing ductal epithelium, and apocrine metaplastic cells with their characteristic granular cytoplasm as well as prominent nucleoli. Certain variants of FCD, namely epithelial proliferation predominant, places the patient at an increased risk for subsequent development of carcinoma. FCD is seen as a triad consisting of cysts (fluid), fibrosis (acellular), or epithelial proliferation (papillomas). Simple FCD, such as illustrated in these images, is composed of cysts and fibrosis.

DeMay RM, The Art & Science of Cytopathology.
Fibrocystic disease (change) of the breast, pp. 859–861.

47. **D** papillary clusters, neoplasm not excluded

Three-dimensional glandular fragments with smooth or scalloped cohesive borders, containing predictable nuclei that maintain polarity throughout the fragment are diagnostic of an intraductal papilloma (IP). These fragments may be associated with bloody discharges, thus hemosiderin-laden macrophages may be present. Most papillomas and subareolar ductal lesions are generally of benign origin, often secondary to mastitis. This central breast lesion should not be confused with papillomatosis (also known as epithelial hyperplasia, and epitheliosis), a peripheral breast lesion associated with ductal epithelial proliferation and fibrocystic disease. Fibrocystic disease is considered a "dysplasia," which places the patient at an increased risk for subsequent development of carcinoma of the breast. Although IP is a common benign disease, its exclusion from papillary carcinoma is not possible, due to their shared cytomorphology. The diagnosis, "papillary clusters, neoplasm cannot be excluded," is preferred until tissue biopsy or ductal excision is performed.

DeMay RM, The Art & Science of Cytopathology.
Intraductal papilloma, p. 295.

48. **A** foam cells

Foam cells represent histiocytic cells that are often associated with physiologic nipple discharges. Their abundant frothy cytoplasm is easily visualized in cytology, and their nuclei are typically round to oval. At times, these cells are multinucleated.

DeMay RM, The Art & Science of Cytopathology.
The cells (foam cells), p. 294.

49. **D** fibroadenoma

Fibroadenomas cytologically present as hypercellular specimens containing sheets or clusters of ductal epithelium and abundant fibroconnective tissue (metachromatic with Romanowsky stain). The background contains copious single, naked, oval nuclei (often myoepithelial in origin) that are spindle-or "cigar"-shaped with bipolar features. Naked oval nuclei are a necessary component in establishing the benign nature of this neoplasm. Care should be taken not to overestimate the importance of rare atypical cells that may sometimes be seen in conjunction with the cellular findings.

DeMay RM, The Art & Science of Cytopathology.
Benign breast neoplasms (fibroadenoma), pp. 862–865

50. **A** lobular carcinoma

Lobular carcinomas present as moderate cellular specimens composed of small, monomorphic epithelial cells with minimal nuclear deviation or pleomorphism. The cells possess scanty cytoplasm, often with signet ring morphology or intracytoplasmic lumens. Nuclear overlapping and eccentric nuclei may be noted on high power. Rare vertebral column formation may be noted. Fibrocollagenous tissue may be interspersed amongst the groups of epithelial cells. Mucin positivity is usually noted. Immunopositivity with E-cadherin (a cell-cohesion protein encoded by a gene on chromosome 16q22.1) may help discriminate between lobular and ductal carcinoma of the breast. Lobular carcinomas lack expression while ductal carcinomas typically express cytoplasmic E-cadherin.

(−) in Lob CA
(+) in Ductal CA

DeMay RM, The Art & Science of Cytopathology.
Lobular carcinoma, p. 882.

Yeh I and Mies C. Application of Immunohistochemistry to Breast Lesions Archives of Pathology and Laboratory Medicine: (2007); Vol. 132, No. 3, pp. 349–358.

51. **B** apocrine metaplastic cells

Apocrine cells are metaplastic ductal cells that resemble oncocytes of the salivary gland or thyroid. These cells present in polygonal forms arranged in sheets and clusters, or found as single cells. The cytoplasm is characteristically coarsely granular, containing central nuclei and often prominent nucleoli. DPAS-positive glycolipid deposits may be present (Lendrum granules).

DeMay RM, The Art & Science of Cytopathology.
The cells (apocrine metaplastic cells), p. 294.

52. **D** **phyllodes tumor**

Phyllodes tumors cytologically mimic their counterpart fibroadenoma, with the exception that these lesions typically present with greater cellularity. The presence of sheets and clusters (often atypical) of epithelial cells and abundant fibroconnective tissue (generally greater than that of fibroadenoma) with associated capillaries is helpful in establishing the diagnosis. Care should be exercised not to overestimate the atypia within the epithelial sheets. The prominent stroma and the lack of single abnormal cells should help to differentiate this neoplasm from ductal carcinoma of the breast. Conversely, malignant phyllodes tumors show abundant stromal overgrowth in sheets, poorly cohesive clusters, and single cells. The stromal cells exhibit nuclear atypia consisting of irregular nuclear membranes, irregular chromatin, multiple nucleoli, and sometimes, intranuclear cytoplasmic inclusions. In malignant phyllodes tumors, osteosarcoma, chondrosarcoma, liposarcoma, angiosarcoma, or neurofibrosarcoma may represent the sarcomatous neoplasm.

DeMay RM, The Art & Science of Cytopathology.
Phyllodes tumors, pp. 865–866.

53. **B** **gynecomastia**

The cellular findings associated with gynecomastia are similar to those found in fibroadenoma. Fibroadenomas cytologically present as hypercellular specimens containing sheets or clusters of ductal epithelium and abundant fibroconnective tissue (metachromatic with Romanowsky stain). The background contains copious single naked oval nuclei (often myoepithelial in origin) that are spindle-or "cigar"-shaped with bipolar features. Naked oval nuclei are a necessary component in establishing the benign nature of this neoplasm.

DeMay RM, The Art & Science of Cytopathology.
Male breast (gynecomastia), p. 890.

Chapter 8

Fine Needle Aspiration

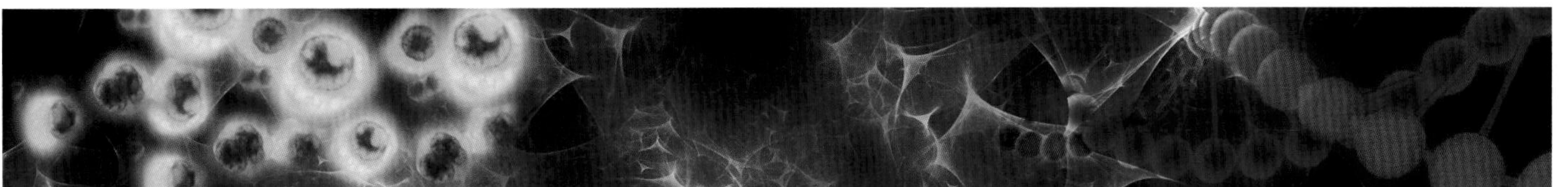

1. A 51-year-old woman presents with an enlarged thyroid. Staining the FNA material with May-Grunwald-Giemsa reveals small uniform cells in monolayers and sheets with honeycombing patterns, circular groups with central material, hemosiderin-laden macrophages, and blood, contained in a background of abundant amorphous material. These cells are diagnostic of:

   A. follicular neoplasm
   B. Hashimoto thyroiditis
   C. colloid goiter
   D. papillary carcinoma

2. A good rule of thumb for identifying an adequate thyroid specimen is the presence of:

   A. colloid
   B. a single follicular cell in every slide
   C. at least 6 clusters of 10 cells over 2 slides
   D. at least 2 clusters on 1 of the slides

3. A 65-year-old man with a history of alcohol abuse and cirrhosis of the liver presents with jaundice. A 2-cm lesion is identified within the liver. FNA reveals a malignant group of glandular cells. ANA staining for bile canaliculi is positive within the malignant cell population. The diagnosis is:

   A. cholangiocarcinoma
   B. hepatocellular carcinoma
   C. metastatic colonic adenocarcinoma
   D. metastatic pancreatic adenocarcinoma

4. HIV-positive patients may suffer from which of the following salivary gland lesions?

   A. basal cell adenomas
   B. benign lymphoepithelial cyst
   C. lipomas
   D. hemangiomas

5. A thyroid aspirate reveals a hypercellular population of follicular cells in acinar formation with enlarged, hyperchromatic nuclei and coarse, irregular chromatin. Macronucleoli are noted. The findings suggest:

   A. follicular adenoma
   B. follicular carcinoma
   C. Hashimoto thyroiditis
   D. papillary carcinoma

6. A 55-year-old man with a history of previous excision of a pleomorphic adenoma presents with a recurrent parotid tumor. FNA reveals sheets and clusters of cells with frothy cytoplasm and hyperchromatic nuclei, irregular chromatin, and macronucleoli. The background could be characterized as proteinaceous and watery. The diagnosis is:

   A. mucoepidermoid carcinoma
   B. polymorphous low-grade adenocarcinoma
   C. acinic cell carcinoma
   D. malignant mixed tumor

7. **Cells secondary to fatty metamorphosis will often have:**

   A. signet ring morphology
   B. papillary morphology
   C. acinar morphology
   D. increased lipofuscin pigment

8. **FNA of a parotid tumor from a 55-year-old man yields a brown doughy substance. Cytology reveals a large population of polygonal cells with eosinophilic granular cytoplasm, central or eccentric nuclei, and prominent nucleoli. The background contains a lymphocytic infiltrate and proteinaceous necrotic debris. The diagnosis is:**

   A. pleomorphic adenoma
   B. oncocytoma
   C. Warthin tumor
   D. monomorphic adenoma

9. **A 35-year-old man with a 3-cm parotid mass evaluated by FNA cytologically presents with a mixture of round cells with foamy cytoplasm, hyperchromatic nuclei, irregular chromatin, and nucleoli. Another smaller cellular component yields cells with dense cytoplasm, pleomorphic cell forms and opaque/India ink nuclear features. A watery background is present. These cells are diagnostic of:**

   A. mucoepidermoid carcinoma, well differentiated
   B. mucoepidermoid carcinoma, poorly differentiated
   C. acinic cell carcinoma, well differentiated
   D. acinic cell carcinoma, poorly differentiated

10. **A malignant minor salivary gland lesion is characterized cytologically as clusters or papillary structures of bland-appearing cuboidal-to-elongated cells with central lumens containing small nuclei, micronucleoli, and vacuolated cytoplasm. Tyrosine-rich crystals are seen. The diagnosis suggests:**

    A. polymorphous low-grade primary adenocarcinoma
    B. adenoid cystic carcinoma
    C. poorly differentiated mucoepidermoid carcinoma
    D. malignant mixed tumor, "benign" metastasizing mixed tumor variant

11. **Should FNA suggest a Warthin tumor but lack the characteristic lymphocytic infiltrate, the diagnosis suggests:**

    A. monomorphic adenoma
    B. acinic cell carcinoma
    C. adenoid cystic carcinoma
    D. oncocytoma

12. **A 51-year-old woman with a painful submaxillary tumor presents for FNA. Cytology reveals a highly cellular smear with bland cells appearing in nests or rosette clusters with central hyaline basement membrane "pink gumball-like" inclusions. Nucleoli are small and inconspicuous. PAS stains are negative. The diagnosis is:**

    A. pleomorphic adenoma
    B. monomorphic adenoma
    C. acinic cell carcinoma
    D. adenoid cystic carcinoma

13. **A 5-year-old boy presents with an enlarged parotid gland. A 2-cm lesion is noted upon examination. FNA reveals a bloody fluid composed of bland spindle cells. The diagnosis is:**

    A. malignant lymphoma
    B. hamartoma
    C. sarcoma
    D. hemangioma

14. **A 60-year-old woman presents with a 2-cm lesion within the minor salivary glands. FNA reveals cohesive clusters of small cells with round to oval dark nuclear features without nucleoli, but with high N/C ratios. These cells are diagnostic of:**

    A. adenoid cystic carcinoma
    B. pleomorphic adenoma
    C. monomorphic adenoma
    D. Mikulicz associated sialadenitis

15. **The most common tumor of the liver is:**

    A. hepatocellular carcinoma
    B. bile duct carcinoma
    C. malignant lymphoma
    D. metastatic carcinoma

16. **Patients suffering from alpha1-antitrypsin deficiency often contain which of the following cytomorphologic features in hepatocytes?**

A. neutral triglycerides
B. hyaline globules
C. Mallory bodies
D. melanin

17. **FNA of a parotid mass reveals a cellular sample containing sheets and clusters of cells with clear to basophilic foamy cytoplasm with PAS-positive granules. Nuclei are uniform with finely granular chromatin. This diagnosis is:**

A. adenoid cystic carcinoma
B. acinic cell carcinoma
C. malignant mixed tumor
D. mucoepidermoid carcinoma

18. **To diagnose follicular carcinoma, which of the following may be helpful?**

A. coarse chromatin
B. vascular or capsular invasion as determined histologically
C. clusters of follicular cells
D. nucleoli

19. **The most common malignancy that often occurs secondary to benign lymphoepithelial lesions or Sjögren syndrome and arises within intraparotid lymph nodes is:**

A. Hodgkin lymphoma
B. lymphangioma
C. adenoid cystic carcinoma
D. non-Hodgkin lymphoma

20. **Which thyroid tumor arises from parafollicular cells?**

A. medullary carcinoma
B. follicular carcinoma
C. papillary carcinoma
D. Hürthle cell carcinoma

21. **A liver aspirate composed of a hypercellular population of bile ductal cells and scattered endothelial cells, fibromyxoid stroma, and adipose tissue is diagnostic of:**

A. cells indigenous to Glisson capsule
B. fatty metamorphosis
C. liver cell adenoma
D. hamartoma

22. **FNA revealed cells in monolayer sheets and single cells with nuclei showing anisonucleosis, irregular membranes, washed out chromatin, and nuclear grooves. Intranuclear cytoplasmic inclusions were noted in many cells. Occasional psammoma bodies were also seen. The diagnosis is:**

A. medullary carcinoma
B. Hashimoto thyroiditis
C. papillary carcinoma
D. follicular neoplasm

23. **A 3-cm neck mass found along the anterior border of the sternocleidomastoid muscle reveals a large population of mature squamous cells, mature lymphocytes, and immunoblasts. These cells are diagnostic of:**

A. branchial cleft cyst
B. cystic hygroma colli
C. parathyroid cyst
D. granuloma

24. **A 55-year-old man presents with a 2×3-cm nodule in the upper pole of the thyroid. FNA reveals numerous spindle to oval cells with fibrillar cytoplasm with dendritic processes. Enlarged eccentric nuclei, multinucleation, and salt-and-pepper chromatin are noted. Intranuclear cytoplasmic invaginations are noted in many of the cells. Macronucleoli are apparent in a large majority of the cells. Amorphous sheets of eosinophilic material are exhibited with the Papanicolaou stain. Immunoperoxidase staining for calcitonin is positive. The diagnosis is:**

A. papillary carcinoma
B. follicular carcinoma
C. anaplastic carcinoma
D. medullary carcinoma

25. A thyroid aspirate reveals large polygonal cells with central and eccentric nuclei, prominent nucleoli, and granular cytoplasm as well as a numerous population of lymphocytes. The diagnosis is:

A. Hürthle cell adenoma
B. Hashimoto thyroiditis
C. follicular neoplasm
D. nodular goiter

26. A thyroid aspiration from a 34-year-old woman with a recent history of mumps consists of small degenerated follicular cells, large multinucleated giant cells surrounding and engulfing colloid, lymphocytes, and epithelioid histiocytes. The diagnosis is:

A. Hashimoto thyroiditis
B. follicular neoplasm
C. Hürthle cell adenoma
D. granulomatous thyroiditis (de Quervain)

27. The most reliable criterion for discriminating liver cell dysplasia from nontrabecular hepatocellular carcinoma by FNA cytology is:

A. monolayer hepatocytes with random atypical cells are found with liver cell dysplasia
B. monolayer hepatocytes with random atypical cells are found with hepatocellular carcinoma
C. absence of atypia in liver cell dysplasia
D. poorly differentiated anaplastic cells are generally found in hepatocellular carcinoma

28. A 35-year-old woman with a history of long-term birth control pill use with a 10-cm liver nodule presents for FNA. No previous history of malignancy is noted. Cytology reveals a hypercellular population of polygonal cells arranged in a monolayers with well-defined cytoplasm. The nuclei are often binucleate, intranuclear inclusions are noted, and chromatin is fine and regular. A low N/C ratio is present. PAS stains are positive. These cells are diagnostic of:

A. liver cell adenoma
B. hepatocellular carcinoma
C. cholangiocarcinoma
D. metastatic melanoma

29. An aspiration of a paramidline neck mass yielded an amorphous fluid containing abundant squamous epithelial cells. The diagnosis is:

A. thyroglossal duct cysts
B. parathyroid cyst
C. epidermoid cysts
D. carotid body tumor

30. A 41-year-old woman presents with a cold 2-cm thyroid nodule. FNA reveals sheets and clusters of small cells with round, uniform nuclei and macronucleoli. Colloid is scarce. These cells are diagnostic of:

A. papillary carcinoma
B. goiter
C. clear cell carcinoma
D. follicular neoplasm

31. Elongated ropy hyaline intracytoplasmic inclusions surrounding the nucleus in hepatocytes associated with alcoholic cirrhosis are called:

A. Councilman bodies
B. Mallory bodies
C. bile
D. lipofuscin

32. A hypercellular population of polygonal cells with eosinophilic granular cytoplasm, round to oval nuclei, and macronucleoli are identified in a thyroid FNA. The background is clean. The diagnosis is:

A. Hashimoto thyroiditis
B. Hürthle cell neoplasm
C. hyalinizing trabecular adenoma
D. Hürthle cell thyroiditis

33. A 77-year-old woman with a large thyroid mass is evaluated with FNA. Cytology shows a highly cellular population of pleomorphic cells with hyperchromasia, irregular chromatin, macronucleoli, and a necrotic background. Giant tumor cells are noted. Immunostaining for keratin, epithelial membrane antigen, thyroglobulin, and thyrocalcitonin are all negative. These cells are diagnostic of:

A. squamous cell carcinoma
B. medullary carcinoma
C. papillary carcinoma
D. anaplastic carcinoma

34. The aspiration of a cystic liver is contraindicated because of the possibility of anaphylaxis when dealing with:

A. *Echinococcus germinosis*
B. *Echinococcus hydatidosis*
C. *Echinococcus cestodosis*
D. *Echinococcus granulosus*

35. CT scan reveals a large nodular lesion in the liver. FNA reveals a hypercellular population of polygonal cells with anisocytosis, binucleation, macronucleoli, intranuclear cytoplasmic invaginations, and numerous bile ductal cells. Mixed chronic inflammation is present. Intracytoplasmic greenish-black globules are identified with Giemsa staining. These findings are suggestive of:

A. hepatocellular carcinoma
B. cholangiocarcinoma
C. cirrhosis
D. metastatic carcinoma

36. FNA biopsy of which of the following lung lesions is considered to be contraindicated?

A. central lesions
B. vascular lesions
C. peripherally located nodules
D. inflammatory lesions

37. A pulmonary aspiration of an upper left lobe peripheral mass shows three-dimensional cell clusters with 20 or more cells, tall columnar in shape, with bland basally located nuclei, increased N/C ratios, and fine, irregular chromatin patterns with large, round, often irregular, centrally located macronucleoli. Intracytoplasmic lumens and occasional intranuclear cytoplasmic invaginations are noted. These cells are diagnostic of:

A. creola bodies
B. pulmonary infarct
C. bronchogenic adenocarcinoma
D. bronchioloalveolar adenocarcinoma

38. A 5-cm lesion extending from the major bronchi to the periphery of the left lower lobe of the lung is examined by fine needle aspiration. Many isolated cells, as well as cells in syncytia with nuclear overlapping, anisocytosis, cyanophilic cytoplasm with little polarity and indistinct borders, and coarse, irregular chromatin, parachromatin clearing, and irregular macronucleoli, are found in a necrotic background. This presentation best describes a diagnosis of:

A. large-cell carcinoma
B. well-differentiated squamous carcinoma
C. chronic interstitial pneumonitis
D. small cell carcinoma, intermediate cell type

39. If one suspects a hematopoietic pathological process, which of the following stains is best for cytologic identification?

A. Romanowsky
B. hematoxylin and eosin
C. oil red O
D. PAS

40. **FNA of a central solitary lesion from a 51-year-old woman shows isolated monotonous cells in sheets, nests, ribbons, and cords. The cells are oval-to-columnar with basophilic cytoplasm and no evidence of terminal bars and/or cilia, and possess uniform nuclei with moderately high N/C ratios containing finely granular, evenly distributed chromatin with inconspicuous nucleoli. These cells are diagnostic of:**

    A. malignant lymphoma
    B. small cell carcinoma
    C. chronic follicular bronchitis
    D. carcinoid tumor

41. **A 66-year-old man presents with a solitary coin lesion measuring 2 cm on CXR. FNA reveals isolated cells in syncytial-like aggregates with nuclear molding. The cytoplasm is scanty, and the nuclei are hyperchromatic with coarse, regular chromatin. The background shows crush artifact, cell ghosts, and necrotic debris. The diagnosis is:**

    A. pulmonary lymphocytic infiltrates
    B. poorly differentiated non-small cell carcinoma
    C. bronchial carcinoid
    D. small cell carcinoma

42. **A 55-year-old woman with a history of gynecologic cancer presents with bilateral lung nodules. FNA reveals spindle to stellate cells with oval, hyperchromatic, fine to coarse chromatin, prominent nucleoli and fibrillar, granular, basophilic cytoplasm. The most likely diagnosis/origin of these cells is:**

    A. squamous cell carcinoma/cervix
    B. teratoma/ovary
    C. adenocarcinoma/fallopian tube
    D. mixed müllerian tumor/uterus

43. **FNA of the lung reveals sheets of monotonous cells with finely granular, evenly distributed chromatin, cells with a spindle appearance and oval nuclei with micronucleoli, and large well-circumscribed structures with eccentrically located nuclei and capillaries. These cells are diagnostic of:**

    A. normal pulmonary constituents
    B. metastatic hepatocellular carcinoma
    C. bronchogenic adenocarcinoma
    D. squamous cell carcinoma

44. **Which of the following may be associated with a false negative fine needle aspiration?**

    A. aspiration of necrotic center
    B. soft nodules
    C. pencil point needles
    D. Chiba needles

45. **FNA of a 4-cm mass reveals snake-like pleomorphic cells, cells with concentric ringing, ink-dot nuclear features, and ghost cells. The diagnosis is:**

    A. spindle cell sarcoma
    B. leiomyosarcoma
    C. squamous carcinoma
    D. large-cell carcinoma

46. **A population of small cells, as well as loose acinar structures with hyperchromasia and prominent nucleoli, were found in an FNA of a lung nodule from a 70-year-old man. Immunostaining for PSA was positive. The diagnosis is:**

    A. small cell carcinoma
    B. adenocarcinoma, kidney
    C. transitional cell carcinoma
    D. adenocarcinoma, prostate

47. **A 44-year-old woman with a known malignancy presents with multiple lung nodules. FNA reveals round-to-oval cells with eccentric nuclei, anisocytosis, and prominent nucleoli with intranuclear cytoplasmic invaginations and intracytoplasmic brownish refractile granules. Staining with HMB-45 is positive. The diagnosis is:**

    A. metastatic hepatocellular carcinoma
    B. hemosiderin-laden macrophages
    C. dust cells
    D. metastatic melanoma

48. **What mediastinal tumor is most common?**

    A. lipoma
    B. neural sheath tumors
    C. parathyroid tumors
    D. lymphangioma

49. **A thyroid aspirate yields a hypercellular population of polygonal cells containing eccentric nuclei, prominent nucleoli, and granular cytoplasm accompanied by numerous lymphocytes. These cellular findings are diagnostic of:**

A. Hashimotos thyroiditis
B. follicular neoplasm
C. colloid goiter
D. lymphocytic lymphoma

50. **FNA of a diffuse lung nodule from an immunocompromised patient reveals GMS-positive structures presenting in "contact lens" shapes, 4-6 mm in diameters with central basophilic intranuclear inclusions among mats of frothy material. The diagnosis is:**

A. *Mycobacterium tuberculosis*
B. *Histoplasma capsulatum*
C. *Pneumocystis carinii*
D. *Cryptococcus neoformans*

51. **A 55-year-old smoker with emphysema presents with a mediastinal shadow on the right lower lobe on CXR. FNA of the area reveals a large inflammatory infiltrate composed of neutrophils, lymphocytes, necrotic detritus, fibrin, macrophages, and blood. The diagnosis is:**

A. osteomyelitis
B. abscess
C. granulomatous disease
D. teratoma

52. **What mediastinal lesion is considered common in infants?**

A. mesenchymal tumors
B. lymphatic cysts
C. gastroenteric cysts
D. seminoma

53. **A 58-year-old man with multicentric lung nodules shows a monomorphic population of cells lying singly containing round cleaved nuclei and coarse chromatin on FNA evaluation. Leu M5 staining was positive. These cells are diagnostic of:**

A. atypical carcinoid
B. malignant lymphoma
C. small cell carcinoma, intermediate cell type
D. normal mesothelial cells

54. **The most common complication associated with pulmonary needle aspirations is:**

A. needle tract tumor seeding
B. infection
C. pneumothorax
D. air embolus

55. **A 44-year-old woman presents with a single nodule in the left upper lobe of the lung. FNA reveals sheets of columnar cells with preserved cellular polarity, cells with large vacuoles with associated capillaries, and cells with eosinophilic cytoplasm, multiple nuclei, and central lacunae. A stringy background is identified. These cells are diagnostic of:**

A. lipoma
B. hamartoma
C. leiomyosarcoma
D. liposarcoma

56. **A 44-year-old man with a history of malignancy presents with multiple lung nodules and a concomitant pleural effusion. FNA of the lung shows a monotonous population of small round to oval cells without cohesion, nuclear grooves, and cleaving with coarse chromatin and frequent nucleoli. These cells are diagnostic of:**

A. small cell carcinoma, oat cell type
B. carcinoid tumor
C. small cell carcinoma, intermediate cell type
D. malignant lymphoma

57. A 55-year-old man with a 3 × 4-cm coin lesion presents for FNA evaluation. Cytology reveals a heterogeneous population of cells including large cells with multiple nuclei and fine regular chromatin with frothy cytoplasm, spindle-appearing cells with oval nuclei and fine chromatin, and lymphocytes. These cells are diagnostic of:

A. giant-cell carcinoma
B. poorly differentiated adenocarcinoma
C. poorly differentiated squamous cell carcinoma
D. granuloma

58. A 45-year-old woman presents with a painless, 3-cm salivary gland mass and complaint of dry eyes and mouth. FNA cytology reveals lymphocytes, plasma cells, and degenerated acinar structures as well as multinucleated giant cells and epithelioid histiocytes. What etiology is associated with the cytological findings?

A. Sjögren syndrome
B. tuberculoma
C. Hashimoto disease
D. sarcoidosis

59. A fine needle aspiration of a 2 × 3-cm lung mass proved difficult due to a strong desmoplastic response surrounding the tumor. An 18-gauge needle yielded a heterogeneous population of cells in three-dimensional groups with mucin positivity. Acinar structures were common. Chromatin was irregular and macronucleoli were present in almost every cell. Based on these findings, the diagnosis is:

A. bronchogenic adenocarcinoma
B. large cell carcinoma
C. squamous cell carcinoma
D. carcinoid tumor

60. A benign salivary disorder, often related to *Staphylococcus aureus,* presenting as lithiasis and acute inflammation and exhibiting the clinical symptom of painful swelling, is referred to as:

A. mucocele
B. sialadenitis
C. pleomorphic adenoma
D. Warthin tumor

61. A small population of single cells with nuclear molding and coarse chromatin were found in an aspirate from a peripheral lung nodule. Special stains with leukocyte common antigen (LCA) will be:

A. positive
B. negative
C. indeterminate
D. peripherally positive

62. A middle mediastinal tumor composed of single cells with hyperchromatic eccentric nuclei and coarse clock-faced peripheral chromatin and binucleated and bizarre multinucleated giant cells is diagnostic of:

A. malignant lymphoma, small cell cleaved
B. malignant lymphoma, large cell non-cleaved
C. plasmacytoma
D. small cell carcinoma, intermediate cell type

63. A malignant anterior mediastinal tumor, often associated with paraneoplastic syndromes that presents cytologically as a biphasic cell pattern of cortical epithelial cells and lymphoid components is:

A. invasive thymoma
B. cystic hygroma
C. neurofibroma
D. schwannoma

64. The most common benign salivary gland neoplasm is:

A. Warthin tumor
B. oxyphilic adenoma
C. pleomorphic adenoma
D. basal cell adenoma

65. A 44-year-old woman presents with a painless, freely movable mass of the parotid. FNA reveals sheets of cells and clusters with well-defined cell borders as well as elongated cells with attenuated ends. A basophilic background is seen with Papanicolaou staining. These cells are diagnostic of:

A. granuloma
B. monomorphic adenoma
C. Warthin tumor
D. pleomorphic adenoma

66. When performing FNA, what recommendation would be suggested for evaluating excessive bloody aspirates?

A. discard and repuncture identical area
B. prepare as is with cell block technique
C. treat with 100% glacial acetic acid
D. treat with Carnoy fixative

67. A multifocal lesion is found in the right lung of a 66-year-old man who has a history of extra-pulmonary cancer. FNA of the nodules reveals large columnar cells in cigar shapes and granular cytoplasm with loss of polarity. The nuclei contain hyperchromatic, fine irregular chromatin with jagged macronucleoli. These cells best describe:

A. metastatic pancreatic carcinoma
B. metastatic squamous carcinoma
C. metastatic colonic adenocarcinoma
D. viral pneumonitis

68. Which of the following is considered a posterior mediastinal malignant lesion?

A. malignant schwannoma
B. thymoma
C. hemangioma
D. parathyroid adenoma

69. A 55-year-old woman with a history of radiation and busulfan therapy for bronchogenic adenocarcinoma is evaluated by FNA due to a shadow seen on chest x-ray. Macrocytes with large, dark nuclei and good cell-to-cell recognition are found. Cellular crowding with terminal bars is seen in the presence of a clean background. The diagnosis is:

A. recurrent bronchogenic adenocarcinoma
B. terminal bronchioloalveolar carcinoma
C. reactive bronchial cells
D. hamartoma

70. In comparison with other pulmonary specimen collection techniques, fine needle aspiration biopsy is most useful for the diagnosis of:

A. central lesions
B. hilar lesions
C. peripheral lesions
D. necrotic lesions

71. A 32-year-old man presents with a nodule located within the vertebral column. FNA reveals multinucleated giant cells (some up to 20 nuclei per cell); spindle cells with predictable cellular features, monomorphic small cells with well-defined borders, granular cytoplasm, and round, eccentric nuclei; and fragments of mature bone in a metachromatic fibrous and bloody background. The diagnosis is:

A. osteosarcoma
B. chondroblastoma
C. osteoblastoma
D. chondrosarcoma

72. FNA of a lung lesion reveals large cells with dense cytoplasm, thick refractile cell walls, and smudgy, greasy-appearing nuclear features, with intracytoplasmic basophilic inclusions. The diagnosis is:

A. creola bodies
B. aspiration pneumonia, plant material
C. squamous cell carcinoma
D. atypical squamous metaplasia

73. A benign lesion ocurring in the epiphysis of the long bones cytologically presents as polygonal cells with dense, glassy ctyoplasm and round to oval nuclei containing grooves. Many cells present with binucleate eccentric features. Multinucleated osteoclasts are found in addition to dense eosinophilic background. These cells are diagnostic of:

A. osteoblastoma
B. chondrosarcoma
C. chondroblastoma
D. giant cell tumor of the bone

74. A 76-year-old man with a previous history of an epithelial malignancy presents with multiple nodules contained within the calvarium. FNA reveals a population of small cells found in repeated microacinar structures with hyperchromatic nuclei, irregular chromatin, and prominent nucleoli. Which special stain would aid in the correlation of his previous disease?

A. prostate-specific antigen (+)
B. Warthin-Starry (+)
C. alcian blue-hyaluronidase (–)
D. amino acid naphthylamidase for bile canaliculi (+)

75. A 67-year-old woman presents with a 2-cm liver nodule located with nuclear magnetic resonance. A history of intrahepatic lithiasis is noted. FNA reveals a hypercellular population containing sheets and microacinar formation, large cells with irregular nuclear membranes, disorderly growth, mild nuclear enlargement, and nuclear crowding. Immunocytochemical analysis shows CEA positivity and alpha-fetoprotein (–). Based on the following, the diagnosis is:

A. hepatocellular carcinoma, well differentiated
B. reactive hepatocytes
C. cholangiocarcinoma, well differentiated
D. normal bile ductal epithelium

76. A cartilaginous tumor affecting individuals between the ages of 40 and 60, occurring within the pelvis or femur, and cytologically composed of anaplastic chondrocytes, chondroblasts, and epithelioid cells among a bright metachromatic myxoid background is diagnostic of:

A. giant cell tumor
B. villonodular synovitis
C. chondroblastoma
D. chondrosarcoma

77. A 14-year-old boy presents with femur pain. FNA reveals slightly cohesive small round cells with granular cytoplasm, coarse chromatin, and rare nucleoli, with cell size about twice that of a lymphocyte. Rosettes are often noted. Which special stain and what diagnosis would confirm your suspicions?

A. PAS(–)/osteogenic sarcoma
B. PAS(+)/Ewing sarcoma
C. neuron-specific enolase (+)/osteosarcoma
D. leukocyte common antigen (+)/small round cell lymphoma

78. A 63-year-old woman with a history of a total hysterectomy without bilateral salpingo-oophrectomy presents with a golf ball-size tumor involving the left ovary. FNA reveals a scanty population of predictable thin spindle-shaped cells with fine regular chromatin. The diagnosis is consistent with:

A. Sertoli cell tumor
B. fibroma
C. interstitial cell tumor
D. granulosa cell tumor

79. FNA of a retroperitoneal tumor consists of pleomorphic vacuolated cells with eccentric nuclei, small round cells, and elongated spindle-shaped, vacuolated cells. A population of multinucleated giant cells containing irregular chromatin and prominent nucleoli with granular cytoplasm arranged in clusters and lacking polarity is also seen. The diagnosis is:

A. proliferative myositis
B. liposarcoma
C. angiosarcoma
D. granulomatous disease

80. Cells in sheets with abundant granular to foamy cyanophilic cytoplasm containing fine yellowish pigment and small eccentric round nuclei with prominent nucleoli in a bloody background when seen in ovarian aspirations are diagnostic of:

A. follicular cyst
B. luteal cyst
C. parovarian cyst
D. Brenner tumor

81. FNA is performed on a 6-cm well-circumscribed kidney mass from an elderly male presenting with hematuria and abdominal pain. Cytology reveals a monotonous population consisting purely of large polygonal cells with abundant granular cytoplasm in loose clusters and as single cells. The cells have small central and eccentrically located nuclei with fine regular chromatin and micronucleoli. The diagnosis is consistent with a:

A. renal cell carcinoma
B. papillary carcinoma
C. collecting duct carcinoma
D. oncocytic neoplasm

82. A 19-year-old boy with a lesion contained within the metaphyseal portion of the distal femur presents for FNA. Cytology reveals a predominant population of cells with plasmacytoid appearance and hyperchromatic nuclei, irregular chromatin, and nucleoli. In addition, multinucleated cells with metachromatic cytoplasmic granules, and central hyaline fibrillar material surrounded by pleomorphic spindle cells are present. The diagnosis is:

A. osteoblastoma
B. osteosarcoma
C. osteoid osteoma
D. osteochondroma

83. A lesion comprised of pleomorphic endothelial cells with coarse irregular chromatin and macronucleoli, associated epithelioid cells, and "erythrophagocytosis" best describes:

A. myositis ossificans
B. benign fibrous histiocytoma
C. malignant fibrous histiosarcoma
D. angiosarcoma

84. Which lesion may commonly present with accompanying granulomatous disease?

A. seminoma
B. asthma
C. encephalitis
D. choroid plexus papillomas

85. FNA of a 5-cm ovarian mass reveals abundant squamous and adnexal material contained within a granular background. These cells are diagnostic of:

A. Sertoli-Leydig cell tumor
B. granulosa cell tumor
C. mature cystic teratoma
D. dysgerminoma

86. An FNA of an ileum mass from a 18-year-old boy reveals a hypercellular population of eosinophils and cells with granular-to-dense cytoplasm with eccentric nuclei and prominent nuclear grooves. Foreign body giant cells, foamy histiocytes, and mature inflammatory components are also identified. The diagnosis is consistent with a (an):

A. callus
B. eosinophilic granuloma
C. aneurysmal bone cyst
D. hemangioma

87. Which statement regarding the FNA of pheochromocytomas is correct?

A. cytology cannot distinguish pheochromocytoma from adrenal cortical adenoma
B. aspiration may precipitate a hypertensive crisis
C. they are associated with decreased urinary catecholamines
D. they are associated with decreased vanillylmandelic acid

88. FNA of an abdominal mass from a patient, status post resection for stage I ovarian adenocarcinoma, reveals epithelioid cells, spindle-appearing cells, and multinucleated cells with frothy cytoplasm, as well as a large population of round structures with Maltese cross birefringence. The diagnosis is:

A. recurrent ovarian adenocarcinoma, poorly differentiated
B. starch granulomatosis
C. recurrent ovarian adenocarcinoma, well differentiated
D. pollen contaminant

89. FNA of an ovarian mass reveals sheets of cells with large overlapping nuclei, coarse, irregular chromatin, prominent nucleoli, clear, lacy cytoplasm with punched-out vacuoles, naked nuclei, and scattered lymphocytes. Epithelioid and multinucleated histiocytes are noted. A tiger-striped background pattern is demonstrated with Diff-Quik. Staining is positive for PAS but negative for alpha-fetoprotein and common leukocyte antigen. The diagnosis is:

A. dysgerminoma
B. lymphoma
C. yolk sac tumors
D. embryonal carcinoma

90. A recent kidney transplant patient presents with a solitary lesion of the lung. FNA evaluation reveals a hypercellular population of cells with large nuclei, macronucleoli, and cilia. Another population of cells shows large nuclei containing intranuclear basophilic inclusions surrounded by halos and chromatic margination. Nuclear molding is absent. These cells are diagnostic of:

A. herpesvirus
B. bronchogenic adenocarcinoma
C. metastatic renal cell carcinoma
D. cytomegalovirus

91. If a Diff-Quik-stained FNA specimen of the lung is negative for malignancy, one should:

A. restain in case of faulty staining technique
B. reaspirate due to faulty sampling technique
C. perform cultures for identification of possible inflammatory process
D. suggest no need for further evaluation

92. A 44-year-old woman presents with a raised pigmented cutaneous lesion on the thigh. FNA reveals well-defined, slender, elongated cells with notched ends and fine regular chromatin, cells with foamy cytoplasm and eccentrically located reniform nuclei, and long slender anatomizing processes containing flattened, peripherally arranged, elongated nuclei. This best describes:

A. hemangioma
B. liposarcoma
C. benign fibrous histiocytoma
D. pleomorphic fibrosarcoma

93. The most common nonneoplastic ovarian cyst is:

A. luteal
B. parovarian
C. endometriotic
D. follicular

94. A 34-year-old woman with an enlarged ovary presents for FNA. Cuboidal cells arranged in clusters as well as monolayered sheets with scanty cytoplasm are seen in conjunction with a population of ciliated cells. Papillary groupings and psammoma bodies are also seen. The diagnosis is:

A. mucinous cystadenoma
B. serous cystadenoma
C. mucinous cystadenocarcinoma
D. serous cystadenocarcinoma

95. FNA of a left ovarian mass yields a sticky mucoid material. Cytology reveals a hypercellular sample with endocervical cell morphology, irregular clusters, single cells, and malignant nuclear features. Deep, basophilic wispy material is demonstrated in the background with Diff-Quik stain.

A. endometriod carcinoma
B. mucinous cystadenocarcinoma
C. dysgerminoma
D. yolk sac tumor

96. FNA of a visceral pleural lung mass from a patient, status post resection for stage II bronchogenic adenocarcinoma, post irradiation therapy, reveals scarce well-defined sheets of cells with spindle-shaped morphology and cytoplasmic streaming, binucleation, and moderate to low N/C ratios. These cells are diagnostic of:

A. recurrent bronchogenic adenocarcinoma
B. granulomatous process
C. spindle cell sarcoma
D. mesenchymal repair

97. An ovarian aspirate from a 32-year-old patient consists of cells with foamy cytoplasm with refractile red pigment and cells with cuboidal morphology, demonstrating regular chromatin arranged in balls and loose clusters. The background consists of fresh and old blood. The diagnosis suggests:

A. luteal cyst
B. sex cord stromal tumor
C. endometriotic cyst
D. mucinous cystadenoma

98. A 44-year-old woman with a 3-cm lesion located by ultrasound submits for FNA. Cytology reveals sheets of cells with abundant cytoplasm and uniform nuclei containing grooves appearing morphologically as "coffee beans." Many cells are arranged in islands with central eosinophilic globules. The diagnosis is:

A. Sertoli-Leydig cell tumor
B. teratoma
C. germinoma
D. Brenner tumor

99. A testicular mass was aspirated from a 22-year-old patient and revealed numerous poorly cohesive large cells with frankly malignant nuclei found in the presence of an interwoven PAS (+) tigroid background. What other cellular population is helpful in establishing which diagnosis?

A. lymphohistiocytic bodies, histiocytic lymphoma
B. benign lymphocytic population, seminoma
C. malignant lymphocytic population, anaplastic seminoma
D. Sertoli cells, benign hydrocele fluid

100. FNA of an enlarged 2×3-cm lymphoid mass reveals multiple intracytoplasmic histiocytic inclusions. Special staining with Giemsa is positive but negative with GMS. Which organism is represented?

A. *Leishmania*
B. *Histoplasma capsulatum*
C. *Pneumocystis carinii*
D. *Coccidioides immitis*

101. An ovarian aspirate reveals single cells and clusters with rounded smooth and folded bean-shaped nuclei and scanty foamy cytoplasm contained within a proteinaceous background. An intact ovum is surrounded by these cells. Carcinoembryonic antigen and alpha-fetoprotein serum levels are minimal. The diagnosis is:

A. follicular cyst
B. luteal cyst
C. serous cystadenoma
D. mucinous cystadenoma

102. FNA of a pelvic lymph node reveals terminal bar-like densities on the apical cytoplasmic borders of the malignant cells. Which of the following may represent a possible primary site/diagnosis?

A. adrenal/pheochromocytoma
B. pancreas/serous cystadenocarcinoma
C. kidney/oncocytic neoplasm
D. colorectal/carcinoma

103. A 44-year-old woman with endometrial hyperplasia presents with an ovarian tumor. FNA of the ovary reveals a hypercellular population of uniform cells in sheets and rosettes surrounding amorphous metachromatic structures. The nuclei are round, have fine regular chromatin, and micronucleoli. The background is clean. These cells are diagnostic of:

A. fibroma
B. germinoma
C. serous cystadenocarcinoma
D. granulosa cell tumor

104. Pancreatic FNA reveals cells in loose sheets with flat sheets with well-defined cell borders, honeycomb appearance, fine regular chromatin, micronucleoli, smooth nuclear membranes, and pale, finely vacuolated cytoplasm. These cells best describe:

A. acinar cells
B. pancreatic adenocarcinoma, well differentiated
C. normal biliary duct
D. pancreatic pseudocyst

105. A gallbladder aspirate reveals sheets of ductal cells with enlarged overlapping nuclei and prominent nucleoli. Few single cells are identified. These cells are diagnostic of:

A. normal gallbladder epithelium
B. acute cholecystitis
C. adenocarcinoma
D. xanthogranulomatous cholecystitis

106. Which criteria are reliable for distinguishing well-differentiated trabecular hepatocellular carcinomas (HCC) from the fibrolamellar variant of HCC?

A. bile ducts are intermingled with the tumor cells in well-differentiated trabecular HCC
B. the cells of the fibrolamellar variant of HCC are larger and more dispersed, with fewer trabeculae
C. the cells of well-differentiated trabecular HCC possess oncocytic cytoplasm with well-defined homogeneous intracytoplasmic pale bodies
D. the cells of the fibrolamellar variant of HCC are morphologically similar to "small blue cell tumors," ie, there is a uniform population of small, round to oval anaplastic cells with high N/C ratios

107. A 55-year old woman presents with abdominal pain and high levels of serum amylase. FNA of the pancreas reveals neutrophils and small clusters of cells with abundant granular cytoplasm, round nuclei, and chromatinic margination. These cells are diagnostic of:

A. microcystic adenoma
B. mucinous cystadenoma
C. papillary epithelial neoplasm
D. pancreatitis

108. Tall columnar mucinous secreting cells (mucicarmine +) as well as signet ring cells with low N/C ratios and stromal cells were identified in a 4-cm mass located in the pancreas of a 44-year-old woman. The background contains abundant metachromatic fibrillary material on Diff-Quik. The diagnosis/method of treatment is:

A. poorly differentiated mucinous adenocarcinoma/surgical resection
B. papillary epithelial carcinoma/no resection required
C. mucinous cystic tumor/surgical resection
D. microcystic adenoma/no resection required

109. A Giemsa-stained aspirate of a pancreatic mass from a 20-year-old woman reveals numerous cellular aggregates consisting of fronds of tissue and fibrovascular stalks with attached monomorphic cells as well as the presence of intracellular metachromatic hyaline globules. These cells are diagnostic of:

A. adenocarcinoma
B. fibrosarcoma
C. papillary epithelial neoplasm
D. mucinous cystadenoma

110. A prostatic aspiration yields a hypercellular population of uniform cells in irregular sheets with well-defined cytoplasmic borders. Microacinar complexes are not identified. No nucleoli are found. These cells are diagnostic of:

A. prostatic adenocarcinoma, well differentiated
B. prostatic adenocarcinoma, poorly differentiated
C. seminal vesicle cells
D. prostatic hyperplasia

111. Pancreatic pseudocysts are a result of:

A. pancreatitis
B. calcification of pancreatic parenchyma
C. granulation tissue scarring
D. fatty metamorphosis

112. What is the correct order for normal lymphocytic differentiation?

A. cleaved => large noncleaved => immunoblastic => plasma cell
B. small round cells => small cleaved => large cleaved => small noncleaved => large noncleaved => immunoblastic => plasma cell
C. small cleaved => large noncleaved => large cleaved => small noncleaved => immunoblastic => plasma cell
D. plasma cell => small noncleaved => small cleaved => large cleaved => immunoblasts

113. Lymphogranular bodies as seen in the FNA of lymph nodes suggest which process?

A. lymphoid
B. malignant
C. metastatic
D. granulomatous

114. A 3-cm mass located in the tail of the pancreas is found to contain a hypercellular population of single cells with round nuclei, coarse chromatin, multiple nucleoli, and increased mitotic figures, with a large population of multinucleated giant malignant cells containing irregular chromatin and irregular nuclear membranes. The diagnosis is:

A. metastatic giant cell carcinoma, lung
B. non-mucus-producing adenocarcinoma, pancreas
C. spindle cell sarcoma
D. anaplastic carcinoma, pancreas

115. A 67-year-old man presenting for a routine annual examination has an elevated serum prostate specific antigen analysis. FNA is performed on a hard, gritty, pea-sized lesion of the prostate. Cytology reveals numerous cells arranged in repeated microacinar formations with small round nuclei, high N/C ratios, and prominent nucleoli. The diagnosis is:

A. malacoplakia
B. well-differentiated adenocarcinoma
C. prostatitis
D. benign prostatic hyperplasia

116. The presence of lymphohistiocytic aggregates in the FNA of lymphadenopathy is usually indicative of:

A. lymphoma
B. metastatic carcinoma
C. reactive condition
D. cat scratch disease

117. The cytomorphologic diagnosis of small round cell lymphoma may be aided by immunocytochemical staining for:

A. common acute lymphocytic leukemia antigen (CALLA/CD10)
B. T-cell and pan-B-cell surface antigens (Leu/CD5)
C. T-cell surface antigens only
D. B-cell surface antigens only

118. The most common benign differential diagnosis of immunoblastic lymphoma is:

A. early reactive lymph node hyperplasia
B. midphase reactive lymph node hyperplasia
C. end-stage lymph node hyperplasia
D. recurrent lymph node hyperplasia

119. A 66-year-old woman with a previously diagnosed malignancy presents with multiple liver nodules. FNA cytology reveals many single cells with well-defined intracytoplasmic eosinophilic inclusions giving the nucleus a targetioid appearance on Diff Quik stain. Some cells are cohesive with vertebral column formation, contain hyperchromatic nuclei with nucleoli, and have frothy cytoplasm. The background was thick and eosinophilic with interspersed fat vacuoles and small fibrous stromal elements. The diagnosis is:

A. colonic adenocarcinoma
B. pancreatic carcinoma
C. ovarian adenocarcinoma
D. breast adenocarcinoma

120. What cell types predominate in late stage lymph node hyperplasia?

A. small round lymphocytes, small cleaved lymphocytes, plasma cells
B. large cleaved and large noncleaved lymphocytes
C. immunoblasts, large cleaved, and large noncleaved lymphocytes
D. plasma cells, large cleaved and small cleaved lymphocytes

121. The predominant cellular population(s) found in the diagnosis of reactive lymph node hyperplasia is (are):

A. small round and small cleaved lymphocytes over large cleaved and noncleaved lymphocytes, lymphohistiocytic aggregates
B. large cleaved and noncleaved lymphocytes over small cleaved and noncleaved lymphocytes, lymphohistiocytic aggregates
C. immunoblasts and plasma cells over small cleaved and large noncleaved lymphocytes
D. immunoblasts and large cleaved lymphocytes over plasma cells and small cleaved lymphocytes

122. A 62-year-old man with dysuria presents for prostatic aspiration. Many pleomorphic cells in loose cohesive clusters with macronucleoli are found. The cytoplasm contains coarse golden brown pigment on Papanicolaou and dark blue-green on Diff-Quik stain. Sperm is noted within the background. These cells are diagnostic of:

A. well-differentiated adenocarcinoma, prostate
B. poorly differentiated adenocarcinoma, prostate
C. a benign cellular component
D. renal cell carcinoma

123. The FNA diagnosis of an axillary lymph node reveals a hypercellular population representing predominantly large single cells with smooth uniform nuclear borders, fine open chromatin patterns, up to three nucleoli per cell, and a scarce population of small cleaved and small round cells with coarse, dense to moderately open chromatin patterns. Lymphogranular bodies are noted. This process is usually:

A. CALLA/CD10 positive
B. Leu1/CD5 positive
C. of monoclonal B cell origin
D. of monoclonal T cell origin

124. Which is true regarding soft tissue tumors?

A. malignant tumors are more common than benign lesions
B. benign lesions are more common than malignant tumors
C. most needle aspirates require the use of 14-gauge needles
D. primary sarcomas of soft tissue are more common than metastatic carcinomas

125. A 72-year-old woman with abdominal pain, weight loss, and jaundice presents with a 10-cm mass located in the head of the pancreas. FNA reveals a hypocellular sample of small clusters of cells with abundant clear cytoplasm. The nuclei are round with fine, regular chromatin. Staining is PAS-positive, PAS-D-negative, and mucicarmine-negative. The diagnosis is:

A. pancreatitis
B. microcystic adenoma
C. mucinous cystic neoplasm
D. pancreatic adenocarcinoma

126. In reactive lymph node hyperplasia, which of the following are seen?

A. a polynuclear population of immature lymphoid cells
B. a population of immunoblasts only
C. a polymorphic population of lymphoid cells
D. a single population of immature lymphocytes

127. The most common subtype of Hodgkin disease found in young adults associated with the cytological diagnosis of mononucleated, nonclassical Reed-Sternberg cells is:

A. lymphocyte predominant type
B. lymphocyte depleted type
C. nodular sclerosing type
D. mixed cellularity type

128. A lymph node aspirate reveals a hypercellular sample that includes neutrophils, debris, histiocytes, and small round lymphocytes. What may be responsible for the cytological findings?

A. viral infection
B. bacterial infection
C. diffuse immunoblastic hyperplasia
D. granulomatous lymphodermitis

129. A 55-year-old African-American man with lymphadenopathy and an enlarged jaw presents for FNA. Small single cells with deep blue, finely vacuolated lipid-positive cytoplasm are observed in the aspirate. Mitotic figures are present in many of the cells. A monoclonal B cell lesion with IgM kappa surface markers is demonstrated with flow cytometry. The diagnosis is:

A. immunoblastic lymphoma
B. lymphoblastic lymphoma
C. small round cell lymphoma
D. Burkitt lymphoma

130. An FNA biopsy of a pancreatic mass from a 70-year-old man with mental weakness, fatigue, and a recent onset of convulsions reveals a monomorphic population of cells with salt-and-pepper chromatin and prominent nucleoli. Intracytoplasmic granules are demonstrated with Diff-Quik, and immunocytochemical staining for chromogranin and insulin is positive. Amyloid is noted within the background. These cells are diagnostic of:

A. islet cell tumor of the pancreas, alpha cell predominance
B. islet cell tumor of the pancreas, beta cell predominance
C. islet cell tumor of the pancreas, G cell predominance
D. islet cell tumor of the pancreas, VIP cell predominance

131. A 58-year-old man presents with an enlarged inguinal lymph node. FNA reveals a large population of small cells with scanty cytoplasm, coarse chromatin patterns, nuclear clefts, and prominent nucleoli as well as a small population of small round cells. Based on the findings, these cells express/are diagnostic of:

A. common acute lymphocytic leukemia antigen/small cell cleaved lymphoma
B. T-cell and pan-B-cell surface antigens/small cell cleaved lymphoma
C. T-cell surface antigens/small cell cleaved lymphoma
D. B-cell surface antigens/small round cell lymphoma

132. What is considered a primary lymphoid granulomatous disease without necrosis?

A. tuberculosis
B. anthrax
C. *Blastomyces dermatitidis*
D. sarcoidosis

133. When confirming the diagnosis of mixed cell lymphoma (MCL) over that of reactive lymph node hyperplasia (RLNH), which cytologic criteria and flow cytometric techniques are helpful?

A. there is an increase in small round cells and immunoblasts in MCL; MCL is polyclonal for light chains
B. there is a lack of small round cells and immunoblasts in MCL; MCL is monoclonal for light chains
C. there is an increase in small round cells and tingible body macrophages in MCL; MCL co-expresses T and B cell surface antigens
D. there is an increase in immunoblasts, tingible body macrophages, and plasma cells in MCL; flow cytometry is not useful in the discrimination of MCL from other lymphomas

134. An FNA of an enlarged cervical lymph node from a 12-year-old boy with fever, unexplained rashes, and recent unexplained weight loss reveals single binucleate cells with large irregular nucleoli. Abundant small round lymphocytes and epithelioid cells are found. These cells are diagnostic of:

A. mixed-cell lymphoma
B. large-cell noncleaved lymphoma
C. immunoblastic lymphoma
D. Hodgkin disease

135. A good indicator for the diagnosis of well-differentiated mucus-producing adenocarcinomas of pancreatic ductal origin is:

A. fine chromatin with macronucleoli
B. drunken honeycombs and goblet cells
C. irregular chromatin and pleomorphism
D. PAS-D negative

136. A pancreatic mass was analyzed using FNA. Cytology reveals a hypercellular population of polygonal cells with granular cytoplasm, eccentric nuclei, irregular chromatin, macronucleoli, and a necrotic background. Serum analysis indicates an increase in amine/peptide products. Staining with neuron-specific enolase was positive. These cells are diagnostic of:

A. oncocytic neuroendocrine carcinoma of the pancreas
B. mucinous cystadenoma
C. pancreatic ductal adenocarcinoma
D. pseudocyst

137. The predominant cell populations seen in the early reactive stages of lymph node hyperplasia are (in descending number):

A. large cleaved lymphocytes, small round lymphocytes, immunoblasts
B. plasma cells, large cleaved lymphocytes, small round lymphocytes
C. large noncleaved lymphocytes, immunoblasts, plasma cells
D. small round lymphocytes, small cleaved lymphocytes, large cleaved lymphocytes, large noncleaved lymphocytes, immunoblasts, plasma cells

138. A 33-year-old woman with axillary lymphadenopathy associated with lymphodermatitis and erythematous papules at the site of the trauma and cytologically seen as epithelioid cells, giant cells, small round lymphocytes and necrosis is associated with a diagnosis of:

A. lipophagic granuloma
B. eosinophilic granuloma
C. cat-scratch disease
D. toxoplasmosis

139. **What lymphoma is characterized histologically as having a "starry sky" pattern?**

A. small cell cleaved lymphoma
B. Burkitt lymphoma
C. large-cell cleaved lymphoma
D. immunoblastic lymphoma

140. **A 58-year-old woman presents with abdominal pain and an 8-cm lesion in the upper pole of the kidney. FNA reveals a hypercellular population of tall columnar cells with wispy, granular-to-frothy cytoplasm staining gossamer blue and floral groups with radiating petal-like projections with a central core. The cells contain large nuclei with fine pale chromatin and cherry-red "stop sign" macronucleoli. Special staining with oil red O is positive. The diagnosis is:**

A. oncocytoma
B. metastatic ovarian adenocarcinoma
C. clear cell renal cell carcinoma
D. sarcomatoid renal cell carcinoma

141. **A 67-year-old woman with multiple liver nodules presents for FNA. Cytology reveals a slightly cohesive monotonous population of single cells attached to fibrocollagenous tissue. The cells have scanty cytoplasm, intracytoplasmic lumens, high N/C ratios, and hyperchromasia. The cellular configuration reveals cells forming a "stack of coins." Special stains reveal the cells are negative for neuron-specific enolase and positive for mucicarmine. Which of the following may represent the cytologic findings?**

A. metastatic breast carcinoma
B. metastatic kidney carcinoma
C. metastatic colon carcinoma
D. metastatic gastrointestinal leiomyosarcoma

142. **The peak incidence of papillary carcinoma of the thyroid occurs:**

A. under 20 years of age
B. 20s–40s
C. 50s–70s
D. over 80 years of age

143. **A 62-year-old woman with a previously established malignancy presents with an increased serum level of carcinoembryonic antigen and multiple liver nodules as demonstrated by CAT scan. FNA of the liver reveals cells with columnar morphology, vacuolated cytoplasm, signet rings, and polar nuclei with coarse, granular chromatin and multiple nucleoli. An extensive necrosis is identified in the background. The diagnosis is most suggestive of:**

A. hepatocellular carcinoma
B. metastatic colonic carcinoma
C. metastatic breast carcinoma
D. metastatic small cell undifferentiated carcinoma of the lung

144. **A 2-year-old boy presents with an 2-cm well-circumscribed solitary liver mass. Serum analysis for alpha-fetoprotein is markedly elevated. FNA of the liver reveals a uniform population of small, round, loosely cohesive cells with scanty cytoplasm and high N/C ratios. The chromatin is fine-to-coarse with micronucleoli. The cellular pattern is suggestive of:**

A. metastatic neuroblastoma
B. adenomatous hyperplasia
C. hepatocellular carcinoma
D. hepatoblastoma

145. A 55-year-old man with a 4-cm minor salivary gland nodule undergoes FNA. These cells represent a highly cellular aspirate. They are diagnostic of:

A. acinic cell carcinoma
B. adenoid cystic carcinoma
C. basal cell adenoma
D. pleomorphic adenoma

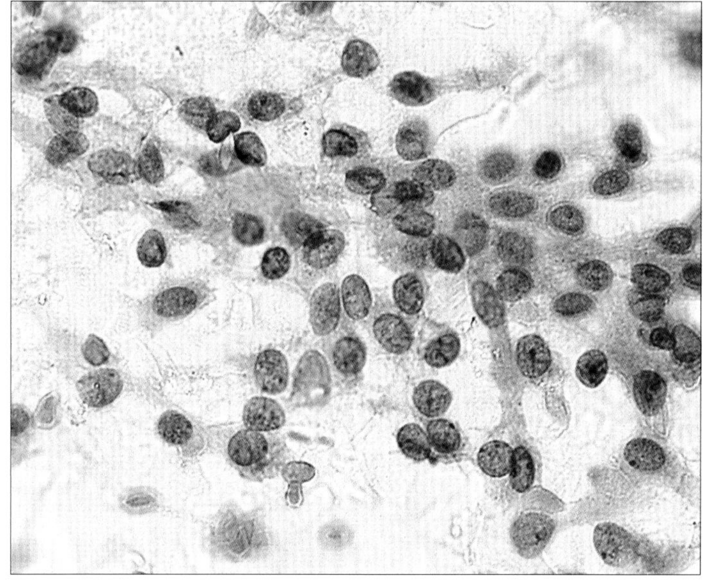

146. An FNA of the thyroid reveals these cells. They are:

A. follicular cells
B. parafollicular cells
C. Hürthle cells
D. macrophages

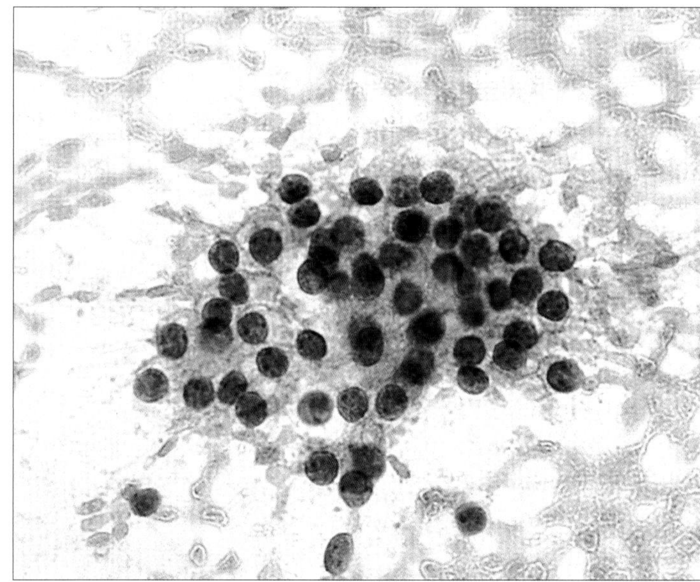

147. A 39-year-old woman with a palpable thyroid nodule undergoes FNA. The depicted cellular process suggests:

A. medullary carcinoma
B. anaplastic carcinoma
C. follicular neoplasm
D. papillary carcinoma

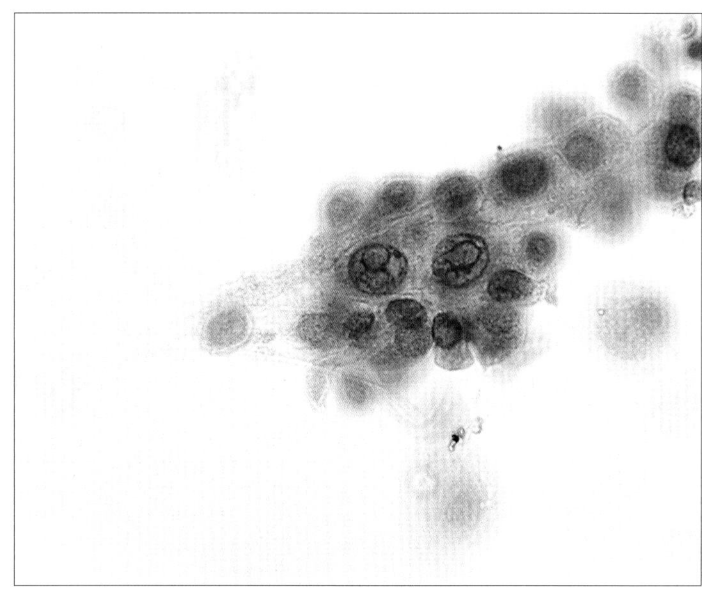

148. Represented is a fine needle aspirate from a 42-year-old woman presenting with a 3-cm parotid mass. These cellular findings represent:

A. mucoepidermoid carcinoma
B. acinic cell carcinoma
C. adenoid cystic carcinoma
D. pleomorphic adenoma

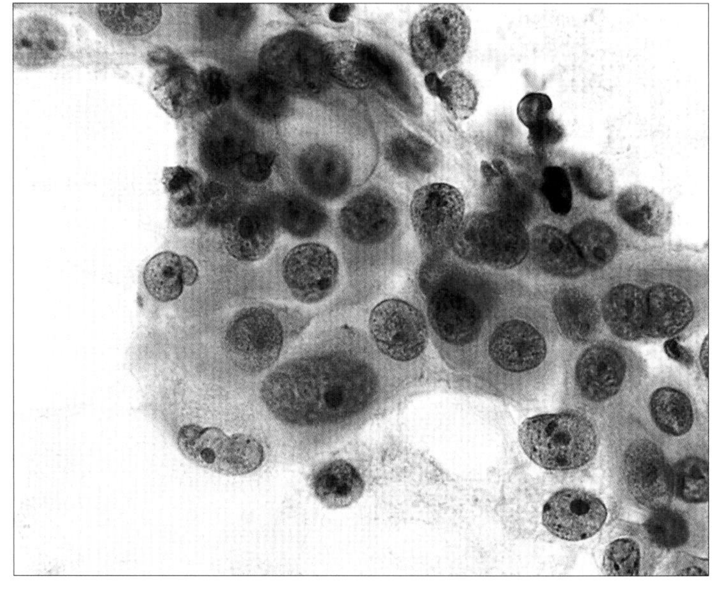

149. These cells are from a 60-year-old woman with a history of thyroiditis. They are:

A. follicular cells
B. parafollicular cells
C. Hürthle cells
D. epithelioid histiocytes

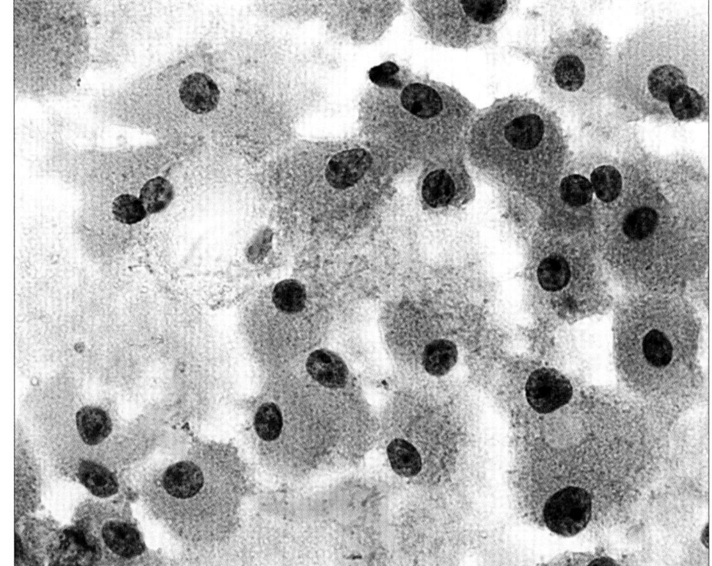

150. This cellular pattern is from a 35-year-old man presenting with painless cervical lymphadenopathy and complaining of a low-grade fever and night sweats. Upon examination, hepatosplenomegaly is noted. FNA of the spleen suggests a diagnosis of:

A. lymphoreticular hyperplasia
B. metastatic sarcoma
C. signet ring adenocarcinoma
D. Hodgkin disease

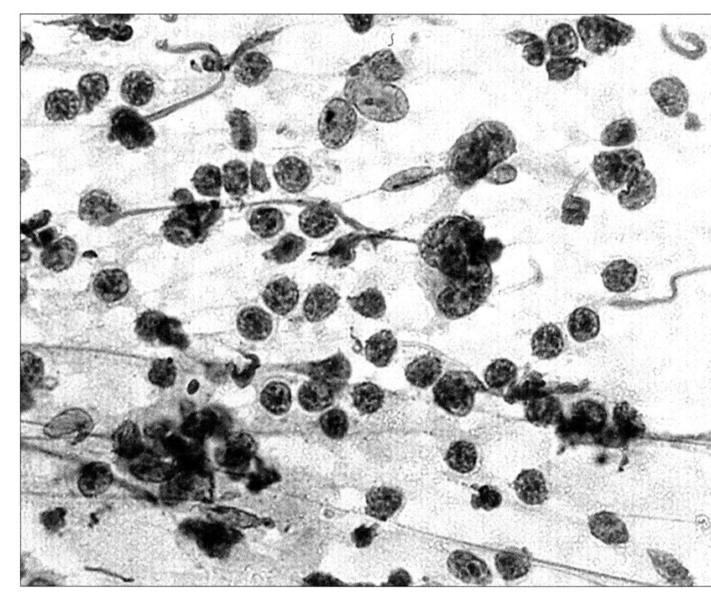

151. A thyroid aspirate from a 56-year-old woman yields these cells. The diagnosis is:

A. de Quervain thyroiditis
B. Hashimoto thyroiditis
C. oncocytoma
D. colloid goiter

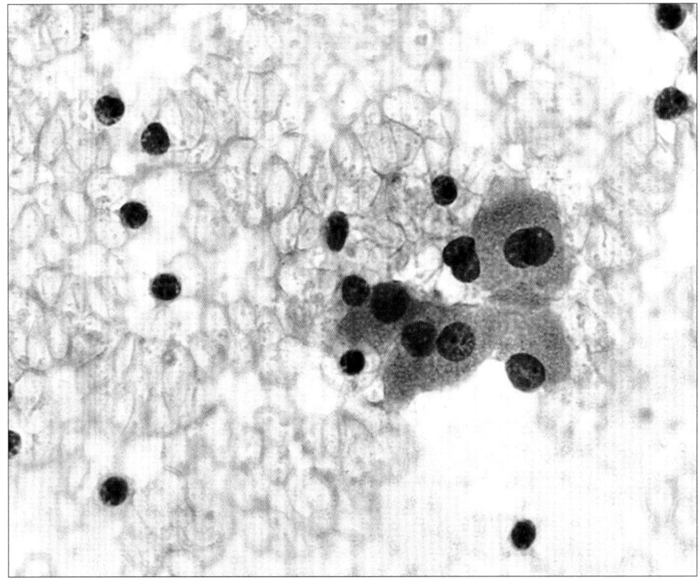

152. A 50-year-old woman with a submandibular mass presents for FNA evaluation. The patient complains of a severe pain during the aspiration procedure. Cytologic findings are suggestive of:

A. acinic cell carcinoma
B. adenoid cystic carcinoma
C. pleomorphic adenoma
D. basal cell adenoma

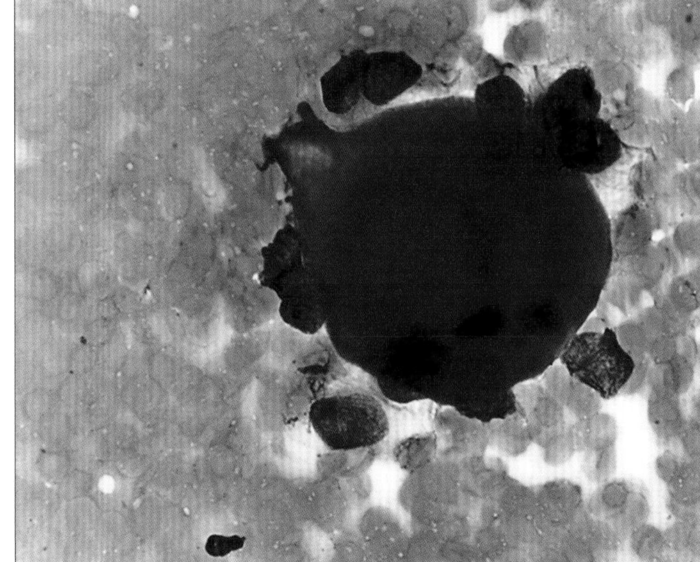

153. FNA of a 4-cm nodule in the cervical region of the neck from a 55-year-old man reveals these cells. These cells were positive for microphtalmia-associated transcription factor (MITF). The cytologic pattern represents:

A. malignant fibrous histiocytoma
B. osteosarcoma
C. metastatic large cell undifferentiated carcinoma
D. metastatic melanoma

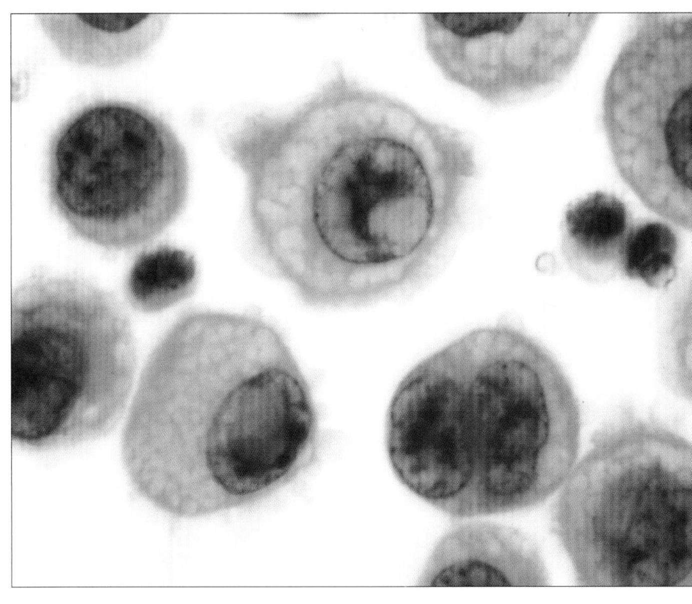

154. A 56-year-old woman with an enlarged palpable thyroid mass that actively takes up radioactive iodine undergoes FNA. The cellular findings are diagnostic of:

A. follicular neoplasm
B. papillary carcinoma
C. nodular goiter
D. medullary carcinoma

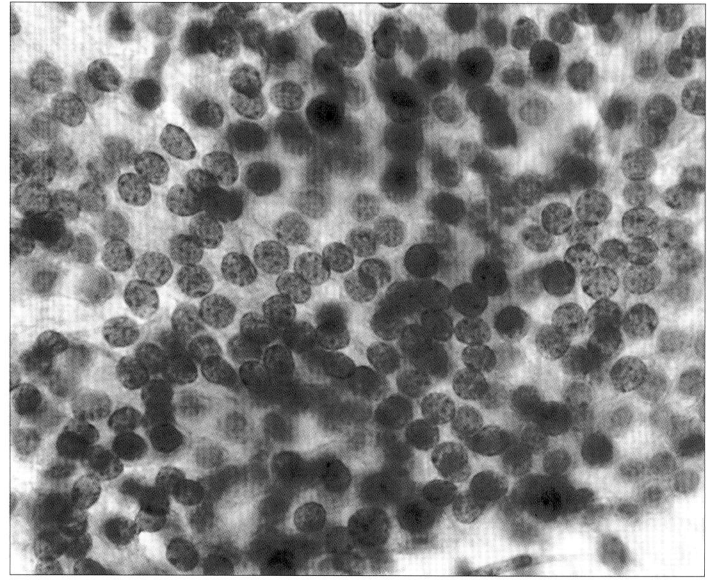

155. A 45-year-old woman presents with an enlarged thyroid. FNA is performed on the mass and yields these cells. The cell at center represents:

A. colloid goiter
B. thyrotoxic goiter
C. giant cell thyroiditis
D. medullary carcinoma

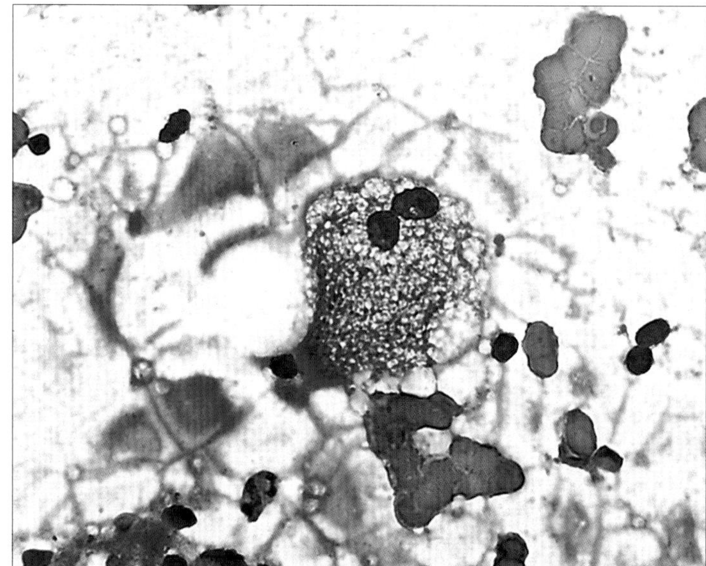

156. A 55-year-old woman presents with bilateral parotid masses. Aspiration cytology confirms the presence of PAS(+) granules within the cytoplasm. The cellular findings are diagnostic of:

A. acinic cell carcinoma
B. monomorphic adenoma
C. adenoid cystic carcinoma
D. lymphoma

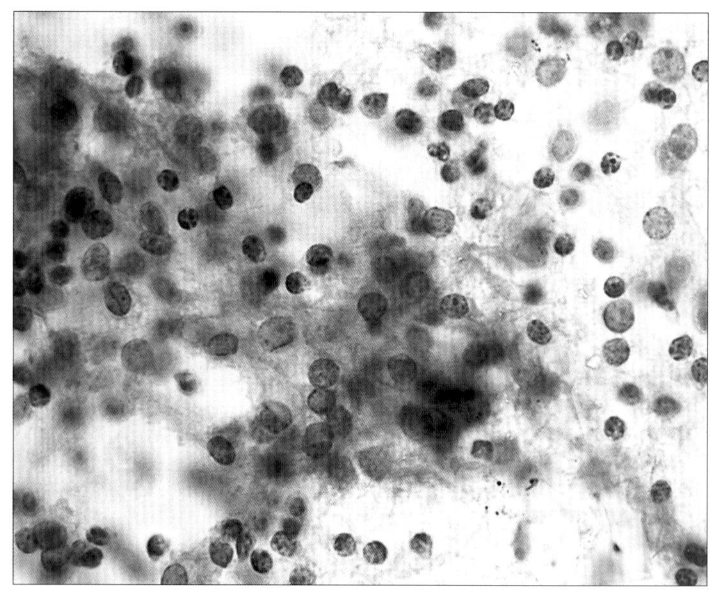

157. **A 67-year-old patient who recently underwent lymphangiography presents with an abdominal lymphoid nodule. The cytologic pattern depicted is:**

A. sinus histiocytosis
B. large-cell cleaved lymphoma
C. end-stage lymphoid hyperplasia
D. lipophagic granuloma

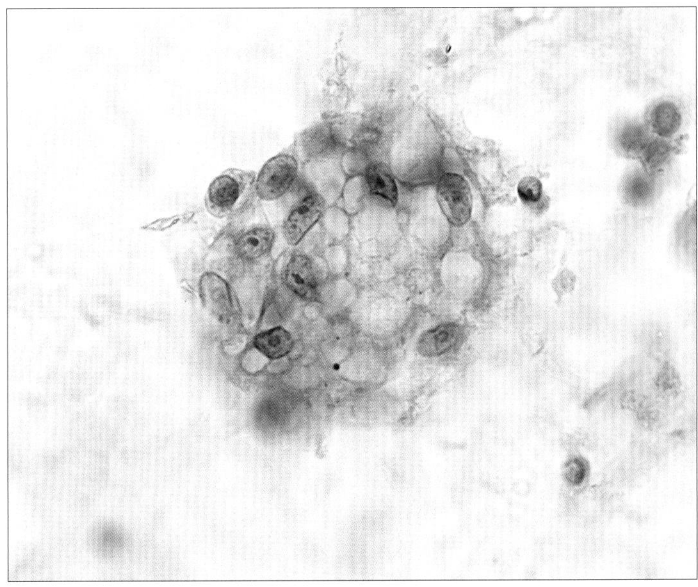

158. **A cervical lymphoid nodule in a 65-year-old woman with an established diagnosis of extralymphatic cancer is evaluated by FNA. The cytologic pattern depicted may represent which of the following?**

A. metastatic melanoma
B. metastatic squamous cell carcinoma
C. metastatic adenocarcinoma, breast
D. granulomatous lymphadenopathy

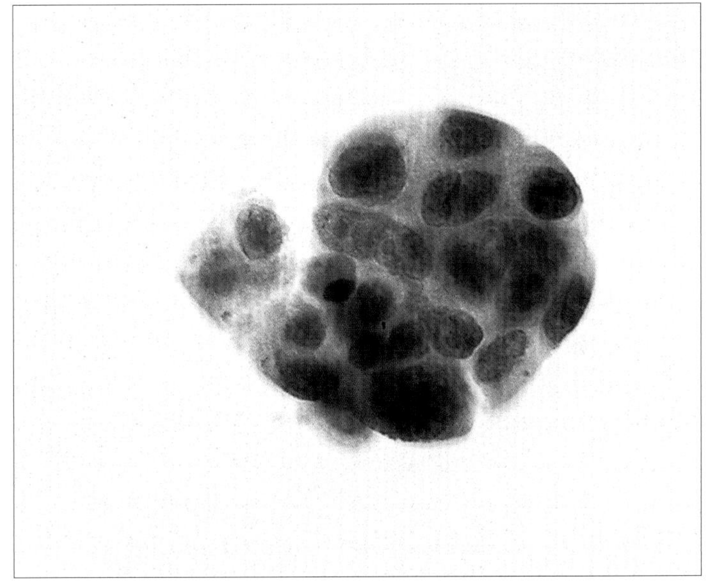

159. **An enlarged thyroid from a 67-year-old man is evaluated with FNA. The cytologic pattern depicted is consistent with:**

A. Hashimoto thyroiditis
B. Hürthle cell adenoma
C. de Quervain thyroiditis
D. lymphoma

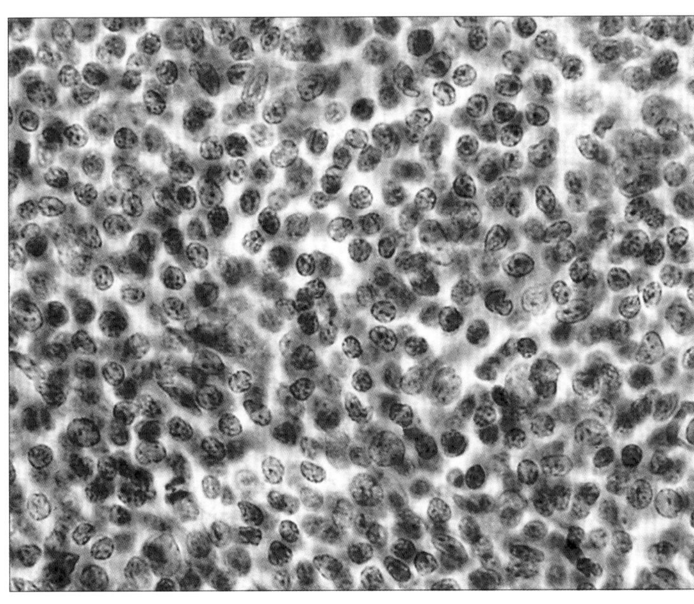

160. **A 16-year-old girl with confirmed viral mononucleosis presents with an enlarged pelvic lymph node. These cells, obtained by FNA, represent:**

A. immunoblastic hyperplasia
B. follicular hyperplasia
C. lymphoblastic lymphoma
D. Hodgkin disease

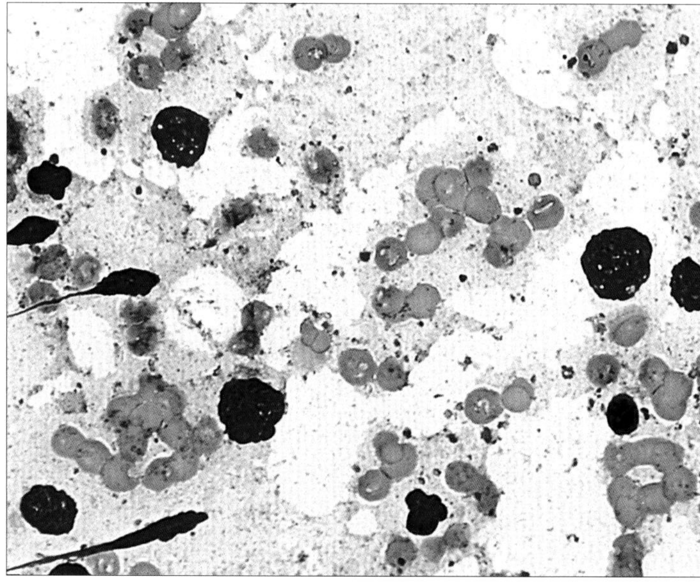

161. **Which thyroid lesion is associated with the findings in this photomicrograph?**

A. follicular neoplasm
B. papillary carcinoma
C. medullary carcinoma
D. metastatic melanoma

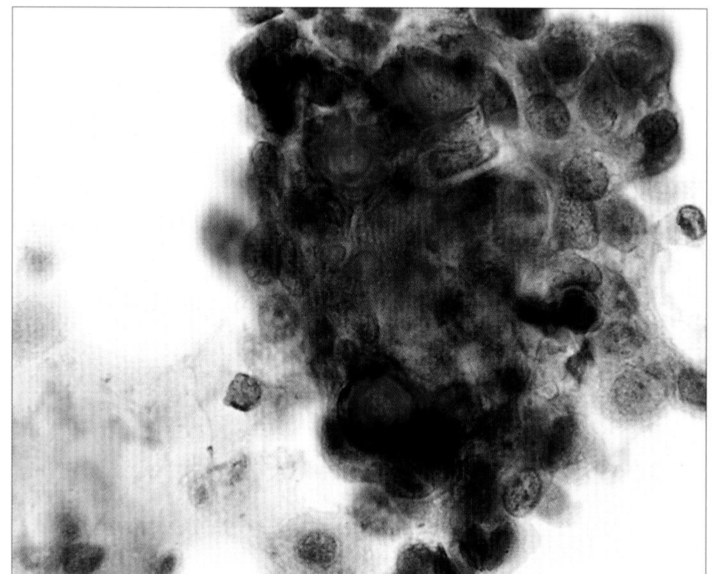

162. **These cells were aspirated from a large painful thyroid mass in an elderly woman. Staining is negative for thyroglobulin and calcitonin, and positive for epithelial membrane antigen. Based on cellular findings and special staining, the diagnosis is:**

A. follicular carcinoma
B. giant cell anaplastic carcinoma
C. medullary carcinoma
D. papillary carcinoma

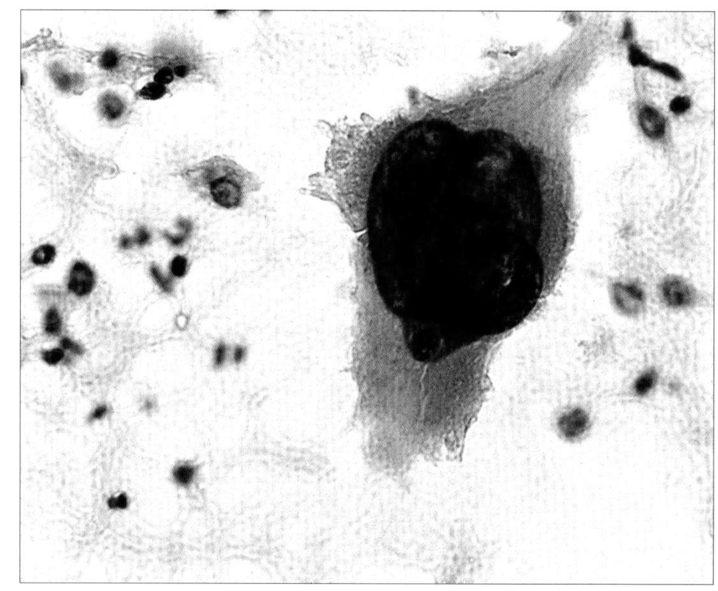

163. These cells are from an umbilical lesion from a 49-year-old woman. The cytologic findings suggest a diagnosis of:

A. lymphoma
B. normal umbilical elements
C. Sister Mary Joseph nodule
D. reactive/reparative changes

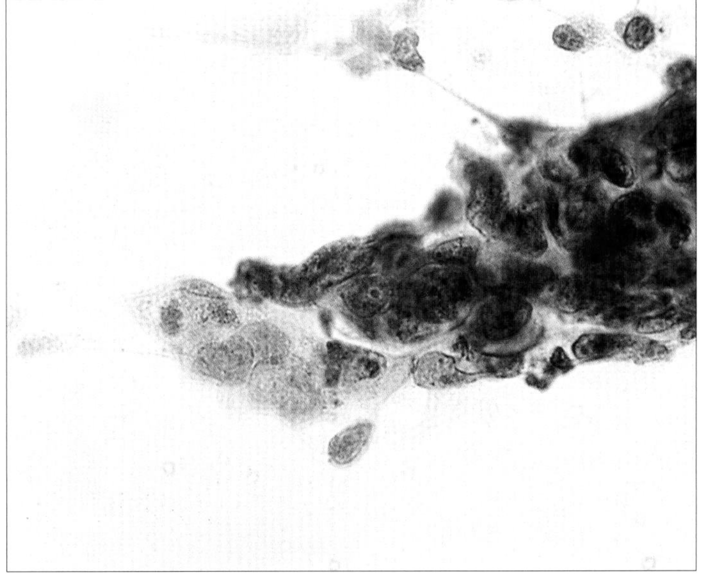

164. These cells are from a cervical lymph node aspirate from a patient with tuberculosis. They are diagnostic of:

A. small cell cleaved lymphoma
B. granulomatous lymphadenitis
C. Burkitt lymphoma
D. midphase lymphoid hyperplasia

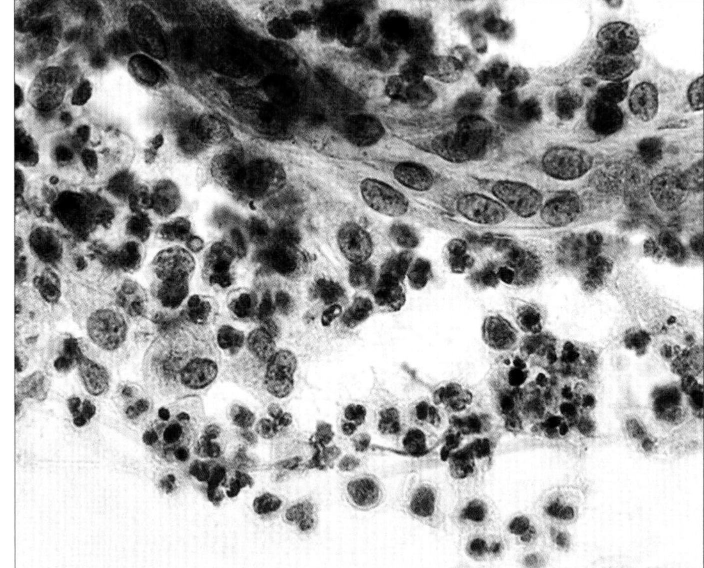

165. A 68-year-old man with an elevated prostate specific antigen (PSA) level presents for FNA evaluation of the prostate. The cytologic pattern depicted is:

A. adenocarcinoma
B. seminal vesicle cells
C. transitional cell carcinoma
D. benign prostatic hyperplasia

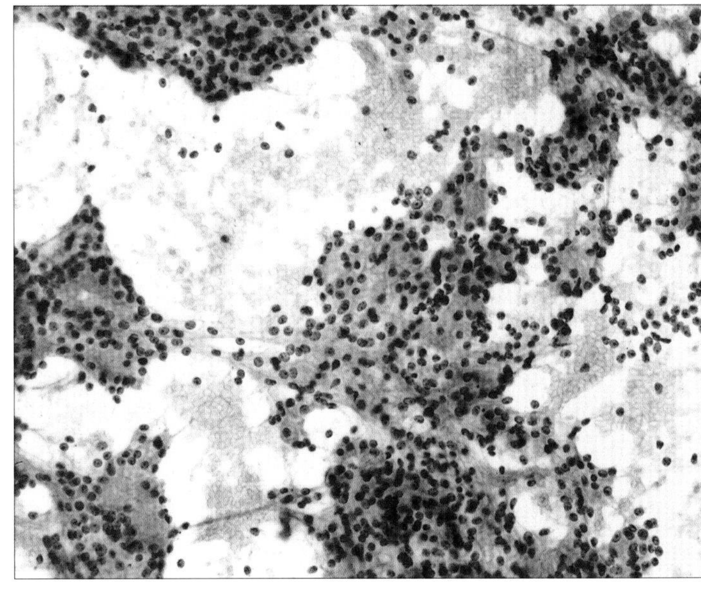

166. These cells are identified in an inguinal lymph node aspirate from a 52-year-old man. Flow cytometry reveals monoclonal serum immunoglobulin. Cytologic correlation suggests:

A. mycosis fungoides
B. large cell lymphoma
C. plasma cell myeloma
D. diffuse immunoblastic hyperplasia

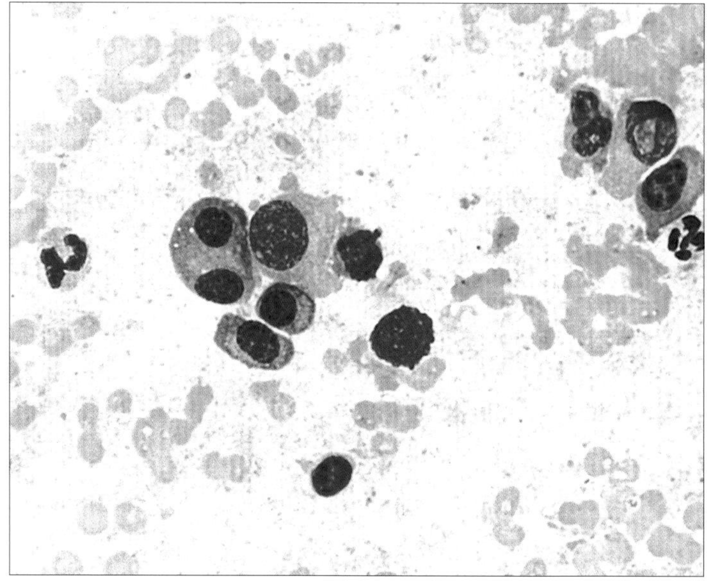

167. A 57-year-old woman with a supraclavicular lymph node enlargement presents for FNA. These cells are identified in the cytologic preparation. The diagnosis is:

A. immunoblastic lymphoma
B. large-cell cleaved lymphoma
C. lymphoblastic lymphoma
D. end-stage lymph node reaction with recurrent antigenic stimulation

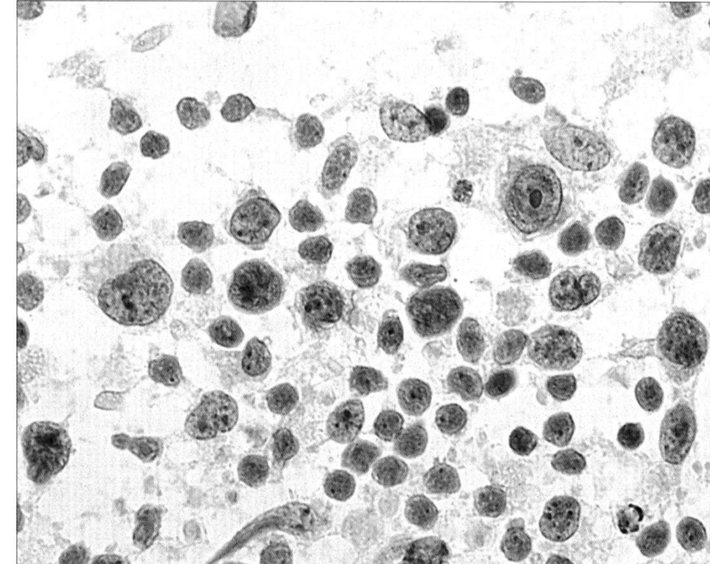

168. A 32-year-old man presents with an enlarged axillary lymph node. FNA reveals:

A. follicular (reactive) hyperplasia
B. granulomatous hyperplasia
C. cat-scratch disease
D. toxoplasmosis

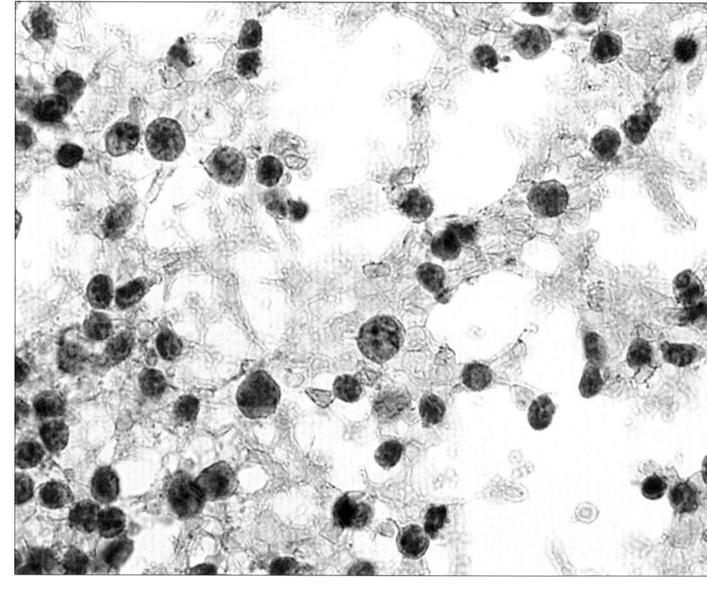

169. **A 44-year-old patient presents with an enlarged inguinal lymph node. Microabscess formation and suppurative necrosis are identified. Which diagnosis is associated with the depicted cellular findings?**

A. toxoplasmosis granulomatosis
B. cat-scratch disease
C. sarcoidosis
D. large-cell cleaved lymphoma

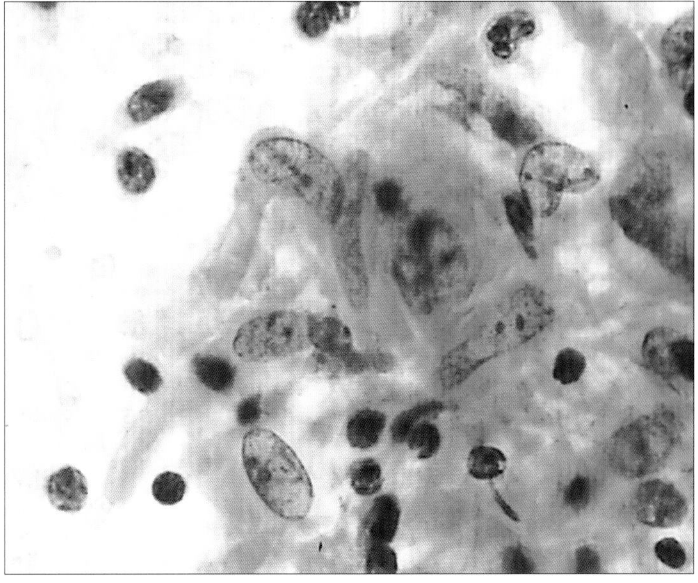

170. **A lesion found within the proximal tibia of a 15-year-old boy is evaluated with FNA. The cytologic pattern depicted is:**

A. osteosarcoma
B. callus
C. giant cell tumor of the bone
D. osteoblastoma

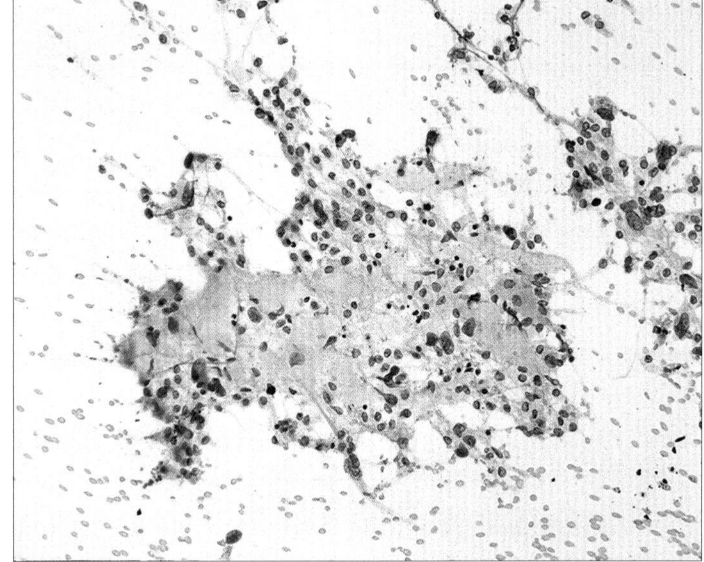

171. **A 55-year-old African American man presents with a markedly enlarged lymph node within the jaw. An FNA specimen is prepared for cytology as well as flow cytometry, which indicates a monoclonal B-cell neoplasm. These cells represent what process?**

A. small round cell lymphoma
B. lymphoblastic lymphoma
C. diffuse immunoblastic hyperplasia
D. Burkitt lymphoma

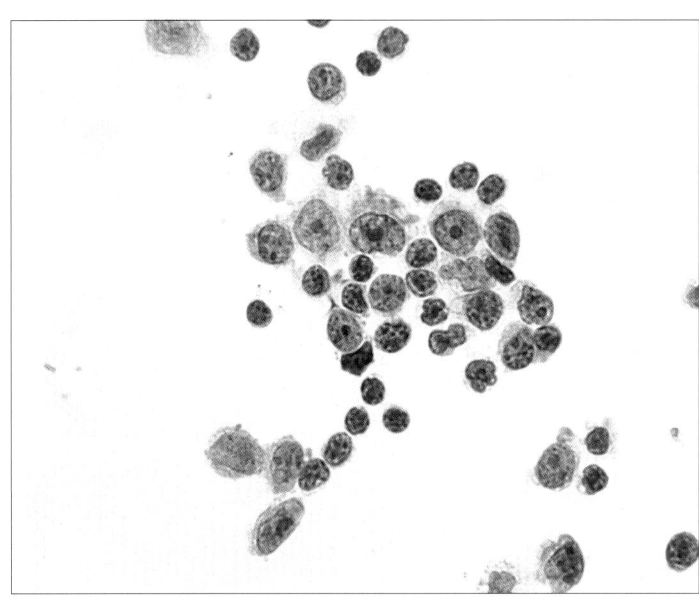

172. **A 52-year-old woman presents with an enlarged cervical lymph node. Based on the cellular findings, the diagnosis is:**

A. small cell noncleaved lymphoma
B. signet ring cell lymphomas
C. follicular hyperplasia
D. mixed small cleaved, large cell lymphoma

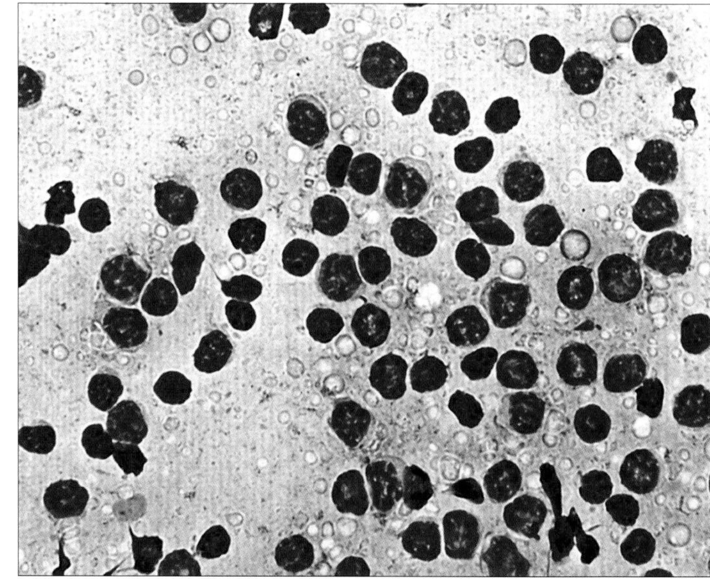

173. **A 55-year-old man with a retroperitoneal soft-tissue mass presents for fine needle aspiration (FNA) evaluation. The cells shown are diagnostic of:**

A. liposarcoma
B. angiosarcoma
C. malignant fibrous histiocytoma
D. hemangioma

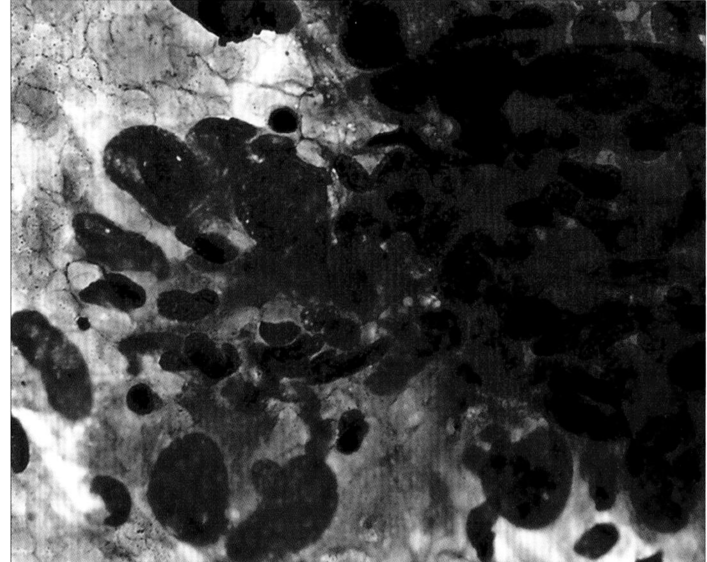

174. **A 16-year-old boy with a history of a testicular tumor presents with a peritoneal lesion. FNA of the pelvic mass reveals these cells. The diagnosis is:**

A. choriocarcinoma
B. seminoma
C. embryonal cell carcinoma
D. endodermal sinus tumor

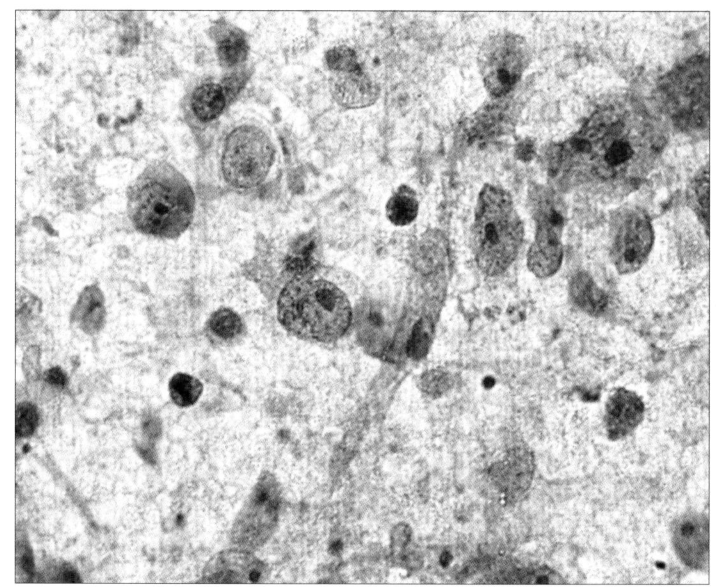

175. A 55-year-old man with a history of multiple lipomas presents with a firm, non-tender nodule in the left thigh (an area resected 5 years earlier). These cells were found in a hypercellular aspirate. The cytologic findings represent:

A. lipoma
B. liposarcoma
C. reactive lymphadenopathy
D. metastatic sarcoma

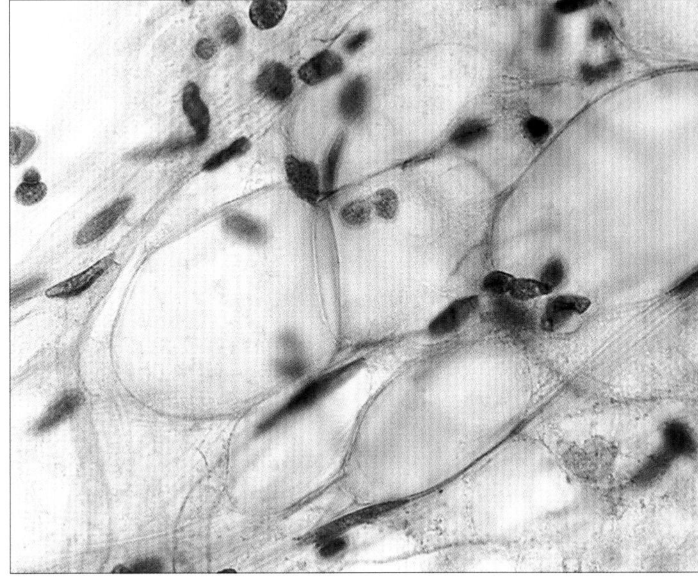

176. A coin lesion of the lung was identified in a 65-year-old man with a history of smoking. FNA cytology reveals:

A. normal bronchial cells
B. metastatic melanoma
C. hemosiderin-laden macrophages
D. hepatocytes, suggest re-aspiration

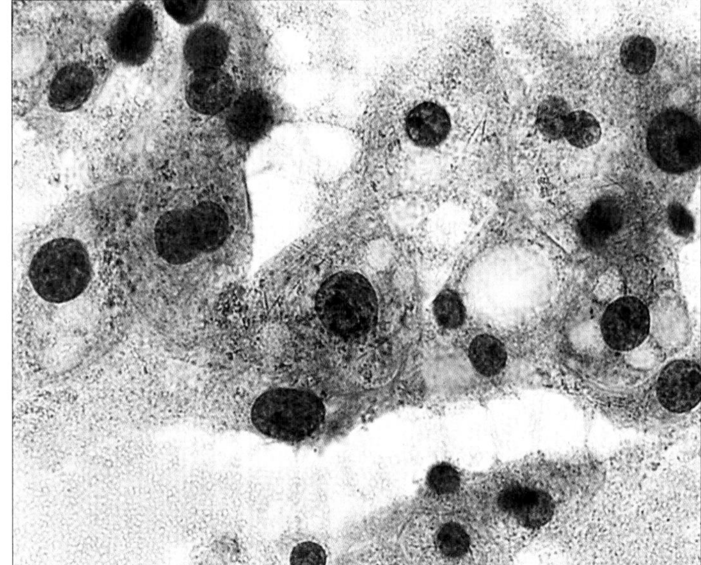

177. Shown is an FNA of a pulmonary lesion, which, when aspirated, may yield a false-negative diagnosis because of:

A. contaminants
B. poor staining quality
C. faulty technique–aspiration of necrotic center
D. vascular nature of the lesion

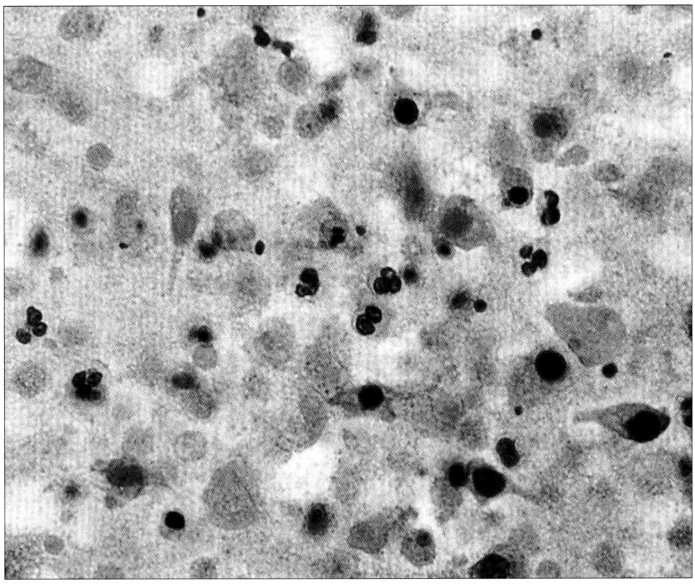

178. A 2-cm nodule located in the renal pelvis is aspirated from a 64-year-old man. These cells were negative when stained with oil red O and mucicarmine. They represent:

A. angiomyolipoma
B. hypernephroma
C. oncocytoma
D. transitional cell carcinoma

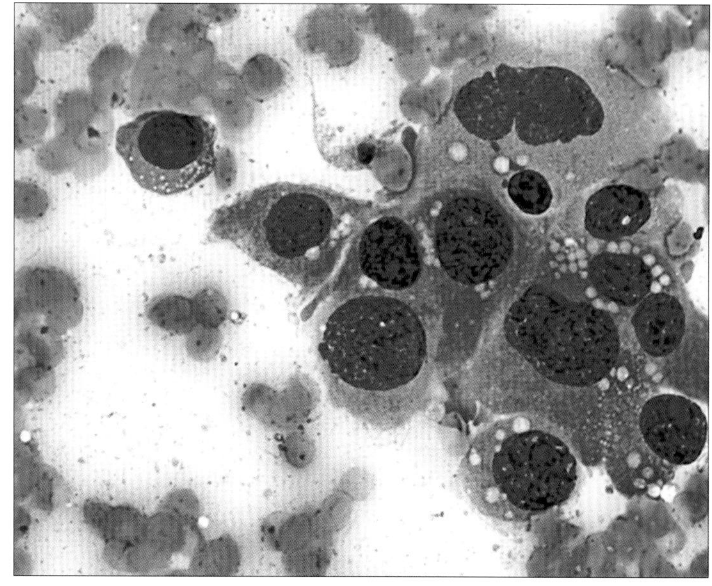

179. The cells in the center of the photomicrograph could arise from:

A. hepatocellular carcinoma
B. melanoma
C. papillary neoplasm of the thyroid
D. any of the above

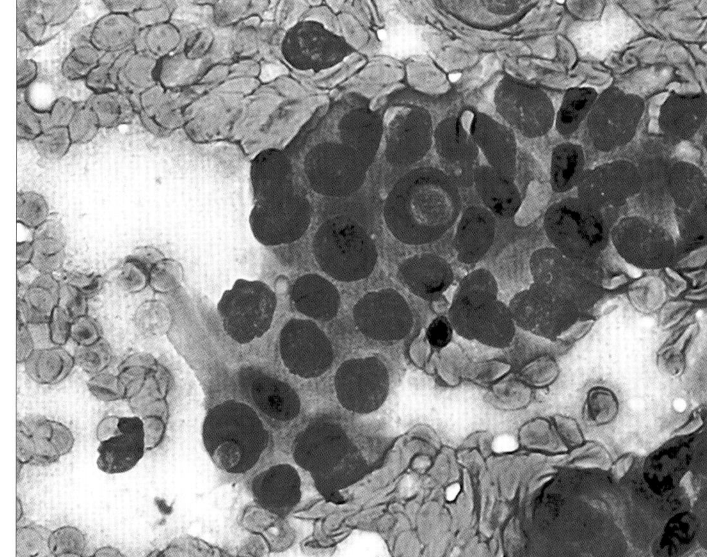

180. What special stain is helpful in establishing the pancreatic islet cell origin of these cells?

A. alpha-fetoprotein
B. S-100
C. chromogranin
D. vimentin

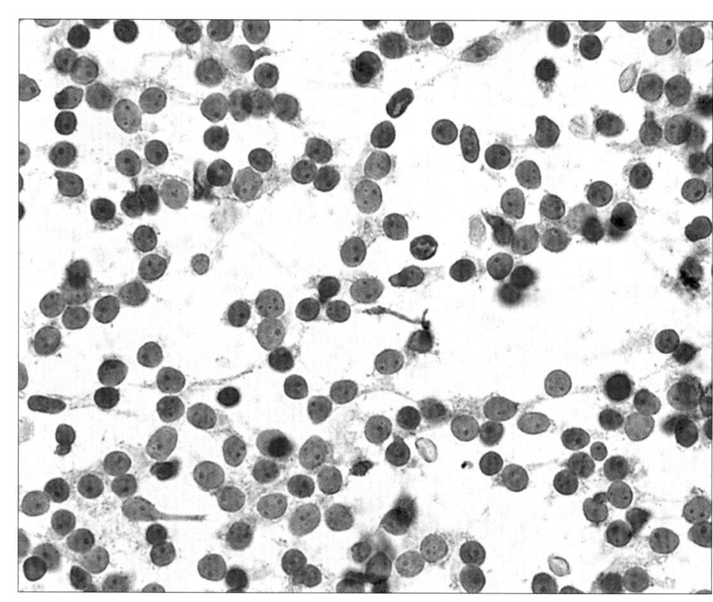

181. A patient develops anaphylaxis when a 3-cm cystic nodule is aspirated. The aspirated material is gritty in nature. This finding is suggestive of:

A. *Strongyloides stercoralis*
B. *Echinococcus granulosis*
C. *Entamoeba histolytica*
D. *Schistosoma mansoni*

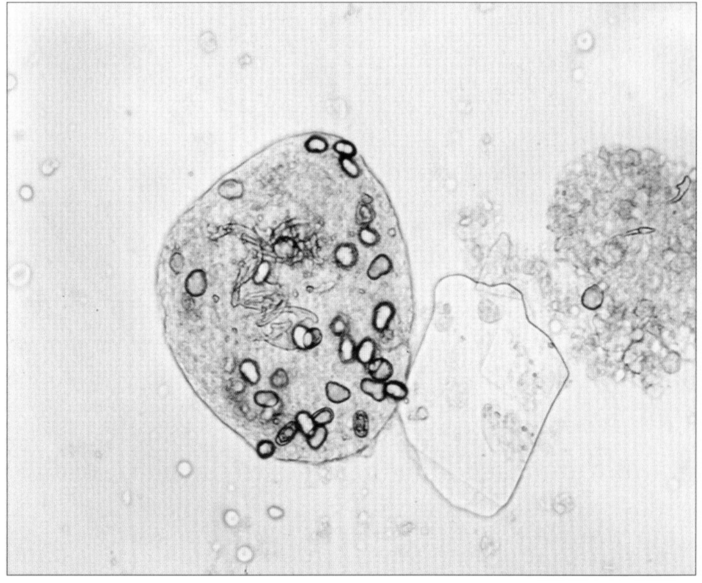

182. A 55-year-old woman with a 4-cm nodule in the head of the pancreas presents for FNA evaluation. Clinical symptoms include jaundice, weight loss, and deep radiating back pain. The cellular findings are diagnostic of:

A. ductal adenocarcinoma
B. microcystic adenoma
C. pancreatitis
D. anaplastic pancreatic carcinoma

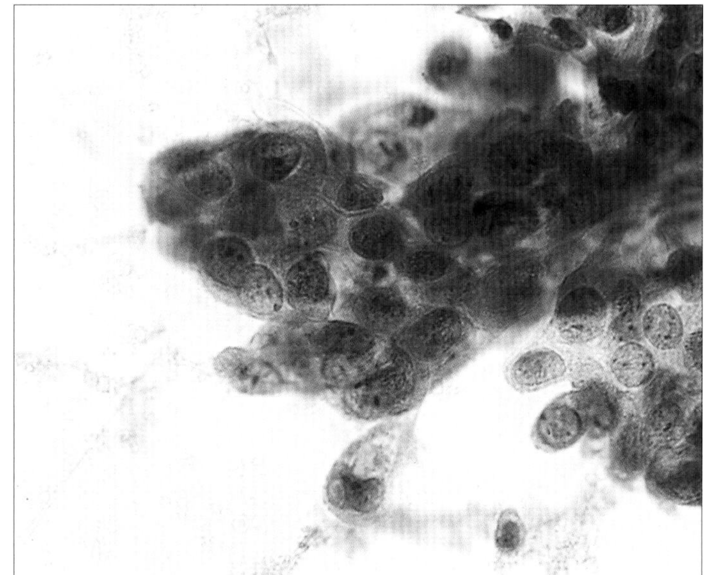

183. A 55-year-old woman with history of pancreatic carcinoma presents with a 1-cm liver nodule. These cells were obtained via aspiration with a 22-gauge needle. Which immunocytochemical results will help establish a diagnosis of metastatic pancreatic carcinoma by differentiating it from primary trabecular hepatocellular carcinoma?

A. alpha-fetoprotein (–), keratin (+)
B. alpha-fetoprotein (+), keratin (–)
C. alpha-fetoprotein (–), keratin (–)
D. alpha-fetoprotein (+), keratin (+)

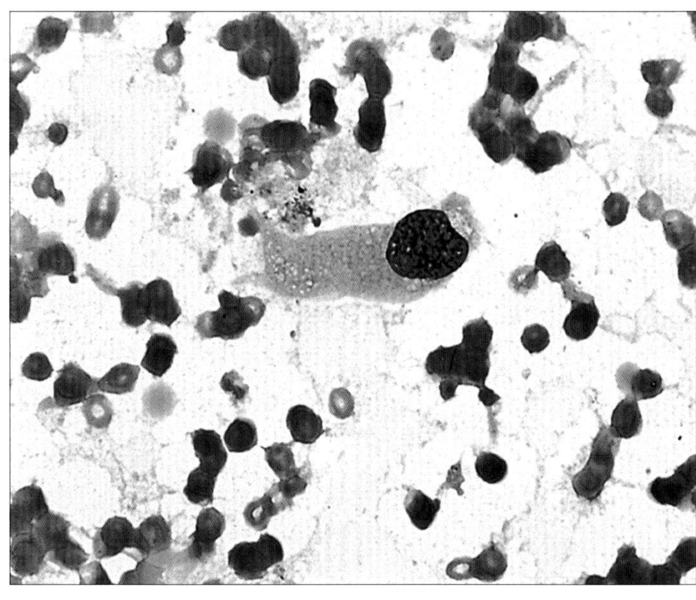

184. **A 33-year-old AIDS patient presents with multiple pigmented erythematous cutaneous lesions of the face and legs. Aspiration cytology of one of the leg lesions reveals these cells. The diagnosis is:**

A. squamous cell carcinoma
B. Kaposi sarcoma
C. melanoma
D. basal cell carcinoma

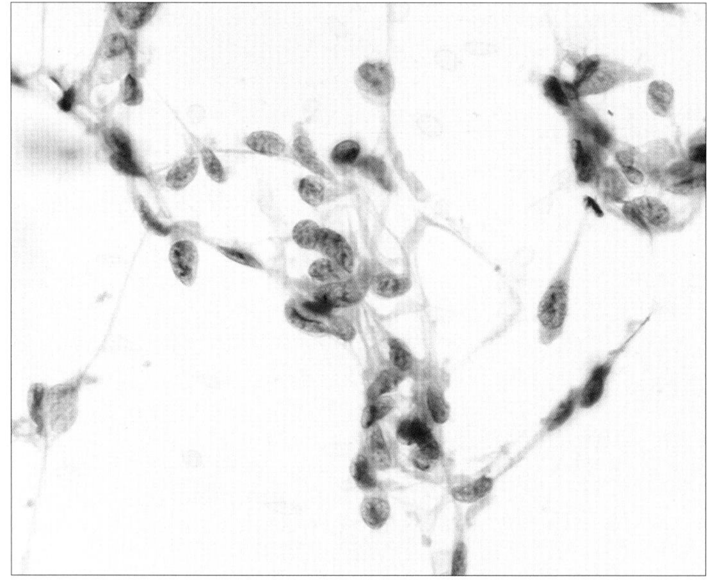

185. **These cells are identified in an aspirate of a 3-cm liver nodule in a 71-year-old man with a history of intrahepatic lithiasis. Immunocytochemical staining for alpha-fetoprotein is negative. The depicted cells represent:**

A. hepatocellular carcinoma
B. cholangiocarcinoma
C. liver cell dysplasia
D. reactive hepatocytes, secondary to lithiasis

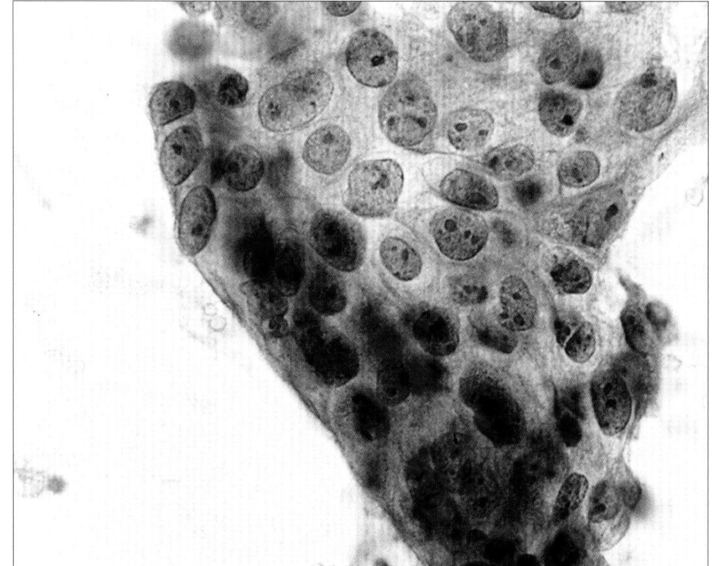

186. **Depicted is an FNA specimen of a 3×4-cm coin lesion in the left upper lobe of the lung. The patient is a 65-year-old man with a 120 pack/yr, 20-year history of smoking. He presents with obstructive pneumonitis and atelectasis. The diagnosis should include:**

A. *Aspergillus* sp., rule out secondary malignancy by re-aspirating from various areas of the mass
B. *Geotrichum candidum,* treat patient for fungal infection
C. *Actinomyces* sp., rule out secondary malignancy by re-aspirating from various areas of the mass
D. saprophytic Phycomycetes, treat patient for fungal infection

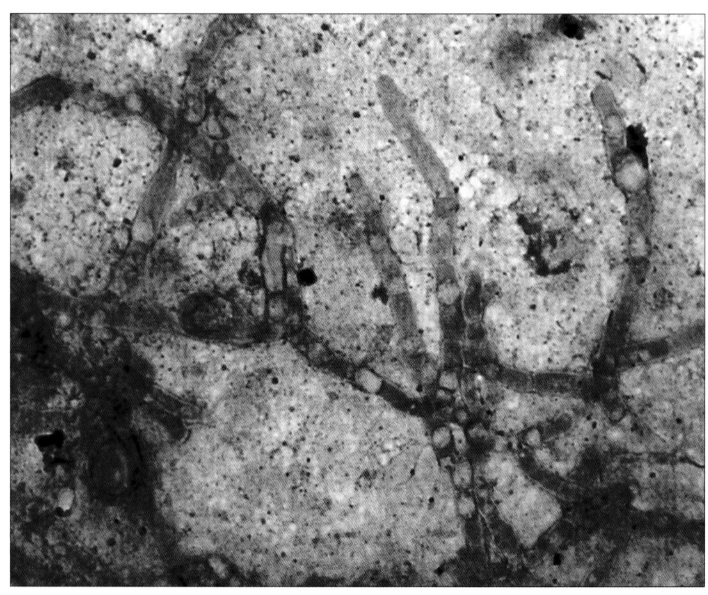

187. **What special stain will positively confirm the interpretation of these aspirated cells from a solitary lung nodule?**

A. chromogranin
B. HMB-45
C. alpha-fetoprotein
D. periodic acid–Schiff

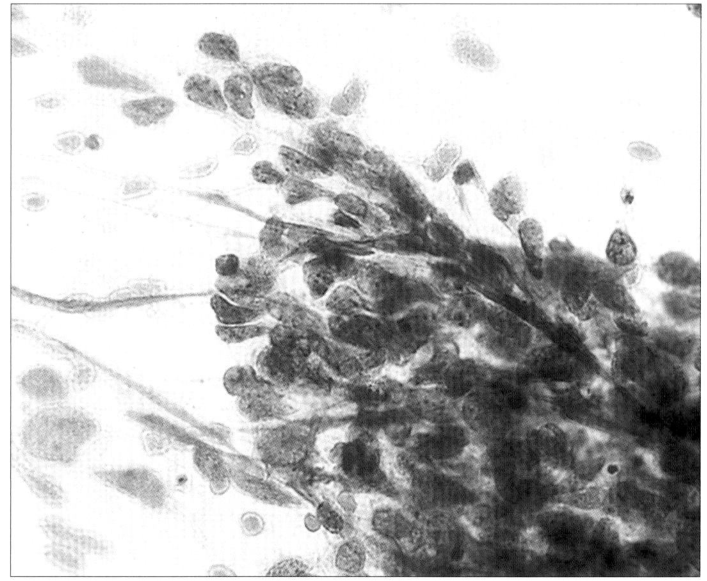

188. **These cells in a purulent supraclavicular lymph node aspirate located near the mandible, are diagnostic of:**

A. diffuse immunoblastic lymphoma
B. follicular hyperplasia
C. acute lymphadenitis
D. sinus histiocytosis

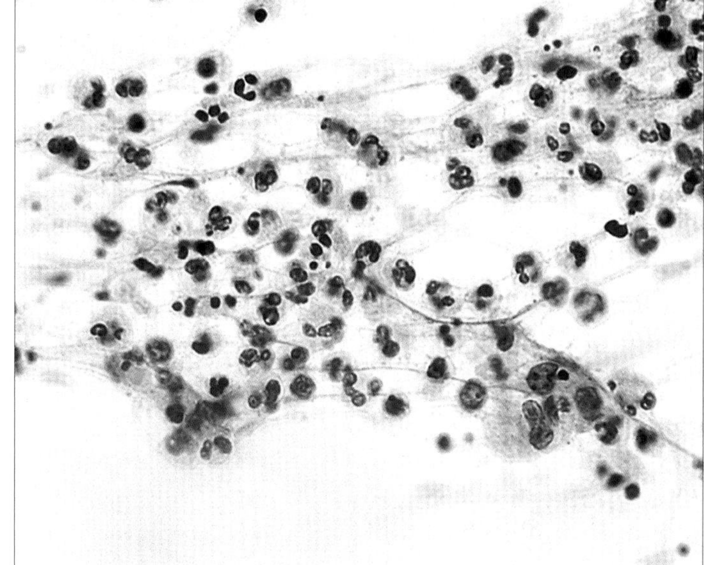

189. **These cells represent an FNA specimen from a patient with no history of a primary tumor but currently presenting with a 4-cm liver lesion and seropositivity for hepatitis B. The diagnosis is:**

A. reactive hepatocytes
B. reactive bile ductal cells
C. cholangiocarcinoma
D. hepatocellular carcinoma

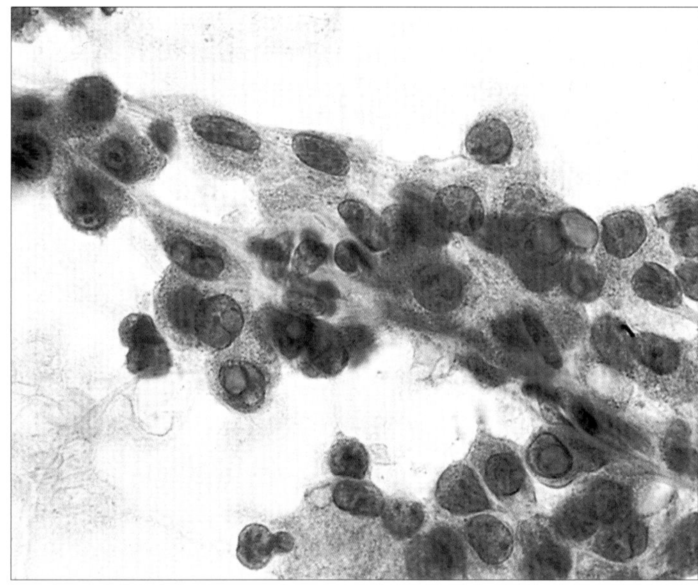

190. **These cells from pulmonary aspirations are:**

A. bronchial cells
B. mesothelial cells
C. fat cells
D. diagnostic of hamartoma

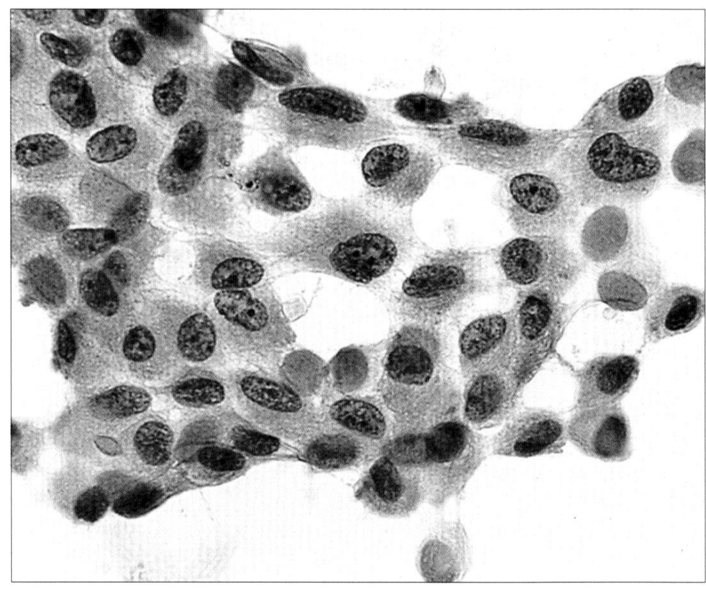

191. **A 23-year-old man with a previously confirmed case of small cell cleaved lymphoma, status post chemotherapy and post irradiation, presents with pneumonitis. FNA is performed to rule out metastatic disease. A GMS stain is performed. The cytologic findings suggest:**

A. metastatic lymphoma
B. *Pneumocystis carinii*
C. *Histoplasma capsulatum*
D. nondiagnostic, suggest repeat aspiration

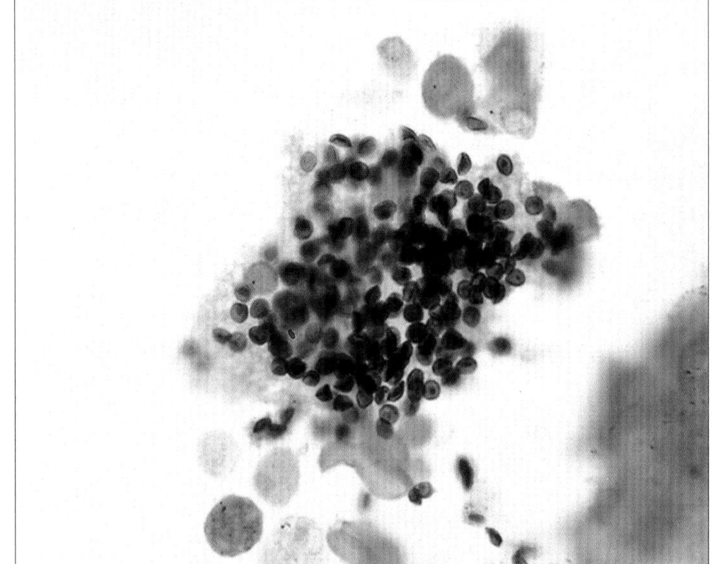

192. **A 66-year-old alcoholic patient with multiple liver nodules undergoes FNA. The depicted cells represent what type of process?**

A. reactive
B. malignant primary
C. metastatic
D. hamartomatous

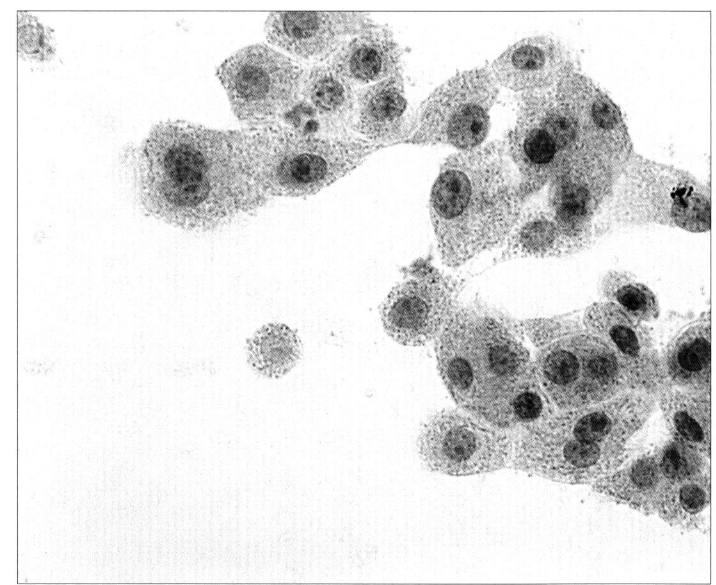

193. A 44-year-old man with a 3-cm lesion of the parotid gland undergoes FNA. A soft mass yields a brownish watery substance. These cells represent:

A. Warthin tumor
B. oxyphilic adenoma
C. pleomorphic adenoma
D. acinic cell carcinoma

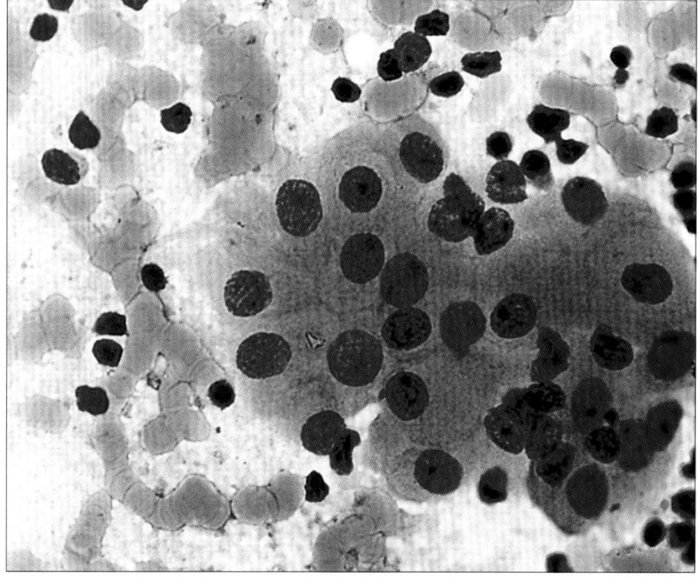

194. These cells from a 5-cm nodule located in the parotid gland suggest a diagnosis of:

A. oncocytoma
B. adenoid cystic carcinoma
C. mucoepidermoid carcinoma
D. pleomorphic adenoma

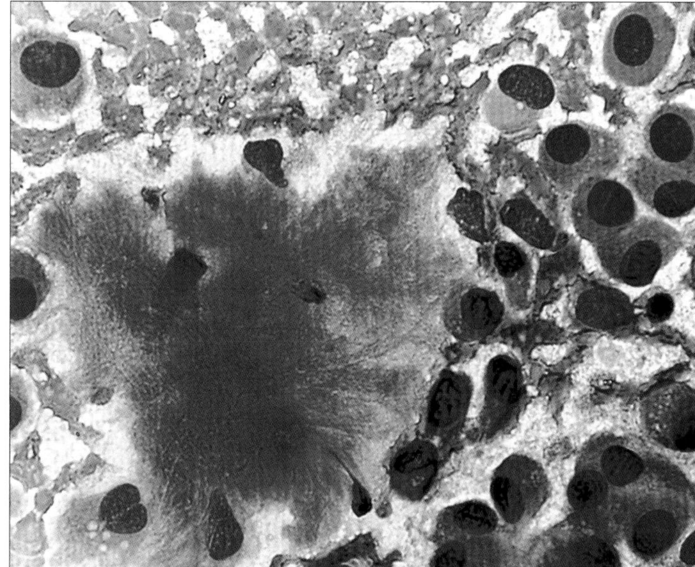

195. These cells represent a transbronchial aspirate from a peripheral 2-cm mass. The cellular findings suggest:

A. adenocarcinoma, poorly differentiated
B. large cell undifferentiated carcinoma
C. squamous cell carcinoma, poorly differentiated
D. adenosquamous carcinoma

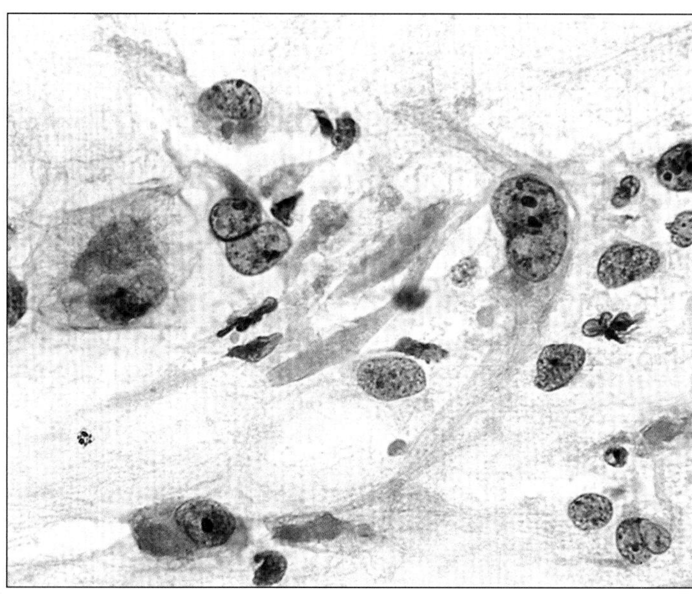

196. A 72-year-old patient with a history of a primary esophageal malignancy presents with multiple solid neck masses. An FNA specimen revealed these cells. The diagnosis is:

A. metastatic squamous cell carcinoma
B. branchial-cleft cyst
C. epidermal inclusion cyst
D. follicular carcinoma, metastatic from the thyroid

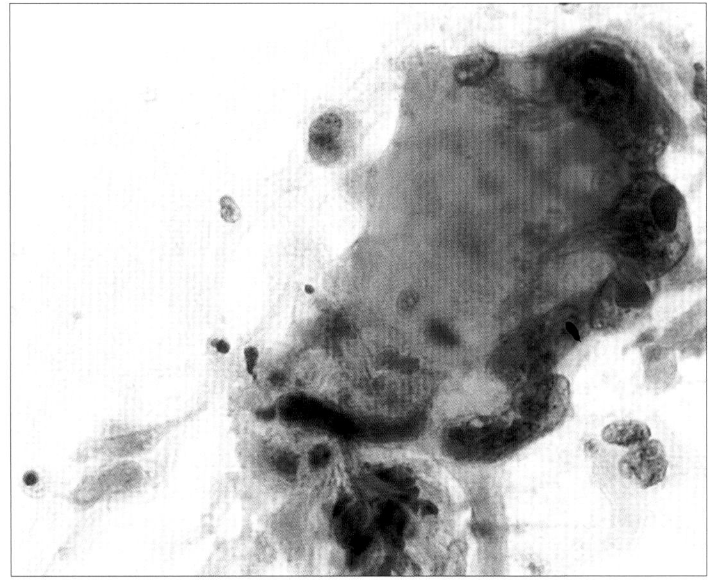

197. These cells are identified in a pancreatic aspirate from a 65-year-old woman with jaundice and Trousseau syndrome. A dilated common bile duct and gallbladder is demonstrated by endoscopic retrograde cholangiopancreatography. Based on the cellular findings, what is the primary diagnosis?

A. secretory ductal carcinoma, pancreas
B. nonsecretory ductal carcinoma, pancreas
C. oncocytic neoplasm, pancreas
D. pancreatoblastoma

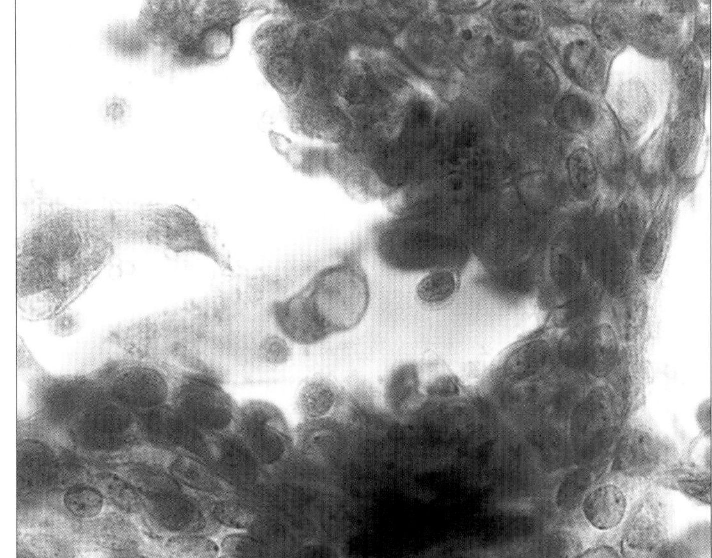

198. A 55-year-old woman with shortness of breath and dyspnea presents with a central cavitating lung lesion as demonstrated by computed tomography. Radiographically guided transbronchial aspiration reveals these cells. Based on the cytologic findings, the diagnosis is:

A. metastatic leiomyosarcoma
B. atypical squamous metaplasia
C. large cell undifferentiated carcinoma
D. squamous carcinoma

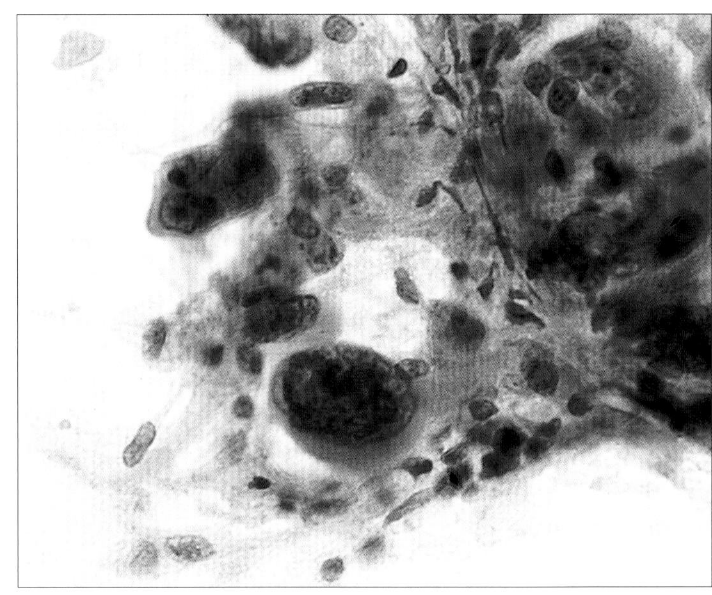

199. A 42-year-old man clinically diagnosed with HIV presents with a 2-cm liver lesion. FNA is performed using a 22-gauge needle. These cells represent:

A. granuloma
B. fat necrosis
C. adenoma
D. liver cell dysplasia

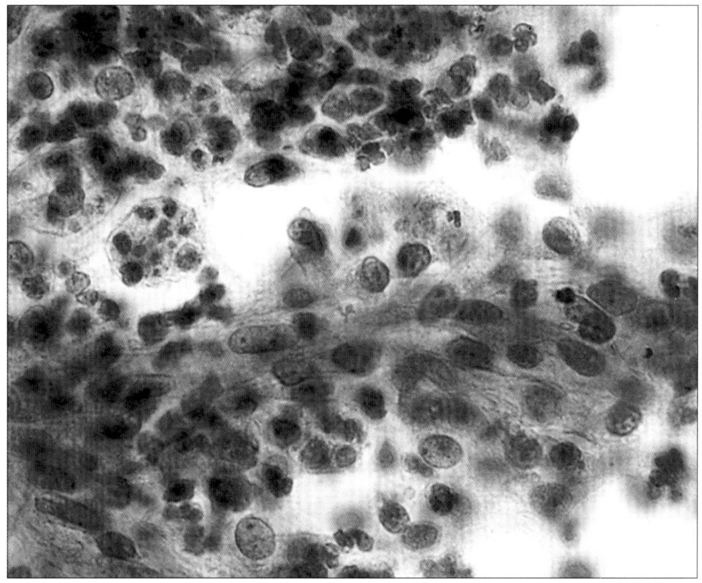

200. These cells from a parotid aspirate are diagnostic of:

A. monomorphic adenoma
B. Warthin tumor
C. oxyphilic adenoma
D. normal parenchyma

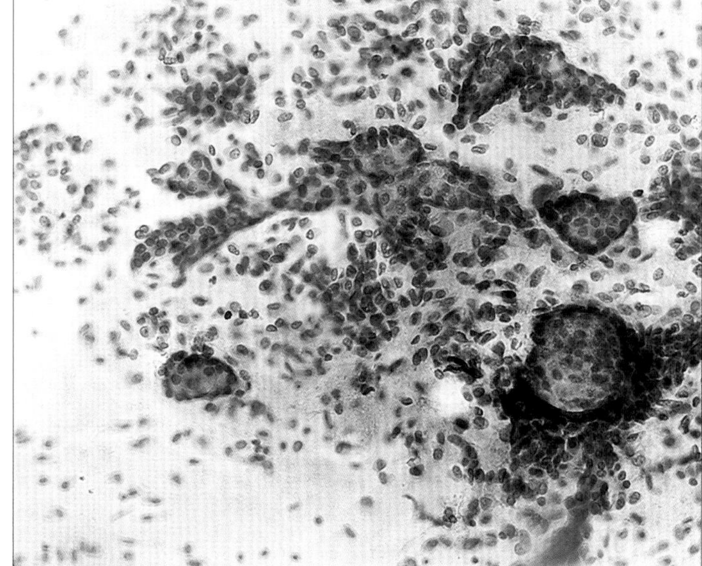

201. A 42-year-old woman with a history of gallstones presents with a cystic pancreas and increased serum amylase levels. FNA evaluation of the pancreas reveals these cells. The diagnosis is:

A. islet cell neoplasm
B. acute pancreatitis
C. microcystic adenoma
D. ductal adenocarcinoma

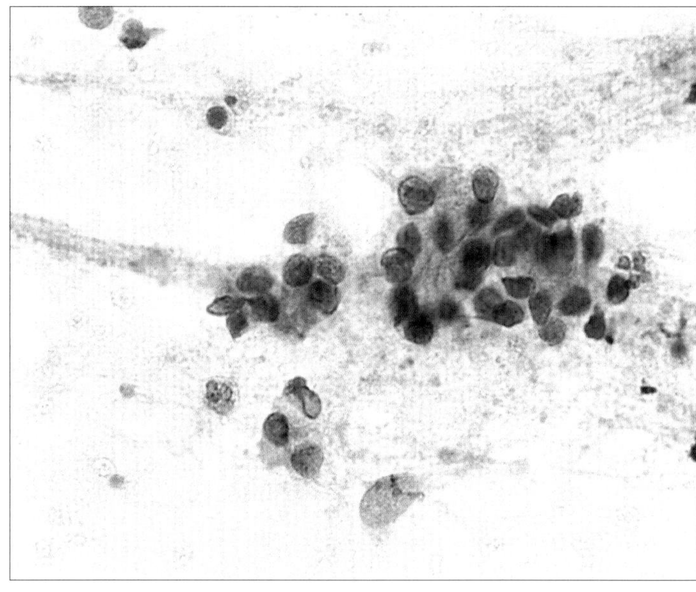

Fine Needle Aspiration *Answer Key*

1. **C colloid goiter**

Benign follicular cells in monolayer or honeycombing sheets in the presence of abundant colloid, appearing as ropy amorphous background material, and associated hemosiderin-laden macrophages and fibroblasts are typical findings associated with the FNA of benign colloid nodules.

DeMay RM, The Art & Science of Cytopathology.
Goiter, pp. 723–724, and FNA biopsy of follicular lesions, pp. 724–728.

2. **C at least 6 clusters of 10 cells over 2 slides**

Thyroid aspirates are hypocellular in nature, containing abundant colloid and blood. The presence of follicular epithelium is necessary to establish the diagnosis of a satisfactory specimen.

DeMay RM, The Art & Science of Cytopathology.
Fine needle aspiration biopsy: The best test, pp. 709–713.

3. **A cholangiocarcinoma**

Well-differentiated cholangiocarcinomas present cytologically as hypercellular specimens containing sheets of cells with slightly enlarged, overlapping nuclei and micronucleoli. Their resemblance to normal ductal cells may cause difficulty in establishing a malignant diagnosis. Careful attention should be given to mild nuclear deviations in light of a radiographically identified neoplasm. Cholangiocarcinomas are negative for alpha-fetoprotein and positive for CEA, whereas hepatocellular carcinomas are positive and negative, respectively.

DeMay RM, The Art & Science of Cytopathology.
Cholangiocarcinoma, pp. 1033–1034.

4. **B benign lymphoepithelial cyst**

Cystic parotid glands are common findings in patients infected with HIV. The cytologic identification of these lesions is based on the finding of a polymorphic population of lymphocytes, tingible body macrophages, and rare keratinizing and nonkeratinizing epithelial cells. Absent from these lesions are oncocytes, therefore, the diagnosis of Warthin tumor may be excluded.

DeMay RM, The Art & Science of Cytopathology.
Benign lymphoepithelial cyst, pp. 667–668.

5. **B follicular carcinoma**

Cells with follicular morphology, possessing numerous classic malignant nuclear features, may suggest follicular carcinoma. Follicular neoplasms cytologically present as a hypercellular population of overlapping follicular cells with cohesive microfollicular or trabecular groupings. Colloid is scanty to absent. The diagnosis of follicular neoplasm is given to those samples in which definitive atypical nuclear features are absent. Follicular adenoma should be reserved for histologic diagnosis only due to the possibility of capsular invasion by these benign-appearing cells and the lack of distinguishable cytologic criteria necessary to differentiate these lesions from well-differentiated carcinomas.

DeMay RM, The Art & Science of Cytopathology.
Follicular neoplasms, pp. 724–729.

6. **D malignant mixed tumor**

These malignant neoplasms may be related to the recurrence of an incompletely excised pleomorphic adenoma, hence it is appropriately named carcinoma ex pleomorphic adenoma. These lesions represent epithelial malignancies arising from pleomorphic adenomas. Cytologically, they present as pure populations of either poorly differentiated adenocarcinoma (most common), squamous cell carcinoma, or adenoid cystic carcinoma.

DeMay RM, The Art & Science of Cytopathology.
Malignant mixed tumors (carcinoma ex pleomorphic adenoma), pp. 680-681.

7. **A signet ring morphology**

Single or multiple clear cytoplasmic vacuoles with sharp borders, often creating a signet ring appearance, are associated with fatty metamorphosis. The absence of classic malignant nuclear features helps distinguish this benign disease from hepatocellular carcinoma. The etiology may be related to increased alcohol consumption, obesity, diabetes mellitus, or liver injuries and metabolic disorders.

DeMay RM, The Art & Science of Cytopathology.
Fatty metamorphosis, p. 1021.

8. **C Warthin tumor**

Warthin tumor (papillary cystadenoma lymphomatosum) cytologically presents with reactive lymphoid populations and oxyphilic/oncocytic epithelial cells. Oncocytes, cytologically presenting as cuboidal cells with eosinophilic granular cytoplasm and central or eccentric nuclei with prominent nucleoli, are suspended within a watery, proteinaceous, or dirty background. The concomitant finding of a lymphocytic infiltrate (representing a germinal center) alongside the oncocytic population excludes the diagnosis of pure oncocytoma or oxyphilic adenoma. Atypical squamous metaplasia (elongated caudate-shaped cells) may be present if the lesion is infarcted or infected; therefore, exercise caution to prevent over interpretation of these lesions as squamous cell carcinoma.

DeMay RM, The Art & Science of Cytopathology.
Warthin tumor, pp. 673–675 and 680–681.

9. **A mucoepidermoid carcinoma, well differentiated**

Mucus-producing columnar cells containing bland nuclei and foamy cytoplasm and a population of benign polygonal intermediate cells define low-grade mucoepidermoid carcinomas of the salivary gland. High-grade lesions present with predominant populations of malignant squamous cells revealing keratinizing features. Differential diagnosis includes a pure keratinizing squamous cell carcinoma, which diagnosis may be preferred in the presence of pearl formations.

DeMay RM, The Art & Science of Cytopathology.
Mucoepidermoid carcinoma, pp. 678–679.

10. **A polymorphous low-grade primary adenocarcinoma**

These terminal duct neoplasms are rare, minor salivary gland lesions that cytologically present as well-differentiated adenocarcinomas. They generally recapitulate gastrointestinal tract neoplasms but rarely metastasize.

DeMay RM, The Art & Science of Cytopathology.
Adenocarcinomas (polymorphous low-grade adenocarcinoma), p. 682.

11. **D oncocytoma**

The cellular evidence of a pure population of oncocytes devoid of a lymphocytic background (as seen in Warthin tumor) is diagnostic of oncocytoma. The cellular groupings, like Warthin tumors, are generally single; however, occasionally three-dimensional microacinar groupings may be seen. Although a lymphocytic infiltrate is not part of the diagnostic spectrum, a few mature lymphocytes may be seen. These lesions are considered rare tumors, usually involving elderly patients.

DeMay RM, The Art & Science of Cytopathology.
Oncocytoma and oncocytic carcinoma, p. 675.

12. **D adenoid cystic carcinoma**

Adenoid cystic carcinomas are frequent submaxillary and minor salivary gland neoplasms arising from the intercalated ducts. These lesions often present as painful lesions due to perineural invasion. Adenoid cystic carcinomas are cytologically identified by the presence of small round epithelial cells in clusters, acinar formations, and three-dimensional tissue fragments in balls or cylinders containing central, eosinophilic, hyaline/homogeneous, fibrillar basement membrane material.

DeMay RM, The Art & Science of Cytopathology.
Adenoid cystic carcinoma, pp. 676–678.

13. **D hemangioma**

These benign vascular lesions are the most common parotid gland neoplasm in children.

DeMay RM, The Art & Science of Cytopathology.
Salivary gland masses in children, p. 685.

14. **C monomorphic adenoma**

Basal cell adenomas are cytologically composed of a pure population of epithelial cells. Small cells as cohesive basaloid cells in cords, aggregates, or irregular clusters with high nuclear-to-cytoplasmic ratios and predictable nuclear features lacking atypia in the presence of copious amounts of metachromatic basement membrane and fibrous stroma are seen in the FNA smears. The absence of neural symptoms may help differentiate these lesions from adenoid cystic carcinomas.

DeMay RM, The Art & Science of Cytopathology.
Monomorphic adenomas (basal cell adenoma), pp. 671–672.

15. **D metastatic carcinoma**

Metastatic carcinomas represent 90% of the liver malignancies. The most common metastatic neoplasms of the liver include colon, stomach, pancreas, breast, lung, and kidney.

DeMay RM, The Art & Science of Cytopathology.
Metastases, pp. 1035-1036.

16. **B hyaline globules**

These eosinophilic intracytoplasmic inclusions may stain PAS positive or negative. They may also be found in cirrhosis, regeneration, or hepatocellular carcinoma.

DeMay RM, The Art & Science of Cytopathology.
Inclusions (hyaline globules), p. 1020.

17. **B** acinic cell carcinoma

Acinic cell carcinomas are considered rare lesions predominantly arising within parotid gland. Cytologically, these lesions may be difficult to interpret except for the lack of typical lobular architecture, their increased cellular size, and the presence of PAS (+) granules within the cytoplasm. However, the presence of a pure population of acinic cells and no recognizable ducts suggests the diagnosis of acinic cell carcinoma. Chronic inflammation may accompany the acinic cells.

DeMay RM, The Art & Science of Cytopathology.
Acinic cell carcinoma, pp. 679–680.

18. **B** vascular or capsular invasion as determined histologically

Although histology is considered the gold standard for determining whether follicular neoplasms have capsular or vascular invasion, up to 3/4 of follicular carcinomas are misdiagnosed in tissue due to interobserver variability. Follicular neoplasms cytologically present as a hypercellular population of overlapping follicular cells with cohesive microfollicular or trabecular groupings. Colloid is scanty to absent. The diagnosis of follicular neoplasm is given to those samples in which definitive atypical nuclear features are absent. The diagnosis of follicular adenoma should be reserved for histologic diagnosis only due to the possibility of capsular invasion by these benign-appearing cells and the lack of distinguishable cytologic criteria necessary to differentiate these lesions from well-differentiated carcinomas.

DeMay RM, The Art & Science of Cytopathology.
Follicular neoplasms, pp. 722–729.

19. **D** non-Hodgkin lymphoma

Lymphomas arising within the salivary gland are of large cell or small cell cleaved B-cell lineage and reveal light chain clonality. Cytology reveals a monotypic population of neoplastic lymphocytes.

DeMay RM, The Art & Science of Cytopathology.
Malignant lymphoma, pp. 683–684.

20. **A** medullary carcinoma

These rare neuroendocrine thyroid lesions that arise from parafollicular or "C" cells actively secrete calcitonin. A familial predilection has been established, related to multiple endocrine neoplasia syndrome. Hypercellular aspirates consist of pleomorphic spindle-appearing cells (often containing intranuclear intracytoplasmic inclusions), lympho/plasmacytoid cells, and Hürthle cells. These cells are suspended within an eosinophilic amorphous background consisting of amyloid, demonstrated by positive apple green birefringence and positive with Congo red. In addition, the tumor cells are immunocytochemically positive for thyrocalcitonin.

DeMay RM, The Art & Science of Cytopathology.
Medullary thyroid carcinoma, pp. 735–737.

21. **D** hamartoma

Bile ductal hamartomas or Meyenburg complexes are composed of embryological bile duct cells and connective tissue constituents. Hepatocytes are absent.

DeMay RM, The Art & Science of Cytopathology.
Bile duct adenomas and hamartomas, p. 1026.

22. **C** papillary carcinoma

Papillary carcinoma generally presents in monolayer sheets or in papillary groupings with fibrovascular cores. The cells contain irregular nuclear membranes with bland chromatin features, nuclear grooves, and intranuclear intracytoplasmic inclusions representing cytoplasmic intranuclear invaginations or nuclear pseudoinclusions. Colloid, foreign body giant cells, and psammoma bodies may accompany these findings. Intranuclear cytoplasmic inclusions (INCIs), or pseudoinclusions, are often found within papillary carcinoma of the thyroid, melanomas, and hepatocellular carcinomas.

DeMay RM, The Art & Science of Cytopathology.
Papillary thyroid carcinoma, pp. 729–735.

23. **A** branchial cleft cyst

These are lymphoepithelial cystic lesions of the neck lined with either mature stratified squamous epithelial cells, glandular cells representing mucin, goblet, or pseudostratified-ciliated types, or both (mucoepidermoid). The presence of reactive lymphoid hyperplasia may accompany these benign cellular findings.

DeMay RM, The Art & Science of Cytopathology.
Branchial cleft and lymphoepithelial cysts, pp. 645–646.

24. **D** medullary carcinoma

These rare neuroendocrine thyroid lesions that arise from parafollicular or "C" cells actively secrete calcitonin. A familial predilection has been established, related to multiple endocrine neoplasia syndrome. Hypercellular aspirates consist of pleomorphic spindle-appearing cells (often containing intranuclear intracytoplasmic inclusions), lympho/plasmacytoid cells, and Hürthle cells. These cells are suspended within an eosinophilic amorphous background consisting of amyloid, demonstrated by positive apple green birefringence and positive with Congo red. In addition, the tumor cells are immunocytochemically positive for thyrocalcitonin.

DeMay RM, The Art & Science of Cytopathology.
Medullary thyroid carcinoma, pp. 735–737.

25. **B** Hashimoto thyroiditis

A predominantly rich heterogeneous population of lymphocytes and follicular center cells with associated Hürthle cells are diagnostic of Hashimoto thyroiditis. Colloid, if present, is scanty.

DeMay RM, The Art & Science of Cytopathology.
Hashimoto thyroiditis, pp. 718–721.

26. **D** granulomatous thyroiditis (de Quervain)

Although of unknown cause, it is postulated that these lesions are linked to systemic viral infections, such as the mumps virus. This lesion is rarely aspirated due to the clinical history; however, it represents one of the most common causes of a painful thyroid.

DeMay RM, The Art & Science of Cytopathology.
Granulomatous thyroiditis, (de Quervain or subacute thyroiditis), pp. 717–718.

27. **A** monolayer hepatocytes with random atypical cells are found with liver cell dysplasia

Nontrabecular hepatocellular carcinomas (HCC) present with numerous cells containing more pronounced nuclear abnormalities and classic malignant features (irregular chromatin with prominent macronucleoli). Although the cellular findings in liver cell dysplasia (LCD) closely resemble those seen in nontrabecular hepatocellular carcinomas, the cytology of LCD shows only random tumor cells, rather than numerous tumor cells. Furthermore, the presence of lipofuscin, iron, or chronic inflammation suggests LCD rather than HCC.

DeMay RM, The Art & Science of Cytopathology.
Cirrhotic nodules: adenomatous hyperplasia, dysplasia, and HCC, pp. 1032–1033.

28. **A** liver cell adenoma

The finding of normal hepatocytes possessing normal-appearing nuclear features in concert with abundant clear (lipid/glycogen +) cytoplasm allows for differentiation of this benign tumor from well-differentiated hepatocellular carcinoma. Bile duct cells are not identified.

DeMay RM, The Art & Science of Cytopathology.
Liver cell adenoma, pp. 1025–1026.

29. **C** epidermoid cysts

These cysts are composed of a pure population of squamous epithelial cells, however, secondary granulomatous changes may be present.

DeMay RM, The Art & Science of Cytopathology.
Dermoid and epidermoid cysts, p. 647.

30. **D** follicular neoplasm

Follicular neoplasms cytologically present as a hypercellular population of overlapping follicular cells with cohesive microfollicular or trabecular groupings. Colloid is scanty to absent. The diagnosis of follicular neoplasm is given to those samples in which definitive atypical nuclear features are absent. The diagnosis of follicular adenoma should be reserved for histologic diagnosis only due to the possibility of capsular invasion by these benign-appearing cells and the lack of distinguishable cytologic criteria necessary to differentiate these lesions from well-differentiated carcinomas.

DeMay RM, The Art & Science of Cytopathology.
Follicular neoplasms, pp. 724–729.

31. **B** Mallory bodies

These cytoplasmic inclusions may be associated with alcoholic cirrhosis and hepatocellular carcinoma.

DeMay RM, The Art & Science of Cytopathology.
Mallory bodies, pp. 1020–1021.

32. **B** Hürthle cell neoplasm

The presence of a pure population of Hürthle cells lacking a lymphocytic infiltrate (Hashimoto thyroiditis) is suggestive of a Hürthle cell neoplasm. As with other follicular neoplasms, the absence of classic malignant nuclear criteria does not preclude the possibility of a well-differentiated carcinoma. Therefore, the diagnosis of "neoplasm" is preferred until histologic confirmation can determine capsular or vascular involvement. Hürthle cells represent mitochondria-rich follicular cells found singly and in clusters, containing abundant, eosinophilic, granular cytoplasm. The nuclei are round to oval and often possess prominent nucleoli. Hürthle cells are also found in Hashimoto thyroiditis, Hürthle cell neoplasms, and benign goiters.

DeMay RM, The Art & Science of Cytopathology.
Hürthle cell neoplasms, pp. 739–740.

33. **D** anaplastic carcinoma

Giant (anaplastic) cell carcinomas of the thyroid are highly anaplastic lesions that comprise between 5% and 10% of thyroid neoplasms.

34. **D** *Echinococcus granulosus*

Hydatid sand is composed of scoleces and hooklets derived from *Echinococcus granulosus*. Aspiration of cystic liver nodules is generally contraindicated due to the possibility of anaphylaxis.

DeMay RM, The Art & Science of Cytopathology.
Hydatid cysts, p. 1023.

35. **C** cirrhosis

Polygonal cells arranged in rows or trabeculae with dense, granular cytoplasm, enlarged central placed bi- or multinucleated cells with smooth nuclear membranes, prominent nucleoli, intranuclear cytoplasmic inclusions, and intracytoplasmic bile pigmentation are diagnostic of reactive hepatocytes. These changes are commonly associated with conditions such as alcoholic cirrhosis or viral hepatitis. Bile duct cells, fibrous connective tissue, and numerous lymphocytes represent concomitant cytologic findings.

DeMay RM, The Art & Science of Cytopathology.
Cirrhosis, pp. 1022–1023.

36. **B** vascular lesions

Vascular lesions, bleeding abnormalities, pulmonary hypertension, uncooperative or debilitated patients, patients with contralateral pneumonectomy, and patients with chronic obstructive pulmonary disease represent some of the possible contraindications for performing pulmonary aspirations.

DeMay RM, The Art & Science of Cytopathology.
Fine needle aspiration biopsy, p. 948.

37. **D** bronchioloalveolar adenocarcinoma

The mucinous variant of bronchioloalveolar adenocarcinoma (BAC) presents cytologically as large tissue fragments with a greater depth of focus than bronchogenic adenocarcinoma. The cells are typically uniform in size and shape and contain round to oval nuclei. Nonmucinous (nm) BAC is cytologically represented in monolayered sheets and pleomorphic nuclei, with large intranuclear cytoplasmic inclusions. In addition, the cells from nm BAC may be accompanied by alveolar macrophages or psammoma bodies.

38. **A** large cell carcinoma

These highly malignant lesions tend to arise within the large bronchi, representing a poorly differentiated non-small cell tumor. Although described as undifferentiated, this diagnosis is reserved for those lesions that, under light microscopy, show neither glandular nor squamous differentiation. However, ultrascopically, these lesions usually show gland formation. Cytologically, these cells are arranged in syncytial-like groupings and lie singly. Nuclei are hyperchromatic, possess coarsely granular, irregularly distributed chromatin, multiple irregular macronucleoli, with marked anisonucleosis. The cytoplasm tends to be basophilic and homogeneous. A variant of this lesion is the so-called giant cell type, which exhibits macrocytic and multinucleated malignant tumor giant cells.

DeMay RM, The Art & Science of Cytopathology.
Large cell undifferentiated carcinoma, p. 970.

39. **A** Romanowsky

If one suspects a hematopoietic neoplasm, the staining of choice may be the Romanowsky, Giemsa, or the modified Wright (Diff-Quik) stain. Because these procedures require air-dried smears, cellular ballooning and gigantism will be accentuated; however, nuclear detail is often lost. Therefore, nuclear criteria utilized for interpreting alcohol-fixed specimens should not be followed.

DeMay RM, The Art & Science of Cytopathology.
Romanowsky stain, pp. 14–15.

40. **D** carcinoid tumor

Carcinoid tumors are slow-growing neuroendocrine tumors which have association with a Kulchitsky (K) cell etiology. These polypoid tumors cytologically present as small cells with N/C ratios and hypochromatic, finely granular, evenly distributed chromatin patterns, with typical oat cell grouping of cords, nest, ribbons, and vertebral column formations. Reactive/reparative cells can be discriminated from these lesions based on the absence of terminal bars and/or cilia with carcinoid lesions. Clinical history (a radiographically detectable lesion) and physiological changes are essential elements in the establishment of carcinoid lesions. Immunocytochemical staining with chromogranin, neuron-specific enolase, or serotonin, as well as histochemical detection of argentaffin or argyrophil, will help establish their neuroendocrine origin. Atypical carcinoid tumors, usually associated with the physiological carcinoid syndrome of right-sided fibrosis of the heart, cyanotic flushing of the skin, and liver metastasis, generally have classical malignant features that may be difficult to distinguish from small cell carcinomas.

DeMay RM, The Art & Science of Cytopathology.
Carcinoid tumors (typical carcinoid), pp. 971–973.

41. **D** small cell carcinoma

Small cell carcinoma is a highly malignant neuroendocrine neoplasm that is ultrastructurally part of the amine precursor uptake and decarboxylation tumors (APUD) due to its cytoplasmic evidence of androgenic amines (membrane-bound granules). These cells contain hyperchromatic, stippled chromatin, coarse clumping, nuclear molding, scanty cytoplasm, and micronucleoli. An important diagnostic feature of small cell carcinoma is the presence of paranuclear cytoplasmic inclusions—blue cytoplasmic globules found indenting the nuclei (best visualized with Diff-Quik staining). The cellular groupings characteristically have vertebral column formation, microbiopsy aggregates, and cords, nests, or ribbons. "Crush artifact," or degenerative nuclear material related to the mechanical crushing associated with the preparation of FNA specimens, is found in the background of most small cell carcinomas. This artifact presents as long clumpy streams of basophilic material. A variant of small cell carcinoma, intermediate cell small cell carcinoma, represents both fusiform and polygonal types which are typically better preserved with open coarse chromatin patterns and enlarged cell areas. Immunocytochemical staining with chromogranin is helpful in establishing the neurosecretory nature of this tumor, but will not differentiate it from carcinoid lesions. Furthermore, the absence of lymphogranular bodies (best demonstrated with the Romanowsky or Diff-Quik stain) will help differentiate these lesions from malignant lymphoid processes.

DeMay RM, The Art & Science of Cytopathology.
Small cell carcinoma, pp. 966–969.

42. **D** mixed müllerian tumor/uterus

The diagnosis of mixed mesodermal/müllerian tumor is determined by the cytologic identification of endometrial adenocarcinoma (usually well-differentiated) with a concomitant homologous or heterologous sarcomatous element.

DeMay RM, The Art & Science of Cytopathology.
Sarcomas, p. 136.

43. **A** normal pulmonary constituents

In addition to bronchial epithelial cells, cells not typically found with conventional exfoliative pulmonary cytology (sputum, bronchoscopy) but found in FNA specimens include sheets of mesothelial cells, fibroconnective tissue elements, fibroblasts, smooth muscle cells, adipose tissue, and hepatocytes.

DeMay RM, The Art & Science of Cytopathology.
The cells, pp. 951–952.

44. **A** aspiration of necrotic center

Aspiration of the center of a lesion yields a specimen composed predominantly of diathesis and necrotic debris. When performing FNA, special attention needs to be given so that multiple sites of neoplasm are aspirated, especially along the peripheral margins (> 10 planes).

DeMay RM, The Art & Science of Cytopathology.
Fine needle aspiration biopsy, p. 949, Complications associated with deep target biopsy, p. 470, and Performing the biopsy, pp. 471–473.

45. **C** squamous carcinoma

Pleomorphic cells with caudate or spindle formations with refractile cytoplasm, anisonucleosis, and opaque ink dot-like nuclei are diagnostic of squamous cell carcinoma. A necrotic background is helpful in establishing this lesion.

DeMay RM, The Art & Science of Cytopathology.
Keratinizing (well-differentiated) SCC, pp. 960–961.

46. **D** adenocarcinoma, prostate

Cells representing prostatic adenocarcinomas present in discohesive sheets, clusters, and microacinar formations with increased nuclear sizes, overlapping nuclei, and the important finding of macronucleoli.

DeMay RM, The Art & Science of Cytopathology.
Adenocarcinoma, pp. 1142–1144.

47. **D** metastatic melanoma

Melanoma typically presents in single cells, aggregates, or as spindle cells with bizarre malignant nuclear features, macronucleoli, intranuclear cytoplasmic inclusions, and possibly intracytoplasmic golden brown pigment. Due to the fact that these diseases may be amelanotic, it may be helpful to confirm this disease process with S-100, HMB-45, Melan A or MITF (microphthlmia-associated transcription factor)—all which preferentially react with melanoma cells.

DeMay RM, The Art & Science of Cytopathology.
Metastasis, pp. 980–981.

Wang JF, Sarma DP, Ulmer P. Diagnostic dilemma: HMB-45 and Melan-A negative tumor, can it be still a melanoma?: MITF (Microphthalmia-associated transcription factor) stain may confirm the diagnosis. The Internet Journal of Dermatology. 2007. Volume 5 Number 1.

48. **B** neural sheath tumors

These lesions are typically paravertebral in origin and arise from the sympathetic or intercostal nerves. They include malignant schwannoma, neurilemoma, and neurofibroma.

DeMay RM, The Art & Science of Cytopathology.
Neurogenic tumors, pp. 1009–1011.

49. **A** Hashimoto thyroiditis

A predominantly rich heterogeneous population of lymphocytes and follicular center cells with associated Hürthle cells are diagnostic of Hashimoto thyroiditis. Colloid, if present, is scanty. Hürthle cells represent mitochondria-rich follicular cells found singly and in clusters, containing abundant eosinophilic, granular cytoplasm. The nuclei are round to oval and often possess prominent nucleoli. Hürthle cells are found in Hashimoto thyroiditis, Hürthle cell neoplasms, and benign goiters.

DeMay RM, The Art & Science of Cytopathology.
Hashimoto thyroiditis, pp. 718–721.

50. **C** *Pneumocystis carinii*

Pneumocystis carinii is considered an opportunistic protozoan that may be seen in immunosuppressed individuals secondary to immunologic disorders, malignancies, or HIV infection, and in premature infants or patients receiving chemotherapy. Cytological identification rests on the presence of frothy mats of eosinophilic material with interspersed "contact lens"-shaped structures containing intranuclear trophozoites.

DeMay RM, The Art & Science of Cytopathology.
Pneumocystis carinii, p. 57.

51. **B** abscess

Abscesses of the lung typically present as cavitating lesions with the cytologic evidence described in the question. These inflammatory processes may be secondary to bacterial invasion, which may be apparent in the background or contained within the cytoplasm of histiocytes. Special stains may be required for differentiation of specific infectious process.

DeMay RM, The Art & Science of Cytopathology.
Abscess, pp. 952–953.

52. **C** gastroenteric cysts

These cystic lesions may arise from the foregut and are cytologically composed of gastric or intestinal epithelial cells.

DeMay RM, The Art and Science of Cytopathology.
Developmental cysts (foregut cysts), p. 1002.

53. **B** malignant lymphoma

These monoclonal neoplasms cytologically present with a predominant population of small cleaved lymphocytes (80%), and a lesser population of small noncleaved/round lymphocytes and large lymphocytes. Their inability to express dual tumor cell marking as seen in small round cell lymphoma (noncleaved, well-differentiated lymphocytic lymphoma) helps differentiate these two lesions.

DeMay RM, The Art & Science of Cytopathology.
Small cleaved (poorly differentiated lymphocytic) lymphoma, pp. 804–805.

54. **C** pneumothorax

Pneumothorax occurs in 5%–50% of the pulmonary aspirations performed. Although most resolve without further intervention, only a minority of the cases (10%) may require a chest tube or therapy. Decreasing the number of FNA passes to only those that are necessary will help decrease the chance of inducing this condition. In addition, there is a decreased chance of pneumothorax if both pleural surfaces are penetrated rapidly without crossing the fissures.

DeMay RM, The Art & Science of Cytopathology.
Complications associated with deep target biopsy, p. 469.

55. **B** hamartoma

Hamartomas of the lung present with groups or sheets of benign epithelial cells, adipocytes, possible cartilage, and a background of fibromyxoid stroma. The cytologic diagnosis of this lesion is similar to that of pleomorphic adenoma of the salivary gland.

DeMay RM, The Art & Science of Cytopathology.
Hamartoma, pp. 955–956.

56. **D** malignant lymphoma

These monoclonal neoplasms cytologically present with a predominant population of small cleaved lymphocytes (80%), and a lesser population of small noncleaved/round lymphocytes and large lymphocytes. Their inability to express dual tumor cell marking as seen in small round cell lymphoma helps differentiate these two lesions.

DeMay RM, The Art & Science of Cytopathology.
Small cleaved (poorly differentiated lymphocytic) lymphoma, pp. 804–805.

57. D granuloma

Elongated, round, or oval cells presenting singly or in syncytial aggregates with oval/reniform nuclei containing finely granular, evenly distributed chromatin and micronucleoli are diagnostic of epithelioid histiocytes. These cells are part of the spectrum of granulomatous inflammation. Other cells associated with granulomatous inflammation include multinucleated histiocytes, fibroblasts, and acute or chronic inflammatory cells.

DeMay RM, The Art & Science of Cytopathology.
Granuloma, p. 953.

58. **A** Sjögren syndrome

This autoimmune disease, related to either Mikulicz disease or Sjögren syndrome, is a benign lymphoepithelial lesion involving the destruction of the salivary gland lymphoid tissue and the lacrimal glands (Mikulicz only). FNA cytology reveals the presence of reactive lymphoid hyperplasia and myoepithelial cell proliferation (benign lymphoepithelial lesion). Similar findings may be seen in human immunodeficiency virus-infected patients or those suffering active acquired immunodeficiency disease.

DeMay RM, The Art & Science of Cytopathology.
Autoimmune sialadenitis, p. 666.

59. **A** bronchogenic adenocarcinoma

Bronchogenic adenocarcinomas cytologically present in two-dimensional acinar clusters with smooth "community" borders and single cells and demonstrate hypochromatic/bland chromatin, or if less well-differentiated, hyperchromasia. The presence of central macronucleoli is helpful in establishing this disease process. These true tissue fragments possess frothy cytoplasm, high N/C ratios, and uniform or lobulated nuclei.

DeMay RM, The Art & Science of Cytopathology.
Adenocarcinoma, pp. 962–964.

60. **B** sialadenitis

The cytology associated with acute sialadenitis reveals degenerated ductal cells, acinar groups, and adipocytes, as well as abundant necrotic debris, polymorphonuclear neutrophils, and macrophages.

DeMay RM, The Art & Science of Cytopathology.
Acute sialadenitis, p. 663.

61. **B** negative

Nuclear molding or cohesion in small cells may be associated with neurosecretory tumors. In contrast, lymphocytic lesions will not demonstrate true cohesive properties—they may "kiss" but do not "hug." Chromogranin or neuron-specific enolase will immunocytochemically identify small cell carcinomas, whereas common leukocyte antigen will positively identify lymphomas.

DeMay RM, The Art & Science of Cytopathology.
Small cell carcinoma, pp. 966–969.

62. **C** plasmacytoma

FNA of plasma cell myelomas reveals cells with "clock face" chromatin, immature cells with fine chromatin and prominent nucleoli, and occasionally binucleated and bizarre multinucleated giant cells. The cytoplasm is generally blue or amphophilic with perinuclear hofs and intranuclear or intracytoplasmic Russell bodies (representing immunoglobulin, usually IgG or IgA).

DeMay RM, The Art & Science of Cytopathology.
Plasma cell myeloma, pp. 821–822.

63. **A** invasive thymoma

Invasive thymomas cytologically present with bland morphologic appearance. Capsular invasion is required before rendering an invasive diagnosis. Paraneoplastic syndromes, such as myasthenia gravis, are commonly found in patients with thymoma.

DeMay RM, The Art and Science of Cytopathology.
Malignant thymoma (invasive thymoma), p. 1005.

64. **C** pleomorphic adenoma

Sheets and clusters of cuboidal cells containing round to oval nuclei and micronucleoli represent the ductal epithelial component of pleomorphic adenoma (benign mixed tumor). Fibromyxoid and chondroid mesenchymal elements (staining bright magenta with Diff-Quik staining) and myoepithelial spindle cells, typically arranged in cords and as single cells, may predominate in the smears.

DeMay RM, The Art & Science of Cytopathology.
Pleomorphic adenoma, pp. 669–671.

65. D pleomorphic adenoma

Sheets and clusters of cuboidal cells containing round to oval nuclei and micronucleoli represent the ductal epithelial component of pleomorphic adenoma (benign mixed tumor). Fibromyxoid and chondroid mesenchymal elements (staining bright magenta with Diff-Quik staining) and myoepithelial spindle cells, typically arranged in cords and as single cells, may predominate in the smears.

DeMay RM, The Art & Science of Cytopathology.
Pleomorphic adenoma, pp. 669–671.

66. D treat with Carnoy fixative

Carnoy fixative may be utilized for bloody specimens, lysing the red blood cells that obscure the cellular detail. A 1:14 mixture of glacial acidic acid to 95% ethanol is appropriate.

67. C metastatic colonic adenocarcinoma

The presence of tall columnar or "cigar-shaped" cells in aggregates with frankly malignant nuclear features, granular cytoplasm, or the presence of malignant signet ring cells may suggest a diagnosis of metastatic adenocarcinoma of the colon. Correlation with the primary lesion is critical.

DeMay RM, The Art & Science of Cytopathology.
Adenocarcinoma, p. 355.

68. A malignant schwannoma

Malignant schwannoma (neurofibrosarcoma), a nerve tissue tumor (of neural sheath) related to von Recklinghausen disease and generally arising within the posterior mediastinum, cytologically presents as monotonous synovial sarcoma. The presence of Verocay bodies, palisading nuclei with "flame-like" cytoplasm, and spindle cells with oval, curved, or twisted nuclei, is an essential component in establishing a primary schwannoma. Immunocytochemistry for S-100 protein and Leu 7 may be positive. Thymoma, hemangioma, and parathyroid adenoma are all considered anterior mediastinal lesions.

DeMay RM, The Art & Science of Cytopathology.
Schwannoma, p. 1010.

69. C reactive bronchial cells

Radiation- and chemotherapy-induced changes characteristically produce macrocytic cells. These reactive cells may share "atypical" nuclear morphology with carcinoma, but the presence of benign products of functional differentiation such as the presence of terminal bars and/or cilia are often seen in these faux "abnormal" cells.

DeMay RM, The Art & Science of Cytopathology.
Therapeutic agents (radiation) (chemotherapy), pp. 221–222.

70. C peripheral lesions

Peripheral lesions, such as bronchioloalveolar carcinomas, generally do not exfoliate in sputum cytology as efficiently as central pulmonary neoplasms. Gaining access to these lesions via bronchoscopy may also prove inadequate. Therefore, the use of FNA in evaluating peripheral (especially small) lung lesions is considered a highly effective diagnostic procedure.

DeMay RM, The Art & Science of Cytopathology.
Fine needle biopsy, p. 950.

71. C osteoblastoma

This vertebral column neoplasm typically presents in children and adolescents.

DeMay RM, The Art & Science of Cytopathology.
Osteoblastoma, pp. 595–596.

72. B aspiration pneumonia, plant material

Vegetable material may falsely give the interpretation of a squamous malignancy; however, their double refractile cell walls and smudged nuclear features help establish this process as plant material. Food particles may be secondary to aspiration pneumonia.

DeMay RM, The Art & Science of Cytopathology.
Aspiration pneumonia, p. 955, and Contaminants (plant cells/food), p. 219.

73. C chondroblastoma

These benign lesions generally arise within the long bones in teenage boys and may involve the knee.

DeMay RM, The Art & Science of Cytopathology.
Chondroblastoma, p. 591.

74. A prostate-specific antigen (+)

Immunocytochemical analysis for prostate-specific antigen (PSA) may be helpful in establishing secondary metastasis of prostatic carcinoma in elderly males.

DeMay RM, The Art & Science of Cytopathology.
Adenocarcinoma, pp. 1142–1143.

75. **C** cholangiocarcinoma, well differentiated

Cholangiocarcinoma of the liver presents in its well-differentiated forms similar to benign ductal epithelium, except for its hypercellularity, minimal anisokaryosis, and nuclear crowding. Lesions may be differentiated from hepatocellular carcinoma by their immunocytochemical positivity with CEA and negativity for alpha-fetoprotein.

DeMay RM, The Art & Science of Cytopathology.
Bile duct carcinomas (cholangiocarcinoma), pp. 1033–1034.

76. **D** chondrosarcoma

Chondrosarcomas are malignant tumors often arising in the axial skeleton, pelvis, femur, or humerus. They typically affect older patients.

DeMay RM, The Art & Science of Cytopathology.
Chondrosarcoma, pp. 591–592.

77. **B** PAS(+)/Ewing sarcoma

These highly anaplastic lesions, of parasympathetic nerve origin, tend to affect the femur, fibula, or tibia in adolescent males. The malignant cells are glycogen-positive (PAS +). In addition, a characteristic dimorphic pattern of large blastemic cells and lymphocytoid cells are seen with Diff-Quik staining.

DeMay RM, The Art & Science of Cytopathology.
Ewing sarcoma, pp. 593–594.

78. **B** fibroma

Fibromas are scirrhous ovarian lesions that yield hypocellular aspirates containing slender spindle fibroblasts. The differential diagnosis is a benign thecoma; however, thecomas cytologically present as pump spindle cells with vacuolated lipid-positive cytoplasm, have an increased cytoplasmic mass, and have irregular nuclei.

DeMay RM, The Art & Science of Cytopathology.
Ovarian fibroma/thecoma, p. 1159.

79. **B** liposarcoma

Pleomorphic liposarcomas are often large in size and arise within the deep soft tissues of the retroperitoneal area or the extremities of middle-aged to older patients.

DeMay RM, The Art & Science of Cytopathology.
Liposarcoma (pleomorphic liposarcoma), p. 576.

80. **B** luteal cyst

FNA of ovarian luteal cysts reveals sheets of luteal cells possessing granular and frothy cytoplasm, low nuclear-to-cytoplasmic ratios, and predictable nuclei with prominent nucleoli. These cells resemble oncocytes as seen in the salivary glands, thyroid, and kidney. A bloody background may include the presence of normal follicular cells, stromal cells, and hemosiderin-laden macrophages.

DeMay RM, The Art & Science of Cytopathology.
Ovarian cysts (corpus luteum cysts) pp. 1163–1164.

81. **D** oncocytic neoplasm

These renal corticol neoplasms represent 5% of all renal tumors. Differentiation between oncocytoma and oncocytic renal cell carcinoma should be reserved until a complete clinical, gross, and microscopic analysis is performed.

DeMay RM, The Art & Science of Cytopathology.
Oncocytoma and oncocytic neoplasms, pp. 1093–1094.

82. **B** osteosarcoma

Osteosarcoma represents the most common primary bone malignancy and typically involves the long bones of adolescent males.

DeMay RM, The Art & Science of Cytopathology.
Osteosarcoma, p. 595.

83. **D** angiosarcoma

These highly malignant vascular lesions often strike the elderly and predominantly arise within the liver, breast, bone, spleen, or the subcutaneous tissues. Immunocytochemical confirmation with Factor VIII antigen may help in the differentiation of these lesions from other soft tissue sarcomas.

DeMay RM, The Art & Science of Cytopathology.
Angiosarcoma, pp. 583–584.

84. **A** seminoma

Seminomas cytologically present as large discohesive germ cells containing irregular chromatin and macronucleoli. The background contains a lymphocytic infiltrate, PAS-positivity, and a "tigroid" pattern demonstrated with Diff-Quik. Granulomas are often seen and serve as a diagnostic clue for seminomas of the testes and dysgerminomas of the ovaries.

DeMay RM, The Art & Science of Cytopathology.
Germinoma (seminoma/dysgerminoma), pp. 1160–1161.

85. **C** mature cystic teratoma

The aspiration of a mature cystic teratoma or dermoid cyst yields squamous epithelial and adnexal components such as anucleate squames, superficial and intermediate cells, hair shafts, and sebaceous fluid. The background is generally granular, amorphous, or basophilic with a proteinaceous precipitate.

DeMay RM, The Art & Science of Cytopathology.
Teratoma (mature cystic teratoma), p. 1162.

86. **B** eosinophilic granuloma

Eosinophilic granulomas are a histiocytosis affecting the skull, ribs, or the spine of children and the ribs, mandible, or clavicle in adults. Cytologically, the presence of multinucleated and mononucleate histiocytes containing kidney bean-shaped indented nuclei (Langerhans), which stain positive for S-100, and an abundant population of normal eosinophils identify the lesion. Tingible body macrophages and Charcot-Leyden crystals may accompany these lesions.

DeMay RM, The Art & Science of Cytopathology.
Eosinophilic granuloma, p. 596.

87. **B** aspiration may precipitate a hypertensive crisis

Pheochromocytomas, the most common adrenal medulla neoplasm, represent chromaffin paragangliomas. A urinary excretion of free catecholamines (norepinephrine and epinephrine) or catecholamine metabolites (vanillylmandelic acid and total metanephrines) or elevated plasma levels of metanephrines are typically the best mechanism for establishing this disease process. There is a possibility of initiating a hypertensive crisis as a result of aspiration biopsy. Nonfunctioning lesions cytologically present as loosely cohesive, pleomorphic, spindle-appearing cells containing intranuclear inclusions, finely granular, regularly distributed chromatin, and prominent nucleoli. Single cells usually predominate in the aspiration of these types of lesions. Another variant of pheochromocytomas may be highly anaplastic. Overall, three diagnostic categories are usually seen: spindle, epithelioid, or ganglion.

DeMay RM, The Art & Science of Cytopathology.
Pheochromocytoma and paragangliomas, pp. 1124–1127.

88. **B** starch granulomatosis

Starch or glove powder contamination (often falsely referred to as talc, which has been replaced by starch in gloves) may cytologically mimic fungal diseases and should be differentiated by its Maltese cross birefringence.

DeMay RM, The Art & Science of Cytopathology.
Arthropods and contaminants, p. 58.

89. **A** dysgerminoma

Sheets and syncytia of cells possessing frothy, vacuolated basophilic cytoplasm, pleomorphic nuclei containing irregularly distributed chromatin, and prominent nucleoli are observed in ovarian dysgerminomas. The presence of a lymphocytic infiltrate is important in defining these lesions as germ cell tumors. Differential diagnoses include yolk sac tumors (YST) and embryonal carcinoma (EC); however, dysgerminomas are characteristically negative for alpha-fetoprotein, whereas YST and EC are typically positive and also lack a lymphoid infiltrate. Granulomas are often seen and serve as a diagnostic clue for germinomas.

DeMay RM, The Art & Science of Cytopathology.
Germinoma (seminoma/dysgerminoma), pp. 1160–1161.

90. **D** cytomegalovirus

Cytomegalovirus infections are herpetic infections found in immunocompromised patients, including those with HIV or cancer.

DeMay RM, The Art & Science of Cytopathology.
Viruses (cytomegalovirus), p. 54.

91. **C** perform cultures for identification of possible inflammatory process

An inaccurate evaluation of inflammatory aspirates may account for false-negative or false-positive cytologic diagnoses. Although the Diff-Quik stain may be helpful in allowing for better cell recovery, a negative aspirate does not rule out the possibility of a bacterial process that must be cultured for microbiologic identification.

DeMay RM, The Art & Science of Cytopathology.
Inflammatory disease (abscess), pp. 952–953.

92. **C** benign fibrous histiocytoma

These lesions are composed of benign-appearing fibroblasts arising from lesions contained within the extremities. The absence of nuclear pleomorphism helps discriminate these cells from malignant fibrous histiocytomas.

DeMay RM, The Art & Science of Cytopathology.
Benign fibrous histiocytoma, p. 571.

93. **D** follicular

Follicular cysts generally present in FNA cytology as hypocellular samples of granulosa and theca cells in clusters or sheets with high nuclear to cytoplasmic ratios and folded bean-shaped nuclei scattered among a proteinaceous or bloody background. If hypercellular samples are seen, the cellular morphology may be quite reactive and mimic malignant features—making differentiation from a malignant neoplasm difficult.

DeMay RM, The Art & Science of Cytopathology.
Ovarian cysts (functional cysts: follicular cysts), p. 1163.

94. **B** serous cystadenoma

Monotonous sheets of epithelial columnar cells with regularly arranged nuclei containing micronucleoli (resembling mesothelial cells) found among a granular background are diagnostic of serous cystadenoma. Their lack of classic malignant nuclear morphology rules out the possibility of a serous cystadenocarcinoma. In addition, the absence of signet ring morphology helps differentiate these lesions from mucinous cystadenomas.

DeMay RM, The Art & Science of Cytopathology.
Ovarian epithelial tumors (serous cystadenomas and carcinomas), p. 1164.

95. **B** mucinous cystadenocarcinoma

Mucinous cystadenocarcinomas (MCAs) resemble colonic carcinomas but lack the extensive necrosis; furthermore, MCAs are generally unilateral while metastatic lesions are often bilateral.

DeMay RM, The Art & Science of Cytopathology.
Ovarian epithelial tumors (mucinous cystadenomas and carcinomas), pp. 1164–1165.

96. **D** mesenchymal repair

Mesenchymal repair, as well as epithelial repair, may be associated with wound healing, trauma, inflammation, chemotherapy or radiation, and ischemic tissue processes.

DeMay RM, The Art & Science of Cytopathology.
Miscellaneous conditions (fibrosis), p. 955.

97. **C** endometriotic cyst

Endometriotic cysts, related to ovarian endometriosis, are often termed "chocolate cysts" on gross examination due to their copious presence of old hemolyzed blood. FNA reveals typical endometrial glandular and stromal cells found among a background consisting of fresh and old blood as well as hemosiderin-laden macrophages.

DeMay RM, The Art & Science of Cytopathology.
Ovarian cysts (endometriotic cyst and endometriosis), p. 1164.

98. **D** Brenner tumor

These solid tumors are composed of sheets of squamoid epithelial cells with regular nuclei containing prominent folds resembling "coffee bean" morphology. Hyalinized eosinophilic globules may be seen with concentrically arranged follicular cells. A differential diagnosis is granulosa cell tumor; however, the cells associated with Brenner tumor are larger with more abundant cytoplasm.

DeMay RM, The Art & Science of Cytopathology.
Ovarian epithelial tumors (Brenner tumor), p. 1164.

99. **B** benign lymphocytic population, seminoma

Seminomas cytologically present as large discohesive germ cells containing irregular chromatin and macronucleoli. The background contains a lymphocytic infiltrate, PAS-positivity, and a "tigroid" pattern demonstrated with Diff-Quik. Granulomas are often seen and serve as a diagnostic clue for seminomas of the testes and dysgerminomas of the ovaries.

DeMay RM, The Art & Science of Cytopathology.
Germinoma (seminoma/dysgerminoma), pp. 1160–1161.

100. **A** *Leishmania*

These intracellular parasites may be differentiated from *Pneumocystis carinii* by their negative reaction with GMS.

DeMay RM, The Art & Science of Cytopathology.
Sinus histiocytosis, pp. 790–791, and Granulomatous lymphadenitis, pp. 792–793.

101. **A** follicular cyst

Follicular cysts may contain mature ova encircled by sheets and clusters of normal follicular cells. Follicular cysts generally present in FNA cytology as hypocellular samples of granulosa and theca cells in clusters or sheets of cells with high nuclear-to-cytoplasmic ratios and folded bean-shaped nuclei scattered among a proteinaceous or bloody background. If hypercellular samples are seen, the cellular morphology may be quite reactive and mimic malignant features—making differentiation from a malignant neoplasm difficult.

DeMay RM, The Art & Science of Cytopathology.
Ovarian cysts (functional cysts: follicular cysts), p. 1163.

102. D colorectal/carcinoma

These faux "terminal bars" represent microvilli manifesting their glycocalyx and "rootlets" that extend into the body of the plasma membrane. Terminal bar-like structures may be seen with gastrointestinal carcinomas, bronchioloalveolar adenocarcinomas, endocervical adenocarcinomas, and mucinous tumors (benign and malignant) of the ovary.

DeMay RM, The Art & Science of Cytopathology.
Glandular cells, pp. 503–504.

103. D granulosa cell tumor

Granulosa cell tumors are estrogen-producing lesions that may be related to the subsequent development of endometrial adenocarcinomas. FNA cytology reveals cells in sheets with uniformly arranged nuclei containing nuclear grooves and micronucleoli. The presence of rosettes (although rare) provides proof of Call-Exner bodies that may contain intra-lumenar eosinophilic material.

DeMay RM, The Art & Science of Cytopathology.
Granulosa cell tumor, p. 1159.

104. C normal biliary duct

Ductal epithelium of the pancreas cytologically presents as monolayer or honeycombing sheets of cells with round, regular, predictable spatially arranged nuclei. These cells resemble endocervical cells.

DeMay RM, The Art & Science of Cytopathology.
Exocrine cells (ductal cells), pp. 1055–1056.

105. C adenocarcinoma

Adenocarcinomas involving the gallbladder present with cytologic features that mirror pancreatobiliary carcinoma. Clinical history usually includes gallstones and is more often seen in Asians and Native Americans than Caucasians or African Americans.

DeMay RM, The Art & Science of Cytopathology.
Gallbladder, p. 1069.

106. B the cells of the fibrolamellar variant of HCC are larger and more dispersed, with fewer trabeculae

The diagnosis of fibrolamellar hepatocellular carcinoma (HCC), although similar to well-differentiated HCC, is based on the cytologic identification of cells with oncocytic cytoplasm, pale intracytoplasmic bodies, and an associated lamellar fibrosis (dense fibrous connective tissue with parallel rows of fibroblasts), which is rare in well-differentiated HCC. As indicated in the question, the cells of fibrolamellar HCC are larger, more dispersed, not commonly arranged in trabeculae, and associated with bile ducts—all factors that contrast with the cytologic identification of well-differentiated trabecular HCC. Clinically, the fibrolamellar variant of HCC is typically seen in younger patients (< 35 years of age), whereas ordinary HCC (> 60 years of age) commonly affects more women than men and carries a better prognosis. Moreover, ordinary HCC is generally associated with an underlying cirrhosis or hepatitis, and fibrolamellar HCC is more likely associated with focal nodular hyperplasia.

DeMay RM, The Art & Science of Cytopathology.
Fibrolamellar varient of hepatocellular carcinoma, pp. 1030–1031.

107. D pancreatitis

A hypocellular sample of degenerated acinar cells in cohesive sheets containing abundant granular cytoplasm, numerous polymorphonuclear neutrophils, and lipid-laden macrophages distributed amongst a background of necrosis is suggestive of acute pancreatitis. Necrotic fat, collagen, neutrophils, reactive mesothelial cells, and fibroconnective tissue may accompany these cellular findings.

DeMay RM, The Art & Science of Cytopathology.
Pancreatitis, pp. 1057–1058.

108. C mucinous cystic tumor/surgical resection

These lesions are considered borderline tumors, which, due to the inadequacy of cytomorphologic criteria to effectively predict their benign or malignant nature, must be resected. As indicated in answer 125, mucinous cystadenomas present with tall columnar morphology and mucus-laden cytoplasm (mucicarmine +), and a fibrillar mucinous background.

DeMay RM, The Art & Science of Cytopathology.
Mucinous cystic neoplasms, pp. 1064–1065.

109. C papillary epithelial neoplasm

Pancreatic papillary epithelial neoplasms are low-grade tumors, most commonly found within the pancreatic tail in young females.

DeMay RM, The Art & Science of Cytopathology.
Solid and papillary epithelial neoplasm, pp. 1065–1066.

110. **D** prostatic hyperplasia

Cells arranged in monolayers and sheets with well-defined honeycomb arrangement, basal cells (resembling myoepithelial cells), and spindle cells are helpful in establishing the diagnosis of benign prostatic hyperplasia.

DeMay RM, The Art & Science of Cytopathology.
Benign prostatic hyperplasia, pp. 1141–1142.

111. **A** pancreatitis

Cytology includes the finding of inflammatory cells and histiocytes contained within a necrotic background. Although epithelial cells are rare to absent, reactive mesenchymal cells may be found demonstrating "atypical" morphology, which must be discriminated from malignancy.

DeMay RM, The Art & Science of Cytopathology.
Pancreatitic pseudocyst, pp. 1058–1059.

112. **B** small round cells => small cleaved => large cleaved => small noncleaved => large noncleaved => immunoblastic => plasma cell

Antigenic stimulation allows for differentiation of the lymphocytes within the lymphoid follicles as indicated.

DeMay RM, The Art & Science of Cytopathology.
Lymphocyte differentiation, pp. 782–784.

113. **A** lymphoid

The presence of lymphogranular bodies as seen with the Romanowsky stain (more difficult with the Papanicolaou stain) will only identify these cells as lymphoid in origin. They cannot be used to differentiate reactive hyperplasia from malignant lymphoma; however, their presence rules out the possibility of a poorly differentiated metastatic epithelial malignancy.

DeMay RM, The Art & Science of Cytopathology.
Other important features of lymph nodes in FNA biopsy (lymphoglandular bodies), pp. 785–786.

114. **D** anaplastic carcinoma, pancreas

Aspirates containing hypercellular populations of single, discohesive, pleomorphic mononucleated cells with classic malignant criteria, multinucleated anaplastic giant cells, and abnormal mitotic figures are diagnostic of pleomorphic giant cell carcinoma of the pancreas.

DeMay RM, The Art & Science of Cytopathology.
Anaplastic carcinoma of the pancreas (pleomorphic giant cell carcinoma), pp. 1061–1062.

115. **B** well-differentiated adenocarcinoma

Cells representing prostatic adenocarcinomas present in discohesive sheets, clusters, and microacinar formations with increased nuclear sizes, overlapping nuclei, and the important finding of macronucleoli. The absence of basaloid cells helps distinguish well-differentiated lesions from dysplastic processes.

DeMay RM, The Art & Science of Cytopathology.
Adenocarcinoma, pp. 1142–1144.

116. **C** reactive condition

Lymphohistiocytic aggregates (not to be confused with lymphogranular bodies) are composed of reticular cells (stellate shaped with oval nuclei), germinal center cells, and tingible body macrophages. Their presence is usually indicative of a reactive lymphoid process.

DeMay RM, The Art & Science of Cytopathology.
Histiocytes (lymphohistiocytic aggregates), pp. 784–785.

117. **B** T cell and pan-B cell surface antigens (Leu/CD5)

These neoplasms may be identified by their co-expression of pan-B and T cell antigen using Leu1/CD5. small cell noncleaved or round cell lymphoma (well-differentiated lymphocytic lymphoma) cytologically presents as a monotonous population composed predominantly of small round cells. The absence of a polymorphic or heterogeneous pattern of mixed lymphocytes differentiates these malignancies from reactive lymphoid hyperplasia. Differentiation from undifferentiated B cell lymphoma/Burkitt or non-Burkitt lymphoma is possible due to the clinical history associated with Burkitt and the presence of lipid-positive cytoplasm associated with Burkitt lymphomas.

DeMay RM, The Art & Science of Cytopathology.
Small (well differentiated) lymphocytic lymphoma, pp. 802–804.

118. **A** early reactive lymph node hyperplasia

Early-phase lymph node reaction (immunoblastic hyperplasia) consists of a polymorphic population of large cleaved and non-cleaved lymphocytes and immunoblasts, and a slightly greater population of small round and cleaved lymphocytes. Lymphohistiocytic aggregates (not to be confused with lymphogranular bodies) composed of reticular cells (stellate shaped with oval nuclei), germinal center cells, and tingible body macrophages are also identified. Early phase reactive lymphoid hyperplasia (EPRLH) may be differentiated from immunoblastic lymphomas (ILs) because EPRLH shows the presence of small round and small cleaved, large noncleaved, and cleaved lymphocytes, whereas ILs do not contain these key elements.

DeMay RM, The Art & Science of Cytopathology.
Immunoblastic lymphoma, pp. 807–808.

119. D breast adenocarcinoma

Lobular carcinomas present as moderately cellular specimens composed of small monomorphic epithelial cells with minimal nuclear deviation or pleomorphism. The cells possess scanty cytoplasm, often with signet ring morphology or intracytoplasmic lumens. Nuclear overlapping and eccentric nuclei may be noted on high power. Rare vertebral column formation may be noted. Fibrocollagenous tissue may be interspersed amongst the groups of epithelial cells. Mucin positivity is usually noted.

DeMay RM, The Art & Science of Cytopathology.
Metastasis, pp. 1035–1036.

120. A small round lymphocytes, small cleaved lymphocytes, plasma cells

Late-stage (end-stage) reactive lymphoid hyperplasia is represented by the finding of a predominant population of small round and cleaved lymphocytes and only scattered immunoblastic or plasmacytoid lymphocytes.

DeMay RM, The Art & Science of Cytopathology.
Chronic lymphadenitis (reactive hyperplasia), pp. 787–792.

121. A small round and small cleaved lymphocytes over large cleaved and noncleaved lymphocytes, lymphohistiocytic aggregates

The follicular hyperplasia variant of chronic lymphadenitis (reactive hyperplasia) presents as a heterogeneous or polymorphic population (in descending percentages) of small round and cleaved lymphocytes, large cleaved and noncleaved lymphocytes, immunoblasts, and plasma cells. This polymorphic pattern should preclude a diagnosis of lymphoma.

DeMay RM, The Art & Science of Cytopathology.
Chronic lymphadenitis (reactive hyperplasia), pp. 787–792.

122. C a benign cellular component

Cells originating from the seminal vesicles cytologically appear as single, often bizarre, "atypical" cells with intracytoplasmic yellow lipofuscin granules. The nuclei of these cells may appear quite abnormal; however, the cytoplasmic pigment should indicate the benignity of these cells.

DeMay RM, The Art & Science of Cytopathology.
Bizarre benign cells, p. 1139.

123. C of monoclonal B cell origin

The immunocytochemical staining confirms the diagnosis of large-cell noncleaved lymphoma (LCNL). LCNL may be differentiated from immunoblastic lymphomas (IL) due to the lack of immunoblastic and plasmacytoid cells in LCNL—necessary components for establishing the diagnosis of IL. The FNA of large-cell lymphomas typically exhibits with a predominant population (80%) of large cells with coarse irregular chromatin and prominent nucleoli. A smaller population of small round or cleaved lymphocytes complete the cytologic picture. The presence of lymphogranular bodies rules out the possibility of a true histiocytic (monocytic) lymphoma.

DeMay RM, The Art & Science of Cytopathology.
Large cell lymphoma (large cell cleaved lymphoma), pp. 806–807.

124. B benign lesions are more common than malignant tumors

The benign to malignant ratio of soft tissue lesions is 100:1.

DeMay RM, The Art & Science of Cytopathology.
Introduction; p. 560.

125. B microcystic adenoma

These lesions commonly affect elderly patients, cytologically presenting as hypocellular specimens containing groups of cuboidal cells with PAS (+), mucicarmine (–) cytoplasm. These lesions may be differentiated from mucinous cystadenomas, which present with tall columnar morphology and mucus-laden cytoplasm (mucicarmine +).

DeMay RM, The Art & Science of Cytopathology.
Serous cystadenoma (microcystic adenoma), p. 1064.

126. C a polymorphic population of lymphoid cells

The follicular hyperplasia variant of chronic lymphadenitis (reactive hyperplasia) presents as a heterogeneous or polymorphic population (in descending percentages) of small round and cleaved lymphocytes, large cleaved and non-cleaved lymphocytes, immunoblasts, and plasma cells. This polymorphic pattern should preclude a diagnosis of lymphoma.

DeMay RM, The Art & Science of Cytopathology.
Chronic lymphadenitis (reactive hyperplasia), pp.787–792.

127. C nodular sclerosing type

The diagnosis of Hodgkin disease rests on the finding of the pathognomonic Reed-Sternberg (RS) cell, a cell with mirror image (binucleated) nuclei, as mononucleated cells ("Hodgkin cells"), lacunar cells (RS cells with clear surrounding cytoplasm), or merely as bare nuclei. The nuclei contain coarsely granular, irregularly distributed chromatin with irregular nuclear membranes and ill-shaped macronucleoli. Associated cellular findings depend on which of the four Rye classification variants are represented: lymphocyte predominant (few RS cells [+/- polylobed RS cells], small round cells, and epithelioid histiocytes), nodular sclerosing (lower cellularity but increased number of mononuclear lacunar RS cells as well as "Hodgkin cells," fibrous connective tissue, small round lymphocytes, plasma cells, eosinophils), mixed cellularity (moderate population of RS cells, abundant eosinophils, neutrophils, plasma cells, small population of small round cells), or the lymphocyte depleted type (abundant polylobed RS, necrosis, and a scanty sample of small round cells and histiocytes).

DeMay RM, The Art & Science of Cytopathology.
Hodgkin disease (lymphocyte-predominant Hodgkin disease), p. 819.

128. B bacterial infection

FNA of lymph nodes harboring acute lymphadenitis presents as a hypercellular population of neutrophils, rare lymphocytes, and tingible body macrophages in a necrotic background. The etiology is generally bacterial in origin and must be cultured for identification.

DeMay RM, The Art & Science of Cytopathology.
Acute lymphadenitis, pp. 786–787.

129. D Burkitt lymphoma

Burkitt lymphomas cytologically present as small non-cleaved lymphomas with intermediate sized nuclei and frothy, vacuolated, lipid-laden cytoplasm. These lesions mimic lymphocytic lymphomas (LLs), with the exception that LLs are T-cell neoplasms which arise in the thymus.

DeMay RM, The Art & Science of Cytopathology.
Small non-cleaved lymphoma: Burkitt and non-Burkitt, pp. 810–811.

130. B islet cell tumor of the pancreas, beta cell predominance

Chromogranin positivity indicates a neurosecretory (islet cell) pancreatic lesion, and the insulin production indicates the diagnosis of an insulinoma—a neoplasm composed predominantly of beta cells.

DeMay RM, The Art & Science of Cytopathology.
Islet cell tumors and carcinoid tumors, pp. 1066–1068.

131. A common acute lymphocytic leukemia antigen/small cell cleaved lymphoma

These monoclonal neoplasms cytologically present with a predominant population of small cleaved lymphocytes (80%) and a lesser population of small noncleaved/round lymphocytes and large lymphocytes. Their inability to express dual tumor cell marking as seen in small round cell lymphoma helps differentiate these two lesions.

DeMay RM, The Art & Science of Cytopathology.
Small cleaved (poorly differentiated lymphocytic) lymphoma, pp. 804–805.

132. D sarcoidosis

The finding of epithelioid macrophages (without intracytoplasmic inclusions), multinucleated histiocytes, and scattered lymphocytes indicates the diagnosis of granulomatous lymphadenitis. The presence of a necrotic background or neutrophilic infiltrate may help in determining whether the etiology is associated with caseous necrosis or suppurative inflammation. The diagnosis of sarcoidosis may only be suggested with the cytologic findings represented in granulomatous disease, generally presenting as a scanty sample and lacking a necrotic background. Schaumann and asteroid bodies may occasionally be seen.

DeMay RM, The Art & Science of Cytopathology.
Granulomatous lymphadenitis (sarcoid), p. 793.

133. B There is a lack of small round cells and immunoblasts in MCL; MCL is monoclonal for light chains

Further differentiation from reactive hyperplasia (RH) is possible due to the full range of heterogeneous cells that are seen in RH, including tingible body macrophages, lymphohistiocytic aggregates, and plasma cells. These elements are virtually absent in mixed lymphomas.

DeMay RM, The Art & Science of Cytopathology.
Mixed lymphoma, pp. 805–806.

134. D Hodgkin disease

The diagnosis of Hodgkin disease rests on the finding of the pathognomonic Reed-Sternberg (RS) cell, a cell with mirror image (binucleated) nuclei, as mononucleated cells ("Hodgkin cells"), lacunar cells (RS cells with clear surrounding cytoplasm), or merely as bare nuclei. The nuclei contain coarsely granular, irregularly distributed chromatin with irregular nuclear membranes and ill-shaped macronucleoli. Associated cellular findings depend on which of the four Rye classification variants are represented: lymphocyte predominant (few RS cells [+/- polylobed RS cells], small round cells, and epithelioid histiocytes), nodular sclerosing (lower cellularity but increased number of mononuclear lacunar RS cells as well as "Hodgkin cells," fibrous connective tissue, small round lymphocytes, plasma cells, eosinophils), mixed cellularity (moderate population of RS cells, abundant eosinophils, neutrophils, plasma cells, small population of small round cells), or the lymphocyte depleted type (abundant polylobed RS, necrosis, and a scanty sample of small round cells and histiocytes).

DeMay RM, The Art & Science of Cytopathology.
Hodgkin disease (lymphocyte-predominant Hodgkin disease), p. 819.

135. B drunken honeycombs and goblet cells

Secretory or mucinous ductal adenocarcinoma of the pancreas cytologically presents as "drunken honeycombs." Goblet cells (mucin positive) resemble benign muciphages. The cells are seen in sheets with increased cytoplasm (low N/C ratios), wobbly cell outlines, and loosely, unevenly spaced nuclei with folds and clefts. The nuclei may have irregular chromatin, and macronucleoli may be present. The differential diagnosis: Cells in a monolayer formation containing overlapping bland nuclei, anisonucleosis, thick-appearing nuclear membranes with prominent nucleoli, a loss of polarity, and crowded sheets represent a well-differentiated nonsecretory pancreatic adenocarcinoma. An inconspicuous population of bizarre malignant tumor cells may accompany these otherwise deceptively malignant cellular findings.

DeMay RM, The Art & Science of Cytopathology.
Ductal adenocarcinoma, pp. 1059–1061.

136. A oncocytic neuroendocrine carcinoma of the pancreas

Oncocytic neuroendocrine carcinomas of the pancreas are confirmed as mentioned in answer 130. However, the neoplastic cells morphologically resemble oncocytes such as those found within the salivary glands, kidneys, and thyroid.

DeMay RM, The Art & Science of Cytopathology.
Islet cell tumors and carcinoid tumors, pp. 1067–1068.

137. D small round lymphocytes, small cleaved lymphocytes, large cleaved lymphocytes, large noncleaved lymphocytes, immunoblasts, plasma cells

Early-phase lymph node reaction (immunoblastic hyperplasia) consists of a polymorphic population of large cleaved and noncleaved lymphocytes and immunoblasts and a slightly greater population of small round and cleaved lymphocytes. Lymphohistiocytic aggregates (not to be confused with lymphogranular bodies) composed of reticular cells (stellate shaped with oval nuclei), germinal center cells, and tingible body macrophages are also identified. Immature plasmacytoid cells with prominent nucleoli help support a diagnosis of infectious mononucleosis. Early-phase reactive lymphoid hyperplasia (EPRLH) may be differentiated from immunoblastic lymphomas (ILs) because EPRLH shows the presence of small round and small cleaved, large noncleaved and cleaved lymphocytes, whereas ILs do not contain these key elements.

DeMay RM, The Art & Science of Cytopathology.
Follicular hyperplasia, pp. 787–788.

138. C cat-scratch disease

Cat-scratch disease differs cytologically from toxoplasmosis due to a predominant population of epithelioid cells, the additional presence of neutrophils and eosinophils, and a possible microabscess-related necrotic background. A Warthin-Starry silver stain will confirm the presence of gram-negative bacterium.

Toxoplasma gondii, on the other hand, may be found in patients who are exposed to feline feces (often from the dust of cat litter). Specimens may indicate the presence of small lymphocytes, immunoblasts, plasma cells, tingible body macrophages, lymphohistiocytic aggregates, and rare epithelioid histiocytes. These cells represent a diagnostic triad of marked follicular hyperplasia, small granulomas, and monocytoid B cells.

DeMay RM, The Art & Science of Cytopathology.
Granulomatous lymphadenitis (cat-scratch disease), pp. 793–794.

139. B Burkitt lymphoma

The starry sky pattern represents tingible body macrophages in the presence of undifferentiated small noncleaved lymphocytes.

DeMay RM, The Art & Science of Cytopathology.
Small non-cleaved lymphoma: Burkitt and nonBurkitt, pp. 810–811.

140. **C** clear cell renal cell carcinoma

The identification of lipid-laden cytoplasm as demonstrated by special staining with oil red O in concert with the described cellular findings is important in establishing the diagnosis of clear cell renal cell carcinoma. These findings may also prove useful in differentiating these lesions from primary transitional cell carcinoma and oncocytoma.

DeMay RM, The Art & Science of Cytopathology.
Renal cell carcinoma (clear cell RCC), pp. 1090–1091.

141. **A** metastatic breast carcinoma

Lobular carcinomas present as moderately cellular specimens composed of small monomorphic epithelial cells with minimal nuclear deviation or pleomorphism. The cells possess scanty cytoplasm, often with signet ring morphology or intracytoplasmic lumens giving the nucleus a targetioid appearance. Cells may be cohesive with vertebral column formation, contain hyperchromatic nuclei with nucleoli, and have frothy cytoplasm. The background is often thick and eosinophilic with interspersed fat vacuoles and small fibrous stromal elements. Nuclear overlapping and eccentric nuclei may be noted on high power. Rare vertebral column formation may be noted. Fibrocollagenous tissue may be interspersed amongst the groups of epithelial cells. Mucin positivity is usually noted.

DeMay RM, The Art & Science of Cytopathology.
Metastases, pp. 1035–1036, and Lobular carcinoma, p. 882.

142. **B** 20s–40s

Papillary carcinoma (PTC) of the thyroid accounts for 75% of all thyroid carcinomas in the US and is two to four times more common in women. This lesion, unlike follicular and anaplastic carcinomas of the thyroid, is etiologically related to iodized salt or radiation exposure. As indicated in the question, the peak incidence is between the ages of 20 and 40; however, PTC is the most common thyroid cancer in young children and may occur at any age. Strictly stated, the younger the patient and the smaller the lesion (< 4 cm), the better the prognosis. Despite being more common in women, men are more likely to have a poorer prognosis.

DeMay RM, The Art & Science of Cytopathology.
Papillary thyroid carcinoma, p. 729.

143. **B** metastatic colonic carcinoma

Metastatic carcinomas represent 90% of the liver malignancies. The most common metastases are adenocarcinomas and gastrointestinal malignancies (colorectal, stomach, pancreatic). Other metastatic lesions include those from the lungs, breast, and kidney followed by gastrointestinal leiomyosarcomas, melanomas, lymphomas, and neuroendocrine tumors. The presence of tall columnar or "cigar-shaped" cells in aggregates with frankly malignant nuclear features, granular cytoplasm, or the presence of malignant signet ring cells may suggest a diagnosis of metastatic adenocarcinoma of the colon. Correlation with the primary lesion is critical.

DeMay RM, The Art & Science of Cytopathology.
Metastases, pp. 1035–1036.

144. **D** hepatoblastoma

Hepatoblastoma (HB) is a rare primary liver lesion usually found in children less than three years of age. This embryonal tumor may be associated with congenital anomalies rather than cirrhosis. HB is third in incidence of the intra-abdominal childhood malignancies, just behind neuroblastoma and Wilms tumor. There are three distinct variants of HB, variants that are epithelial, epithelial and mesenchymal (mixed), or anaplastic; however, these epithelial cells may have anaplastic, embryonal, or fetal differentiation. In this question, the anaplastic variant of HB is described, a lesion that is similar to other "small blue cell tumors." Cells of embryonal differentiation are cytologically identified as more mature, arranged in cords or ribbons with typical malignant nuclear features. The fetal type cells are even larger than the anaplastic or embryonal types, possess granular or clear cytoplasm (often containing fat, glycogen, or bile), typical malignant nuclear features, and lower N/C ratios than the other cell types. These cells are loosely cohesive, and arranged in sheets, acini, or three-dimensional structures (disorganized trabeculae). The fetal cells of HB may also be associated with extramedullary hematopoiesis (megakaryocytes and immature red and white blood cells). Lastly, the mesenchymal variant of HB has undifferentiated cells, osteoid, or metaplastic components such as squamous cells, skeletal tissue, muscle, or cartilage.

DeMay RM, The Art & Science of Cytopathology.
Hepatoblastoma, p. 1033.

145. **C** basal cell adenoma

Basal cell adenomas (BCAs) are cytologically composed of a pure population of epithelial cells. Small cohesive basaloid cells in cords, aggregates, or irregular clusters with high nuclear-to-cytoplasmic ratios and predictable nuclear features (lacking atypia) in the presence of copious amounts of metachromatic basement membrane are diagnostic of BCA. However, the fibrous stroma component necessary for the diagnosis of pleomorphic adenoma is absent in these lesions. Clinically, the absence of neural symptoms may also help differentiate BCA from adenoid cystic carcinomas.

DeMay RM, The Art & Science of Cytopathology.
Monomorphic adenomas (basal cell adenoma), pp. 671–672.

146. **A** follicular cells

Follicular cells present as small cells with uniform nuclei found in clusters with or without associated colloid and as monolayer sheets with honeycombing (resembling endocervical cells). Single cells may be observed.

DeMay RM, The Art & Science of Cytopathology.
Follicular cells, pp. 713–714.

147. **D** papillary carcinoma

Papillary carcinoma generally presents in monolayer sheets or in papillary groupings with fibrovascular cores. The cells contain irregular nuclear membranes with bland chromatin features, nuclear grooves, and intranuclear intracytoplasmic inclusions representing cytoplasmic intranuclear invaginations or nuclear pseudoinclusions. Colloid, foreign body giant cells, and psammoma bodies may accompany these findings.

DeMay RM, The Art & Science of Cytopathology.
Papillary thyroid carcinoma, pp. 729–735.

148. **A** mucoepidermoid carcinoma

High-grade mucoepidermoid carcinomas (MECs) of the salivary gland present with predominant populations of malignant squamous cells revealing typical nonkeratinizing or keratinizing features. Mucus-producing columnar cells containing bland nuclei and foamy cytoplasm and a population of benign polygonal intermediate cells define low-grade MEC. The differential diagnosis of a high-grade MEC includes a pure keratinizing squamous cell carcinoma, a diagnosis that may be preferred in the presence of pearl formations.

DeMay RM, The Art & Science of Cytopathology.
Mucoepidermoid carcinoma, p. 678.

149. **C** Hürthle cells

Hürthle cells represent mitochondria-rich follicular cells found singly and in clusters, containing abundant, eosinophilic, granular cytoplasm. The nuclei are round to oval and often possess prominent nucleoli. Hürthle cells are found in Hashimoto thyroiditis, Hürthle cell neoplasms, and benign goiters.

DeMay RM, The Art & Science of Cytopathology.
Hürthle cells, p. 714.

150. **D** Hodgkin disease

The diagnosis of Hodgkin disease rests on the finding of the pathognomonic Reed-Sternberg (RS) cell, a cell with mirror image (binucleated) nuclei, as mononucleated cells ("Hodgkin cells"), lacunar cells (RS cells with clear surrounding cytoplasm), or as bare nucleoli. The nuclei contain coarsely granular, irregularly distributed chromatin with irregular nuclear membranes and ill-shaped macronucleoli. Associated cellular findings depend on which of the four Rye classification variants are represented: lymphocyte predominant (few RS cells [+/-polylobed RS cells], small round cells and epithelioid histiocytes), nodular sclerosing (lower cellularity but increased number of mononuclear lacunar RS cells as well as "Hodgkin cells," fibrous connective tissue, small round lymphocytes, plasma cells, eosinophils), mixed cellularity (moderate population of RS cells, abundant eosinophils, neutrophils, plasma cells, small population of small round cells), or the lymphocyte-depleted type (abundant polylobed RS, necrosis, and a scanty sample of small round cells and histiocytes).

DeMay RM, The Art & Science of Cytopathology.
Hodgkin disease, pp. 816–821.

151. **B** Hashimoto thyroiditis

A predominantly rich heterogeneous population of lymphocytes and follicular center cells with associated Hürthle cells are diagnostic of Hashimoto thyroiditis. Colloid, if present, is scanty.

DeMay RM, The Art & Science of Cytopathology.
Hashimoto thyroiditis, pp. 718–721.

152. **B** adenoid cystic carcinoma

Adenoid cystic carcinomas are cytologically identified by the presence of small round epithelial cells in clusters, acinar formations, and three-dimensional tissue fragments in balls or cylinders containing central, eosinophilic, hyaline/homogeneous, fibrillar basement membrane material. Adenoid cystic carcinomas are frequent submaxillary and minor salivary gland neoplasms arising from the intercalated ducts. These lesions often present as painful lesions due to perineural invasion.

DeMay RM, The Art & Science of Cytopathology.
Adenoid cystic carcinoma, pp. 676–678.

153. **D** metastatic melanoma

Melanoma typically presents in single cells, aggregates, or as spindle cells with bizarre malignant nuclear features, macronucleoli, intranuclear cytoplasmic inclusions, and possibly intracytoplasmic golden brown pigment. Due to the fact that these diseases may be amelanotic, it may be helpful to confirm this disease process with S-100, HMB-45, Melan A or MITF (microphthalmia-associated transcription factor)—all which preferentially react with melanoma cells.

Wang JF, Sarma DP, Ulmer P. Diagnostic dilemma: HMB-45 and Melan-A negative tumor, can it be still a melanoma?: MITF (Microphthalmia-associated transcription factor) stain may confirm the diagnosis. The Internet Journal of Dermatology. 2007. Volume 5 Number 1.

154. **A** follicular neoplasm

Follicular neoplasms cytologically present as a hypercellular population of overlapping follicular cells with cohesive microfollicular or trabecular groupings. Colloid is scanty to absent. The diagnosis of follicular neoplasm is given to those samples in which definitive atypical nuclear features are absent. Follicular adenoma should be reserved for histologic diagnosis only due to the possibility of capsular invasion by these benign-appearing cells and the lack of distinguishable cytologic criteria necessary to differentiate these lesions from well-differentiated carcinomas.

DeMay RM, The Art & Science of Cytopathology.
Follicular neoplasms, pp. 724–729.

155. **A** colloid goiter

Benign follicular cells in monolayer or honeycombing sheets in the presence of abundant colloid (appearing as ropy amorphous background material) and (as seen) associated hemosiderin-laden macrophages and fibroblasts are typical findings associated with the FNA of benign colloid nodules.

DeMay RM, The Art & Science of Cytopathology.
Goiter, pp. 723–724, and FNA biopsy of follicular lesions, pp. 724–728.

156. **A** acinic cell carcinoma

Hypercellular specimens composed of acinic cells (without ducts) in sheets, acini, or tubules containing uniform to slightly enlarged central or eccentric nuclei, nucleoli, and clear or granular (PAS +) cytoplasm with intracytoplasmic granules are representative of acinic cell carcinoma. Fibrofatty stroma is absent while a lymphocytic infiltrate may be common. Acinic cell carcinomas are considered rare lesions predominantly arising within the parotid gland.

DeMay RM, The Art & Science of Cytopathology.
Acinic cell carcinoma, pp. 679–680.

157. **D** lipophagic granuloma

Lipid-laden macrophages predominate in aspiration biopsy specimens in patients who have received lymphangiography. Special staining with oil red O may help elucidate the benign nature of these cells.

DeMay RM, The Art & Science of Cytopathology.
Granulomatous lymphadenitis (foreign body granulomas), p. 794.

158. **C** metastatic adenocarcinoma, breast

Metastatic carcinomas represent the most common lymph node malignancy, even more common than primary lymphoid neoplasms. FNA of this lymph node shows an infiltrating ductal carcinoma of the breast, a tumor that presents as hypercellular epithelial cells in well-formed microacini with malignant nuclear characteristics. Cohesive clusters of "foreign" cells are helpful in establishing a diagnosis of metastatic carcinoma.

DeMay RM, The Art & Science of Cytopathology.
Metastatic malignancy, pp. 794–795.

159. **D** lymphoma

Large cell or histiocytic lymphoma accounts for the most common primary lymphoma of the thyroid. These cells present as a predominant population of large lymphocytes with irregular nuclear membranes and coarse, irregular chromatin patterns with prominent nucleoli, as well as small cleaved lymphocytes with similar nuclear features. The presence of lymphogranular bodies as seen with the Romanowsky stain will help identify these cells as being of lymphoid origin, differentiating the process from poorly differentiated malignancies. Lymphomas involving the thyroid may be primary or represent metastatic neoplasms.

DeMay RM, The Art & Science of Cytopathology.
Hematopoietic neoplasms, pp. 742–743.

160. **A** immunoblastic hyperplasia

Early-phase lymph node reaction (immunoblastic hyperplasia) consists of a polymorphic population of large cleaved and noncleaved lymphocytes and immunoblasts and a slightly greater population of small round and cleaved lymphocytes. Lymphohistiocytic aggregates (not to be confused with lymphogranular bodies) composed of reticular cells (stellate shaped with oval nuclei), germinal center cells, and tingible body macrophages are also identified. Immature plasmacytoid cells with prominent nucleoli help support a diagnosis of infectious mononucleosis. Early phase reactive lymphoid hyperplasia (EPRLH) may be differentiated from immunoblastic lymphomas (ILs) because EPRLH shows the presence of small round and small cleaved, large noncleaved and cleaved lymphocytes, whereas ILs do not contain these key elements.

DeMay RM, The Art & Science of Cytopathology.
Paracortical, or diffuse immunoblastic, hyperplasia, pp. 789–790.

161. **B** papillary carcinoma

Papillary carcinoma generally presents in monolayer sheets or in papillary groupings with fibrovascular cores. The cells contain irregular nuclear membranes with bland chromatin features, nuclear grooves, and intranuclear intracytoplasmic inclusions representing cytoplasmic intranuclear invaginations or nuclear pseudoinclusions. Colloid, foreign body giant cells, and psammoma bodies may accompany these findings.

DeMay RM, The Art & Science of Cytopathology.
Cytology of PTC, pp. 731–732.

162. **B** giant cell anaplastic carcinoma

These lesions generally affect elderly females and present cytologically as anaplastic giant pleomorphic tumor cells with classic nuclear morphology. Abundant diathesis and abnormal mitotic figures are common findings in these aspirations.

DeMay RM, The Art & Science of Cytopathology.
Giant and spindle cell (anaplastic) carcinoma, pp. 737–738.

163. **C** Sister Mary Joseph nodule

These tumors represent metastatic gastric or colonic carcinomas. For related information, see chapter 5, Gastrointestinal Tract.

Holladay EB, Cytopathology Review Guide.
Gastrointestinal Tract, pp. 205–228.

164. **B** granulomatous lymphadenitis

The finding of epithelioid macrophages (without intracytoplasmic inclusions), multinucleated histiocytes, and scattered lymphocytes indicates the diagnosis of granulomatous lymphadenitis. The presence of a necrotic background or neutrophilic infiltrate may help in determining whether the etiology is associated with caseous necrosis or suppurative inflammation.

DeMay RM, The Art & Science of Cytopathology.
Granulomatous hyperplasia (tuberculosis), pp. 792–794.

165. **A** adenocarcinoma

Cells representing prostatic adenocarcinomas present in discohesive sheets, clusters, and microacinar formations with increased nuclear sizes, overlapping nuclei, and the important finding of macronucleoli. The absence of basaloid cells helps distinguish well-differentiated lesions from dysplastic processes.

DeMay RM, The Art & Science of Cytopathology.
Adenocarcinoma, pp. 1142–1144.

166. **C** plasma cell myeloma

FNA of plasma cell myelomas reveal cells with "clock face" chromatin, immature cells with fine chromatin and prominent nucleoli, and occasionally binucleated and bizarre multinucleated giant cells. The cytoplasm is generally blue or amphophilic with perinuclear hofs and intranuclear or intracytoplasmic Russell bodies (representing immunoglobulin, usually IgG or IgA).

DeMay RM, The Art & Science of Cytopathology.
Plasma cell myeloma, pp. 821–822.

167. **B** large cell cleaved lymphoma

Large cell cleaved lymphomas typically present as a predominant population (80%) of large cleaved cells with coarse irregular chromatin and prominent nucleoli. A smaller population of small round or cleaved lymphocytes complete the cytologic picture. Differentiation from immunoblastic lymphomas is based on the absence of large immunoblasts and plasmacytoid cells as well as the absence of mature lymphocytes. The presence of lymphogranular bodies rules out the possibility of a true histiocytic (monocytic) lymphoma.

DeMay RM, The Art & Science of Cytopathology.
Large cell lymphoma (large cell cleaved lymphoma), pp. 806–807.

168. **A** follicular (reactive) hyperplasia

The follicular hyperplasia variant of chronic lymphadenitis (reactive hyperplasia) presents as a heterogeneous or polymorphic population (in descending percentages) of small round and cleaved lymphocytes, large cleaved and noncleaved lymphocytes, immunoblasts, and plasma cells. This polymorphic pattern should preclude a diagnosis of lymphoma.

DeMay RM, The Art & Science of Cytopathology.
Chronic lymphadenitis (reactive hyperplasia) follicular hyperplasia, pp. 787–789.

169. **B** cat-scratch disease

Cat-scratch disease is marked by a predominant population of epithelioid cells, the additional presence of neutrophils and eosinophils, and a possible microabscess-related necrotic background. A Warthin-Starry silver stain will confirm the presence of gram-negative bacteria. Alternatively, *Toxoplasma gondii* may be found in patients who are exposed to feline feces (often from the dust of cat litter). Specimens may indicate the presence of small lymphocytes, immunoblasts, plasma cells, tingible body macrophages, lymphohistiocytic aggregates, and rare epithelioid histiocytes. These cells represent a diagnostic triad of marked follicular hyperplasia, small granulomas, and monocytoid B cells.

DeMay RM, The Art & Science of Cytopathology.
Granulomatous lymphadenitis (cat-scratch disease), pp. 793–794.

170. **A** osteosarcoma

Osteosarcoma cytologically presents as round to polygonal cells with pleomorphic sarcomatous cytoplasm in the company of an eosinophilic (metachromatic with Romanowsky stain) osteoid matrix. Multinucleated giant tumor cells are common findings.

DeMay RM, The Art & Science of Cytopathology.
Metastatic malignancy, p. 795.

171. **D** Burkitt lymphoma

Burkitt lymphomas cytologically present as small noncleaved lymphomas with intermediate nuclei and frothy, vacuolated, lipid-laden cytoplasm. These lesions mimic lymphocytic lymphomas (LLs) with the exception that LLs are T-cell neoplasms that arise in the thymus.

DeMay RM, The Art & Science of Cytopathology.
Small, non-cleaved lymphoma: Burkitt and nonBurkitt, pp. 810–811.

172. **A** small cell noncleaved lymphoma

Small cell noncleaved or round cell lymphomas (well-differentiated lymphocytic lymphoma) cytologically present as a monotonous population composed predominantly of small round cells. The absence of a polymorphic or heterogeneous pattern of mixed lymphocytes and the presence of a positive staining reaction with Leu-1/CD5 differentiate these malignancies from reactive lymphoid hyperplasia. Differentiation from undifferentiated B cell lymphoma/Burkitt or non-Burkitt lymphoma is possible due to the clinical history associated with Burkitt and the presence of lipid-positive cytoplasm associated with Burkitt lymphomas.

DeMay RM, The Art & Science of Cytopathology.
Small (well differentiated) lymphocytic lymphoma, pp. 802–804.

173. **C** malignant fibrous histiocytoma

Soft tissue aspirations containing bizarre giant tumor cells with classic malignant nuclear morphology and spindle-shaped and polygonal fibroblasts occurring singly and in overlapping fashion, seen in combination with a lymphocytic infiltrate, are diagnostic of malignant fibrous histiocytoma.

DeMay RM, The Art & Science of Cytopathology.
Malignant fibrous histiocytoma, p. 571.

174. **B** seminoma

Seminomas cytologically present as large discohesive germ cells containing irregular chromatin and macronucleoli. The background contains a lymphocytic infiltrate, PAS-positivity, and a "tigroid" pattern demonstrated with Diff-Quik. Granulomas are often seen and serve as a diagnostic clue for seminomas of the testes and dysgerminomas of the ovaries.

DeMay RM, The Art & Science of Cytopathology.
Germinoma (seminoma/dysgerminoma), pp. 1160–1161.

175. **A** lipoma

Lipomas are characterized in cytology by the presence of mature adipose tissue in sheets with "chicken wire" appearance. The cells have eccentrically located nuclei, single large lipid droplets within the cytoplasm, and anatomizing capillaries. Oily material may "bead up" on Diff-Quik preparations.

DeMay RM, The Art & Science of Cytopathology.
Lipoma, pp. 573–574.

176. **D** hepatocytes, suggest re-aspiration

This inadequate or unsuccessful lung aspirate reveals normal hepatocytes that are identified as polygonal cells arranged in monolayer formations. The cytoplasm is described as granular with bile inclusions, while the nuclei are generally round to oval with prominent nucleoli. Many cells are binucleated while others may contain intranuclear cytoplasmic inclusions. Care should be exercised to prevent confusion of these cells with indigenous pulmonary mucosa.

DeMay RM, The Art & Science of Cytopathology.
Miscellaneous cells, p. 951.

177. **C** faulty technique–aspiration of necrotic center

Represented is a necrotic center of a centrally detected squamous cell carcinoma of the lung. Aspiration of the center of this lesion yielded a specimen composed predominantly of diathesis and necrotic debris. When performing FNA, special attention needs to be given so that multiple sites of neoplasm are aspirated, especially along the peripheral margins (>10 planes).

DeMay RM, The Art & Science of Cytopathology.
Fine needle aspiration biopsy, p. 949, Complications associated with deep target biopsy, p. 470, and Performing the biopsy, pp. 471–473.

178. D transitional cell carcinoma

Cells possessing eccentric, hyperchromatic, and round to oval nuclei, anisonucleosis, irregular nuclear membranes, and irregular chromatin distribution with macronucleoli, arranged in loose aggregates, and containing dense, granular cytoplasm with scattered vacuoles are diagnostic of high grade primary transitional cell carcinoma of the kidney. Negative reactions for intracytoplasmic fat and mucicarmine rule out the possibility of a renal cell carcinoma.

DeMay RM, The Art & Science of Cytopathology.
Transitional cell carcinoma of the renal pelvis, pp. 1094–1095.

179. D any of the above

Intranuclear cytoplasmic inclusions (INCIs), or pseudoinclusions, are often found within papillary carcinoma of the thyroid, melanomas, and hepatocellular carcinomas. The presence of INCIs are helpful in confirming these malignant diseases, however, they have been reported in benign lesions as well, such as benign liver conditions.

DeMay RM, The Art & Science of Cytopathology.
Combined glandular and squamous differentiation, p. 505.

180. C chromogranin

Islet cell tumors (pancreatic endocrine neoplasms) present as loosely cohesive clusters or rosettes and as single cells containing eccentrically located nuclei and sparsely fine, red granular cytoplasm demonstrated on Diff-Quik. The chromatin is described as salt-and-pepper. Immunocytochemical studies for chromogranin, neuron-specific enolase, insulin, gastrin, or argyrophilic positivity may help identify these neuroendocrine tumors.

DeMay RM, The Art & Science of Cytopathology.
Islet cell tumors and carcinoid tumors, pp. 1066–1068.

181. B *Echinococcus granulosus*

Hydatid sand is composed of scoleces and hooklets derived from *Echinococcus granulosus.* Aspiration of cystic liver nodules is generally contraindicated due to the possibility of anaphylaxis.

DeMay RM, The Art & Science of Cytopathology.
Hydatid cysts, p. 1023.

182. A ductal adenocarcinoma

Cells in a monolayer formation containing overlapping bland nuclei, anisonucleosis, thick-appearing nuclear membranes with prominent nucleoli, a loss of polarity, and crowded sheets represent a well-differentiated nonsecretory pancreatic adenocarcinoma. An inconspicuous population of bizarre malignant tumor cells may accompany these otherwise deceptively benign cellular findings.

DeMay RM, The Art & Science of Cytopathology.
Ductal adenocarcinoma, pp. 1059–1061.

183. A alpha-fetoprotein (–), keratin (+)

Hepatocellular carcinoma (HCC) will stain positive for alpha-fetoprotein, whereas pancreatic carcinomas are negative. Both lesions are positive for low (CAM 5.2) and high (AE1/AE3) molecular weight keratin. The morphologic presence of "tombstome cells" (tall columnar) helps support a diagnosis of pancreatic carcinoma rather than HCC.

DeMay RM, The Art & Science of Cytopathology.
Ductal adenocarcinomas, pp. 1059–1061.

184. B Kaposi sarcoma

The FNA of Kaposi sarcoma presents with bland, slender, spindle-shaped cells arranged in sheets and bundles with hyperchromatic nuclei. A very important component of this diagnosis is the presence of hemorrhagic background and the finding of hemosiderin contained within the cytoplasm of the cells. PAS-positive nonspecific hyaline globules may be identified. Kaposi sarcoma most likely does not represent a malignant process, but rather a proliferative or hyperplastic process (Gallo). Its natural history typically has a fatal outcome within 6 months.

DeMay RM, The Art & Science of Cytopathology.
Kaposi sarcoma, pp. 582–583.

185. B cholangiocarcinoma

Well-differentiated cholangiocarcinomas present cytologically as hypercellular specimens containing sheets of cells with slightly enlarged, overlapping nuclei and micronucleoli. Their resemblance to normal ductal cells may cause difficulty in establishing a malignant diagnosis. Careful attention should be given to mild nuclear deviations in light of a radiographically identified neoplasm. Cholangiocarcinomas are negative for alpha-fetoprotein and positive for CEA, whereas hepatocellular carcinomas are positive and negative, respectively.

DeMay RM, The Art & Science of Cytopathology.
Cholangiocarcinoma, pp. 1033–1034.

186. **A** *Aspergillus* sp., rule out secondary malignancy by re-aspirating from various areas of the mass

Mycotic infections (aspergillosis, blastomycosis, or others) secondary to malignant processes are often due to a cancer causing post obstructive pneumonitis. These coexisting secondary infections are often peripherally located to the malignancy; therefore, thorough sampling becomes an important aspect in the evaluation of lung masses. The presence of fungal elements may not preclude the possibility of a primary lesion that was missed due to improper sampling. *Aspergillus* sp. present as thick hyphae with dichotomous branching occurring at 45-degree angles.

DeMay RM, The Art & Science of Cytopathology.
Nonkeratinizing (poorly differentiated) SCC, p. 962.

187. **A** chromogranin

Small cell carcinoma is a highly malignant neuroendocrine neoplasm that is ultrastructurally part of the amine precursor uptake and decarboxylation tumors (APUD) due to its cytoplasmic evidence of androgenic amines (membrane-bound granules). These cells contain hyperchromatic, stippled chromatin, coarse clumping, nuclear molding, scanty cytoplasm, and micronucleoli. An important diagnostic feature of small cell carcinoma is the presence of paranuclear cytoplasmic inclusions—blue cytoplasmic globules found indenting the nuclei (best visualized with Diff-Quik staining). The cellular groupings have vertebral column formation, microbiopsy aggregates, and cords, nests, or ribbons. "Crush artifact," or degenerative nuclear material related to the mechanical crushing associated with the preparation of FNA specimens, is found in the background of most small cell carcinomas. This artifact presents as long clumpy streams of basophilic material. A variant of small cell carcinoma, intermediate cell small cell carcinoma, represents both fusiform and polygonal types, which are typically better preserved with open coarse chromatin patterns and enlarged cell areas. Immunocytochemical staining with chromogranin is helpful in establishing the neurosecretory nature of this tumor, but will not differentiate it from carcinoid lesions. Furthermore, the absence of lymphogranular bodies (best demonstrated with the Romanowsky or Diff-Quik stain) will help differentiate these lesions from malignant lymphoid processes.

DeMay RM, The Art & Science of Cytopathology.
Small cell carcinoma, pp. 966–968.

188. **C** acute lymphadenitis

FNA of lymph nodes harboring acute lymphadenitis presents as a hypercellular population of neutrophils, rare lymphocytes, and tingible body macrophages in a necrotic background. The etiology is generally bacterial in origin and must be cultured for identification.

DeMay RM, The Art & Science of Cytopathology.
Acute lymphadenitis, pp. 786–787.

189. **D** hepatocellular carcinoma

Trabecular (well-differentiated) hepatocellular carcinomas present with confluent trabeculating structures on low power analysis. Hyperchromatic nuclei with overlapping features revealing high N/C ratios are unlike those found with poorly differentiated nontrabecular lesions. Hepatocytes arranged in cords and circumscribed by endothelium are typically found in well-differentiated hepatocellular carcinoma. Poorly differentiated lesions present with pronounced nuclear abnormalities and lack the trabecular organization. Elevated alpha-fetoprotein may be demonstrated by serum analysis.

DeMay RM, The Art & Science of Cytopathology.
Hepatocellular carcinoma, pp. 1026–1030.

190. **B** mesothelial cells

Mesothelial cells representing nondiagnostic elements from the visceral or parietal pleura appear in sheets with regularly spaced, round to oval uniform nuclei, often containing intranuclear grooves.

DeMay RM, The Art & Science of Cytopathology.
Mesothelial cells, p. 951.

191. **B** *Pneumocystis carinii*

Pneumocystis carinii is considered an opportunistic protozoan which may be seen in immunosuppressed individuals secondary to immunologic disorders, malignancies, or HIV infection, and in premature infants or patients receiving chemotherapy. Cytological identification rests on the presence of frothy mats of eosinophilic material with interspersed "contact lens"-shaped structures containing intranuclear trophozoites.

DeMay RM, The Art & Science of Cytopathology.
Pneumocystis carinii, p. 57.

192. **A** reactive

Polygonal cells arranged in rows or trabeculae with dense, granular cytoplasm, enlarged centrally placed bi- or multinucleated cells with smooth nuclear membranes, prominent nucleoli, intranuclear cytoplasmic inclusions, and intracytoplasmic bile pigmentation are diagnostic of reactive hepatocytes. These changes are commonly associated with conditions such as alcoholic cirrhosis or viral hepatitis. Bile ductal cells, fibrous connective tissue, and numerous lymphocytes represent concomitant cytologic findings.

DeMay RM, The Art & Science of Cytopathology.
Diffuse liver diseases, pp. 1022–1023.

193. **A** Warthin tumor

Warthin tumor (papillary cystadenoma lymphomatosum) cytologically presents with reactive lymphoid populations and oxyphilic/oncocytic epithelial cells. Oncocytes, cytologically presenting as cuboidal cells with eosinophilic granular cytoplasm and central or eccentric nuclei with prominent nucleoli, are suspended within a watery, proteinaceous, or dirty background. The concomitant finding of a lymphocytic infiltrate (representing a germinal center) alongside the oncocytic population excludes the diagnosis of pure oncocytoma or oxyphilic adenoma. Atypical squamous metaplasia (elongated, caudate-shaped cells) may be present if the lesion is infarcted or infected; therefore, exercise caution to prevent overinterpretation of these lesions as squamous cell carcinoma.

DeMay RM, The Art & Science of Cytopathology.
Warthin tumor, pp. 673–675.

194. **D** pleomorphic adenoma

Sheets and clusters of cuboidal cells containing round to oval nuclei and micronucleoli represent the ductal epithelial component of pleomorphic adenoma (benign mixed tumor). Fibromyxoid and chondroid mesenchymal elements (staining bright magenta with Diff-Quik staining) and myoepithelial spindle cells, typically arranged in cords and as single cells, may predominate in the smears.

DeMay RM, The Art & Science of Cytopathology.
Pleomorphic adenoma, pp. 669–671.

195. **A** adenocarcinoma, poorly differentiated

Poorly differentiated adenocarcinomas may be difficult to separate from other poorly differentiated malignancies, including squamous cell carcinoma and large-cell undifferentiated carcinoma. Aspirates yield hypercellular samples containing a heterogeneous population of single cells and slightly cohesive fragments. Anisokaryosis, fine to coarsely granular, irregularly distributed chromatin patterns, multiple macronucleoli, and elevated nuclear/cytoplasmic ratios are common findings. The hallmark for identifying these lesions as glandular in origin is the identification of frothy, lacy, vacuolated to granular cytoplasmic textures.

DeMay RM, The Art & Science of Cytopathology.
Adenocarcinoma, pp. 962–964.

196. **A** metastatic squamous cell carcinoma

Squamous cell carcinoma cytologically resembles those neoplasms identified in their primary esophageal location. Pleomorphic, keratinizing cells with irregular chromatin, keratinizing pearls, and cellular cannibalism represent many of the features that are found amongst a necrotic background. Poorly differentiated lesions will display classic malignant nuclear features and homogeneous, dense cytoplasm.

DeMay RM, The Art & Science of Cytopathology.
Squamous cell carcinoma, p. 338.

197. **A** secretory ductal carcinoma, pancreas

Secretory or mucinous ductal adenocarcinoma of the pancreas cytologically presents as "drunken honeycombs." Goblet cells (mucin positive) resemble benign muciphages. The cells are seen in sheets with increased cytoplasm (low N/C ratios), wobbly cell outlines, and loosely, unevenly spaced nuclei with folds and clefts. The nuclei may have irregular chromatin and macronucleoli may be present.

DeMay RM, The Art & Science of Cytopathology.
Ductal adenocarcinomas, pp. 1060–1061.

198. **D** squamous carcinoma

Pleomorphic cells with caudate or spindle formations with refractile cytoplasm, anisonucleosis, opaque ink dot-like to vesicular nuclei, and coarsely granular, irregularly distributed chromatin are representative of squamous cell carcinoma. A necrotic background is helpful in establishing this lesion.

DeMay RM, The Art & Science of Cytopathology.
Squamous cell carcinoma, pp. 960–962.

199. **A** granuloma

Liver granulomas may be cytologically identified by the presence of single and multinucleated giant cells, epithelioid histiocytes, lymphocytes, and plasma cells. Fibrous connective tissue may be interspersed amongst the inflammatory cellular findings.

DeMay RM, The Art & Science of Cytopathology.
Granuloma, p. 1023.

200. **D** normal parenchyma

Cells representing normal acinar structures composed of serous and mucous glandular fragments are seen in the photomicrograph. These cells are cuboidal in shape with granular (serous) or vacuolated (mucinous) cytoplasm and eccentrically located nuclei. Interspersed adipose tissue is also a common finding in normal salivary gland aspirates. Rarely, ductal cells and myoepithelial cells are seen.

DeMay RM, The Art & Science of Cytopathology.
Acinic cells, p. 660.

201. **B** acute pancreatitis

A hypocellular sample of degenerated acinar cells in cohesive sheets containing abundant granular cytoplasm, numerous polymorphonuclear neutrophils, and lipid-laden macrophages distributed among a background of necrosis is suggestive of acute pancreatitis. Necrotic fat, collagen, neutrophils, reactive mesothelial cells, and fibroconnective tissue may accompany these cellular findings.

DeMay RM, The Art & Science of Cytopathology.
Pancreatitis, p.1057.

Chapter 9

Cytopreparatory Techniques/ Lab Operations

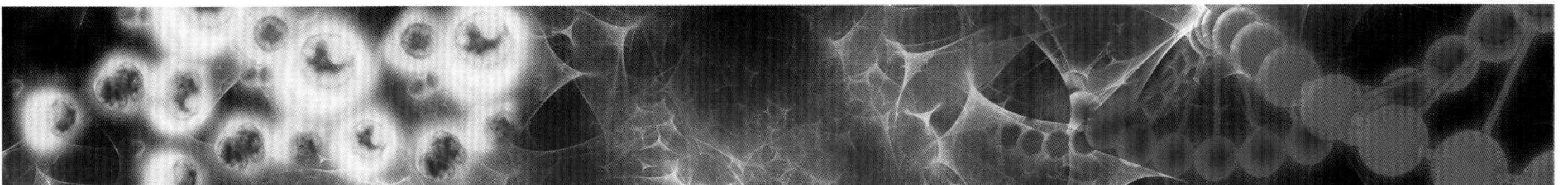

1. **Which of the following is considered a hazardous chemical?**

   A. ethanol
   B. saline
   C. Scott's water
   D. lithium carbonate

2. **What will allow for increased adherence of cerebrospinal fluids and urines to the glass slides?**

   A. Hanks balanced salt solution
   B. polylysine coated slides
   C. non-albuminized slides
   D. 95% ethanol

3. **What type of fire extinguisher is to be used for burning liquids?**

   A. A
   B. C
   C. B
   D. D

4. **Which statement regarding thionin blue is true?**

   A. it must be dissolved in 100% ethanol
   B. it will not stain red blood cells
   C. the formula requires normal acetic acid
   D. it is a synonym for toluidine blue

5. **All of the following are components of the material safety data sheets except:**

   A. date material was prepared
   B. permissible exposure limits
   C. emergency first aid procedures
   D. type of gloves required for clean up

6. **If sputum specimens must be preserved before cytopreparation, which fixative is best?**

   A. 100% ethanol
   B. 95% ethanol
   C. 70% ethanol
   D. 50% ethanol

7. **AutoPap®, a primary screening system for use with cervical smears, has an FDA-approved "sort rate" (those slides defined by the user that require no further review) of:**

   A. 10%
   B. 25%
   C. 50%
   D. 75%

8. **What chemicals should not be stored together because of their incompatibility?**

   A. acetic acid and acetone
   B. ammonia and acetic acid
   C. flammable liquids and nitric acid
   D. chlorine with any flammable liquids

9. **What is considered an alternative processing method (in lieu of the centrifugation/sediment method) for preparing cell blocks?**

A. plasma thrombin method
B. saponin method
C. Hanks method
D. thionin method

10. **When handling chemicals:**

A. reuse all unlabeled vials to prevent wastefulness
B. label all containers with common name only
C. dispose of gloves at the end of each day to prevent contamination
D. pour acid into water, never water into acid

11. **What may reduce the water contamination in xylene, thus preventing a milky cellular appearance?**

A. filtering the xylene weekly
B. increasing the HCl concentration in the regressive Papanicolaou staining process
C. adding 0.1% Hanks' balanced salt solution to the xylene
D. adding siliacic acid to the final absolute alcohol rinse

12. **The earliest action required in the event of a fire is:**

A. tell visitors to exit
B. telephone the switchboard
C. pull the fire alarm and rescue burning people
D. contain the fire with a fire blanket

13. **After performing FNA, a sound methodology for preparing the smears, which will ensure adequate cytologic evaluation, is:**

A. express a minimum of 10 mL, let air material air dry, then forcibly crush the aspirated material with a second slide to ensure material is adequately broken up; fix slides immediately (as needed)
B. express 10 drops on the edge of the slide, then place a cover slip on top; proceed with staining
C. spray the specimen through the air onto the slide. Air dry all slides
D. express a small drop near the frosted end of the slide, then place a second slide on top and quickly pull slides apart; fix a designated number of slides immediately, and purposely air dry others

14. **Screening errors may be attributed to:**

A. inadequate sampling
B. good sampling preparation
C. well-established quality control
D. atrophy in postmenopausal females

15. **The fire extinguisher that can be used for burning wood, paper, or refuse and is also considered general purpose is type:**

A. B
B. D
C. A
D. C

16. **Should a chemical come in contact with your skin, you should:**

A. rinse the contaminated clothing with water
B. flush the area with 95% ETOH
C. clean the area with neutralizing agents or ointments
D. read material safety data sheets and wash the chemical off with soap and water if possible

17. **When processing fine needle aspiration specimens, one should:**

A. process all smears with the Papanicolaou stain; air-dried smears should never be used unless necessary for possible lymphopoietic malignancies
B. process a few fixed smears with the Papanicolaou stain and a few air-dried smears with a compatible stain (Romanovsky or Diff-Quik)
C. process a few air-dried smears with the Papanicolaou stain and a few alcohol-fixed smears with a compatible stain (Romanovsky or Diff-Quik)
D. process all smears with the Papanicolaou stain; batch FNA slides with the general processing of Pap smears, this will insure optimal staining for most pathologic processes

18. **What is a sound procedure for a dealing with a small chemical spill?**

A. evacuate the building
B. evacuate all people from the building
C. use the "spill up" kit available
D. solid spills must be diluted with water before cleaning up

19. **The optimal thickness of the coverslip used for cytology is:**

A. 0.5
B. 1.0
C. 1.5
D. 2

20. **When handling hazardous materials one must make sure to:**

A. inform the laboratory workers by word of mouth
B. keep the material safety data sheet within the laboratory procedure manual
C. conduct weekly employee information training
D. maintain warning labels and common chemical names on all materials

21. **Which of the following describes the advantages of using the Saccomanno technique over the "pick and smear" or direct spreading technique for processing sputum specimens?**

A. Saccomanno technique is the method of choice for preparing fresh sputum specimens
B. using the Saccomanno technique allows the entire sputum specimen to be sampled; it yields slides with a uniform, even distribution of the cells, and eliminates the mucus within the specimen
C. when using the Saccomanno technique, it is not necessary to have cells prefixed in polyethylene glycol and alcohol solution, as is the case with the direct smear method
D. the Saccomanno technique allows for better cytologic identification of cellular groupings and clusters

22. **One of the best methods for preventing the spread of infectious agents while working in the laboratory is:**

A. wearing adhesive bandages
B. hand washing
C. washing all counters with Hanks balanced salt solution
D. wearing a cloth lab coat

23. **When using the Cytospin centrifugation technique for preparing transudative fluids (such as urines and cerebrospinal fluids), which of the following processing methodologies will help ensure specimen adequacy?**

A. add 1 mL of Saccomanno fixative if preparing for the Pap stain, place 10-15 drops of specimen into the chamber, and centrifuge at 100 rpm for 10-15 minutes
B. add a few drops of Saccomanno fixative if preparing for the Pap stain, place 2-5 drops of specimen into the chamber, and centrifuge at 500-600 rpm for 4-5 minutes
C. add 10 mL of Saccomanno fixative if preparing for the Pap stain, place 10 mL (equal volumes) of specimen into the chamber, and centrifuge at 1,500-2,000 rpm for 10 minutes
D. do not add Saccomanno fixative (regardless of the staining technique to be used), place 5 mL of specimen into the chamber, and centrifuge at 1,000-1,500 rpm for 4-5 minutes

24. **For a cancer screening program to become successful, which of the following is considered a prerequisite?**

A. the disease must affect a small percentage of the population
B. a suitable test must be at no cost to be effective
C. the physical and psychological harm of the test and treatment should outweigh the benefit
D. the cost benefit analysis should show the screening is economically beneficial

25. **What is considered a universal precaution?**

A. pregnant or nursing mothers should never be allowed to process cytological specimens
B. make sure to recap all needles prior to discarding
C. use biological safety hoods for processing gynecologic specimens
D. decontaminate the work area at least once per shift with an appropriate germicide

26. **The primary reason for using a liquid-based monolayer specimen preparation system for Papanicolaou smears is it:**

A. provides a cleaner background and helps prevent overlapping and crowding of cells
B. allows an identical number of cells to be aliquoted every time for each slide prepared
C. uses fixatives that enlarge the cells, making it easier to visualize small cell lesions and diagnose abnormal conditions
D. spreads a monolayer of cells over the entire glass slide, increasing the surface area of the slide utilized and the number of cells that can be diagnosed

27. **The fixative of choice for preparing cell blocks is:**

A. 30% formalin
B. 10% formalin
C. 25% glacial acetic acid
D. 1:1 diethyl ether in 95% ethyl alcohol

28. **A slide should be "fixed" for:**

A. 15–30 minutes
B. 45–60 minutes
C. 5–10 minutes
D. a minimum of 1 hour

29. **Fresh body fluids, those without added fixatives, are suggested for cytopreparation because:**

A. alcohol acts as a tissue culture medium, cultivating bacterial growth, which may interfere with cytopreparation
B. prefixed specimens cannot be de-stained if needed
C. fresh specimens stain more readily with eosin Y
D. alcohol coagulates proteins, rendering processing of the specimen difficult

30. **Which applies regarding the Papanicolaou staining process?**

A. filter stains weekly
B. check the percent of lithium blue each day when using the regressive staining procedure
C. maintain the alkalinity of the bluing solution when using the progressive staining procedure
D. store all stains in clear bottles to minimize oxidation

31. **The cytologic evaluation of urine specimens is most optimal when the urine is:**

A. preserved with alcohol
B. refrigerated
C. fresh
D. preserved with carbowax

32. **Regarding cytologic fixatives, which of the following is true?**

A. 100% ethanol has many advantages over 95% ethanol
B. 95% ethanol is suitable only for gynecological smears
C. 100% methanol produces less cell shrinkage
D. 80% isopropanol is unacceptable for cytologic fixation

33. **What is a suitable lysing agent for excessively bloody specimens?**

A. 1:14 glacial acetic acid in 95% ethanol
B. 10 mol urea
C. 1:1 hydrochloride in 95% ethanol
D. 1:50 glacial acetic acid in 95% ethanol

34. **Which EA stain is most useful in helping to distinguish endometrial adenocarcinomas from endocervical adenocarcinomas?**

A. EA-35
B. EA-36
C. EA-50
D. EA-65

35. **To achieve the best results, the pH of the EA solution should be:**

A. 1.5–2.0
B. 2.5–3.0
C. 3.0–4.0
D. 4.5–5.0

36. **A dull-appearing cellular specimen may be related to:**

A. not enough water within the clearing solutions
B. stains are changed too often
C. HCl concentration is too high
D. residual polyethylene glycol on the cells

37. **What method can be used to remove excess blood from an extremely bloody (previously air-dried) glass slide or in a cell fluid?**

A. Saccomanno method
B. thionin method
C. egg-albumin method
D. saponin method

38. **If nuclear overstaining occurs:**

A. HCl concentration is too dilute; increase the concentration
B. ammonium hydroxide concentration is too weak; increase the concentration
C. air dry the slide completely before staining
D. decrease the fixation time before staining

39. **If the oven temperature is excessively high during the preparation of a cell block slide, what effect may occur?**

A. slides are too blue
B. darker nuclei
C. slides are yellow
D. lighter nuclei

40. **What coating fixative is best for specimens which must be transported?**

A. commercial hair spray
B. 95% ethanol
C. polyethylene glycol
D. 2% glacial acetic acid

41. **With regard to centrifugation, cells sediment best at what centrifugal force and for how long?**

A. 300g, 15 minutes
B. 500g, 5 minutes
C. 600g, 10 minutes
D. 1,200g, 10 minutes

42. **The total surface area covered by the pores of Nucleopore filters is roughly:**

A. 2%
B. 10%
C. 20%
D. 50%

43. **Which is true regarding the progressive Papanicolaou staining process?**

A. hydrochloric acid (HCl) removes excess hematoxylin
B. nuclei are overstained then de-stained
C. lithium carbonate is used to blue or set the hematoxylin
D. nuclei are understained then blued with HCl

44. **If the nuclei appear too pale after staining:**

A. decrease the alkalinity of the tap water rinse
B. increase the alkalinity of the tap water rinse
C. decrease time in hematoxylin
D. change the stains daily

45. **Water in the xylene will cause:**

A. excessive basophilia
B. excessive eosinophilia
C. a milky haze on the slide
D. dark nuclear features

46. **Which EA stain contains half the original amount of light green?**

A. EA-65
B. EA-50
C. EA-36
D. EA-35

47. **In order to minimize the possibility of "floaters" found in cerebrospinal fluid specimens, one should:**

A. delete the OG
B. separate equipment and staining dishes
C. use polycarbonate filters only
D. use cellulosic filters only

48. **What is an effective fire safety precaution?**

A. make sure to store incompatible chemicals together
B. have your evacuation plan memorized
C. store flammable liquids in glass bottles
D. keep all chemicals on the workbench

49. **What solvent has a detrimental effect on both polycarbonate and cellulosic filters?**

A. 1-propanol
B. 100% ethanol
C. chloroform
D. 3N ammonium hydroxide

50. **A stain useful for rapid examination of non-fixed fluids is:**

A. EA-65
B. Papanicolaou
C. toluidine blue
D. Hanks

51. **What produces the "hill and valley" effect on cellulosic filters?**

A. expanding in 100% ETOH
B. expanding in 100% acetone
C. expanding in methyl alcohol
D. not expanding in 95% ETOH

52. **If the cytoplasm appears too green, one should:**

A. increase eosin or decrease the staining time in the EA
B. increase the light green concentration in the EA
C. increase the staining time in EA
D. change the EA more often

53. **In regressive Papanicolaou staining, the nuclei are:**

A. understained
B. overstained
C. stained to desired intensity
D. stained after the cytoplasmic stains

Cytopreparatory Techniques/Lab Operations *Answer Key*

1. **A** ethanol

   Examples of other hazardous chemicals include chloroform, ammonium hydroxide, and bleach.

   Keebler CM, Somrak TM, The Manual of Cytotechnology. *Chemical safety, p. 372.*

2. **B** polylysine coated slides

   The coating on these slides will increase the cellular yield in normally hypocellular specimens.

   Keebler CM, Somrak TM, The Manual of Cytotechnology. *Slide preparation after centrifugation, p. 425.*

3. **C** B

   For related information, see question 15.

   Keebler CM, Somrak TM, The Manual of Cytotechnology. *Fire extinguishers, p. 374.*

4. **B** it will not stain red blood cells

   Thionin blue, methylene blue, and toluidine blue are all stains that allow for rapid examination of wet specimens. For related information, see question 50.

   Keebler CM, Somrak TM, The Manual of Cytotechnology. *Thionin blue, p. 433.*

5. **D** type of gloves required for clean up

   Material Safety Data Sheets (MSDS) must be kept for all laboratory chemicals. The date the MSDS was prepared, chemical identity, hazard emergency information, physical hazards, first-aid protocols, disposal methods, and the common chemical name are some of the important informative data found for each chemical.

   Keebler CM, Somrak TM, The Manual of Cytotechnology. *Material Safety Data Sheets, p. 372.*

6. **C** 70% ethanol

   70% ethanol is preferred for collecting sputum specimens over 95% ethanol due to its possibility for mucoprotein coagulation.

   Keebler CM, Somrak TM, The Manual of Cytotechnology. *Prefixed specimens, pp. 427–428.*

7. **B** 25%

   The maximum sort rate for primary review by the AutoPap® computer (without human interface) is set by the FDA at 25%.

   Screening Errors and Reporting. International Consensus Conference on the Fight Against Cervical Cancer. Chicago, 2000.

8. **C** flammable liquids and nitric acid

   A list of chemicals that may and may not be stored together should be posted in clear sight of the storage area for the benefit of all laboratory personnel.

   Keebler CM, Somrak TM, The Manual of Cytotechnology. *Appendix, p. 375.*

9. **A** plasma thrombin method

   The plasma thrombin clot (PTC) method may be used as an alternative to the conventional fixed sediment (FS) methodology for cell block preparation. In the PTC method, equal drops of plasma and thrombin are added to the centrifugate to allow for a clot to form. The clot is placed onto lens paper and processed using conventional histologic processing techniques. Another alternative to the FS method is the bacterial agar methodology. This method uses Bouin fluid as a fixative (centrifugate is allowed to sit in fixative for 2 hours). The supernatant is poured off, the sediment is removed and placed on tissue paper, cut in half, and placed into a petri dish with melted agar. After the agar hardens, the specimen is placed onto tissue paper, loaded into a cassette, and processed using conventional histologic processing.

   Keebler CM, Somrak TM, The Manual of Cytotechnology. *Fixatives for cell block technique, pp. 413–414, Smear preparation, p. 243, and Cell block preparation, p. 247.*

10. **D** pour acid into water, never water into acid

    This information is key in the proper disposal of acid.

    Keebler CM, Somrak TM, The Manual of Cytotechnology. *Proper handling and disposal of hazardous chemicals, pp. 372–373.*

11. **D** adding siliacic acid to the final absolute alcohol rinse

    For related information, see question 45.

    Keebler CM, Somrak TM, The Manual of Cytotechnology. *Appendix: Troubleshooting guidelines, p. 443.*

12. **C pull the fire alarm and rescue burning people**

Pull the alarm to notify others in danger, remove visitors, and if possible, contain the fire with an appropriate extinguisher.

Keebler CM, Somrak TM, The Manual of Cytotechnology.
Fire prevention, pp. 373–374.

13. **D express a small drop near the frosted end of the slide, then place a second slide on top and quickly pull slides apart: fix a designated number of slides immediately, and purposely air dry others**

In preparing FNA smears for cytologic interpretation, it is important to express a tiny drop of the harvest onto the slide, being careful not to spray the specimen through the air, which may create aerosols that are potentially infectious. The spreader slide must be gently lowered onto the diagnostic slide in a crosswise fashion over the droplet and pulled down over the length (taking care not to spread to the edges) of the diagnostic slide with a smooth motion.

DeMay RM, The Art & Science of Cytopathology.
Preparing the smears, pp. 473–474.

14. **A inadequate sampling**

It is estimated that 2/3 to 1/2 of the screening errors that occur in gynecologic cytopathology are related to inadequate samples or poor specimen preparation of the smear-taker, and up to 1/2 of the false negative cases are related to the laboratory (inadequate screening, poor quality control, inadequate interpretation). Errors in each area are in the range of 5%–10%.

DeMay RM, The Art & Science of Cytopathology.
Failure of the Pap smear, pp. 141–146.

15. **C**

"B" extinguishers are for burning liquids, and "C" extinguishers should be used in the event of an electrical fire.

Keebler CM, Somrak TM, The Manual of Cytotechnology.
Fire extinguishers, p. 374.

16. **D read material safety data sheets and wash the chemical off with soap and water if possible**

Removing the contaminated clothing and flushing the affected area with water, when appropriate as determined by MSDS instructions, followed by cleaning with soap and water is important. Always immediately seek medical care.

Keebler CM, Somrak TM, The Manual of Cytotechnology.
Chemical spills, p. 373.

17. **B process a few fixed smears with the Papanicolaou stain and a few air-dried smears with a compatible stain (Romanovsky or Diff-Quik)**

Preparing a few air-dried slides allows for staining with a compatible stain such as Romanovsky or Diff-Quik. Air drying the cells has many advantages, and contrary to popular belief, provides essential information that often cannot be appreciated with the conventional fixed-based Papanicolaou stain. In addition to increasing cell adherence to the slide, staining air-dried slides allows for the cytologic visualization of extracellular substances (mucin, ground substance, colloid) and enhances the ability to appreciate cytoplasmic pleomorphism, gland and lymphoreticular differentiation, and microbiologic agents.

DeMay RM, The Art & Science of Cytopathology.
Preparing the smears, pp. 473–474, and Stains, pp. 14-15.

18. **C use the "spill up" kit available**

After seeking information from the MSDS, spill pillows and silicone absorbent may be used to clean up the spill. Proper disposal is imperative.

Keebler CM, Somrak TM, The Manual of Cytotechnology.
Chemical spills, p. 373.

19. **B 1.0**

The refractive index of the mounting media together with a maximum coverslip thickness of 0.96-1.06 mm will allow for the most effective microscopy in cytology (based on the corrective figure of 0.17 mm-0.18 mm objectives). Cytologic specimens are generally thicker than tissue sections; therefore, a 1.5 mm coverslip may be used.

Keebler CM, Somrak TM, The Manual of Cytotechnology.
Glass slides and coverslips, p. 418.

20. **D maintain warning labels and common chemical names on all materials**

Warning labels must describe the common chemical name, potential health hazards, and manufacturer's address. The warning diamond, designed by the National Fire Protection Association), is divided into four sections and graded from 0-4. The left side of the diamond (blue in color) is the health hazard section: 0—normal material, 1—slightly hazardous, 2—hazardous, 3—extreme danger, and 4—deadly. The top section of the diamond (red in color) is fire hazard (flash points): 0—will not burn, 1—not exceeding 200 degrees F, 2—above 100 degrees F, 3—below 100 degrees F, 4—below 73 degrees F. The far right side of the diamond (yellow) is reactivity/instability: 0—stable, 1—unstable as heated, 2—violent chemical change, 3—shock and heat, 4—may detonate. The bottom section of the diamond (white) refers to specific hazards: ACID—acid, ALK—alkali, COR—corrosive, OXY—oxidizer, P— polymerization, radioactive symbol ( )—radioactive, W (crossed by an X)—use no water.

Keebler CM, Somrak TM, The Manual of Cytotechnology.
Proper handling and disposal of hazardous chemicals, p. 372.

21. **B using the Saccomanno technique allows the entire sputum specimen to be sampled; it yields slides with a uniform, even distribution of the cells, and eliminates the mucus within the specimen**

The Saccomanno technique is the methodology of choice for prefixed sputum specimens (polyethylene glycol and 70% ethanol). The advantages are as listed in the answer; however, the disadvantage of this technique (when compared to the direct or "pick and smear" technique) is that cellular groupings are often disassociated in the blending process. For instance, the cytologic diagnosis of small cell neuroendocrine carcinoma (which possesses cells in molding groups or in streaks) may be more difficult, as well as adenocarcinomas that present in tight cohesive clusters. If either are suspected, one should blend the specimen at lower speeds or prepare the sputum by gently crushing an aliquot of the specimen between two slides, separate the slides, and equally distribute the smeared material over both slides with an applicator slick (direct smear method). Excessively mucoid or bloody specimens prepared by the direct smear technique may be treated with mucolex, the saponin method, or sputolysin.

Keebler CM, Somrak TM, The Manual of Cytotechnology.
Processing respiratory tract specimens, p. 427, and Saccomanno blending technique, p. 441.

22. **B hand washing**

Proficient and efficient hand washing will reduce the possibility of contracting disease or contaminating the workplace.

Keebler CM, Somrak TM, The Manual of Cytotechnology.
Biosafety hazards, p. 374.

23. **B add a few drops of Saccomanno fixative if preparing for the Pap stain, place 2-5 drops of specimen into the chamber, and centrifuge at 500-600 rpm for 4-5 minutes**

When preparing specimens for cytocentrifugation with the Cytospin, Saccomanno fixative should be added for slides that are to be stained with the Pap stain. Only a few drops of the specimen need to be added (using a disposable pipette) to the cytofunnel chamber to achieve optimal results. Four drops are usually sufficient for body fluids and bronchial or gastrointestinal washings, 2 drops for urines, and 4-6 drops for patients with known infectious disease. Centrifugation should be performed at 500 rpm for 5 minutes (cerebrospinal fluid) or 600 rpm for 4 minutes (all others); if performed any faster or longer, the specimens are at risk for air drying or cell lysis.

Keebler CM, Somrak TM, The Manual of Cytotechnology.
Cytocentrifugation using Cytospin 2, p. 440.

24. **D the cost benefit analysis should show the screening is economically beneficial**

In order to help ensure a successful screening program, the disease has to represent an important health problem with a known natural history and recognizable early stage, be of moderate cost, and be effectively managed if treated at an early stage.

Screening, Screening Errors and Reporting. International Consensus Conference on the Fight Against Cervical Cancer. Chicago, 2000.

25. **D decontaminate the work area at least once per shift with an appropriate germicide**

Taking universal precautions, such as wearing barrier protection, masks, gloves, face shield, disposable fluid-resistant gowns, and the practice of safe cytopreparatory techniques under biological fume hoods will help decrease the possibility of exposure of yourself or others to infectious diseases, especially hepatitis B or the human immunodeficiency virus.

Keebler CM, Somrak TM, The Manual of Cytotechnology.
Universal precautions, pp. 374–375.

26. **A provides a cleaner background and helps prevent overlapping and crowding of cells**

Additional advantages of liquid-based monolayer systems for cytopreparation (such as ThinPrep® or Autocyte Prep®) are that they help to minimize the amount of blood and inflammatory cells present in the specimen, as well as decrease any protein or mucus that may interfere with the ability of the diagnostician to render a satisfactory or adequate diagnosis.

Aponte-Cipriani SL, Teplitz C, Rorat E, et al, Acta Cytologica. 1995;34(4).

27. B 10% formalin

Alcohol shrinks and hardens tissue, making microtomy quite difficult. Fixation with a 1:9 solution of 40% formaldehyde and water creates a 10% formalin solution. Formalin should be neutral (pH 7.0) and be stored in the dark to prevent the formation of formic acid.

Keebler CM, Somrak TM, The Manual of Cytotechnology.
Fixatives for cell block preparation, pp. 413–414.

28. A 15–30 minutes

Fixing cells less than 15 minutes may create undesirable effects such as lack of crisp nuclear detail or pale nuclei. A minimum of 15 minutes is required to remove the wax cellular coating (2% carbowax) used to preserve the cells for transport. Fixation longer than 30 minutes has not been shown to provide additional benefit.

Keebler CM, Somrak TM, The Manual of Cytotechnology.
Wet fixation, p. 412.

29. D alcohol coagulates proteins, rendering processing of the specimen difficult

Fresh body fluids are preserved in their own culture medium, which helps to prevent cellular degeneration. Performing membrane filtration is easier with unfixed fluids due to the ease with which soluble proteins pass through the filter. Alcohol denatures these proteins, often clogging the membrane and creating difficulty in filtration.

Keebler CM, Somrak TM, The Manual of Cytotechnology.
Cell samples fixed in the laboratory, p. 413.

30. C maintain the alkalinity of the bluing solution when using the progressive staining procedure

The color change will not occur at a pH less than 8.0. If the laboratory is using running tap water to blue its nuclei, the pH should be tested to ensure its feasibility. Chlorine may also cause cellular fading; therefore, these levels should also be tested if using tap water as a blueing agent.

Keebler CM, Somrak TM, The Manual of Cytotechnology.
Nuclear stain, pp. 414–416.

31. C fresh

For related information, see question 4.

Keebler CM, Somrak TM, The Manual of Cytotechnology.
Genitourinary tract specimens, p. 422.

32. C 100% methanol produces less cell shrinkage

This effect allows for better cell preservation. Hospitals that do not have a license to buy ethanol may choose to use this fixative in place of ethanol.

Keebler CM, Somrak TM, The Manual of Cytotechnology.
Wet fixation, p. 412.

33. A 1:14 glacial acetic acid in 95% ethanol

Glacial acetic acid diluted 1:14 (modified Carnoy) is an excellent lysing agent for hemolyzing red blood cells and allowing for the enhancement of the cellular foreground.

Keebler CM, Somrak TM, The Manual of Cytotechnology.
Lysing Fixatives, p. 413, and Lysing fixatives for bloody cell samples, p. 430.

34. D EA-65

EA-65 will often stain endocervical adenocarcinomas (granular cytoplasm) eosinophilic and endometrial adenocarcinomas (frothy, vacuolated cytoplasm) basophilic or cyanophilic.

Keebler CM, Somrak TM, The Manual of Cytotechnology.
Cytoplasmic stains, pp. 416–417.

35. D 4.5–5.0

Maintaining a consistent pH between 4.5 and 5.0 will allow for optimal color consistency.

Keebler CM, Somrak TM, The Manual of Cytotechnology.
Appendix: Troubleshooting guidelines T35.14, p. 443.

36. D residual polyethylene glycol on the cells

For related information, see written question 28.

Keebler CM, Somrak TM, The Manual of Cytotechnology.
Appendix: Troubleshooting guidelines T35.14, p. 443.

37. D saponin method

The saponin method may be used for most types of bloody specimens, those either already air-dried, or in a cell fluid. The method uses a 1% saponin solution (0.2% sodium p-hydroxybenzoate) and 3% calcium gluconate. After centrifugation, the red blood cells are lysed leaving a predominant population of non-erythrocytes. Alternatively, less bloody specimens may be treated with Carnoy fixative (2mol/L urea, 0.5 glacial acetic acid:7.0 95% ethanol, and 1 drop hydrochloric acid:500mL 95% ethanol).

Keebler CM, Somrak TM, The Manual of Cytotechnology.
Lysing bloody air-dried specimens, p. 425, Saponin method, p. 441, and Lysing fixatives for bloody cell samples, pp. 425 and 430.

38. A HCl concentration is too dilute; increase the concentration

If the HCl is too dilute, the hematoxylin removal may be inadequate, resulting in over stained nuclei.

Keebler CM, Somrak TM, The Manual of Cytotechnology.
Appendix: Troubleshooting guidelines T35.14, p. 443.

39. C slides are yellow

Once the slides are yellow (due to a much higher temperature than necessary to bake the tissue section onto the slide[s] before staining) the condition is irreversible.

Keebler CM, Somrak TM, The Manual of Cytotechnology.
Appendix: Troubleshooting guidelines T35.14, p. 443.

40. C polyethylene glycol

2% polyethylene glycol (carbowax) and 95% ethanol is a cellular fixative that coats the cells with a waxy substance that helps to prevent air drying during transport of the specimen.

Keebler CM, Somrak TM, The Manual of Cytotechnology.
Coating fixatives, p. 412.

41. C 600g, 10 minutes

Whole cells sediment most efficiently at 600g for 10 minutes. The centrifugal speed may be determined by measuring (in centimeters) the center of the centrifuge head to the bottom of the specimen holder. This number can then be applied to a centrifugal force chart that will read the optimal number of rpm necessary to spin the sample.

Keebler CM, Somrak TM, The Manual of Cytotechnology.
Centrifugation, p. 424.

42. A 2%

These pores are visible when viewing polycarbonate (Nucleopore) filters under the microscope unless the pores are dissolved with chloroform. Nucleopore filters may also be used to make imprint smears.

Keebler CM, Somrak TM, The Manual of Cytotechnology.
Membrane filters, pp. 425–426.

43. C Lithium carbonate is used to blue or set the hematoxylin

Blueing is necessary to change the nuclear stain color from red to blue using an alkaline solution such as lithium carbonate, ammonium hydroxide, or Scott's tap water. Running water may also be used as long as the pH is above 8.0.

Keebler CM, Somrak TM, The Manual of Cytotechnology.
Papanicolaou staining method, pp. 414–417.

44. B increase the alkalinity of the tap water rinse

A deep blue can be attained if the alkalinity of the blueing agent (progressive staining) is above 8.0.

Keebler CM, Somrak TM, The Manual of Cytotechnology.
Appendix: Troubleshooting guidelines T35.14, p. 443.

45. C a milky haze on the slide

Care should be exercised to drain the slides properly between steps, thus preventing the possibility of water contamination in the clearing solution. The addition of siliacic acid pellets to the previous 100% ethanol may alleviate this problem.

Keebler CM, Somrak TM, The Manual of Cytotechnology.
Appendix: Troubleshooting guidelines T35.14, p. 443.

46. A EA-65

EA-65 may be preferred for non-glycogenated preparations. EA-36 was Papanicolaou's original stain and EA-50 uses a different solvent.

Keebler CM, Somrak TM, The Manual of Cytotechnology.
Cytoplasmic stains, pp. 416–417.

47. B separate equipment and staining dishes

"Floaters" are considered cross-contaminated cells from one specimen to the glass slide of another specimen. Their presence on a different focal plane or field when viewing the slide, as well as the morphologic recognition of like cells in another specimen, will help determine their origin as a contaminant. Cytopreparatory steps that may help reduce the possibility of "floaters" include gentle agitation during the staining process, performing toluidine blue wet preparations before processing cells to determine the possibility of malignant cells, and daily filtering of all stains.

Keebler CM, Somrak TM, The Manual of Cytotechnology.
Cerebrospinal fluids, pp. 422 and 424.

48. B have your evacuation plan memorized

In the event of a fire, there may be no time to consider a possible evacuation plan. An evacuation plan should be placed in clear view and all employees should familiarize themselves with the escape route.

Keebler CM, Somrak TM, The Manual of Cytotechnology.
Fire prevention, pp. 373–374.

49. B 100% ethanol

Absolute ethanol will dissolve both polycarbonate and cellulose membrane filters. For related information, see written question 51.

Keebler CM, Somrak TM, The Manual of Cytotechnology.
Membrane filters, pp. 425–426.

50. C toluidine blue

This stain may be used on centrifuged or other specimens for quick examination of the cellularity/diagnosis. One drop of toluidine blue on the unfixed specimen allows for excellent cell examination. This technique may be used for quick diagnosis or to decrease the possibility of unidentified "floaters."

Keebler CM, Somrak TM, The Manual of Cytotechnology.
Wet preparations, pp. 426–427.

51. D not expanding in 95% ETOH

Expanding cellulose filters in 95% ethanol before using them will reduce the "hill and valley" effect often encountered when microscopically viewing membrane filters. Additionally, flattening the filter onto the slide and mounting media by rolling a wooden applicator stick over the surface of the freshly stained filter helps to keep the cells on the filter in the same focal plane.

Keebler CM, Somrak TM, The Manual of Cytotechnology.
Membrane filters, pp. 425–426.

52. A increase eosin or decrease the staining time in the EA

The desired amount of green cytoplasm may be determined based on these principles. Conversely, when all green disappears, the stain is exhausted and should be replaced.

Keebler CM, Somrak TM, The Manual of Cytotechnology.
Appendix: Troubleshooting guidelines T35.14, p. 443.

53. B overstained Pap

Regressive staining requires over staining with an unacidified hematoxylin followed by the removal of the excess hematoxylin with hydrochloric acid. Next, a running bath is necessary to stop the action of the hydrochloric acid. This may be a contraindication when staining non-gynecologic slides due to the possibility of decreased cellular adhesion when the slides are soaking in a running water bath.

Keebler CM, Somrak TM, The Manual of Cytotechnology.
Papanicolaou staining method, pp. 414–417.

Chapter 10

Liquid-Based Cytology

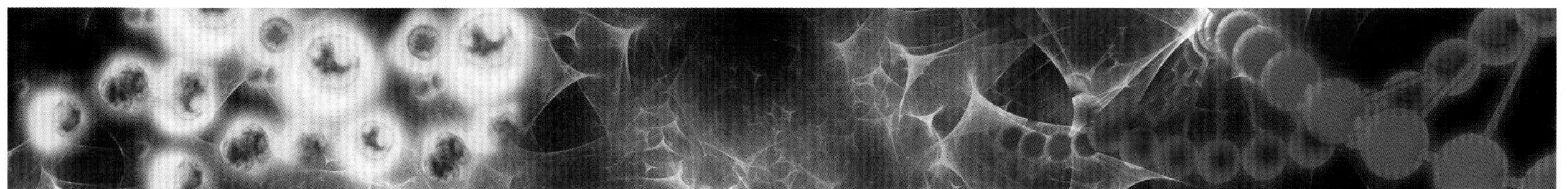

1. **The ThinPrep Pap test is a liquid-based preparation system that allows for a uniform distribution of a single layer of cervical epithelial cells into a 20-mm circle on a glass slide. PreservCyt, the fluid preservative within the vial, is predominantly composed of what base for fixation purposes?**

   A. ethanol
   B. methanol
   C. isopropanol
   D. formalin

2. **Once collected, the storage limit for all liquid-based Pap specimen vials prior to processing is:**

   A. 1 week
   B. 3 weeks
   C. 2 months
   D. 6 months

3. **What is the rationale for the "holes" that may be seen in specimens prepared with the ThinPrep processor?**

   A. blood/mucus or large epithelial fragments that do not disperse during preparation by the processor blocking the filter pores
   B. lack of epithelial cells in sample vial
   C. breaks in the membrane filter that occur during preparation
   D. microbial contaminants blocking the filter pores

4. **Which of the following is considered a key difference between liquid-based cytology and conventional Pap smears?**

   A. cell shape
   B. cell membrane characteristics
   C. cell size
   D. presence of endocervical component

5. **Which of the following morphologic criteria are not as pronounced in liquid-based preparations as compared with conventional Pap smears?**

   A. hyperchromasia
   B. cell membrane
   C. microbiology
   D. nucleoli

6. **Which are the most important criteria for identifying an abnormality in a liquid-based Pap specimen?**

   A. extreme hyperchromasia
   B. presence of nucleoli
   C. presence of mitotic figures
   D. increased N/C ratios, irregular cellular groupings

7. **Which of the following features is typically seen on slides prepared with liquid-based preparation systems?**

   A. reduction in white blood cell population
   B. reduction in koilocytic changes
   C. reduction in transformational zone component
   D. reduction in high-grade squamous intraepithelial lesion cells

8. **Tumor diathesis, or necrosis associated with malignant squamous processes, is described as which of the following when analyzing liquid-based cytology specimens?**

   A. watery, cloudy
   B. refractile, metachromatic
   C. cotton candy-like, "ratty"
   D. tumor diathesis cannot be visualized in liquid-based preparations due to the removal of the products during the automated preparation process

9. **Which of these cellular processes require more vigilance by the cytologist when reviewing liquid-based Pap tests?**

   A. endometrial cells
   B. mature squamous cells
   C. *Candida* sp. infections
   D. low-grade squamous intraepithelial lesions

10. **Which of the following diagnoses are cytologically different when comparing liquid-based and conventional preparations?**

   A. atrophic vaginitis
   B. LSIL
   C. HSIL
   D. squamous cell carcinoma

11. **Based on Bethesda 2001, how many cells must be confirmed on a liquid-based Pap slide to establish a satisfactory specimen for diagnosis?**

   A. 1,000
   B. 2,500
   C. 5,000
   D. 10,000

12. **Based on Bethesda 2001, how many transformational zone cells must be confirmed on a liquid-based Pap slide to establish an adequate specimen?**

   A. 5
   B. 10
   C. 20
   D. 0

13. **Liquid-based preparations exhibit less air-drying than conventional smears. This alters the appearance of:**

   A. cell size
   B. cell quantity
   C. N/C ratio
   D. nuclear membrane

14. **A common feature of conventional slides not seen in liquid-based preparations is:**

   A. sheet formation of endocervical cells
   B. metaplastic cells having cytoplasmic extensions
   C. streaming of cells in mucus
   D. background of inflammatory cells

15. **Compared with liquid-based preparations, smeared cells may appear more:**

   A. rounded and clustered
   B. flattened and elongated
   C. rounded and single
   D. layered in depth of focus

16. **In matched pairings of conventional smears and liquid-based preparations from the same patient, the background elements of inflammation, blood, and mucus in the liquid-based Paps are:**

   A. more visible
   B. absent
   C. reduced
   D. increased

17. **Compared with conventional smears, the nuclear borders of HSIL in liquid-based Paps are:**

   A. not evident
   B. identical
   C. more rounded
   D. more irregular

18. **Compared with conventional smears, the nuclear chromatin of liquid-based Paps shows:**

   A. more detail
   B. less detail
   C. more smudging
   D. more opacity

19. **Compared with conventional smears, tumor diathesis seen in liquid-based Paps is often:**

   A. absent
   B. clinging to cells
   C. found at the periphery of the preparation
   D. obscuring cellular material

20. Compared with liquid-based Paps, metaplastic cells in conventional smears appear to have:

A. thicker cytoplasm
B. more cytoplasm
C. increased cyanophilia
D. increased eosinophilia

21. Compared with conventional smears, endocervical cells in liquid-based Paps may appear:

A. more flattened
B. more elongated
C. more hypochromatic
D. more hyperchromatic

22. Endocervical component, as seen in liquid-based preparations, is composed of:

A. mature superficial squamous cells
B. endometrial cells
C. endocervical and/or squamous metaplastic cells
D. cervical mucus

23. Compared with conventional smears, cells in liquid-based Paps demonstrate:

A. larger nuclear diameter
B. smaller nuclear diameter
C. paler staining
D. more atypia

24. An important feature in distinguishing cells of HSIL from small metaplastic cells in liquid-based Paps is the presence of:

A. hyperchromasia
B. higher N/C ratios
C. irregular nuclear borders
D. homogeneous chromatin distribution

25. The greatest cause of false-negative Paps, both conventional and liquid-based, is attributed to:

A. screening locator error
B. screening interpretation error
C. slide preparation error
D. sampling error

26. Compared with conventional smears, liquid-based Paps statistically report fewer interpretations of:

A. limited cellularity
B. LSIL and HSIL
C. endocervical adenocarcinoma
D. *Trichomonas* infection

27. Following an interpretation of atypical glandular cells of undetermined significance (AGUS) in a liquid-based Pap, compared with AGUS in a conventional smear, the follow-up diagnosis of the cervical biopsy is more often:

A. carcinoma in situ
B. reactive endocervical epithelium
C. glandular pathology
D. normal

28. Compared with conventional smears, red blood cells seen in liquid-based Paps are usually:

A. better preserved
B. lysed
C. absent
D. nucleated

29. Compared with conventional smears, the cell groups of adenocarcinoma as seen in liquid-based Paps show:

A. greater depth of focus
B. flattening of cell sheets
C. larger clusters
D. less nuclear overlap

30. Compared with conventional smears, the cells of squamous cell carcinoma as seen in liquid-based Paps may:

A. show increased orangeophilia and keratinization
B. lack orangeophilia and keratinization
C. exhibit more tadpole forms
D. be larger in size

31. The incidence of infectious organisms in liquid-based Paps, compared with conventional smears, is:

A. higher
B. lower
C. identical
D. infectious organisms cannot be diagnosed with liquid-based Paps

32. A 38-year-old female with a history of radiation and chemotherapy for carcinoma of the uterine cervix presents with diplopia and severe headaches. The following cells represent a CSF specimen processed with the Thin Prep 2000. The diagnosis is:

A. reactive lymphocytes associated with meningitis
B. metastatic cervical cancer
C. leptomeningeal cells
D. large cell lymphoma

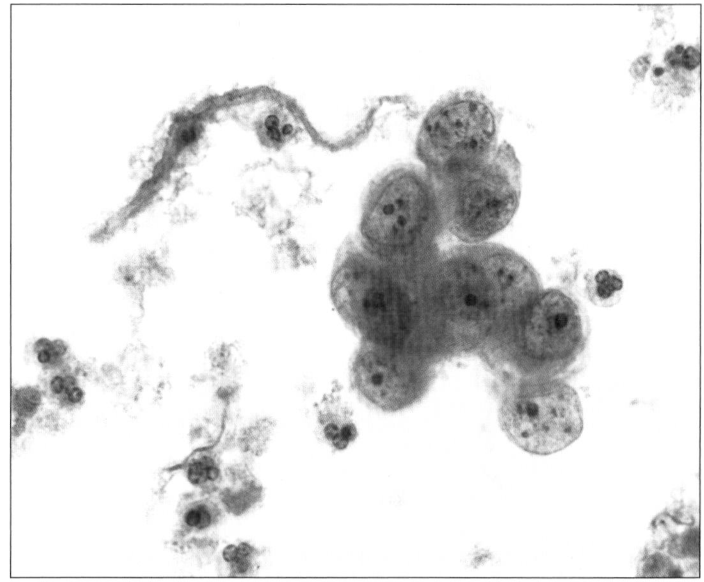

33. A 26-year-old post partum (post 8 weeks) female presents to the clinician for a repeat Thin Prep Pap test after a previous ASCUS diagnosis during the first trimester. The HPV test was negative. The diagnosis is:

A. atypical atrophy
B. HSIL
C. NIL
D. AGUS, favor neoplastic

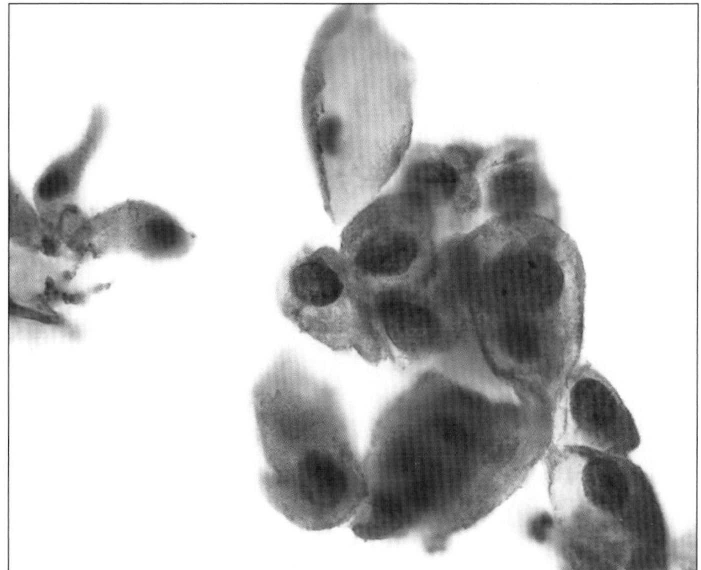

34. A 58-year-old postmenopausal female with complaints of vaginal bleeding presents to the clinician for a pelvic examination. At the time of visual inspection, a vaginal cuff specimen was taken and processed with the Thin Prep 3000. The cells are diagnostic of:

A. adenocarcinoma, ovarian primary
B. vaginal adenosis
C. adenocarcinoma, endometrial origin
D. benign endometrial cells

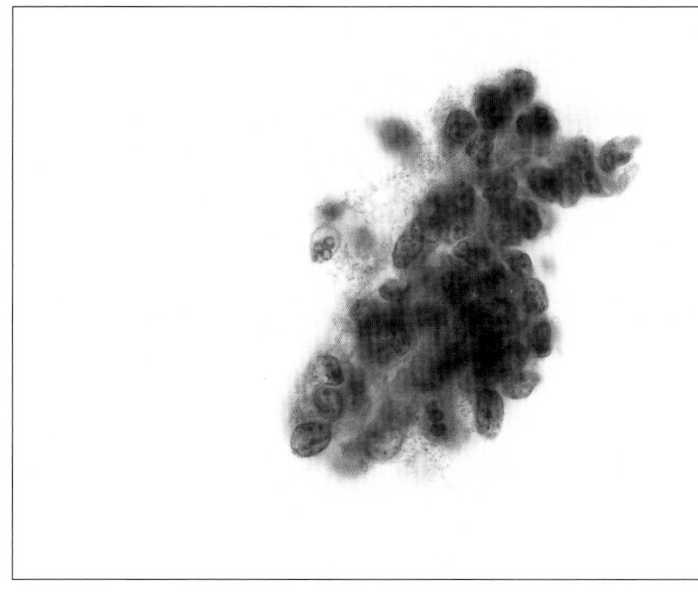

35. **An 18-year-old female, LMP 3 weeks prior, presents for annual Pap test. Based on the cells shown, what is the diagnosis and the appropriate clinical management?**

A. ASCUS, repeat Pap test in 6 months
B. ASCUS, recommend colposcopy
C. LSIL, recommend colposcopy
D. LSIL, repeat Pap test in 12 months

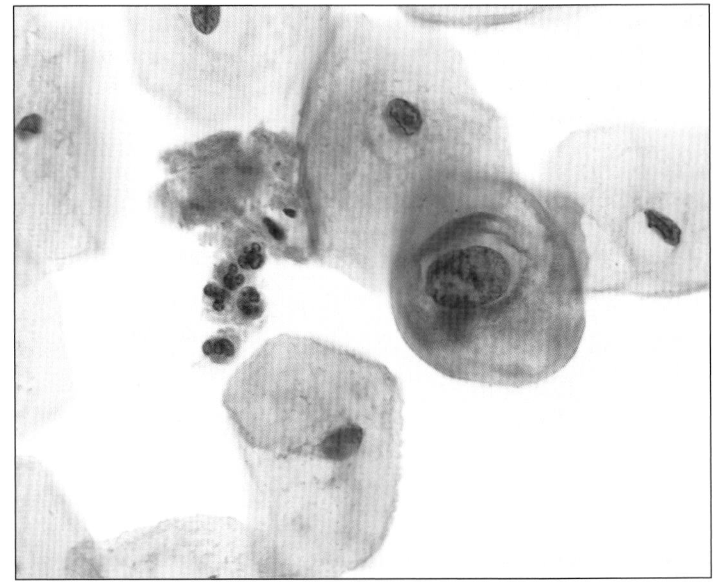

36. **A 45-year-old female presents to the clinician with postcoital bleeding. Her last Pap test was 10 years prior, in her first trimester or pregnancy. The cells are diagnostic of:**

A. HSIL
B. squamous cell carcinoma, nonkeratinizing type
C. AGUS, endometrial origin
D. ASC-US

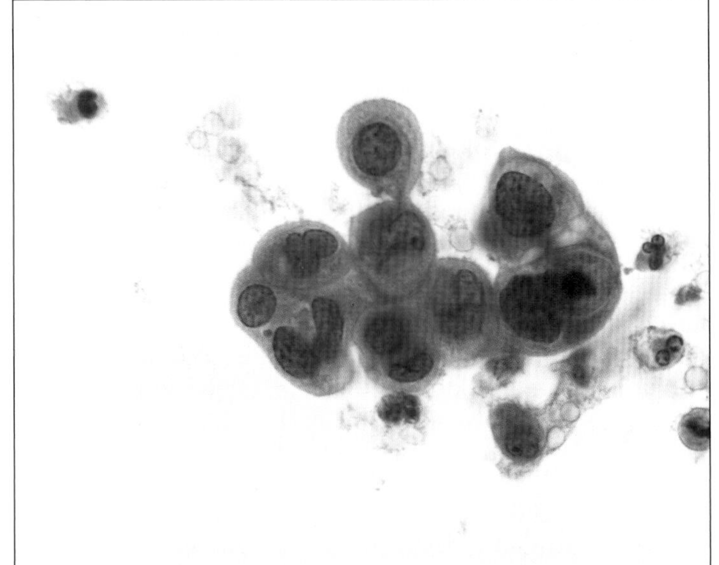

37. **A 62-year-old female presents with intermittent bleeding. Endometrial curettings are negative. The following cells from a ThinPrep Pap test were subsequently stained for p16 immunomarkers. The diagnosis is:**

A. adenocarcinoma, endometrial type
B. small cell squamous carcinoma
C. adenocarcinoma, endocervical type
D. adenocarcinoma in situ; endocervix

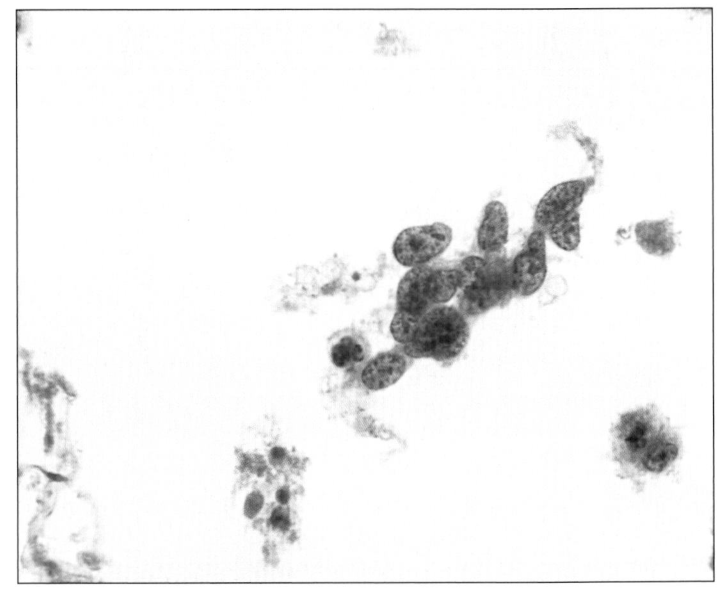

38. **A 41-year-old female with a 2 year history of atypical Pap tests presents for a follow-up Pap after 6 months. High-risk HPV testing was positive. The cells are from a ThinPrep Pap test. The diagnosis is:**

A. AGUS, endometrial
B. NIL, Reactive endocervical cells
C. small cell carcinoma
D. adenocarcinoma in situ, endocervical type

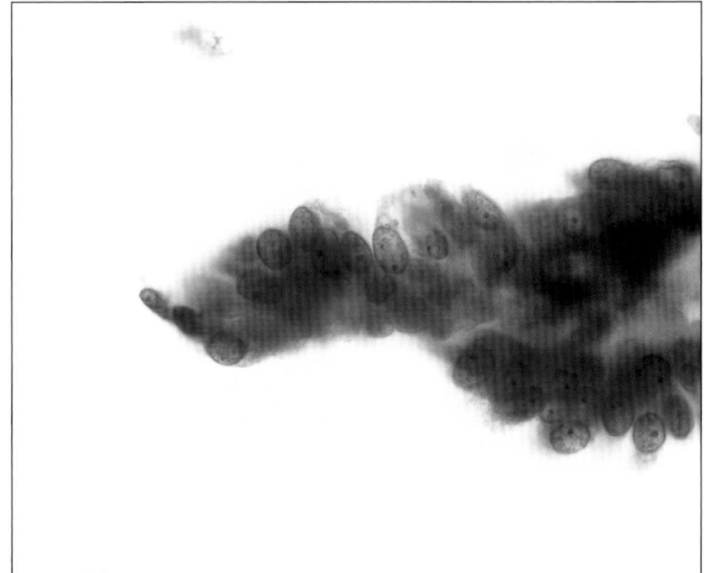

39. **The following cells represent a routine Pap test from a 28-year-old female, day 18. The diagnosis is:**

A. small cell carcinoma
B. HSIL
C. NIL; inflammatory cells
D. endometrial hyperplasia

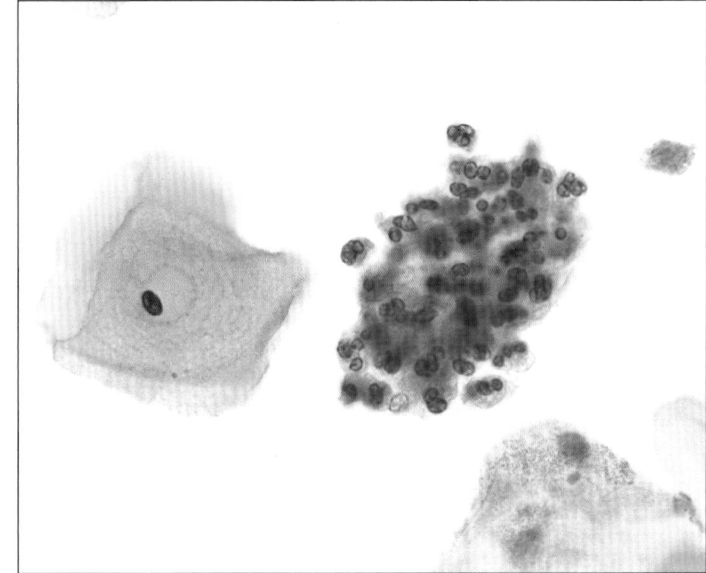

40. **These cells are from a cervical scrape and an endocervical brushing from a 23-year-old woman, 4 months pregnant. The clinical management should be:**

A. colposcopy
B. repeat Pap in 12 months
C. perform HPV testing
D. vaginal delivery should be avoided

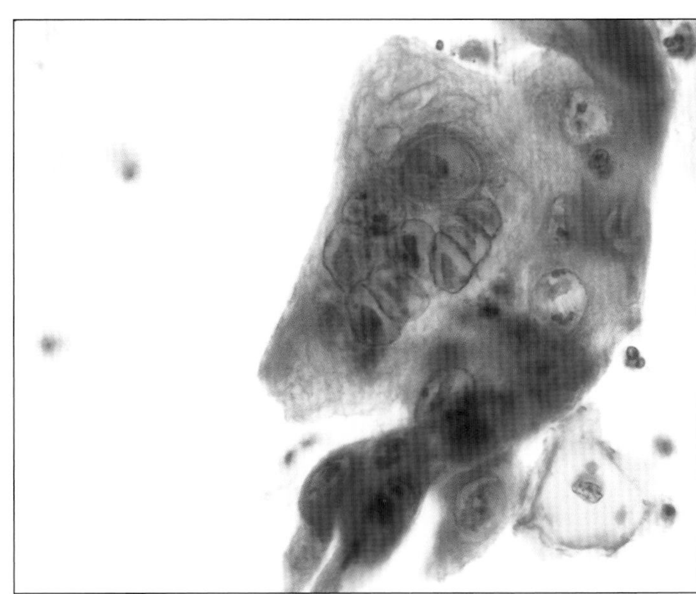

41. **The following represents a pelvic washing from a 45-year-old female, post surgery for a Sertoli-Leydig cell tumor of the ovary. The diagnosis is consistent with:**

A. Sertoli-Leydig cell tumor
B. malignant mesothelioma
C. endometriosis
D. benign collagen balls

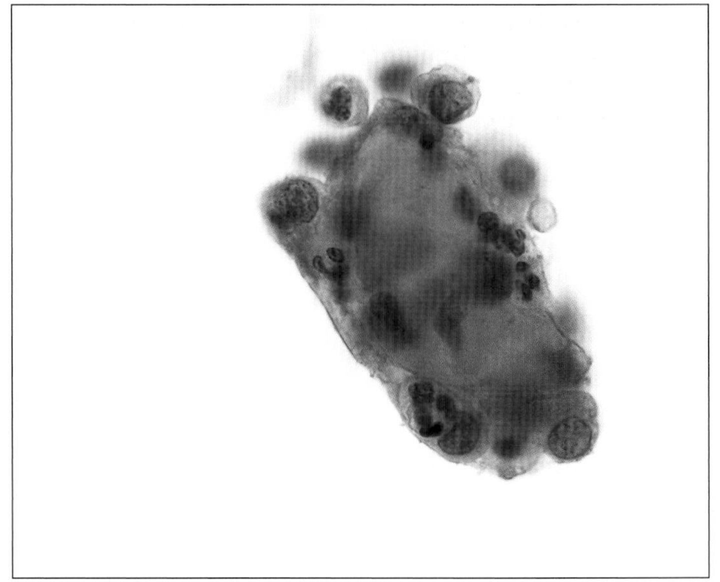

42. **The patient represented in question 42 above also had the following cellular components represented in the ThinPrep processed specimen of the pelvic washing. Based on the previous, the diagnosis is:**

A. reactive mesothelial cells
B. Sertoli-Leydig cell tumor
C. endometriosis
D. malignant mesothelioma

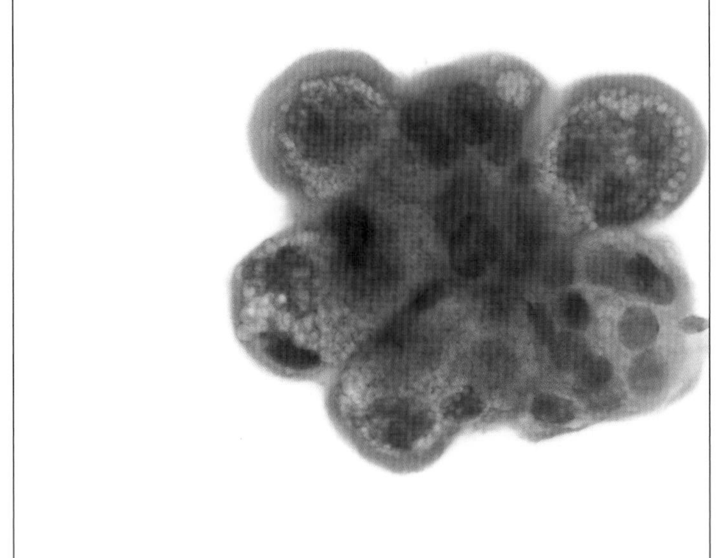

43. **A 66-year-old obese nulliparous female with a previous history of a gynecologic malignancy two years ago (treated with hysterectomy, radiation and chemotherapy) presents to the clinician with vaginal bleeding. Visual inspection of the vagina reveals a 3-cm mass in the cul de sac. A direct scraping of the lesion was immersed into ThinPrep vial containing 20 mL of fluid. The diagnosis is:**

A. reactive endocervical cells
B. primary adenocarcinoma of the vagina
C. metastatic endometrial stromal sarcoma
D. HSIL

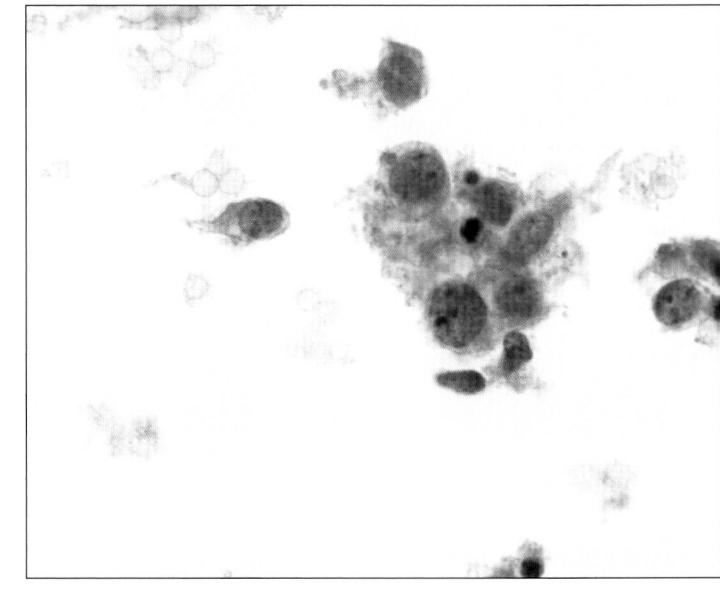

44. **These cells were found in a 48-year-old female with a rectal vaginal fistula of previous unknown etiology. A Thin Prep Pap of the vagina/cervix was performed. The cells are diagnostic of:**

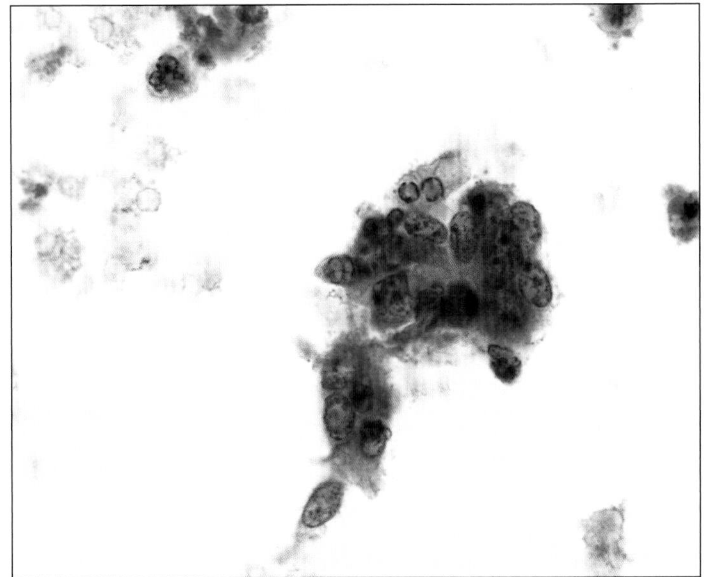

A. metastatic colon cancer
B. reactive endocervical cells
C. AGUS; endocervical
D. primary adenocarcinoma, endocervix

Liquid-Based Cytology *Answer Key*

1. **B methanol**

   Although conventional Pap smears are traditionally fixed with 95% ethanol, the ThinPrep Pap Test uses predominantly methanol as a preservative for fixation.

   Lee KR, et al, Obstet Gynecol. 1997;90(2), pp. 278–284.

2. **B 3 weeks**

   After three weeks, the vials must be properly discarded. The FDA does not approve testing or slide preparation for clinical purposes after this time period.

   Lee KR, et al, Obstet Gynecol. 1997;90(2), pp. 278–284.

3. **A blood/mucus or large epithelial fragments that do not disperse during preparation by the processor blocking the filter pores**

   Although infrequent, these "halos" or "holes" are caused by sample biology.

   Lee KR, et al, Obstet Gynecol. 1997;90(2), pp. 278–284.

4. **C cell size**

   Wet fixation, or liquid-based cytology, where cells are immersed into a liquid fixative, can cause cells to round up and shrink somewhat as compared with conventional Pap smears, where cells are somewhat air-dried before they are coated with an ethanol spray fixative.

   Lee KR, et al, Obstet Gynecol. 1997;90(2), pp. 278–284.

5. **A hyperchromasia**

   Although present in aneuploidy cells, hyperchromasia is not as pronounced in liquid-based (LB) preparations due to the immediate fixation of the cervical broom or cervix brush. Hyperchromasia is accentuated in conventional smears due to the additive degenerative effect of the less-rapid fixation time. Chromatin detail is better with immediate fixation as well, providing more detail about the true DNA texture and dispersion of the nucleus.

   Lee KR, et al, Obstet Gynecol. 1997;90(2), pp. 278–284.

6. **D increased N/C ratios, irregular cellular groupings**

   Increased nuclear-to-cytoplasmic (N/C) ratios over that of the reference normal parent cell and the non-polarity of cellular groupings are the most important features for determining true abnormality in a liquid-based Pap test specimen.

   Lee KR, et al, Obstet Gynecol. 1997;90(2), pp. 278–284.

7. **A reduction in white blood cell population**

   White blood cells, mucus, and thick cellular areas are reduced in liquid-based preparation systems providing for a "cleaner" background and allowing the cytologist better visualization of the cellular material. This factor increases the possibility of identifying significant abnormal cells (as compared with conventional Pap smears).

   Lee KR, et al, Obstet Gynecol. 1997;90(2), pp. 278–284.

8. **C cotton candy-like, "ratty"**

   The pulled cotton candy or gritty/ratty background is maintained in malignant squamous processes prepared with liquid-based cytology.

   Lee KR, et al, Obstet Gynecol. 1997;90(2), pp. 278–284.

9. **A endometrial cells**

   Endometrial cells, metaplastic cells, and cells from high-grade squamous intraepithelial lesions are often quite small and require great vigilance on the part of the cytologist to correctly identify and diagnose. Endometrial cells lack polarity even as a normal feature and often prompt the cytologist to falsely diagnose normal cells as abnormal. Ghost lysed red blood cells in the background may be a clue to the significance of endometrial cells, and the clinical history (LMP, etc) is a valuable tool for correctly identifying these cells.

   Lee KR, et al, Obstet Gynecol. 1997;90(2), pp. 278–284.

10. **A atrophic vaginitis**

    Due to the lack of degenerative air-drying artifact in liquid-based specimens, the "blue blobs," "mummified cells," and bare nuclei commonly seen with conventional Pap smears are not seen. Instead, well-preserved parabasal cells in sheets with requisite inflammatory cells are present for diagnostic confirmation.

    Lee KR, et al, Obstet Gynecol. 1997;90(2), pp. 278–284.

11. **C** 5,000

A minimum of 5,000 cells are required to render a liquid-based Pap specimen adequate for evaluation, whereas 8,000-12,000 cells are considered optimal for analyzing conventional Pap smears.

Solomon D, et al, JAMA. 2002;287(16), pp. 2114–2119.

12. **B** 10

The presence or absence of a transformational zone component should be reported in the specimen adequacy section of the cytology report and a minimum of 10 well-preserved transformation zone cells (endocervical and/or squamous metaplastic cells) as individuals and/or groups. Mucus or parabasal cells do not count in this computation.

Solomon D, et al, JAMA. 2002;287(16), pp. 2114–2119.

13. **A** cell size

Cells immersed in a liquid-based medium have a tendency to lose their surface tension; thus rounding up of the cell size is more common when compared with conventional Pap smears.

Douglass K, ThinPrep Pap Test: Morphology Reference Manual.

14. **C** streaming of cells in mucus

Cells are often trapped in pools of mucin in conventional Pap smears whereas liquid-based preparations show uniform dispersion of transformation zone components throughout the slide.

Douglass K, ThinPrep Pap Test: Morphology Reference Manual.

15. **B** flattened and elongated

Smeared cells "lie down" in a more flattened proportion when compared with the "rounding up" associated with liquid-based preparation systems.

Douglass K, ThinPrep Pap Test: Morphology Reference Manual.

16. **C** reduced

Blood, mucus, inflammatory cells, and cellular debris are reduced in liquid-based preparation systems and allow the cytologist to better visualize the morphologic detail of the majority of the cells present.

Ashfaq R, et al, Acta Cytol. 1996;40(5), p. 1047.

17. **D** more irregular

Nuclear detail is better preserved, therefore irregular nuclear membranes may have more clarity when visualizing liquid-based Pap tests. The degree of nuclear membrane irregularity increases with significance of cervical disease.

Wilbur DC, et al, Diagn Cytopathol. 1996;14(3), pp. 201–211.

18. **A** more detail

The chromasia is clearer and the distribution of the chromatin pattern is better visualized with liquid-based Pap tests.

Wilbur DC, et al, Diagn Cytopathol. 1996;14(3), pp. 201–211.

19. **B** clinging to cells

Although reduced when compared with conventional smears, the key difference when analyzing tumor necrosis or diathesis in liquid-based Pap tests is the appearance of ratty material clinging to the cells throughout the preparation.

Wilbur DC, et al, Diagn Cytopathol. 1996;14(3), pp. 201–211.

20. **A** thicker cytoplasm

A denser and thicker cytoplasm is common in parabasal and metaplastic cells with conventional Pap smears.

Douglass K, ThinPrep Pap Test: Morphology Reference Manual.

21. **D** more hyperchromatic

Due to the small cell size as well the lack of air-drying features, the nuclei of endocervical cells may appear at first impression darker; however, closer inspection of the cytoplasmic polarity (honeycombing, picket fence) and well-delineated cell borders that push the cells apart (as if someone "erased" in between the cells, thus allowing the observer the perception that he/she can "cut them out" with scissors) verifies the benignity of these cells.

Evans SK, Wilbur DC, Acta Cytol. 1993;37(5), p. 776.

22. **C** endocervical and/or squamous metaplastic cells

Cells found in the endocervical canal are both squamous metaplastic and endocervical glandular type.

Corkill M, et al, Acta Cytologica. 1997;41(1), pp. 39–44.

23. **B** smaller nuclear diameter

Liquid-based preparations tend to "shrink" the overall cell and nuclear size when compared with the air-drying typically seen with conventional Pap smears.

Douglass K, ThinPrep Pap Test: Morphology Reference Manual.

24. **C** irregular nuclear borders

Nuclear-to-cytoplasmic ratios and the irregular nuclear borders are important features for confirming the presence of a significant cervical disease process.

Wilbur DC, et al, Diagn Cytopathol. 1996;14(3), pp. 201–211.

25. **D** sampling error

Sampling error accounts for ½ to ¾ of all the false-negative Pap test diagnoses reported in the literature.

Linder J, Zahniser D, Arch Pathol Lab Med. 1998;122(2), pp. 139–144.

26. **A** limited cellularity

Obscuring cellular elements are commonplace when analyzing conventional Pap smears; however, these factors are minimized in liquid-based preparation systems, thus providing the morphologist with a decreased probability that the slide has limited cellularity.

Lee KR, et al, Obstet Gynecol. 1997;90(2), pp. 278–284.

27. **C** glandular pathology

Better morphologic visualization of the atypical features (nuclear stratification and cellular feathering) is seen when analyzing true glandular abnormalities in liquid-based preparation systems. This correlates with fewer false-positive diagnoses and a higher propensity for a biopsy proven lesion.

Ashfaq R, et al, Acta Cytol. 1999;43(1), pp. 81–85.

28. **B** lysed

In liquid-based Paps, red blood cell casts are dispersed throughout the slide and don't preclude the visualization of other cells as compared with the likelihood that obscuring blood will cover important cells (as often seen in conventional Pap smears).

Douglass K, ThinPrep Pap Test: Morphology Reference Manual.

29. **A** greater depth of focus

True tissue fragments with community borders, such as those seen with adenocarcinoma, will round up in liquid-based preparations and have a greater depth of focus as compared with the flattening of the cells seen in conventional Pap smears.

Ashfaq R, et al, Acta Cytol. 1999;43(1), pp. 81–85, and Roberts JM, et al, Acta Cytol. 1999;43(1), pp. 74-90.

30. **B** lack orangeophilia and keratinization

Orangeophilia and keratinization are often exaggerated in degenerative specimens, such as those that allow for more degeneration to occur after the cells are removed from the patient (as conventional Paps). The diagnosis of squamous cell carcinoma in liquid-based Pap specimens is more akin to that seen in freshly prepared specimens, such as effusions and fine-needle aspirations. It is important to point out that the diagnosis of squamous cell carcinoma is best determined by the degree of pleomorphism, rather than simply the color of the cell.

Douglass K, ThinPrep Pap Test: Morphology Reference Manual.

31. **C** identical

The incidence and identification of microorganisms in liquid-based specimens is comparable to that seen with conventional Papanicolaou smears. Although the amount and number of microorganisms may be reduced in liquid-based Pap tests, the likelihood for identification remains good owing to the decreased inflammatory background in these specimens.

Evans SK, Wilbur DC, Acta Cytol. 1993;37(5), p. 776.

32. **B** metastatic cervical cancer

These cells represent endocervical adenocarcinoma that has metastasized to the subarachnoid space. The cells appear in acinar formation and possess cohesive features, thus ruling out a benign or malignant lymphoid process. The cells associated with metastatic adenocarcinoma of the cervix in the CSF, albeit rare, may present in rosettes with granular cytoplasm and elongated, hyperchromatic nuclei with prominent multiple nucleoli. Primary malignancies of the CNS are extremely uncommon as compared to metastatic carcinomatosis.

33. **A** atypical atrophy

The diagnosis of atypical squamous cells of undetermined significance (ASC-US) includes an alteration in the normal squamous nuclear size, possibly 2–3 times greater than that of a normal intermediate cell nucleus. The chromatin is finely granular, regularly distributed, and generally hypochromatic (normochromatic). A true ASC-US is a non-inflammatory related change that may be related to subclinical or early manifestations of the human papillomavirus infection or dysplasia; however, ASC-US may also involve immature squamous epithelial cells as well as basal and parabasal cells found in atrophic conditions. Based on the cytologic diagnosis and the negative HPV test, the appropriate management for this patient should be a repeat Pap test in 12 months.

DeMay RM, The Art & Science of Cytopathology.
Atypical squamous cells of undetermined significance, pp. 94–97.

34. **C** adenocarcinoma, endometrial origin

Endometrial adenocarcinomas have diffusely vacuolated cytoplasm and often contain engulfed polymorphonuclear cells. Endometrial adenocarcinomas often present with fewer numbers of cells on the slide (as opposed to endocervical adenocarcinomas), cell clusters with scalloping borders and three-dimensional tissue fragments, high nuclear-to-cytoplasmic ratios, and frothy, delicate, lacy, vacuolated cytoplasm. Finally, the presence of a watery diathesis with associated lipophages may be helpful in discriminating endometrial adenocarcinomas from other epithelial malignancies.

DeMay RM, The Art & Science of Cytopathology.
Differential diagnosis of endocervical and endometrial adenocarcinoma, p. 129 and Endometrial adenocarcinoma, pp. 125–127.

35. **D** LSIL; repeat Pap in 12 months

Adolescents (women under 20) with a cytologic diagnosis of LSIL have a high rate of regression; however, immunologic clearance, followed by regression, may take several years. Because of the regressive feature of LSIL in adolescents, follow-up with annual cytologic testing is only recommended. Upon annual follow up, only those adolescents with a cytologic diagnosis of HSIL or greater should be referred to colposcopy.

Wright TC Jr, Massad LS, Dunton CJ, et al. 2006 American Society for Colposcopy and Cervical Pathology-sponsored Consensus Conference. 2006 consensus guidelines for the management of women with abnormal cervical cancer screening tests. Am J Obstet Gynecol. 2007 Oct;197(4):346-355

36. **B** squamous cell carcinoma, nonkeratinizing type

Syncytial fragments, and cannibalism, nuclei exhibiting hyperchromasia and coarse irregular chromatin with macronucleoli are diagnostic criteria of nonkeratinizing squamous cell carcinoma of the uterine cervix. A tumor diathesis, presenting as "cotton candy" like frothy material found in the background is commonly seen with liquid based preparations as compared with the granular diathesis typical represented in conventional Pap preparations.

DeMay RM, The Art & Science of Cytopathology.
Nonkeratinizing squamous cell carcinoma, pp. 84–85.

37. **B** small cell squamous carcinoma

p16 is a cyclin-dependent kinase-4 inhibitor that is expressed in HPV-associated lesions, including invasive squamous carcinomas. Endometrial cells/lesions are negative for p16. Small cell carcinomas may be poorly differentiated squamous lesions or neuroendocrine tumors, both of which arise within the endocervical canal. Poorly differentiated squamous carcinomas, such as this case from a postmenopausal patient, are composed of small cells with high N/C ratios, uniform cellular sizes with well-defined borders, coarse chromatin with nucleoli, but little-to-absent "crush" artifact. An abnormal host response or necrotic tumor diathesis often accompanies these squamous lesions. Conversely, and as depicted in this photomicrograph, neuroendocrine small cell tumors reveal fine chromatin, inconspicuous nucleoli, and distinguished vertebral-like arrangements and nuclear molding, recapitulating their lung counterparts. These cells contain hyperchromatic stippled chromatin, coarse clumping, nuclear molding, scanty cytoplasm, and micronucleoli. They have characteristic vertebral column formation, microbiopsy aggregates, cords, nests, or ribbons. In 1/3 of the cases, neuroendocrine differentiation may be demonstrated by immunocytochemical staining with chromogranin, neuron-specific enolase, or synaptophysin. Neuroendocrine differentiation (argyrophilia) may also be demonstrated.

DeMay RM, The Art & Science of Cytopathology.
Small cell squamous carcinoma, p. 84.

38. **D** adenocarcinoma in situ, endocervical type

The diagnosis of endocervical adenocarcinoma in situ (AIS) may often be difficult to differentiate from squamous carcinoma in situ (CIS) with the exception that AIS often possesses feathering or pseudostratified syncytial-like fragments, stratified strips, or rosettes. The maintenance of columnar morphology may also be a key feature in establishing the diagnosis of an atypical endocervical process.

DeMay RM, The Art & Science of Cytopathology.
Early endocervical glandular neoplasia, pp. 129–131.

39. **C** NIL; inflammatory cells

These cells represent normal polymorphonuclear neutrophils found in a "cannonball" formation. This phenomenon is often seen as a result of the processing associated with liquid-based Thin Prep specimens. Although the majority of inflammation is eliminated with from liquid based Pap tests, a notable quantity is still represented in patients with severe inflammation. The aggregation of inflammatory cells is found in a mucous wisp and allows the reviewer to comment on acute inflammation.

40. **D** vaginal delivery should be avoided

A caesarian section recommended due to the diagnosis of herpesvirus. The presence of "ground glass" chromatin, chromatinic margination, multinucleation, and nuclear molding, with or without intranuclear eosinophilic Cowdry Type A inclusions, suggests a diagnosis of herpesvirus. Grossly, these lesions appear as erythematous papules or ulcerations. They must be distinguished from other multinucleated cells found within a liquid-based Pap test.

DeMay RM, The Art & Science of Cytopathology.
Specific infections, p. 112.

41. **D** benign collagen balls

Bland mesothelial cell nuclei arranged around a hyaline globule of collagen are described as "collagen balls." The use of peritoneal washings can help determine subclinical peritoneal dissemination by non-serous ovarian tumors.

DeMay RM, The Art & Science of Cytopathology.
Miscellaneous Findings, p. 266.

42. **A** reactive mesothelial cells

Aka (reactive hyperplasia) shows papillae and pseudoacini with knobby borders instead of true community borders, and single cells with "windows" between adjacent cells—a result of Thin Prep processing—and maintenance of the cytoplasmic brush border. The finding of a brush border infers benignity, and is often described as indistinct or fuzzy in appearance. The nuclei of these cells is round and centrally located with well-defined, regular nuclear membranes and finely granular, regularly distributed chromatin with nucleoli. The cytoplasmic morphology is homogeneous and dense with peripheral fading, often demonstrating an endo-ectoplasmic demarcation. The density of the cytoplasm may give a false "atypical" impression of hyperchromatic nuclei; however, when the nuclear intensity is compared with that of the cytoplasm, there is little divergence.

DeMay RM, The Art & Science of Cytopathology.
Reactive changes in mesothelial cells, p. 263.

43. **C** metastatic endometrial stromal sarcoma

Endometrial stromal sarcoma is a homologous sarcoma found as small cells or groups with high N/C ratios and coarse hyperchromatic oval nuclei, spindle-shaped cells with frothy wispy cytoplasm. Since a secondary lesion has developed, direct scrapings will likely produce a diathesis similar to the original primary lesion.

DeMay RM, The Art & Science of Cytopathology.
Sarcomas, p. 137.

44. **A** metastatic colon cancer

The diagnosis of metastatic colon cancer in gynecological specimens is related to the presence of abundant abnormal palisading cells with basophilic granular cytoplasm and cigar-shaped nuclei. Presence of finely granular, regularly distributed chromatin is important in the diagnosis of this disease. A diathesis may be visualized if the tumor has metastasized by direct extension or seeded within the vagina. The diagnosis of this lesion may be difficult to distinguish from endocervical adenocarcinoma; therefore, a history of normal pelvic examinations may be necessary.

DeMay RM, The Art & Science of Cytopathology.
Metastasis, p. 137.

Chapter 11

Molecular Techniques and Special Stains

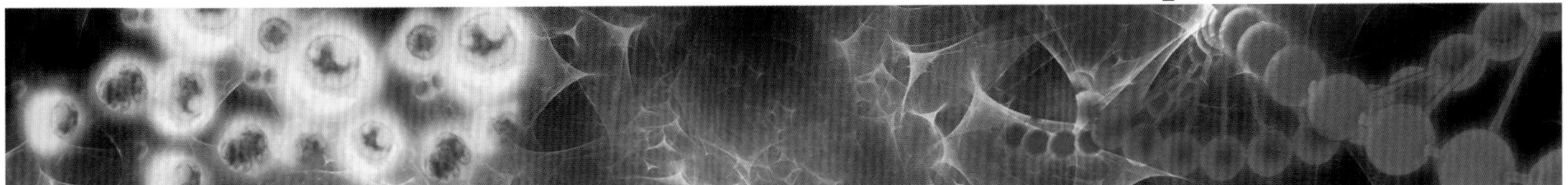

1. **One of the principal preparation differences between the Romanovsky and the Papanicolaou stains is:**

   A. air-drying artifact is associated with the Romanovsky stain
   B. increased cell adherence to the slide is associated with the Romanovsky stain
   C. alcohol fixation is mandatory for Romanovsky staining
   D. an increased propensity for "floaters" within the Romanovsky stain due to cells falling off the prepared slides

2. **Which of the following cellular elements are best visualized with the Romanovsky stain when compared with the Papanicolaou stain?**

   A. mucin
   B. keratin
   C. viral changes
   D. euchromatin

3. **Which of the following describes the role of molecular diagnostics as it relates to the practice of cytopathology?**

   A. no value as an adjunctive testing modality for establishing the diagnosis of precancerous disease
   B. increasing number of molecular techniques are available for infectious diseases and tumor diagnostics
   C. a poor reflex for equivocal morphology
   D. often difficult to standardize procedures and an overall lack of automation

4. **What morphologic enhancements does the Romanovsky stain have over the Papanicolaou stain?**

   A. the Romanovsky stain enables better differentiation of nuclear chromasia
   B. the Romanovsky stain is more helpful when analyzing three-dimensional tissue fragments
   C. the cellular morphology demonstrated with the Romanovsky stain is akin to that seen with H&E
   D. the Romanovsky stain is a metachromatic stain enabling better visualization of various mucins, neurosecretory granules, and stromal elements

5. **Which of the following special stains may prove useful when differentiating plasmacytomas from small cell cleaved lymphomas?**

   A. rhodanine
   B. Congo red
   C. PAS
   D. methyl green pyronine

6. **Which statements regarding the utility of cotesting cytopathology with molecular diagnostics are considered true?**

   A. cotesting may impede service/patient care due to decreased turn around time
   B. cotesting is often cost prohibitive due to poor reimbursement
   C. cytology professionals are not educated to perform molecular testing
   D. integrating reporting enhances the overall standard of care

7. **A 63-year-old male with a 50-year history of moderate alcohol intake now presents with multiple liver nodules. Cellular morphology reveals cells that suggest a diagnosis of cholangiocarcinoma over hepatocellular carcinoma. Which of the following enzyme reactions would help confirm this suspicion?**

   A. aminopeptidase
   B. acid phosphatase
   C. aryl sulfatase
   D. lysozyme

8. **A 55-year-old female with a prior history of partial colonectomy for rectal cancer now presents with a 1.5-cm solitary lung mass. Cellular morphology reveals cells that more closely resemble bronchogenic adenocarcinoma rather than metastatic colonic adenocarcinoma. Which of the following enzyme reactions will confirm lung primary over a metastatic colonic carcinoma?**

   A. alcian blue
   B. Congo red
   C. alkaline phosphatase
   D. lysosyme

9. **Rare abnormal cells with atypical features suggesting a high-grade intraepithelial lesion were found in a liquid-based cytology preparation. DNA analysis for low- and high-risk HPV DNA was inconclusive. Polymerase chain reaction (PCR), using a universal consensus oligonucleotide primer for high-risk HPV DNA types 16, 18, 31, 33, 35, 41, and 45, was used to test the residual cellular material from the vial. Dot blot analysis revealed a positive reaction. Which of the following statements apply?**

   A. colposcopy is likely to reveal a high-grade squamous intraepithelial lesion
   B. PCR is not useful in confirming HPV DNA
   C. high-risk primers comprise HPV types 6 and 11
   D. PCR is the most useful tool for evaluating gynecologic material

10. **Which of the following molecular assays are least commonly used as adjunctive tests in cytopathology?**

    A. fluorescent in situ hybridization (FISH)
    B. Hybrid Capture 2
    C. polymerase chain reaction
    D. strand displacement amplification

11. **A consensus universal primer is designed to show cross reactivity for common nucleic acid sequences. For purposes of testing HPV in vitro, these primers are grouped into low- and high-risk genotype sequences in order to separate those patients with low potential for developing cervical intraepithelial neoplasia from those at high risk who need to be triaged into colposcopy or biopsy. Which of the following statements is true regarding these universal primers?**

    A. low-risk types include 16, 18, 31, 33, 35, 45, 51, 52, 56, 58, 59, and 68
    B. high-risk types include 6, 11, 42, 43, and 44
    C. a quantitative index of viral load is provided when using consensus primers
    D. specimens are considered positive if any of the low-risk or high-risk viral infections are found within each respective probe cocktail

12. **One of the advantages of using in situ hybridization testing for HPV DNA is:**

    A. it can be performed on archival tissue specimens
    B. it can be performed on circulating peripheral blood
    C. it is more sensitive than a Pap test
    D. it is more sensitive than polymerase chain reaction

13. **Which of the following statements represents the molecular function of Hybrid Capture 2 testing?**

    a. antibodies attach to captured hybrids reacting with a substrate to emit an amplified chemiluminescent signal
    b. specimens are morphologically analyzed with fluorescent in situ hybridization (FISH)
    c. specimens are morphologically analyzed with bright field microscopy using chromogenic detection
    d. cleavage-based amplification is utilized for the reaction

14. **Flow cytometry of Pap tests with suspected cytologic changes of cervical intraepithelial neoplasia will help the pathologist determine:**

    A. DNA aneuploidy confirms high-grade lesions
    B. DNA aneuploidy confirms low-grade lesions
    C. DNA aneuploidy is strongly associated with non-oncogenic, non-transforming episomal HPV infections
    D. flow cytometry cannot be used to analyze cervical samples owing to its inability to distinguish polyploidy from aneuploidy in any cervical intraepithelial lesion

15. **The periodic acid-Schiff (PAS) stain verifies the presence of:**

    A. keratohyalin granules
    B. hyaluronic acid
    C. carbohydrate moieties
    D. neutral mucin

16. **Which of the following special stains is useful when determining muscle fibers?**

A. argentaffin silver stain
B. oil red O
C. methyl green pyronine
D. Masson trichrome

17. **Epithelial lesions are immunocytochemically positive for which of the following intermediate filaments?**

A. keratin
B. vimentin
C. desmin
D. actin

18. **An advantage of coupling in situ hybridization with cytopathology in the interpretation of precancerous or equivocal cytopathology specimens is:**

A. true replication/cloning of oligonucleotide targeted endogenous genetic aberrations allows for amplification of a single genetic copy
B. conventional microscopy (bright field) can be used to interpret genetic signals
C. genetic signals are measured by a luminometer
D. restriction fragment length polymorphisms (RFLPs) may provide confirmation of equivocal morphologic interpretations

19. **The molecular assay which utilizes/amplifies specific targets by adding dideoxynucleotides (ddATP, ddCTP, ddGTP, and ddTTP) to four separate DNA synthesis reactions containing oligonucleotides, template and DNA polymerase is referred as:**

A. signal amplification for Hybrid Capture 2
B. in situ hybridization
C. polymerase chain reaction (PCR)
D. branched DNA amplification

20. **Immunocytochemical markers are helpful because:**

A. they are specific for specific tumor types
B. the FDA must approve them for use before testing begins
C. they often aid in the diagnosis of lesions that are difficult to classify
D. they do not require confirmation by additional diagnostic studies

21. **Melanomas may react to all of the following immunocytochemical markers, except:**

A. S-100
B. epithelial membrane antigen
C. vimentin
D. Factor VIII

22. **Which of the following applications describes a signal amplification system which targets nucleic acids using a series of probes binding to a target, producing an overlap that is cut by an enzyme, where the addition of a complementary FRET probe with a reporter molecule located in the proximity of a quencher molecule subsequently binds to a signal probe producing a flap (which is cut by the earlier enzyme) releasing the reporter molecule from the quencher molecule ultimately producing a quantifiable signal?**

A. Qß-replicase assay
B. ligase chain reaction
C. strand displacement amplification
D. invader (cleavage-based) amplification

23. **Which of the following special stains may be helpful in differentiating spindle cell neoplasms?**

A. melanin
B. phosphotungstic acid-hematoxylin
C. orcein stain
D. Congo red

24. **Which of the following intermediate filament immunocytochemical markers will help identify the possibility of a rhabdomyosarcoma?**

A. desmin
B. vimentin
C. glial fibrillary acidic protein (GFIP)
D. neurofilament

25. **Which of the following molecular assays can be used for determining oncogenic HPV from liquid-based specimens?**

A. Western blots
B. invader (cleavage-based) amplification
C. mitochondrial DNA polymorphisms
D. cycling probe assays

26. **A ThinPrep Pap test from a 44-year-old female with no previous history of abnormal cytology reveals few rare immature metaplastic cells with high N/C ratios, hyperchromasia, and irregular nuclear membranes. Based on these findings, which of the following may be recommended?**

A. PCR testing for low-risk HPV
B. loop electrosurgical excision procedure (LEEP)
C. Hybrid Capture 2 testing for high-risk HPV
D. repeat Pap test in 1 year

27. **The most important aspect of Hybrid Capture 2 testing is the:**

A. negative predictive value
B. positive predictive value
C. specificity
D. sensitivity in CIN I

28. **Carcinoid tumors may be confirmed with which of the special stains?**

A. PAS
B. argentaffin
C. rubeanic acid
D. alcian blue

29. **Hybrid Capture 2, the only commercially available HPV test approved by the Food and Drug Administration for use with liquid-based Pap tests, is a nucleic acid signal amplification based assay that hybridizes a RNA probe with the target HPV DNA gene in vitro. How does the system allow for visualization of a positive product?**

A. captured RNA–DNA hybrids with alkaline phosphatase conjugated antibodies are detected with a chemiluminescent substrate and signaled by a luminometer
B. it is a quantitative assay that uses type-specific primers that hybridize with RNA–DNA hybrids and are detected with ethidium bromide
C. it uses a Southern blot analysis of DNA hybrids that are visualized with radioactive 32P via autoradiography
D. it uses tissue in situ hybridization of cellular and viral nucleic acid sequences visualized by biotinylated probes

30. **An advantage of Hybrid Capture 2 assays, as compared to other molecular assays, is its:**

A. ability to differentiate integrated from episomal viral infections
B. ability to provide specific virus genotyping
C. specificity for high-risk viral types
D. sensitivity for HSIL and cancer

31. **Cervical squamous intraepithelial lesions have a progressive dysfunction of proliferative ability where proliferating cells and mitotic figures increase as a factor of increasing CIN grades. Which of the following immunocytochemical markers may be useful markers of proliferation?**

A. HPV E6/E7
B. p53
C. Rb
D. Ki-67

32. **An advantage of in situ hybridization, as compared to other molecular assays for diagnosing precancerous cervical lesions, is its:**

A. excellent tissue or cytology localization of HPV-infected cells
B. labeling as an analyte-specific reagent
C. increased sensitivity over Hybrid Capture 2
D. use of a thermal cycler to clone low-signal viral copies to help the gynecologist predict the likelihood for a clinically visible lesion in the future

33. **High-molecular-weight keratin is expressed in which of the following lesions?**

A. dysgerminoma
B. endodermal sinus tumor
C. squamous cell carcinoma
D. malignant lymphoma

34. **Flow cytology was performed on a bronchial washing specimen from a 66-year-old male with a history of smoking but nondiagnostic cytology. A high S phase fraction was determined, which may indicate:**

A. reactive bronchial alveolar cells
B. idiopathic pulmonary hemosiderosis
C. hamartoma
D. bronchogenic carcinoma

35. **Which molecular assay has increased sensitivity and specificity over immunohistochemistry for determining overexpression of the Her2/neu gene (chromosome 17 (17q11.2-q12) in breast cancer?**

A. fluorescent in situ hybridization (FISH)
B. RFLP typing
C. bisulfite DNA sequencing
D. single strand conformation polymorphism (SSCP)

36. **Which assay will allow for increased sensitivity (as compared to cytology) for establishing the diagnosis of low-grade malignant tumors from benign urothelial cells?**

a. Hybrid Capture 2
b. pyrosequencing
c. fluorescent in situ hybridization (FISH)
d. cleavage-based amplification

37. **Electron microscopy was performed due to the unknown histogenesis of a liver lesion thought to be metastatic. Features revealed intracellular lumens forming flocculent-filled acini lined by microvilli. Which of the following lesions is likely?**

A. squamous cell carcinoma
B. adenocarcinoma
C. sarcoma
D. lymphoma

38. **For purposes of CLIA '88, HPV testing is considered:**

A. low complexity
B. moderate complexity
C. high complexity
D. CLIA '88 does not rule on the complexity of HPV testing in the laboratory

39. **Which special stain is used for Barr body identification?**

A. Biebrich-Scarlet
B. PAS
C. Feulgen
D. Giemsa

40. **Which special stain will help elucidate a hepatocellular process?**

A. Prussian blue
B. Sudan black
C. Shorr
D. Fouchet method

41. **The distinction of hemosiderin-laden macrophages from malignant melanoma may be aided by:**

A. Nile blue sulfate
B. iron stain
C. GMS
D. alcian blue

42. **Which FDA-approved urologic assay uses a multi-color test that detects aneuploidy for chromosomes 3,7, 9p21, and 17?**

A. Urovision® (Abbott Molecular, Inc.)
B. BTA TRAK test (Polymedco, Inc.)
C. APTIMA® (Gen-Probe, Inc.)
D. NMP22 (Matritech, Inc.)

43. **The identification of lipid is best achieved with what special stain?**

A. Nile blue sulfate
B. Sudan black
C. Giemsa
D. Feulgen

44. **Which stain is helpful in determining fetal maturity?**

A. Nile blue sulfate
B. Shorr
C. Janus green
D. Feulgen

45. **Which disease/genetic mutation/and adjunctive molecular assay can assist fine needle aspiration cytology to classify genetic mutations that can aid in stratifying aggressive versus less aggressive tumors?**

A. retinoblastoma/p53/PCR
B. pancreatic cancer/RET tyrosine kinase domain (RETTK)/PCR
C. thyroid (papillary) cancer/ K-ras mutations/PCR
D. neuroblastoma/N-myc/fluorescent in situ hybridization (FISH)

46. **Which of the following oncogenes is considered a tumor suppressor protein (which normally functions to prevent cells from dividing in the absence of an appropriate signal) where its deletion or inactivation can be used as a biomarker for tumor progression in many types of cancer, including esophagus, head and neck, bladder, colon, lung, melanoma and cervix?**

A. p16
B. K-ras
C. BRCA 1 and 2
D. N-myc

47. **When differentiating metastatic hepatocellular carcinoma (HCC) from melanoma, alpha-fetoprotein would stain:**
   A. positive for HCC, negative for melanoma
   B. negative for HCC, positive for melanoma
   C. positive for both
   D. negative for both

48. **Which special stain may aid in the diagnosis of metastatic melanoma?**
   A. keratin
   B. neuron-specific enolase
   C. S-100
   D. LCA

49. **What special stain is most helpful in identifying *Pneumocystis carinii?***
   A. iron
   B. Feulgen
   C. GMS
   D. mucicarmine

50. **Well-differentiated mucus-producing adenocarcinomas may be distinguished from poorly differentiated squamous cell carcinomas by using:**
   A. mucicarmine
   B. Giemsa
   C. Gram-Weigert
   D. Feulgen

51. **The identification of fungi may be determined best with what special stain?**
   A. GMS
   B. oil red O
   C. Biebrich-Scarlet
   D. iron

52. **Biomarkers targeted at MSH2 and MLH1 genes (normally involved in correcting replicative errors, ie, mismatched error in DNA bases) can help determine which patients are at risk for Lynch syndrome or hereditary nonpolypoid colorectal cancer. The aberrant molecular process is referred as:**
   A. gene rearrangement
   B. somatic hypermutation
   C. microsatellite instability
   D. loss of heterozygosity

53. **The Feulgen reaction is used for the identification of:**
   A. DNA
   B. melanin
   C. fat
   D. glycogen

54. **Which special stain may aid in differentiating histiocytes from mesothelial cells?**
   A. Feulgen
   B. Prussian blue
   C. Rakoff
   D. neutral red-Janus green

55. **What immunocytochemical stain will help differentiate malignant lymphoma from a neuroendocrine tumor?**
   A. keratin; lymphoma is positive, neuroendocrine tumors are negative
   B. HMB-45; lymphoma is positive, neuroendocrine tumors are negative
   C. leukocyte common antigen; lymphoma is positive, neuroendocrine tumors are negative
   D. PAS; lymphomas are negative, neuroendocrine tumors are positive

56. **Immunocytochemistry might be helpful in differentiating pancreatic adenocarcinoma (PAC) from hepatocellular carcinoma (HCC) by staining with:**
   A. keratin; HCC is positive, PAC is negative
   B. alpha-fetoprotein; HCC is positive, PAC is negative
   C. keratin; HCC is negative, PAC is positive
   D. immunocytochemistry is not helpful in distinguishing these tumors

57. **Differentiating anucleate squamous cells from nucleated squamous cells is possible with the:**
   A. Gram and Gram-Weigert
   B. Prussian blue and Feulgen
   C. PAS and mucicarmine
   D. Shorr and Rakoff

58. **Which of the following cancers are associated with translocations resulting in the chromosomal abnormality t(14;18), t(8;14)?**
   A. follicular lymphoma
   B. acute lymphocytic leukemia
   C. multiple myeloma
   D. Waldenström macroglobinemia

59. **What immunocytochemical stain will have a positive staining reaction and help in the confirmation of a metastatic sarcoma?**

A. keratin
B. vimentin
C. alpha-fetoprotein
D. neuron-specific enolase

60. **Metastatic colonic adenocarcinoma to the liver could be differentiated from primary hepatocellular carcinoma (HCC) by using what immunocytochemical stain?**

A. keratin–low molecular weight (CAM 5.2); HCC is strongly positive, colonic adenocarcinoma is negative
B. keratin–high molecular weight (AE1/AE3); HCC is negative to weakly positive, colonic adenocarcinoma is strongly positive
C. HMB-45; HCC is positive, colonic adenocarcinoma is negative
D. S-100; HCC is negative, colonic adenocarcinoma is positive

61. **Most fungi will stain positive with which of the following special stains?**

A. PAS
B. Nile blue sulfate
C. Shorr
D. Rakoff

62. **Immunocytochemical staining for chromogranin is helpful for the identification of:**

A. lymphoma
B. adenocarcinoma
C. squamous carcinoma
D. carcinoid tumors

63. **Small cell carcinoma may be differentiated from malignant lymphoma by using what special stain?**

A. chromogranin
B. S-100
C. HMB-45
D. alpha-fetoprotein

64. **If staining for glycogen, which special stain is required?**

A. mucicarmine
B. PAS
C. Nile blue sulfate
D. neutral red

65. **Which of the following statements regarding molecular diagnostics is false?**

A. over 5000 diseases have direct genetic causes
B. provides a high sensitivity and increased specificity for most tests and adds diagnostic utility
C. may provide a viable reflex for equivocal morphology
D. turnaround time of FDA approved tests may prohibit use in gynecologic cytopathology

66. **What immunocytochemical stain might help in differentiating metastatic pleomorphic carcinoma of the pancreas from metastatic fibrous histiocytoma (MFH) in liver aspirations?**

A. keratin; positive for carcinoma, negative for MFH
B. keratin; negative for carcinoma, positive for MFH
C. HMB-45; positive for carcinoma, negative for MFH
D. HMB-45; negative for carcinoma, positive for MFH

67. ***Cryptococcus* may be identified best with what special stain?**

A. mucicarmine
B. Gram
C. PAS-D
D. Janus green

68. **HMB-45 may be a useful marker for determining the presence of:**

A. undifferentiated squamous carcinoma
B. hepatocellular carcinoma
C. poorly differentiated adenocarcinoma
D. metastatic melanoma

69. **A helpful stain for the identification of hematopoietic and lymphoid cells is:**

A. Gram
B. PAS
C. Romanovsky
D. mucicarmine

70. A ThinPrep Pap specimen taken from a 44-year-old female immunologically stained for the p16[INK4a] protein. Which of the following represents the most appropriate clinical management?

A. recommend follow-up Pap test every 6 months to determine if progression to adenocarcinoma in situ occurs
B. immediate colposcopy
C. hysterectomy
D. HPV testing in 12 months

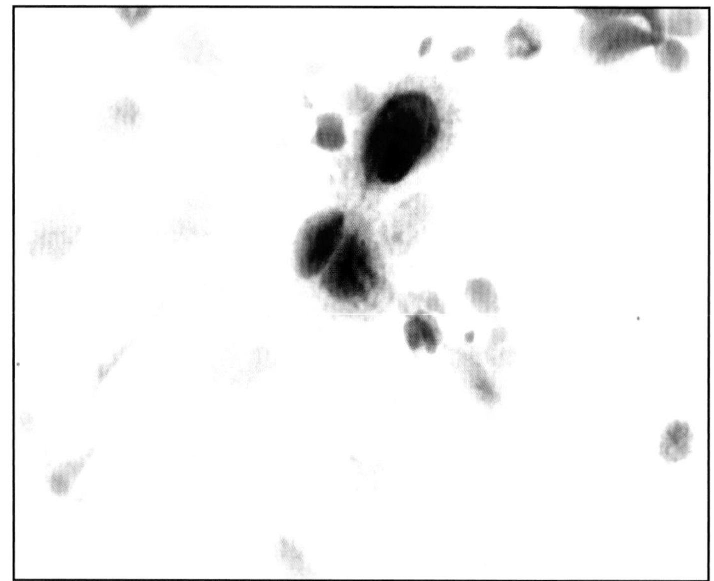

71. A 66-year-old, former Hall of Fame pitcher for the Chicago Cubs, with a history of orpharyngeal cancer presents with a 2-cm cervical neck mass of unknown etiology. The cells illustrated were extracted from the mass and fixed in ethanol and processed for the Papanicolaou stain and in situ hybridization (ISH) using Inform HPV III Family 16 probe (Ventana Medical Systems). ISH stains revealed dark blue to black nuclear dots. The diagnosis is consistent with:

A. reactive lymphoid hyperplasia
B. branchial cleft cyst
C. metastatic squamous cell carcinoma
D. sialadenitis

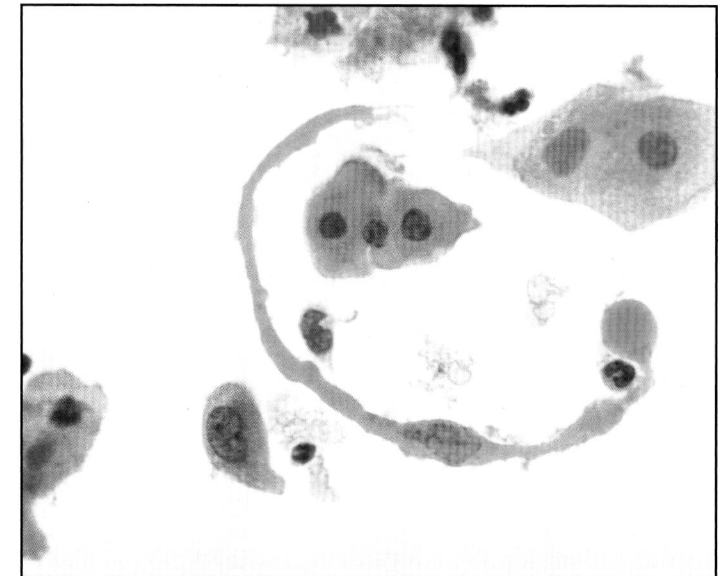

72. A 58-year-old female with a previous history of a breast malignancy presents with difficulty in breathing and a blood-streaked sputum. A liquid-based sputum sample was processed with a modified Pap stain and a fresh sample was submitted for FISH analysis. A multi-target FISH probe to the centromeric region of chromosome 6 and to the 5p15, 8q24 (site of the MYC gene) and 7p12 (site of the EGFR gene) loci revealed 5 cells with multiple gains. These cells represent the Pap-stained cytology. The diagnosis is:

A. metastatic breast cancer (ductal)
B. metastatic colon cancer
C. primary lung cancer (squamous cell carcinoma)
D. benign respiratory epithelium

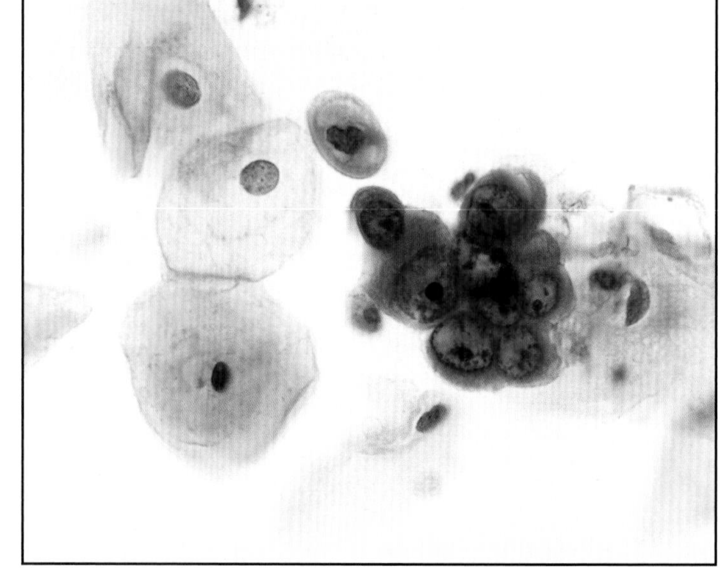

Molecular Techniques and Special Stains *Answer Key*

1. **B increased cell adherence to the slide is associated with the Romanovsky stain**

   Air drying is generally the first step in the Romanovsky or Diff Quik stains, allowing for better cellular adhesion to the slide and decreasing the likelihood that cells will "fall off" the slide, as will often occur when immersing fresh specimens into the alcoholic medium for fixation for compatibility with the Papanicolaou stain. It should be noted, however, that Romanovsky staining is compatible with alcohol-fixed material, yields excellent cytoplasmic detail, and helps with visualization of stromal components.

   DeMay RM, The Art & Science of Cytopathology.
   Romanovsky stain, p. 14.

2. **A mucin**

   For related information, see answer to question 1.

   DeMay RM, The Art & Science of Cytopathology.
   Romanovsky stain, p. 14.

3. **B increasing number of techniques for infectious diseases and tumor diagnostics**

   The use of molecular tests has become invaluable, as adjunctive assays for establishing the diagnosis of precancerous cervical disease are now considered an important reflex for equivocal cellular morphology (ASC-US). Within the past 5 years, myriad platforms have been developed that have helped standardize the reliability of companion molecular diagnostics using semi-automation—increasing the overall sensitivity of testing.

   Schmitt FC, Longatto-Filho A, Valent A, Vielh P. Molecular techniques in cytopathology practice. Journal of Clinical Pathology. 2008 Mar;61(3):258-67.

4. **D the Romanovsky stain is a metachromatic stain enabling better visualization of various mucins, neurosecretory granules, and stromal elements**

   For related information, see answer to questions 1 and 2.

   DeMay RM, The Art & Science of Cytopathology.
   Romanovsky stain, p. 14

5. **D methyl green pyronine**

   Methyl green pyronine (MGP) binds to the cytoplasm and/or nucleus of cells with abundant RNA (endoplasmic reticulum or pronounced nucleoli). Cell markers such as leukocyte common antigen (LCA) are usually negative with plasma cells and therefore may also be helpful in differentiating these two malignancies.

   DeMay RM, The Art & Science of Cytopathology.
   Other special stains, p. 16.

6. **D integrating reporting enhances the overall standard of care**

   Cotest results are now the standard of care for reporting atypical gynecologic Pap tests (ASC-US) under the 2006 ASCCP Guidelines for the management of abnormal cervical lesions. In addition, the efficiency of testing (turn around time of results) is not compromised using the latest generation of molecular assays.

   Schmitt FC, et al. Molecular techniques in cytopathology practice. Clinic Pathol. 2008;61(3):258-67.

7. **A aminopeptidase**

   Aminopeptidase positivity suggests bile duct, kidney, bladder, or stomach origin rather than hepatocellular carcinoma. Negative staining with alpha-fetoprotein, an oncofetal glycoprotein, may be helpful in this case but does not necessarily exclude hepatocellular carcinoma. Antinuclear staining for bile canaliculi may also have utility. For related information, see question 42 in the FNA chapter.

   DeMay RM, The Art & Science of Cytopathology.
   Enzyme reactions, p. 16.

8. **C alkaline phosphatase**

   Alkaline phosphatase, although nonspecific, reacts with adenocarcinomas including those from the lung, ovary, endometrium, or kidneys but does not react with lesions of gastrointestinal tract origin. In this case, a positive reaction would exclude the probability that the patient has a metastatic colonic adenocarcinoma and may verify a new primary malignancy. Aryl sulfatase, on the other hand, would react just the opposite, failing to react with the suspected bronchogenic tumor. If it were suspected that the cells were metastatic from the colon, a positive reaction would be seen.

   DeMay RM, The Art & Science of Cytopathology.
   Enzyme reactions, p. 16.

9. **A colposcopy is likely to reveal a high-grade squamous intraepithelial lesion**

   Confirmation of high-risk HPV DNA is possible with PCR. Quantitative RT-PCR may be even more useful in determining RNA transcripts in cervical infections with low viral copy number. However, PCR is not without its inherent limitations, including the relatively costly nature of performing the tests and the possibility of false-positive results due to laboratory contamination or procedural errors.

   DeMay RM, The Art & Science of Cytopathology.
   Polymerase chain reaction, p. 22.

10. D strand displacement amplification

Common molecular tests in cytopathology include Hybrid Capture 2, in situ hybridization (co-testing for the cytologic diagnosis of ASC-US) and fluorescent in situ hybridization (useful for determining recurrent bladder cancer and prognostic markers for breast cancer).

Schmitt FC, et al. Molecular techniques in cytopathology practice. Clinic Pathol. 2008;61(3):258-267.

11. D specimens are considered positive if any of the low-risk or high-risk viral infections are found within each respective probe cocktail

The probe cocktails simply indicate which patients are at low risk (probes that can hybridize to any of HPV types 6, 11, 42, 43, and 44) or high risk (types 16, 18, 31, 33, 35, 45, 51, 52, and 56).

Manos MM, et al, Identifying women with cervical neoplasia: Using human papillomavirus DNA testing for equivocal Papincolaou results. JAMA. 1999;281(17), pp. 1605–1610.

12. A it can be performed on archival tissue specimens

In situ hybridization can be performed on fresh unstained or archival (paraffin-embedded) formalin-fixed tissues as well as archived cervical smears or samples.

Liang XM, et al, In situ hybridization with human papillomavirus using biotinylated DNA probes on archival cervical smears. J Histochem Cytochem. 1991;39(6), pp. 771–775.

13. A antibodies attach to captured hybrids reacting with a substrate to emit an amplified chemiluminescent signal

The specimen is initially hybridized with RNA probe (assume target sequence is present), captured by an RNA probe to detect hybrids, followed by conjugation with antibodies that attach to the captured hybrids ultimately reacting with a substrate to emit an amplified chemiluminescent signal.

Dehn D, Torkko KC, Shroyer KR. Human papillomavirus testing and molecular markers of cervical dysplasia and carcinoma. Cancer. 2007; 111(1):1-14.

14. A DNA aneuploidy confirms high-grade lesions

DNA aneuploidy in cervical lesions is regarded as a true precursor for cervical cancer. Aneuploidy is absent in low-grade lesions and thereby may help clinicians determine which patients need treatment. In addition, DNA aneuploidy in post irradiation cervicovaginal smears after cervical carcinoma may indicate recurrence

Wright TC, et al, Blaustein's Pathology for the Female Genital Tract, pp. 229–277; and Davey DD, Zaleski S, Sattich M, et al. Cancer. 1998;25;84(1): pp. 11–16.

15. C carbohydrate moieties

For related information, see answer to question 61.

DeMay RM, The Art & Science of Cytopathology.
Other special stains, p. 15.

16. D Masson trichrome

Masson trichrome stains will help identify skeletal or smooth muscle differentiation versus non-muscle fibers.

DeMay RM, The Art & Science of Cytopathology.
Other special stains, p. 15.

17. C desmin

Epithelial tumors are generally positive for keratin and soft tissue tumors are positive for vimentin, but not exclusively. Certain tumors of both categories such as renal cell carcinoma and synovial sarcoma as well as Wilms tumor and mesotheliomas are some of the lesions that cross-react with both immunocytochemical stains.

DeMay RM, The Art & Science of Cytopathology.
Brown stains and "magic markers" (immunocytochemistry), p. 16.

18. B conventional microscopy (bright field) can be used to interpret genetic signals

In addition to the specificity of in situ hybridization, an added advantage is that the molecular signal can be compared with the cytomorphology such that the interpreter can view a microscopic signal in situ for comparative purposes.

Guo M, et al. A human papillomavirus testing system in women with abnormal Pap results: a comparison study with follow-up biopsies. Acta Cytol. 2007;51(5):749-54.

19. C polymerase chain reaction (PCR)

PCR is the prototypical method for cloning and amplifying target nucleic acid in a rapid fashion (hours) such that the gene of interest can be detected in vitro.

Buckingham, L and Flaws M. Molecular diagnostics; fundamentals, methods, & clinical applications. F.A. Davis 2007.

20. C they often aid in the diagnosis of lesions that are difficult to classify

Immunocytochemical stains are useful but are often not specific. It is reasonable that other diagnostic procedures be performed to rule on the sensitivity of immunocytochemical markers. They can often be as misleading as they are useful.

DeMay RM, The Art & Science of Cytopathology.
Brown stains and "magic markers" (immunocytochemistry), p. 16.

21. D Factor VIII

Factor VIII marks endothelial components only.

DeMay RM, The Art & Science of Cytopathology.
Brown stains and "magic markers" (immunocytochemistry), p. 17.

22. D invader (cleavage-based) amplification

Targets for this application include cystic fibrosis, factor V Leiden, and high-risk human papillomavirus.

Buckingham, L and Flaws M. Molecular diagnostics; fundamentals, methods & clinical applications. F.A. Davis 2007.

23. A melanin

Spindle cell melanomas and clear cell sarcoma can be differentiated from other spindle cell or pleomorphic sarcomas owing to their melanin positivity.

DeMay RM, The Art & Science of Cytopathology.
Other special stains, p. 15.

24. C glial fibrillary acidic protein (GFIP)

Vimentin is found in mesenchymal cells and sarcomas, desmin is found in all kinds of muscle tissue but is more sensitive to skeletal muscle, neurofilaments are found in neuronal tumors, and glial acidic proteins mark glial supportive cells of the central nervous system.

DeMay RM, The Art & Science of Cytopathology.
Brown stains and "magic markers" (immunocytochemistry), p. 16.

25. B invader (cleavage-based) amplification

Targets for this application include cystic fibrosis, factor V Leiden, and high-risk human papillomavirus.

Wong AK, et al. Human papillomavirus (HPV) in atypical squamous cervical cytology: the Invader HPV test as a new screening assay. Clinic Microbiol. 2008;46(3):869-875.

26. C Hybrid Capture 2 testing for high-risk HPV

It may be appropriate to perform HPV testing for high-risk (transforming) virotypes to determine if atypical cells of undetermined significance (ASC-US) or (ASC-H) are significant cytologic findings. If the HPV test is positive, colposcopy and biopsy are recommended (ALTS trial data, Shiffman and Solomon, National Cancer Institute). If the HPV high-risk test is negative, the patient will be asked for a repeat Pap in 6 months or return to routine surveillance. Triage of atypical cells may help reduce unnecessary colposcopy on patients with equivocal Pap tests by determining which patients are truly at risk for progressive cervical intraepithelial disease. Between 10% and 20% of equivocal Pap tests confirmed positive for high-risk HPV may prove to be high-grade disease at colposcopy.

Ferenczy A, Int J Gynecol Cancer.
1995;5(5), pp. 321–328.

27. A negative predictive value

Hybrid Capture 2 represents an FDA-approved assay for the detection of high risk HPV. The sensitivity for detecting CIN 2 or higher is 83-96% and the negative predictive value is 98%.

Dehn D, et al. Cancer. 2007;111(1):1-14.

28. B argentaffin

Silver stains may be useful when demonstrating neurosecretory granules from neuroendocrine lesions such as carcinoid tumors, small cell carcinomas, islet cell tumors, medullary carcinomas, paragangliomas, and neuroblastomas. However, immunocytochemical staining with neuron-specific enolase or chromogranin may prove more useful.

DeMay RM, The Art & Science of Cytopathology.
Other special stains, p. 15.

29. A captured RNA–DNA hybrids with alkaline phosphatase conjugated antibodies are detected with a chemiluminescent substrate and signaled by a luminometer

Hybrid Capture 2 is the only commercially approved in vitro HPV test for determining low- or high-risk infections. The test uses microplates for capturing RNA hybrids and has an analytical sensitivity of 1.0 pg/mL (5,000 HPV genomes per test). The test is approved direct to vial or can be tested off liquid-based medium.

Manos MM, et al, JAMA.
1999;281(17), pp. 1605–1610.

30. D sensitivity for HSIL and cancer

Hybrid Capture 2 represents an FDA-approved assay for the detection of high risk HPV. The sensitivity for detecting CIN 2 or higher is 83-96% and the negative predictive value is 98%.

Dehn D, et al. Cancer. 2007;111(1):1-14.

31. D Ki-67

Studies have shown that expression of the proliferation marker Ki-67 in normal, metaplastic, and dysplastic changes. The MIB1 monoclonal antibody shows progressively increased Ki-67 positive cells as CIN grades increase. Other studies have used Ki-67 to discriminate HSIL from atypical atrophy

al-Saleh W, Proliferation in the normal cervix and in preinvasive cervical lesions. J Clin Pathol. 1995;104(2), pp. 154–160; and Bulten J, de Wilde PC, Schijf C et al. Decreased expression of ki-67 in atrophic cervical epithelium of post-menopausal women. J Pathol. 2000;190(5): pp. 545–553.

32. A excellent tissue or cytology localization of HPV-infected cells

In addition to the specificity of in situ hybridization, an added advantage is that the molecular signal can be compared with the cytomorphology such that the interpreter can view a microscopic signal in situ for comparative purposes.

Guo M, et al. Acta Cytol. 2007;51(5):749-754.

33. C squamous cell carcinoma

High-molecular-weight keratin is expressed in squamous cell carcinomas and mesotheliomas, whereas low-molecular-weight keratins are expressed in all cell lines with epithelial differentiation, such as endodermal, neuroectodermal, mesenchymal, or germ cell tumors.

DeMay RM, The Art & Science of Cytopathology.
Brown stains and "magic markers" (immunocytochemistry), p. 16.

34. D bronchogenic carcinoma

Aneuploidy or high S phase fraction may assist in the confirmation of a malignant neoplastic disease. Flow cytometry may also prove useful in the diagnosis of high-grade dysplasia from ulcerative colitis, carcinoma in situ in urothelial tumors, metastatic carcinomatous in cerebral spinal fluid specimens, and carcinoma of the breast via fine-needle aspiration. It also has prognostic utility with hematopoietic lesions, neuroblastoma, medulloblastoma, and acute lymphoblastic leukemia.

DeMay RM, The Art & Science of Cytopathology.
Flow cytometry, p. 21.

35. A fluorescent in situ hybridization (FISH)

HER2 overexpression is associated with clinically aggressive breast tumors which have a higher recurrence rate and poorer prognosis. The use of a quantifiable FISH technique is considered more sensitive and specific when compared to the subjective interpretation of an immunohistochemical stain.

Sińczak-Kuta A, Tomaszewska R, Rudnicka-Sosin L, et al. Evaluation of HER2/neu gene amplification in patients with invasive breast carcinoma; Comparison of in situ hybridization methods. Polish Journal of Pathology. 2007;58(1):41-50.

36. C fluorescent in situ hybridization (FISH)

Although the sensitivity of cytology is good for establishing the diagnosis of high-grade urothelial tumors, low-grade tumors are difficult and often impossible to distinguish from benign urothelial cells. In addition, bladder cancer commonly recurs, and early recurrence is often difficult to detect cytologically with cystoscopic specimens. Utilization of FISH can help identify both low-grade neoplasms and recurrent transitional cell carcinoma of the bladder.

Daniely M, Rona R, Kaplan T, et al. Combined morphologic and fluorescence in situ hybridization analysis of voided urine samples for the detection and follow-up of bladder cancer in patients with benign urine cytology. Urol Oncol. 2008;26(3):332.

37. B adenocarcinoma

In contrast to adenocarcinomas and lymphomas, squamous cell carcinomas would reveal tonofilaments such as intercellular bridges (desmosomes) and microvilli attached at their tips by desmosomes.

DeMay RM, The Art & Science of Cytopathology.
Uranyl acetate and lead citrate stain (electron microscopy), p. 19.

38. C high complexity

The CLIA laboratory and staff must be approved for high complexity testing.

Manos MM, et al, JAMA.
1999;281(17), pp. 1605–1610.

39. A Biebrich-Scarlet

The Barr body or sex chromatin body will stain nicely eosinophilic against a green nuclear background.

Koss LG, Diagnostic Cytology.
Cytologic techniques/principles of operation of a laboratory of cytology, pp. 1492–1505.

40. **D Fouchet method**

Fouchet method stains for bile pigment. The intracytoplasmic pigment will stain olive green.

Koss LG, Diagnostic Cytology.
Cytologic techniques/principles of operation of a laboratory of cytology, pp. 1492–1505.

41. **B iron stain**

PAS stains for hemosiderin and may prove useful in discriminating hemosiderin-laden macrophages from melanoma. These benign cells are also immunocytochemically negative for S-100, HMB-45, Melan A and MITF (Microphthalmia-associated transcription factor)—all which are positive in a high percentage of melanomas.

DeMay RM, The Art & Science of Cytopathology.
The cytoplasm, p. 47.

Wang JF, Sarma DP, Ulmer P. Diagnostic dilemma: HMB-45 and Melan-A negative tumor, can it be still a melanoma?: MITF (Microphthalmia-associated transcription factor) stain may confirm the diagnosis. The Internet Journal of Dermatology. 2007. Volume 5 Number 1.

42. **A Urovision® (Abbott Molecular, Inc.)**

Although the sensitivity of cytology is good for establishing the diagnosis of high-grade urothelial tumors, low-grade tumors are difficult and often impossible to distinguish from benign urothelial cells. In addition, bladder cancer commonly recurs, and early recurrence is often difficult to detect cytologically with cystoscopic specimens. Utilization of FISH can help identify both low grade neoplasms and recurrent transitional cell carcinoma of the bladder.

Daniely M, et al. Urol Oncol. 2008;26(3):332.

43. **B Sudan black**

Sudan black will stain phospholipids black.

DeMay RM, The Art & Science of Cytopathology.
Other special stains, p. 15.

44. **A Nile blue sulfate**

Nile blue sulfate will differentially stain only cells of sebaceous gland origin; therefore, an estimation of fetal maturity may be established based on the presence of these differentiated cells.

Koss LG, Diagnostic Cytology.
Cytologic techniques/principles of operation of a laboratory of cytology, pp. 1492–1505.

45. **D neuroblastoma/n-myc/ fluorescent in situ hybridization (FISH)**

In addition to overexpression of n-myc in the PI3K-mediated VEGF regulation of neuroblastoma cells, p53 oncoproteins have been identified in up to 50% of all cancers, K-ras mutations have been found in pancreatic cancer, and the RET tyrosine kinase domain (RETTK) is overexpressed in papillary carcinoma of the thyroid.

Kang J, Rychahou PG, Ishola TA, Mourot JM, Evers BM, Chung DH. N-myc is a novel regulator of PI3K-mediated VEGF expression in neuroblastoma. Oncogene. 2008 Feb 18.

46. **A p16**

Overexpression of $p16^{INK4a}$ protein indicates infection and genomic integration of high-risk human papillomavirus (high-risk HPV) and may be useful for determining the progression of abnormal cervical lesions to carcinoma.

Holladay EB, Logan S, Arnold J, Knessel B and Smith DG. A Comparison of the Clinical Utility of p16INK4a Immunolocalization to the Presence of Human Papillomavirus by Digene Hybrid Capture 2 for the Detection of Cervical Dysplasia/Neoplasia. Cancer Cytopathology. Vol. 108, (6) (31 October 2006).

47. **A positive for HCC, negative for melanoma**

Alpha-fetoprotein will positively distinguish hepatocellular carcinoma from melanoma but will not differentiate liver cell dysplasias and germ cell neoplasms.

DeMay RM, The Art & Science of Cytopathology.
Oncofetal antigens, p. 18.

48. **C S-100**

S-100, HMB-45, Melan A or MITF (microphthalmia-associated transcription factor) all preferentially react with melanoma cells.

Wang JF, et al. The Internet Journal of Dermatology. 2007. (5)1.

49. **C GMS**

Gomori methenamine silver stains for fungi and *Pneumocystis carinii.* These infectious agents will stain characteristically gray to black.

DeMay RM, The Art & Science of Cytopathology.
Fungi, p. 57.

50. A mucicarmine

Mucicarmine stains for intracellular mucin, found within mucus-producing glandular lesions. Mucin will stain rose to red in color.

DeMay RM, The Art & Science of Cytopathology.
Other special stains, p. 15.

51. A GMS

For related information, see answer to question 49.

DeMay RM, The Art & Science of Cytopathology.
Fungi, pp. 56–57.

52. C microsatellite instability

Lynch Syndrome is an inherited condition that accounts for 5% of all colon cancers.

Buckingham and Flaws. Molecular diagnostics; fundamentals, methods, & clinical applications. F.A. Davis 2007.

53. A DNA

The Feulgen reaction will positively stain double-stranded nucleic acid deep red to purple in color. RNA does not stain with Feulgen.

Koss LG, Diagnostic Cytology.
Cytologic techniques/principles of operation of a laboratory of cytology, pp. 1492–1505.

54. D neutral red-Janus green

Neutral red-Janus green, a supravital stain that must be performed on nonfixed specimens, will positively identify white blood cells and histiocytes from mesothelial cells.

Koss LG, Diagnostic Cytology.
Cytologic techniques/principles of operation of a laboratory of cytology, pp. 1492–1505.

55. C leukocyte common antigen; lymphoma is positive, neuroendocrine tumors are negative

For related information, see answer to questions 62 and 63.

DeMay RM, The Art & Science of Cytopathology.
Other cell markers, p. 18.

56. B alpha-fetoprotein; HCC is positive, PAC is negative

For related information, see answer to question 47.

DeMay RM, The Art & Science of Cytopathology.
Oncofetal antigens, p. 18.

57. D Shorr and Rakoff

Shorr and Rakoff will differentiate anucleate squames (orange or red) and nucleated squamous cells (pale in superficial cells, green in intermediate, parabasal, and basal cells).

Koss LG, Diagnostic Cytology.
Cytologic techniques/principles of operation of a laboratory of cytology, pp. 1492–1505.

58. A follicular lymphoma

Translocations often given rise to the development of hematological malignancies, such as chronic myelogenous leukemia and follicular lymphoma.

Buckingham and Flaws. Molecular diagnostics; fundamentals, methods, & clinical applications. F.A. Davis 2007.

59. B vimentin

Vimentin will strongly express positivity in cells of mesenchymal origin.

DeMay RM, The Art & Science of Cytopathology.
Filaments, p. 16.

60. B keratin–high-molecular-weight (AE1/AE3); HCC is negative to weakly positive, colonic adenocarcinoma is strongly positive

Only high-molecular-weight (MW) keratin is effective in discriminating these lesions. Low-MW keratin will positively identify both neoplasms with equal intensity.

DeMay RM, The Art & Science of Cytopathology.
Filaments, p. 16.

61. A PAS

Periodic acid–Schiff stain will color fungi, carbohydrates, and glycogen as magenta red.

DeMay RM, The Art & Science of Cytopathology.
Other special stains, p. 15.

62. D carcinoid tumors

Neuroendocrine tumors such as carcinoid tumors, small cell carcinomas, neuroblastomas, medullary tumors of the thyroid, and pituitary tumors may stain positive with chromogranin or neuron-specific enolase.

DeMay RM, The Art & Science of Cytopathology.
Hormones, p. 18.

63. **A** chromogranin

Lymphomas are positive for common leukocytic antigen. For related information, see answer to question 62.

DeMay RM, The Art & Science of Cytopathology.
Hormones, p. 18.

64. **B** PAS

For related information, see answer to question 61.

DeMay RM, The Art & Science of Cytopathology.
Other special stains, p. 15.

65. **D** turn around time of FDA approved tests may prohibit use in gynecologic cytopathology

The efficiency of testing (turn around time of results) is not compromised using the latest generation of molecular assays. In addition, co-testing cytology and high risk HPV molecular results are now considered the standard of care for reporting atypical gynecologic Pap tests (ASC-US).

Schmitt FC, et al. Clinic Pathol. 2008;61(3):258-267.

66. **A** keratin; positive for carcinoma, negative for MFH

Keratin intermediate filaments will identify pancreatic carcinomas as epithelial lesions but will not stain malignant fibrous histiocytoma. However, keratin may be co-expressed in muscle sarcomas, synovial sarcomas, epithelioid sarcomas, and Wilms tumors.

DeMay RM, The Art & Science of Cytopathology.
Filaments, p. 16.

67. **A** mucicarmine

The mucinous capsule of *Cryptococcus neoformans* will stain rose to red.

DeMay RM, The Art & Science of Cytopathology.
Fungi, p. 56.

68. **D** metastatic melanoma

For related information, see answer to question 48.

DeMay RM, The Art & Science of Cytopathology.
Other cell markers, p. 19.

69. **C** Romanovsky

The Romanovsky stains may be used to analyze lymphoreticular and hematopoietic specimens that are air-dried. This stain may prove particularly useful when differentiating lymphopoietic malignancies.

DeMay RM, The Art & Science of Cytopathology.
Romanovsky stain, pp. 14–15.

70. **B** immediate colposcopy

Overexpression of p16^{INK4a} protein indicates infection and genomic integration of high-risk human papillomavirus (high-risk HPV) and may be useful for determining the progression of abnormal cervical lesions to carcinoma.

Holladay EB, et al. Cancer Cytopathol. 2006;108, (6).

71. **C** metastatic squamous cell carcinoma

These cells represent a metastasis from a primary orpharyngeal carcinoma. A necrotic background lacking lympho proliferative elements with keratinizing debris with scattered pleomorphic squamous cells possessing smudged opaque nuclei are represented. Intranuclear signals as confirmed via molecular confirmation with ISH assists with the diagnosis. Even in the absence of malignant morphology, the presence of true squamous elements and confirmation with ISH may help establish the diagnosis of metastatic carcinoma.

72. **A** metastatic breast cancer (ductal)

FISH allows for the differentiation of true neoplastic glandular cells from reactive atypia. These cells, representing ductal carcinoma of the breast, present as hypercellular epithelial cells arranged in well-formed microacini with pleomorphic nuclei, nuclear crowding and overlapping, hyperchromasia, irregular nuclear membranes, irregular chromatin and prominent nucleoli.

Spasenija S, Glatz K, Schoenegg R, et al--. Chest. 2006;129:1629-1635.

Chapter 12

Laboratory Management and Administration

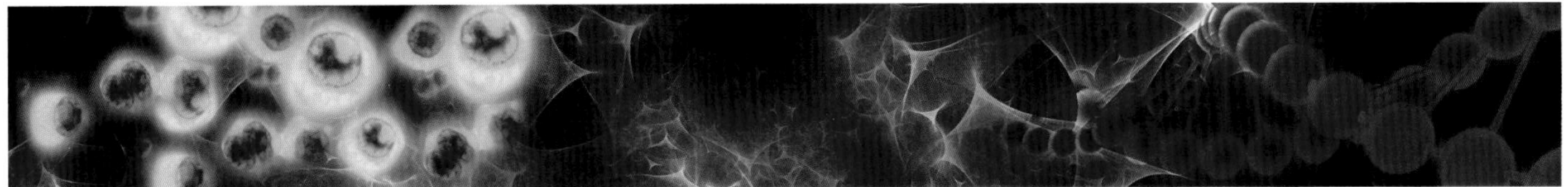

1. The acceptable deviation of a determined laboratory analysis from its true value is its:

   A. standard deviation
   B. allowable error
   C. predictive value
   D. coefficient of variance

2. According to Maslow's Hierarchy of Needs, which of the following is a primary need and thus serves as a prime motivator in the workplace?

   A. acceptance by peers
   B. recognition for accomplishments
   C. job security
   D. job satisfaction

3. In a criterion-based job description, what factor is important to task completion but has little impact on outcomes if the task is performed incorrectly?

   A. critical task
   B. essential task
   C. outcome metrics
   D. key job area

4. What common term is defined as the official acknowledgment of technical or professional competence?

   A. peer assurance
   B. credentialing
   C. registration
   D. regulation

5. Analysis of what type of costs enables the measurement of productivity in terms of fluctuations in the cost to produce a given service?

   A. unit
   B. direct
   C. indirect
   D. mixed

6. Which of the following measures of group effectiveness is defined by the ratio of outputs to inputs?

   A. production
   B. adaptiveness
   C. development
   D. efficiency

7. Which federal agency regulates market entry of medical devices, laboratory instruments, reagents, and systems?

   A. Centers for Disease Control
   B. Health Care Financing Administration
   C. Food and Drug Administration
   D. Department of Defense

8. Which of the following facilities would be subject to the regulations of the National Labor Relations Act?

   A. a VA hospital with annual receipts of $1,000,000
   B. a nursing home with annual receipts of $90,000
   C. a for-profit adult day care center with annual receipts of $125,000
   D. a not-for-profit hospital with annual receipts of $300,000

9. **When negligence appears so obvious that the court shifts the burden of proof to the defendant, the concept is referred to as:**

A. *negligence ipso facto*
B. *res ipsa loquitor*
C. *negligence per se*
D. *respondeat superior*

10. **A manager following McGregor's theory-Y leadership style would do which of the following?**

A. require employees to set their own goals and objectives
B. closely supervise and control staff work responsibilities
C. motivate staff with financial reward for good performance
D. structure workflow according to published standards

11. **Costs that are sensitive to changes in test volume are called:**

A. fixed
B. variable
C. direct
D. indirect

12. **Which agency investigates alleged discrimination cases under Title VII?**

A. National Labor Relations Board
B. Equal Employment Opportunity Commission
C. US Department of Labor
D. Affirmative Action

13. **Which method of costing (cost accumulation) attempts to allocate indirect costs to the hospital laboratory?**

A. direct
B. standard
C. variance
D. full

14. **According to Herzberg's Two Factor motivation theory, what two factors contribute to strong motivation of employees?**

A. hygiene factors and satisfiers
B. interpersonal factors and motivators
C. good feelings and personal factors
D. recognition and expectation

15. **A technologist commits a major error in laboratory testing that results directly in the death of a patient. The family of the patient brings suit against the technologist, the pathologist, and the hospital administrators. What is the legal premise that gives them the right to sue the hospital administrators?**

A. *res ipsa loquitor*
B. *respondeat superior*
C. *procedenti ab utroque*
D. *locum tenens*

16. **Which one of the following questions can be legally asked on an employment application?**

A. Have you ever been arrested?
B. Do you have any relatives employed by this company?
C. Do you have a disability?
D. Do you prefer to be addressed as Ms., Mrs., or Mr.?

17. **What set of laws and regulations pertains to labor relations in the private sector?**

A. Civil Service Reform Act
B. National Labor Relations Act
C. state labor laws
D. local jurisdiction laws

18. **In plotting statistical tests of method comparison data, what calculation is a measure of proportional bias?**

A. slope of the line
B. intercept of the line
C. standard error
D. correlation coefficient

19. **What is the most commonly cited reason for conducting a performance appraisal?**

A. documentation of disciplinary action
B. behavior modification
C. salary and promotion decisions
D. competency assessment

20. **In the context of employee performance appraisal, a standard may be defined as a:**

A. reference for the formation of judgments
B. clear definition of what constitutes good or bad performance
C. mutual consent to specified goals
D. measure to which like objects are expected to conform

21. **The Age Discrimination in Employment Act (ADEA) protects employees against discrimination in terms of paid benefits and continued employment to workers over what age?**

A. 18
B. 21
C. 40
D. 70

22. **What agency is responsible for oversight of labor relations in the federal sector?**

A. National Labor Relations Board
B. Equal Employment Opportunity Commission
C. Merit Systems Protection Board
D. Federal Labor Relations Authority

23. **According to Herzberg's Two Factor motivation theory, a marginal employee will be more likely to perform at unacceptable levels when what factors are absent?**

A. motivators
B. hygiene
C. interpersonal
D. expectation

24. **Which of the following quality improvement tools is best for determining the significance of data?**

A. Pareto diagram
B. fishbone diagram
C. scatter diagram
D. affinity diagram

25. **Which legal doctrine holds an employer liable for the actions of an employee?**

A. *res ipsa loquitor*
B. *respondeat superior*
C. *negligence per se*
D. *compar sit laudatio*

26. **What method of process control can be used to assess the repeatability and accuracy of test results?**

A. reference sample
B. control sample
C. gold standard
D. predictable standard

27. **According to French and Raven's bases of power model, a manager who is able to lead by the charisma of her personality demonstrates what type of power of influence?**

A. reward
B. expert
C. referent
D. legitimate

28. **What factor is the most common reason for CLIA proficiency testing failure?**

A. imprecision
B. inaccuracy
C. bias
D. internal coefficient of variation

29. **What is the most important management decision in the implementation of a Westgard process control system?**

A. number of controls analyzed
B. desirable error detection rate
C. acceptable rejection rate
D. acceptable standard deviation

30. **A member of the laboratory team likes to work alone, prefers to solve new problems, likes analysis and putting things into logical order, and works best following a predetermined plan. What Myers-Briggs Type is this person most likely to be?**

A. introvert, intuiting, thinking, judging
B. extrovert, sensing, feeling, perceiving
C. introvert, sensing, thinking, judging
D. extrovert, intuiting, feeling, judging

31. **The ability of a laboratory analysis to measure or detect a given test outcome consistently over time refers to the test's:**

A. sensitivity
B. specificity
C. precision
D. accuracy

32. **The ability of a laboratory analysis to detect the smallest amount of an element or analyte is a measure of its:**

A. specificity
B. sensitivity
C. precision
D. accuracy

33. **In examining Levy-Jennings Process control charts, a change in the precision of a test would be reflected as a:**

A. dispersion
B. trend
C. shift
D. cluster

34. **Which term refers to governmental control over an economic market?**

A. accreditation
B. certification
C. licensure
D. regulation

35. **Laboratories in which of the following settings are exempt from CLIA '88 regulation?**

A. physician office
B. Pap smear laboratories
C. skilled nursing facilities
D. Department of Defense drug surveillance facilities

36. **What individual is qualified as General Supervisor under CLIA '88?**

A. PhD degree with 1 year of experience in cytopathology
B. MS degree with 5 years of experience, 1 in cytopathology
C. BS degree with 5 years of experience, 2 in cytopathology
D. BS degree with 3 years of experience, 2 in cytopathology

37. **Under CLIA '88 guidelines, a cytotechnologist may evaluate:**

A. 120 slides per day
B. 200 slides per day
C. a total number established by the Technical Supervisor, not to exceed 100
D. a total number established by the General Supervisor, not to exceed 100

38. **What is considered a necessary component of an annual report?**

A. cytology-histology correlation
B. number of patients requesting information
C. needs assessment of the personnel benefits
D. the square footage of the cytotechnologist's workspace

39. **Cytopreparatory technicians, those individuals responsible for the preparation of cytologic material, are required to meet what CLIA regulation?**

A. cytology degree, certification by the American Society for Clinical Pathology
B. cytology degree, certification by the American Society for Cytotechnologists
C. high school degree, supervision by the General Supervisor
D. no degree required, only supervision by General Supervisor

40. The maximum number of slides allowed per 24-hour period for primary reviewing by the cytotechnologist under CLIA '88 is:

A. 80
B. 100
C. 120
D. 150

41. CLIA '88 regulations require that original requisitions be kept for a minimum of:

A. 2 years
B. 5 years
C. 10 years
D. 20 years

42. All of the following are considered important managerial responsibilities, except:

A. adhering to the laboratory procedure manual
B. planning a weekly budget
C. organization of staff
D. development of internal and external quality control and quality assurance

43. Optimally, each cytotechnologist participates in continuing education:

A. at least 1 hour per year
B. in house as well as through professional societies
C. through all of the professional agencies at least 5 times per month
D. a minimum of 10 hours per week

44. Under CLIA '88, the Technical Supervisor is defined as:

A. the cytotechnologist supervisor
B. the cytotechnologist in charge of the laboratory
C. the pathologist in charge of cytology
D. both the cytotechnologist supervisor and the pathologist in charge of cytology

45. Under CLIA '88, copies of final reports must be kept for a minimum of:

A. 2 years
B. 5 years
C. 10 years
D. 20 years

46. Which statement is correct regarding specimen preparation?

A. gynecologic specimens must be stained separately from nongynecologic specimens
B. staining quality should be checked weekly
C. all stains and solutions must be dated by the laboratory supervisor
D. all solutions must be filtered a minimum of once per month

47. When ordering laboratory supplies, one may:

A. jointly purchase supplies with the histology laboratory
B. make sure to accumulate inventory
C. order 3 years in advance
D. order supplies after the solution runs out to avoid oversupplying

48. Accreditation of a cytotechnology program in the United States is determined by:

A. American Society for Clinical Pathology
B. American Society of Cytopathology
C. American Society for Cytotechnology
D. American Pathology Association

49. The CLIA regulations stipulate that glass slides must be kept for a minimum of:

A. 2 years
B. 5 years
C. 10 years
D. 20 years

50. Should a cytotechnology laboratory vacancy occur, the best mechanism to compensate until the position if filled is to:

A. maximize the total number of specimens each cytotechnologist can review
B. increase productivity
C. stagger work hours/split shifts to cover the laboratory operations
D. train individuals on the job until it can be filled by a qualified individual

51. The maximum number of slides allowed per 24-hour period (both primary and re-screen) that a cytotechnologist can review under CLIA '88 is:

A. 80
B. 100
C. 120
D. primary review cannot exceed 80 but there is no limit on the number of re-screen cases

52. A primary cytotechnologist diagnostic error is defined as:

A. missing by one grade, ASCUS to LGSIL
B. failing to determine specimen type
C. incorrect judgment of specimen adequacy
D. missing an obvious malignancy

53. The purpose of quality control and quality assurance protocols is:

A. to ensure that the job gets done right the first time
B. to ensure that the job eventually gets done correctly
C. to increase revenues for the laboratory
D. to identify strengths so that administration can see that the laboratory is doing a good job

54. A uniform, strict set of guidelines that apply to all laboratories reimbursable by Medicare/Medicaid are referred to as:

A. Clinical Laboratory Improvement Amendments of 1988 (CLIA '88)
B. Occupational Safety and Health regulations
C. Bethesda System terminology
D. interlaboratory comparison regulations

55. CLIA '88 requires:

A. 10% review of focused or high-risk cases as well as random review
B. 10% random review only
C. 10% focused or high-risk only
D. 10% of abnormal diagnoses

56. Quality assurance is defined as:

A. collecting the data to determine efficacy of the individual and/or laboratory
B. determining patterns or trends in test accuracy with the collected data
C. reexamination of the negative material
D. performing a 10% review on all gynecologic cases

57. Which are considered important budgetary considerations for laboratory operations?

A. calculating the direct and indirect costs associated with laboratory operations
B. cost of equipment maintenance on a 5-year basis
C. deflation of supplies
D. enforcing the 100-slide limit on each cytotechnologist to maximize profit

58. Regarding laboratory procedure manuals, which of the following statements are correct?

A. laboratory manual must be kept, reviewed periodically, and signed by the Technical Supervisor
B. laboratory manual must be kept, reviewed periodically, and signed by the General Supervisor
C. laboratory manuals are not required under CLIA '88
D. laboratory manuals must be updated each week as required by CLIA '88

59. What is an important employee record to maintain for each of the laboratory personnel?

A. employee's future job plans
B. employee's education
C. accidents occurring at home
D. outside income

60. On the average, (1) how many women are diagnosed with cervical cancer annually, (2) how many die of the disease, and (3) how does this compare with the incidence and mortality data from 50 years ago?

A. 2,500; 1,300; decrease of 90%
B. 5,000; 2,500; decrease of 30%
C. 13,000; 5,000; decrease of 70%
D. 26,000; 13,000; decrease of 25%

61. **When conducting appraisal of new employees, one should consider:**

A. not performing an interview to rule out possible biases
B. emphasizing their negative attributes only to increase their productivity
C. measuring specific variables
D. emphasizing their positive attributes to keep the laboratory from any possible employee litigation

62. **A process by which a nongovernmental agency recognizes a program or laboratory as competent is termed:**

A. accreditation
B. licensure
C. OSHA
D. Clinical Laboratory Improvement Act of 1988

63. **What is considered methodology to ensure productivity?**

A. review of the individual's workload every 6 months by the Technical Supervisor
B. maximizing the governmental slide limits
C. performing 20% re-screen on all focused cases
D. identifying the number of malignancies missed per week

64. **When conducting quality control on gynecologic cases:**

A. the laboratory supervisor should pick a number and each cytotechnologist should re-evaluate his/her own specimens
B. the Technical Supervisor must review 10% of each cytotechnologist's workload for that particular day
C. a blind or random sampling method should be conducted independently of each cytotechnologist's work
D. 10% of the cytotechnologist's abnormal diagnoses should be reviewed by the Technical Supervisor

65. **The governing agency responsible for overseeing safety is referred to as:**

A. CLIA
B. JCAHO
C. OSHA
D. ASCP

66. **In the workload log record each cytotechnologist should include all of the following, *except:***

A. number of cases/slides reviewed
B. number of discrepancies
C. workload limit
D. number of well-preserved slides

67. **The process by which a public authority grants permission to an individual or organization to engage in professional practice is called:**

A. accreditation
B. certification
C. licensure
D. articulation

68. **The Clinical Laboratory Improvement Amendments of 1988 (CLIA '88) require all of the following conditions, *except:***

A. all cases of atypical squamous cells of undetermined significance (ASCUS) are considered part of the 5-year retrospective review process
B. a diagnosis of a high-grade squamous intraepithelial lesion mandates follow-up of the patient
C. daily record of the number of slides reviewed as well as the amount of time spent reviewing the slides must be kept for each cytotechnologist
D. board-certified pathologists may not perform primary review of more than 100 cytology slides in any 24-hour period

69. **According to most organizational theorists, the administrative process includes:**

A. planning and organizing
B. clerical work and proofreading
C. specimen processing and bench work
D. buying and selling

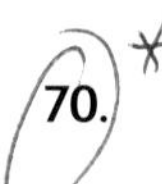

70. **The maximum number of cytology slides allowed per 24-hour period (both primary and re-screen) for a pathologist under CLIA '88 is:**

A. 80 total, regardless if primary or re-screen
B. 100 primary, 100 re-screen
C. 100 total
D. 100 primary, unlimited re-screens

71. **In forecasting inventory needs, which method is more responsive to change?**

A. moving average
B. regression analysis
C. exponential smoothing
D. base index

72. **Which rate-setting technique is best suited to departments in which the cost of supplies is high in relation to the cost of labor?**

A. hourly rate
B. surcharge
C. weighted-value
D. per diem

73. **What budgeting process identifies resources for budget items such as buildings and major equipment purchases?**

A. physical plant
B. revenue
C. operational
D. capital

74. **Which measure of CAP Workload productivity will reflect a potential personnel shortage?**

A. paid productivity
B. worked productivity
C. specified productivity
D. unspecified productivity

75. **In the CAP Workload Recording Method of determining labor costs, what calculation represents the mean number of workload units required to perform a procedure once?**

A. unit volume per procedure
B. raw count
C. item for count
D. unit for count

76. **Which coding system provides the reasoning and justification for ordering and performing laboratory procedures?**

A. Current Procedural Terminology
B. HCFA Common Procedural Coding System
C. International Classification of Diseases–9
D. International Classification of Functioning, Disability and Health

77. **Practices that result in failure to comply with governmental regulations involving intentional deception for personal gain are considered:**

A. fraud
B. abuse
C. misdemeanor
D. battery

78. **The ratio of the average annual investment return for a capital purchase to the initial investment cost defines its:**

A. present value
B. time-adjusted return
C. payback
D. average rate of return

79. **Which method of cost accounting examines only those additional costs required to perform potential increases in test volume?**

A. macro
B. micro
C. mini
D. incremental

80. **What element of negligence requires that damages be shown to be the direct result of a negligent act?**

A. duty
B. breach of duty
C. standard of care
D. proximate cause

81. What type of budget allows periodic negotiation and adjustment without requiring sanctions from external authorities?

A. appropriation
B. fixed forecast
C. variable
D. limited term

82. In a quality systems design, what documents that a procedure performs at preset specifications?

A. proficiency testing
B. process validation
C. calibration
D. process control

83. What are the basic output units for analyzing productivity in the CAP Laboratory Management Index Program (LMIP)?

A. billable and total test
B. labor and FTE
C. consumable and equipment
D. discharges and outpatient visits

84. What type of budget report plots budgeted revenue and collections against expenses?

A. departmental trend summary
B. fund-balance statement
C. profit and loss statement
D. cost reports

85. What type of witness to a legal proceeding is permitted to offer an opinion based on "reasonable scientific certainty"?

A. ordinary
B. expert
C. fact
D. reasonable

86. Which LMIP measure represents the ratio of on-site testing to outsourced testing?

A. on-site billable per technical FTE
B. on-site billable per total billable tests
C. on-site billable per total FTE
D. worked to paid hours

87. In examining LMIP data to manage cost effectiveness, which ratio can be expected to increase as the total number of billable tests increases?

A. total laboratory expenses per discharge
B. total labor expense per on-site billable test
C. labor and direct expense per on-site billable test
D. consumable and direct expense per on-site billable test

88. Besides OSHA, which of the following federal agencies regulates laboratory operations?

A. Federal Bureau of Investigation
B. Central Intelligence Agency
C. Department of Transportation
D. Social Security Administration

Laboratory Management and Administration ***Answer Key***

1. **B** allowable error

Allowable error defines how far from the true value a test result can be and remain acceptable.

Snyder JR, Wilkinson DS, eds., Management in Laboratory Medicine.
Process control and method evaluation, p. 302.

2. **C** job security

Primary needs are physiologic (food, clothing, shelter) and safety (from harm, disease, disaster). In the workplace, money is a motivator to satisfy physiologic needs, and such things as insurance benefits and job security satisfy safety needs. Acceptance, recognition, and job satisfaction are motivators to satisfy secondary needs in Maslow's Hierarchy.

Snyder JR, Wilkinson DS, eds., Management in Laboratory Medicine.
Motivation—Managerial assumptions and effects, pp. 97–98.

3. **A** critical task

Critical tasks are those that are significant in the completion of a task but have little impact on outcomes when performed poorly. Essential tasks are those involving the utmost attention to detail and accuracy. Outcome metrics evaluate the performance, cost effectiveness, quality, and quantity of a task. Key job areas define major job roles and responsibilities.

Snyder JR, Wilkinson DS, eds., Management in Laboratory Medicine.
Staffing and scheduling of laboratory personnel, p. 232.

4. **B** credentialing

Credentialing is the common term applied to the official acknowledgment of professional or technical competence. Peer assurance defines a voluntary process of subjecting to oversight by an external professional constituent organization; registration usually occurs at the state level and involves filing name and qualifications of a professional to practice; regulation refers to governmental control of an economic market.

Snyder JR, Wilkinson DS, eds., Management in Laboratory Medicine.
Laboratory regulation, certification, and accreditation, p. 375.

5. **A** unit

Examining unit costs identifies changes in the cost to produce a unit of service and enables monitoring of productivity.

Snyder JR, Wilkinson DS, eds., Management in Laboratory Medicine.
Introduction to laboratory financial management, p. 465.

6. **D** efficiency

Efficiency is the ratio of outputs to inputs. Production refers to a laboratory's ability to meet the organization's needs in terms of quality and quantity of laboratory testing. Adaptiveness relates to a laboratory's response to internal and external change forces. Development refers to operations investment over the long term.

Snyder JR, Wilkinson DS, eds., Management in Laboratory Medicine.
Leadership styles and group effectiveness, p. 127.

7. **C** Food and Drug Administration

The Food and Drug Administration regulates market entry of medical devices, laboratory instruments, and reagents and supplies under the Food, Drug and Cosmetic Act.

Snyder JR, Wilkinson DS, eds., Management in Laboratory Medicine.
Laboratory regulation, certification, and accreditation, p. 385.

8. **D** a not-for-profit hospital with annual receipts of $300,000

Amendments to the National Labor Relations Act apply to hospitals with annual receipts exceeding $250,000, nursing homes with receipts over $100,000 per year, and to voluntary not-for-profit health care institutions with receipts of $300,000 or more annually to NLRA regulation.

Snyder JR, Wilkinson DS, eds., Management in Laboratory Medicine.
Labor relations and the clinical laboratory, p. 271.

9. **B** *res ipsa loquitor*

Res ipsa loquitor or "the thing speaks for itself" refers to negligence so apparent that the court shifts the burden of proof from the plaintiff to the defendant. *Negligence per se* exists when a practice is in direct violation of a state law or federal regulation that establishes a standard of care. *Respondeat superior* or "look to the one higher up" is the legal doctrine by which plaintiffs can sue an employer for the negligent actions of an employee. *Negligence ipso facto* is nonsense.

Snyder JR, Wilkinson DS, eds., Management in Laboratory Medicine.
Medicolegal concerns in laboratory medicine, p. 412.

10. A require employees to set their own goals and objectives

Theory-Y managers motivate staff by allowing them to direct and control themselves. Theory-X managers structure, control, and closely supervise their staff under the assumption that they are incapable of doing it for themselves.

Snyder JR, Wilkinson DS, eds., Management in Laboratory Medicine.
Managerial assumptions and effects, p. 101.

11. B variable

Fixed costs remain unchanged over time while variable costs fluctuate in proportion to volume. Direct costs include all those that can be specifically associated with a test while indirect cost or overhead are the costs included in the expense of operating a laboratory.

Snyder JR, Wilkinson DS, eds., Management in Laboratory Medicine.
Introduction to laboratory financial management, pp. 463–465.

12. B Equal Employment Opportunity Commission

Title VII of the Civil Rights Act guarantees equality to all people and is enforced by the Equal Employment Opportunity Commission. Affirmative Action refers to programs designed to reverse the effects of discrimination.

Snyder JR, Wilkinson DS, eds., Management in Laboratory Medicine.
Interviewing and employee selection, p. 198.

13. D full

As methods for accumulating direct and indirect costs of operation, direct costing allocates all direct costs to the laboratory while full costing assigns indirect costs to the laboratory. Standard costs indicate the total cost of efficient operation.

Snyder JR, Wilkinson DS, eds., Management in Laboratory Medicine.
Introduction to laboratory financial management, p. 465.

14. A hygiene factors and satisfiers

The combination of hygiene factors and satisfiers tends to produce strong employee motivation.

Snyder JR, Wilkinson DS, eds., Management in Laboratory Medicine.
Motivation—Managerial assumptions and effects, pp. 99–100.

15. B *respondeat superior*

Respondeat superior is the legal doctrine by which employers are responsible for the actions of employees. Res ipsa loquitor addresses negligence that is so obvious that the court shifts the burden of proof away from the plaintiff and toward the defendant. Locum tenens is a temporary substitute for a doctor or clergy member. Procedenti ab utroque is a phrase from a Latin hymn.

Snyder JR, Wilkinson DS, eds., Management in Laboratory Medicine.
Medicolegal concerns in laboratory medicine, p. 413.

16. B Do you have any relatives employed by this company?

It is legal to inquire about relatives who may work for the same company in order to abide by requirements of nepotism policies. It is not legal to ask for the names of family members specifically, except to ask whom to notify in case of emergency. It is legal to inquire about convictions, but not arrests. Employers may ask about impairments that would interfere with ability to perform the job, but not about disabilities in general. Questions as to form of address can be construed as attempts to identify marital status or gender, both of which are unlawful questions.

Snyder JR, Wilkinson DS, eds., Management in Laboratory Medicine.
Interviewing and employee selection, p. 201.

17. B National Labor Relations Act

Labor relations are regulated through the National Labor Relations Act for the private sector and through the Civil Service Reform Act for the federal sector.

Snyder JR, Wilkinson DS, eds., Management in Laboratory Medicine.
Labor relations and the clinical laboratory, p. 269.

18. A slope of the line

The slope of the regression line reflects proportional bias. The Y-intercept of the line detects constant bias and the standard error determines the scatter of plots about the line. The correlation coefficient is not well suited for method comparison studies in the clinical lab, owing to its variability with the distribution of data.

Snyder JR, Wilkinson DS, eds., Management in Laboratory Medicine.
Process control and method evaluation, p. 317.

19. **C** salary and promotion decisions

The most commonly cited reason for conducting employee performance evaluation is as a means to make decisions related to salary and promotion.

Snyder JR, Wilkinson DS, eds., Management in Laboratory Medicine.
Standards and appraisals of laboratory performance, p. 246.

20. **D** measure to which like objects are expected to conform

A standard is a measure to which like objects are expected to conform. A criterion is a reference used in forming judgments.

Snyder JR, Wilkinson DS, eds., Management in Laboratory Medicine.
Interviewing and employee selection, pp. 195–219.

21. **C** 40

The ADEA provides protection against age discrimination to workers over 70 years of age and eliminates mandatory retirement. Amendments also protect workers over age 40 from discriminatory practices related to paid benefits or continued employment.

Snyder JR, Wilkinson DS, eds., Management in Laboratory Medicine.
Interviewing and employee selection, p. 199.

22. **D** Federal Labor Relations Authority

Collective bargaining in the federal sector is overseen by the Federal Labor Relations Authority.

Snyder JR, Wilkinson DS, eds., Management in Laboratory Medicine.
Labor relations and the clinical laboratory, p. 270.

23. **B** hygiene

Hygiene or environmental factors are related to dissatisfaction, the absence of which encourages unacceptable performance. Motivators are related to job satisfaction and encourage performance above accepted levels.

Snyder JR, Wilkinson DS, eds., Management in Laboratory Medicine.
Motivation—Managerial assumptions and effects, pp. 99–100.

24. **A** Pareto diagram

A Pareto diagram is best suited for use in determining the significance of data. Fishbone or cause and effect diagrams are useful in distinguishing the true cause of an observed effect from randomly associated causes. Scatter diagrams plot two characteristics on an X and Y axis to determine the existence of relationship between the characteristics. Affinity diagrams are useful in defining groups of items from among large quantities of descriptive or verbal data.

Snyder JR, Wilkinson DS, eds., Management in Laboratory Medicine.
Problem solving—The decision-making process, p. 69.

25. **B** *respondeat superior*

Respondeat superior or "look to the one higher up" is the legal doctrine by which plaintiffs can sue an employer for the negligent actions of an employee. *Res ipsa loquitor* or "the thing speaks for itself" refers to negligence so apparent that the court shifts the burden of proof from the plaintiff to the defendant. *Negligence per se* exists when a practice is in direct violation of a state law or federal regulation that establishes a standard of care. *Compar sit laudatio* is a phrase from a Latin hymn.

Snyder JR, Wilkinson DS, eds., Management in Laboratory Medicine.
Medico legal concerns in laboratory medicine, p. 413.

26. **A** reference sample

The reference sample method assesses laboratory performance by examining the results of tests repeated on same and different days for the ability to repeat identical and accurate results consistently.

Snyder JR, Wilkinson DS, eds., Management in Laboratory Medicine.
Process control and method evaluation, p. 293.

27. **C** referent

Referent power arises solely from a leader's personality. Reward power uses the expectation of gaining substantial gain. Expert power results from the use of specialized cognitive knowledge or technical skill. Legitimate power is the authority arising from the formal organizational structure.

Snyder JR, Wilkinson DS, eds., Management in Laboratory Medicine.
Leadership styles and group effectiveness, p. 130.

28. **C** bias

Failure to control for bias is the most common reason for CLIA PT failure.

Snyder JR, Wilkinson DS, eds., Management in Laboratory Medicine.
Process control and method evaluation, p. 310.

29. **D** acceptable standard deviation

In the development of a Westgard process control system, managers must decide on a number of factors including error rate, false rejection rate, and number of controls, but the most important decision is setting the standard deviation for the analysis, as it determines acceptance or rejection of data.

Snyder JR, Wilkinson DS, eds., Management in Laboratory Medicine.
Process control and method evaluation, p. 300.

30. **A** introvert, intuiting, thinking, judging

The personality described is that of an intuiting, thinking, judging introvert.

Snyder JR, Wilkinson DS, eds., Management in Laboratory Medicine.
Leadership styles and group effectiveness, pp. 138–141.

31. **C** precision

The ability of a laboratory test to detect minute amounts of an analyte is a measure of the test's sensitivity. Specificity refers to the ability of an analysis to reliably detect a specific element in the presence of possible confounding factors. Accuracy refers to how close to the true value of an analyte a test can measure. Precision relates to the ability of a test to consistently measure at the same value with repeated performance over time.

Snyder JR, Wilkinson DS, eds., Management in Laboratory Medicine.
Process control and method evaluation, p. 319.

32. **B** sensitivity

The ability of a laboratory test to detect minute amounts of an analyte is a measure of the test's sensitivity. Specificity refers to the ability of an analysis to reliably detect a specific element in the presence of possible confounding factors. Accuracy refers to how close to the true value of an analyte a test can measure. Precision relates to the ability of a test to consistently measure at the same value with repeated performance over time.

Snyder JR, Wilkinson DS, eds., Management in Laboratory Medicine.
Process control and method evaluation, p. 319.

33. **A** dispersion

Data points tend to be either dispersed or contracted with a change in precision. Trends are seen when the testing conditions worsen over time, and shifts may be caused by changes in method or reagents.

Snyder JR, Wilkinson DS, eds., Management in Laboratory Medicine.
Process control and method evaluation, p. 298.

34. **D** regulation

Regulation is the term applied to the governmental control of an economic market for the purpose of public protection.

Snyder JR, Wilkinson DS, eds., Management in Laboratory Medicine.
Laboratory regulation, certification, and accreditation, p. 371.

35. **D** Department of Defense drug surveillance facilities

Facilities subject to regulation by the Substance and Mental Health Services Administration are exempt from CLIA '88, including drug surveillance facilities in the Department of Defense.

Snyder JR, Wilkinson DS, eds., Management in Laboratory Medicine.
Laboratory regulation, certification, and accreditation, p. 378.

36. **D** BS degree with 3 years of experience, 2 in cytopathology

Gen. Supervisor

For related information, see answer to question 8.

Keebler CM, Somrak TM, The Manual of Cytotechnology.
General supervisor, p. 337.

37. **C** a total number established by the Technical Supervisor, not to exceed 100

The Technical Supervisor must establish the total number of slides that each cytotechnologist may review daily. Furthermore, he or she must reevaluate this established rate on a periodic basis (at least every 6 months).

Keebler CM, Somrak TM, The Manual of Cytotechnology.
Microscopy, pp. 340–341.

38. **A** cytology-histology correlation

Annual Reports

Some of the annual statistics required by cytopathology laboratories include the cytotechnologist worklogs, workload statistics, quality control data and quality assurance guidelines, total number of specimens processed, and a breakdown of number of specimens by diagnosis.

Keebler CM, Somrak TM, The Manual of Cytotechnology. *Record-keeping practices, p. 338.*

39. **D** no degree required, only supervision by General Supervisor

Cytopreparatory technicians must meet no minimal education requirements. On the job training is acceptable.

Keebler CM, Somrak TM, The Manual of Cytotechnology. *Support personnel, p. 337.*

40. **B** 100

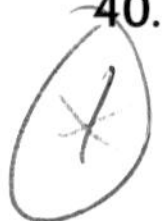

One hundred slides, whether primary or review, gynecological or non-gynecological, is the total number of slides that a cytotechnologist may review in any given 24-hour period. This number is estimated for a typical 8-hour day. However, if prorated, a cytotechnologist may not exceed 12.5 slides per hour.

Keebler CM, Somrak TM, The Manual of Cytotechnology. *Quality control practices, pp. 340–342.*

41. **A** 2 years

These requisitions may be kept in hard files or on microfilm with accompanying biopsy or autopsy reports if applicable.

Keebler CM, Somrak TM, The Manual of Cytotechnology. *Record-keeping practices, pp. 338–340.*

42. **B** planning a weekly budget

A yearly or biannual long-range budget should be developed based on the patterns or trends from past budgets and predictions for the upcoming year. Before developing a budget, a complete cost analysis for performing the laboratory tests (supplies, equipment/instrument or capital purchases, continuing education costs, etc.) should be developed to include direct and indirect costs, and personnel costs need to be determined (including possible increases in salary or differential pay). Periodic reassessment throughout the year is necessary to establish the baseline necessary to determine requirements for future budgetary processes.

Keebler CM, Somrak TM, The Manual of Cytotechnology. *Budget process, pp. 358–362.*

43. **B** in house as well as through professional societies

Continuing education is essential for each cytotechnologist to keep abreast of the evolving nature of diagnostic cytopathology. Key considerations include developing in-house workshops; attending regional, state, or national meetings; subscribing to the American Society of Cytopathology teleconferencing series; purchasing the numerous ASCP educational programs (Check Sample, Chapter 12: Laboratory Management and Administration Answer Key 419 etc.); subscribing to the ASCP GYN PTTM slide program; or participating in the College of American Pathologists Interlaboratory Comparison program.

Keebler CM, Somrak TM, The Manual of Cytotechnology. *Continuing Education, p. 362.*

44. **C** the pathologist in charge of cytology

Tech Supervisor

For related information, see answer to question 58.

Keebler CM, Somrak TM, The Manual of Cytotechnology. *Technical supervisor, p. 337.*

45. **C** 10 years

These reports must be available as hard copies for a minimum of 10 years.

Keebler CM, Somrak TM, The Manual of Cytotechnology. *Record-keeping practices, pp. 338–340.*

46. **A** gynecologic specimens must be stained separately from nongynecologic specimens

Gynecologic processing must be performed independently of nongynecologic specimens due to the possibility of "floaters."

Keebler CM, Somrak TM, The Manual of Cytotechnology. *Specimen preparation, p. 340.*

47. **A** jointly purchase supplies with the histology laboratory

Bulk discounts may be realized if the laboratory has the potential to jointly purchase supplies with the histology laboratory.

Keebler CM, Somrak TM, The Manual of Cytotechnology. *Laboratory supplies, p. 361.*

CLIA 88

Orig req. 2yrs
Final report 10 yrs
Glass slides 5 yrs

CAP

48. **B** **American Society of Cytopathology**

Other cytopathological accrediting bodies include the International Academy of Cytology (IAC), the College of American Pathologists, and the Joint Commission on Accreditation of Healthcare Organizations. The IAC and the American Society of Cytopathology are the only accreditation bodies that evaluate the education and practice of cytopathology.

Keebler CM, Somrak TM, The Manual of Cytotechnology.
Laboratory accreditation, p. 334.

49. **B** **5 years**

All glass slides must be kept for a minimum of 5 years, regardless of whether they are normal or abnormal, gynecologic or non-gynecologic.

Keebler CM, Somrak TM, The Manual of Cytotechnology.
Record-keeping practices, pp. 338–340.

50. **C** **stagger work hours/split shifts to cover the laboratory operations**

Overtime scheduling may be needed to maintain productivity and ensure timely patient diagnoses. Flexible time shifts may provide some support when recruiting for vacant positions.

Keebler CM, Somrak TM, The Manual of Cytotechnology.
Position vacancy, p. 361.

51. **B** **100**

For related information, see answer to question 40.

Keebler CM, Somrak TM, The Manual of Cytotechnology.
Quality control practices, pp. 340–342.

52. **D** **missing an obvious malignancy**

A primary error is a misdiagnosis that would have changed the clinical management of the patient. This error must be originally made by the cytotechnologist who screened the specimen. The error should be noted in the personnel file for determination of a possible plan of action.

Keebler CM, Somrak TM, The Manual of Cytotechnology.
Primary error, p. 363.

53. **A** **to ensure that the job gets done right the first time**

Eliminating mistakes begins by establishing a stringent set of guidelines that each cytotechnologist must follow. Updated and current procedure manuals that reflect the current practice of the laboratory and identify the expected role of the cytotechnologist will help ensure quality and performance within the workplace. Timely appraisal of individual performance standards ensures that if mistakes do occur, they are eliminated with the utmost efficiency.

Keebler CM, Somrak TM, The Manual of Cytotechnology.
Quality management, p. 365.

54. **A** **Clinical Laboratory Improvement Amendments of 1988 (CLIA '88)**

The CLIA '88 regulations attempt to regulate all laboratories to ensure quality patient care.

Keebler CM, Somrak TM, The Manual of Cytotechnology.
Laboratory accreditation, p. 334.

55. **A** **10% review of focused or high-risk cases as well as random review**

For related information, see answer to question 56 and 64.

Keebler CM, Somrak TM, The Manual of Cytotechnology.
Personnel performance, p. 342, and Productivity issues, p. 364.

56. **B** **determining patterns or trends in test accuracy with the collected data**

Quality control is the collection of the data necessary to establish statistical information needed to evaluate the efficacy of the laboratory. Quality assurance is using the collected data to establish patterns or trends that the laboratory can use to improve its operation.

Keebler CM, Somrak TM, The Manual of Cytotechnology.
Quality assurance/quality control measures and practices, pp. 353–355.

57. **A** **calculating the direct and indirect costs associated with laboratory operations**

For related information, see answer to question 42.

Keebler CM, Somrak TM, The Manual of Cytotechnology.
Budget process, pp. 358–362.

58. A laboratory manual must be kept, reviewed periodically, and signed by the Technical Supervisor

The Technical Supervisor of the laboratory must be a board-certified pathologist. Subspecialization in cytopathology is not mandated by CLIA '88. The cytotechnology supervisor is regarded as the General Supervisor. This individual must possess at least 3 years of experience. In addition, only cytotechnologists who qualify for General Supervisor status under CLIA '88 are permitted to perform intralaboratory quality control or 10% re-screen.

Keebler CM, Somrak TM, The Manual of Cytotechnology.
Record-keeping practices, pp. 338–340.

59. B employee's education

An employee's education and experience are two important records that should be maintained for each cytotechnologist. Other records include his or her attendance, productivity, reliability, professionalism, and diagnostic accuracy.

Keebler CM, Somrak TM, The Manual of Cytotechnology.
Personnel issues, pp. 362–365.

60. C 13,000; 5,000; decrease of 70%

The incidence of cervical cancer has decreased overall 70% since the test was implemented (1950s). It stands today as the most successful cancer screening test in medicine.

American Cancer Society Facts and Figures;
2002: http://cancer.org.

61. C measuring specific variables

Measuring specific variables allows the interviewer to evaluate each of the candidates fairly with relatively unbiased interpretations. Collected data can be kept on file should the future necessitate.

Keebler CM, Somrak TM, The Manual of Cytotechnology.
Performance standards, p. 365.

62. A accreditation

Accreditation is awarded to institutions, whereas licensure is awarded to individuals.

Keebler CM, Somrak TM, The Manual of Cytotechnology.
Laboratory accreditation, p. 334.

63. A review of the individual's workload every 6 months by the Technical Supervisor

The Technical Supervisor, a cytopathologist who is the typically the Director of the Cytology Laboratory, must review the productivity of each cytotechnologist within the laboratory to determine his or her competency and productivity levels.

Keebler CM, Somrak TM, The Manual of Cytotechnology.
Productivity issues, p. 363.

64. C a blind or random sampling method should be conducted independently of each cytotechnologist's work

CLIA '88 regulations require that a 10% random and focused review be performed blindly without the knowledge of which case will be re-reviewed by a General Supervisor level cytotechnologist.

Keebler CM, Somrak TM, The Manual of Cytotechnology.
Productivity issues, p. 364.

65. C OSHA

The Occupational Safety and Health Administration establishes guidelines and monitors compliance with chemical and biohazardous regulations.

Keebler CM, Somrak TM, The Manual of Cytotechnology.
Chemical safety, p. 372.

66. D number of well-preserved slides

Each cytotechnologist must strictly comply with the CLIA '88 guidelines to ensure quality of patient care. For related information, see answer to question 33.

Keebler CM, Somrak TM, The Manual of Cytotechnology.
Productivity issues, pp. 363–364.

67. C licensure

Licensure is the legal process governing the right to professional practice. Certification is the process by which a peer group or governmental agency recognizes that an organization or individual has met certain requirements. Articulation refers to terms of agreement between educational institutions relating to student placement.

Snyder JR, Wilkinson DS, eds., Management in Laboratory Medicine.
Laboratory regulation, certification and accreditation, p. 371.

68. A all cases of atypical squamous cells of undetermined significance (ASCUS) are considered part of the 5-year retrospective review process

The only cases warranting a 5-year retrospective review are those currently diagnosed as high-grade intraepithelial lesions or above.

Keebler CM, Somrak TM, The Manual of Cytotechnology.
Quality control practices, pp. 340–342.

69. A planning and organizing

The administrative process includes planning, organizing, directing, and controlling.

Snyder JR, Wilkinson DS, eds., Management in Laboratory Medicine.
The nature of management in laboratory medicine, p. 10.

70. D 100 primary, unlimited re-screens

If a pathologist is acting as the primary screener, he or she may not exceed the CLIA limits established for cytotechnologists (see answer to question 40). The number of reevaluated slides, or those previously evaluated by a cytotechnologist, that a cytopathologist may evaluate is unlimited.

Keebler CM, Somrak TM, The Manual of Cytotechnology.
Quality control practices, pp. 340–342.

71. C exponential smoothing

Exponential smoothing responds to trends better than the moving average approach because its weights are based on historical data.

Snyder JR, Wilkinson DS, eds., Management in Laboratory Medicine.
Inventory management and cost containment, pp. 557–559.

72. B surcharge

The surcharge or cost-plus technique is useful for departments in which supply costs exceed labor costs to provide a service. The hourly rate method is better suited to departments in which there is a good association between the service provided and the time required to provide the service. In the weighted-value approach, relative-value of a procedure is assigned depending upon the direct cost of performing it.

Snyder JR, Wilkinson DS, eds., Management in Laboratory Medicine.
Budgeting laboratory resources, p. 490.

73. D capital

The capital budget identifies resources for the acquisition and maintenance of physical resources such as buildings and major equipment.

Snyder JR, Wilkinson DS, eds., Management in Laboratory Medicine.
Budgeting laboratory resources, p. 480.

74. C specified productivity

Specified productivity reflects activities not included in calculations of CAP Workload unit time and therefore may better reflect the need for additional personnel.

Snyder JR, Wilkinson DS, eds., Management in Laboratory Medicine.
Laboratory cost accounting, pp. 502–504.

75. A unit volume per procedure

Unit volume per procedure is the mean number of workload units required to perform a procedure one time. Raw count is a total of the items to be counted and item for count specifies what is to be counted.

Snyder JR, Wilkinson DS, eds., Management in Laboratory Medicine.
Laboratory cost accounting, p. 494.

76. C International Classification of Diseases–9

The International Classification of Disease–9 provides the coding framework for justifying laboratory testing. Current Procedural Terminology codes identify services for Medicare, Medicaid, and many third-party reimbursement payers.

Snyder JR, Wilkinson DS, eds., Management in Laboratory Medicine.
Coding, billing, and reimbursement management, pp. 509–514.

77. A fraud

Fraud is a felony offense involving intentional misrepresentation to knowingly gain personal benefit. Abuse is considered a misdemeanor offense and involves practices that fail to follow standard practice and result in improper reimbursement. Battery is the infliction of nonconsensual touching.

Snyder JR, Wilkinson DS, eds., Management in Laboratory Medicine.
Coding, billing, and reimbursement management, pp. 509–515.

78. **D** average rate of return

The average rate of return for a capital purchase is the average annual investment return divided by the initial investment cost. Payback analysis determines the time in the life of the instrument when cash flows can recover the original investment. The present value of an item is what it would cost at some future point if the present cost were invested and earned returns equal to a specific amount. The time-adjusted return method is a calculation of the rate at which the net present value totals zero.

Snyder JR, Wilkinson DS, eds., Management in Laboratory Medicine.
Budgeting laboratory resources, pp. 483–485.

79. **D** incremental

The incremental method examines the additional costs associated with increases in test volume. The macro method assigns direct cost to the appropriate cost center, whereas the micro method examines the cost per test of direct and indirect labor, materials, instrumentation, and overhead.

Snyder JR, Wilkinson DS, eds., Management in Laboratory Medicine.
Laboratory cost accounting, pp. 494–500.

80. **D** proximate cause

The plaintiff must show proximate cause, or that the injury or damage resulted directly from the negligent act.

Snyder JR, Wilkinson DS, eds., Management in Laboratory Medicine.
Medicolegal concerns in laboratory medicine, p. 412.

81. **B** fixed forecast

Fixed forecast budgets permit renegotiation of budget elements without external sanctioning. Appropriation budgets from governmental agencies are apportioned periodically from central agencies and cannot be renegotiated during a given budget period.

Snyder JR, Wilkinson DS, eds., Management in Laboratory Medicine.
Budgeting laboratory resources, p. 475.

82. **B** process validation

Process validation ensures that a new procedure will perform according to preset specifications. Process control enables identification of opportunities to reduce error and decrease variation.

Snyder JR, Wilkinson DS, eds., Management in Laboratory Medicine.
Quality management in the laboratory, p. 400.

83. **A** billable and total test

The billable and total tests are the basic output units of productivity, while labor, FTE, and financial costs represent basic input units.

Snyder JR, Wilkinson DS, eds., Management in Laboratory Medicine.
Assessing laboratory operating performance: The laboratory management index program, p. 452.

84. **C** profit and loss statement

Profit and loss statements reflect budgeted revenue and actual collections vs. actual expenses.

Snyder JR, Wilkinson DS, eds., Management in Laboratory Medicine.
Budgeting laboratory resources, pp. 479–480.

85. **B** expert

Only an expert witness may offer an opinion based on reasonable scientific certainty. An ordinary or fact witness may offer only an opinion based on his or her own experience.

Snyder JR, Wilkinson DS, eds., Management in Laboratory Medicine.
Medico legal concerns in laboratory medicine, p. 417.

86. **B** on-site billable per total billable tests

On-site billable per total billable tests measures the percentage of tests performed in-house vs. that sent to reference laboratories.

Snyder JR, Wilkinson DS, eds., Management in Laboratory Medicine.
Assessing laboratory operating performance: The laboratory management index program, p. 456.

87. **A** total laboratory expenses per discharge

The total laboratory expense per discharge can be expected to increase as the total number of billable tests increases. The other three measures listed can be expected to decrease as the total number of billable tests increases.

Snyder JR, Wilkinson DS, eds., Management in Laboratory Medicine.
Assessing laboratory operating performance: The laboratory management index program, pp. 456–457.

88. **C** Department of Transportation

The Department of Transportation regulates laboratory operations related to safe practices in packaging, transporting, and handling biologic materials.

Snyder JR, Wilkinson DS, eds., Management in Laboratory Medicine.
Laboratory regulation, certification, and accreditation, p. 389.

Chapter 13
2001 Bethesda System and ASCCP 2006 Consensus Guidelines

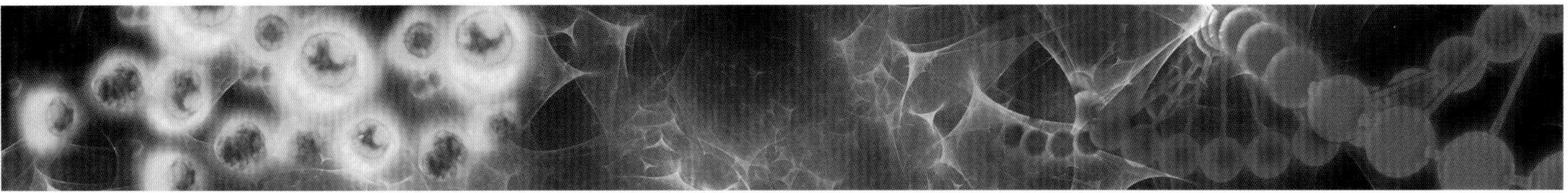

All questions in this section assume exclusive use of the 2001 Bethesda System (http://bethesda2001.cancer.gov/terminology.html) and ASCCP 2006 Consensus Guidelines (http://www.asccp.org/consensus/histological.shtml) terminology, definitions, and classifications, except as specifically noted otherwise.

1. **Which of the following are considered pertinent for issuing a final report of "satisfactory for evaluation?"**

   A. at least 2 microscopic fields of squamous cells found in liquid-based preparation
   B. presence or absence of endocervical/transformation zone component
   C. specimen not processed
   D. inflammation obscures all but 2% of squamous cells in a conventional slide

2. **Which of the following is considered acceptable terminology when rendering a diagnosis of benign or negative?**

   A. Class 1
   B. Benign cellular changes
   C. WNL; Within Normal Limits
   D. NIL; Negative for Intraepithelial Lesion or Malignancy

3. **Which of the following statements is acceptable terminology classification of GYN cytology slides?**

   A. satisfactory, but limited by lack of endocervical cell component
   B. benign cellular changes (as a separate category)
   C. "other" category to include endometrial cells in women at least 40 years of age
   D. atypical squamous cells of undetermined significance (ASCUS), favor reactive

4. **Which of the following statements is acceptable terminology for classification of GYN cytology slides?**

   A. ASCUS, favor neoplastic
   B. endocervical adenocarcinoma in situ
   C. atypical glandular cells of undetermined significance (AGUS), favor reactive
   D. AGUS, favor dysplasia

5. **Which of the following is an acceptable report category for classification of GYN cytology slides?**

   A. hormonal evaluation
   B. ancillary testing
   C. organisms and other non-neoplastic findings mandatory under "negative for intraepithelial lesion or malignancy"
   D. conventional cytological review

6. **The presence of endometrial cells on cervical cytology in women who are at least 45 years of age is more often associated with endometrial hyperplasia or even adenocarcinoma as opposed to benign endometrium.**

   A. true
   B. false

7. **The Pap test is reliable for the detection of endometrial lesions and can be used to evaluate suspected endometrial abnormalities.**

   A. true
   B. false

8. **If automated computer systems are used to scan slides, the type of system used and the result should be reported.**

A. true
B. false

9. **How many cells must be confirmed on a liquid-based Pap slide to establish a satisfactory specimen for diagnosis?**

A. 1,000
B. 2,500
C. 5,000
D. 10,000

10. **How many transformational zone cells must be confirmed on a liquid-based Pap slide to establish an adequate specimen?**

A. 5
B. 10
C. 20
D. 0

11. **Which is considered unsatisfactory for evaluation under the specimen adequacy clause of the Bethesda System?**

A. 50% of the cellular material is obscured by inflammation
B. air drying that obscures evaluation of at least 75% of the epithelial cells
C. air drying that obscures evaluation of at least 30% of the epithelial cells
D. 25% of the cells are obscured by blood

12. **Which professional organization sets the guidelines for the management of women with abnormal cervical cancer screening tests?**

A. ASCCP
B. ACOG
C. ASC
D. ASCP

13. **Which of the following management recommendations is appropriate for women with an initial diagnosis of atypical squamous cells of undetermined significance (ASC-US):**

A. high-risk HPV test(-); repeat cytology at 6 and 12 months
B. high-risk HPV test(-) repeat cytology in 12 months
C. triage to colposcopy, regardless of HPV test status
D. high-risk HPV test(+); perform conization

14. **Which of the following is the appropriate management algorithm for patients with ASC-US?**

A. high-risk HPV test (+); requires repeat in HPV test in 6 months
B. high-risk HPV test (+); requires colposcopy
C. ASC-US requires immediate colposcopy regardless of HPV risk status
D. 3 consecutive cytologic diagnoses of ASC-US diagnoses at 6, 12 and 18 months are recommended before colposcopy.

15. **A patient with ASCUS and a positive HPV test was referred to colposcopy. The colposcopy was negative; therefore, the appropriate follow-up would be:**

A. repeat cytology at 6 and 12 months or HPV test in 12 months
B. immediate conization
C. immediate repeat high-risk HPV test
D. repeat high-risk HPV in 6 months

16. **A patient with an initial diagnosis of ASC-US was eventually referred to colposcopy due to a co-test HPV result that was high-risk positive. Colposcopy showed CIN I. The management paradigm should be:**

A. repeat HPV test
B. repeat cytology at 6 and 12 months or HPV test in 12 months
C. perform diagnostic excision procedure
D. return the patient to routine cytologic testing in 12 months

17. **What is the appropriate management for women with a cytologic diagnosis of LSIL?**

A. immediate colposcopy
B. perform diagnostic excision procedure
C. confirm with HPV test, if HPV test is positive, perform LEEP
D. repeat Pap in 6 months

18. What is the management for women with LSIL that are confirmed as negative by colposcopy and for which the endocervical curettings (ECC) were negative?

A. repeat cytology at 6 and 12 months or HPV test in 12 months
B. repeat colposcopic examination
C. repeat immediately with an HPV test, if HPV test is positive, perform a LEEP
D. routine screening in 12 months

19. What is the management for women who have LSIL and confirmed by colposcopy as CIN I (with a negative ECC)?

A. perform an HPV test, if HPV test is positive, perform a LEEP
B. repeat colposcopic examination
C. repeat cytology at 6 and 12 months or HPV test in 12 months
D. routine screening in 12 months

20. What is the management for women who have LSIL that are confirmed by colposcopy as CIN 2 or 3?

A. hysterectomy
B. repeat colposcopy in 6 months to determine regression of disease
C. repeat immediately with an HPV test, if HPV test is positive, perform a loop electrosurgical excision (LEEP)
D. loop electrosurgical excision (LEEP) with ECC

21. What is the recommended management for women under 20 with a cytologic diagnosis of ASC-US?

A. repeat Pap in 6 months
B. repeat Pap in 12 months
C. immediate colposcopy
D. high-risk HPV test recommended, if positive, immediate colposcopy

22. What is the recommended management for women under 20 with a cytologic diagnosis of LSIL?

A. repeat Pap in 6 months
B. repeat Pap in 12 months
C. immediate colposcopy
D. high-risk HPV test recommended, if positive, immediate colposcopy

23. Which of the following statements is correct regarding an 18-year-old female with LSIL and a positive HPV test?

A. repeat Pap in 6-months; if LSIL, perform immediate colposcopy
B. immediate colposcopy
C. 2 consecutive positive HPV tests are required in adolescents with LSIL at 6 month intervals before colposcopy is warranted
D. inadvertent HPV test should be ignored regardless of positivity; colposcopy is not warranted; repeat Pap in 12 months

24. What is the recommended management for women under 20 with a cytologic diagnosis of HSIL?

A. repeat Pap test in 6 months
B. colposcopy
C. immediate loop electrosurgical excision (LEEP)
D. high-risk HPV test recommended, then follow as clinically indicated

25. What of the following is a recommended management for women with a cytologic diagnosis of atypical squamous cells of undetermined significance; cannot rule out high-grade (ASC-H) who has received a negative colposcopy?

A. immediate HPV test
B. repeat colposcopy
C. HPV testing in 12 months
D. conization

26. What is the recommended management for women with a cytologic diagnosis of atypical squamous cells of undetermined significance; cannot rule out high-grade (ASC-H) who has received colposcopy that showed CIN I?

A. immediate HPV test
B. HPV testing in 12 months
C. repeat colposcopy
D. conization

27. **What is the preferred method for a 30-year-old pregnant patient with a cytologic diagnosis of LSIL?**

A. colposcopy
B. perform HPV Testing post partum
C. repeat Pap at 6 weeks post partum
D. immediate loop electrosurgical excision (LEEP)

28. **What is the preferred management for a 16-year-old female with a cytologic diagnosis of HSIL followed by a negative colposcopic evaluation?**

A. D & C
B. repeat colposcopy in 3 months
C. repeat colposcopy and cytology in 3 and 6 months
D. repeat colposcopy and cytology in 6-month intervals for up to 2 years

29. **What is that management paradigm for a 17-year-old patient with HSIL, followed by a negative colposcopy at 6 and 12 months, but with an HSIL cytologic diagnosis that persists for a year?**

A. conization
B. HPV testing to confirm HSIL
C. repeat colposcopy in 3 months
D. biopsy

30. **What is the appropriate management for a 34-year-old patient with a cytologic diagnosis of atypical glandular cells of undetermined significance (AGC); endocervical cells NOS?**

A. follow up Pap every 6 months to determine if progression to adenocarcinoma in situ occurs
B. colposcopy with ECC, HPV Testing
C. immediate loop electrosurgical excision (LEEP)
D. HPV testing in 12 months

31. **What is the appropriate management for a 48-year-old patient with a cytologic diagnosis of atypical glandular cells of undetermined significance (AGC); endometrial cells favor neoplastic?**

A. follow up Pap every 6 months to determine if progression to adenocarcinoma in situ occurs
B. endometrial and endocervical sampling
C. immediate loop electrosurgical excision (LEEP)
D. hysterectomy

32. **What is the appropriate management for a 37-year-old patient with a cytologic diagnosis of atypical glandular cells of undetermined significance (AGC); glandular cells, NOS ?**

A. follow up Pap every 6 months to determine if progression to adenocarcinoma in situ occurs
B. immediate loop electrosurgical excision (LEEP)
C. colposcopy with ECC, HPV testing, endometrial sampling
D. hysterectomy

33. **What is the appropriate management for a 29-year-old patient with an initial cytologic diagnosis of adenocarcinoma in situ (AIS)?**

A. HPV testing followed by colposcopy
B. hysterectomy
C. repeat Pap in 6 months; If AIS persists by cytology, perform a conization
D. diagnostic excisional procedure

34. **What is the appropriate management for a 37-year-old patient who received co-testing with HPV as a primary screening tool where the cytology is negative but the HPV test is positive?**

A. immediate colposcopy
B. repeat HPV test immediately
C. repeat HPV and Pap test every 6 months
D. repeat HPV and Pap test at 12 months

35. **After appropriate follow up of a 37-year-old patient with negative cytology and a positive HPV test, a repeat HPV test proved negative but the cytology was ASC-US. What is the appropriate management for the patient at this point?**

A. repeat cytology at 12 months
B. colposcopy
C. repeat HPV test immediately
D. immediate loop electrosurgical excision (LEEP)

2001 Bethesda System and ASCCP 2006 Consensus Guidelines *Answer Key*

1. **B** presence or absence of endocervical/ transformational zone component

The 2001 Bethesda System includes specific statements about specimen adequacy. As compared to the 1991 Bethesda system, "satisfactory" and "unsatisfactory" are retained in Bethesda 2001, but "satisfactory but limited by" is eliminated. This 1991 category proved confusing to clinicians and may have led to unnecessary repeat testing. Studies have not proven that a lack of transformation zone components (in a specimen that would otherwise be diagnosed as negative) places the patient at a subsequent higher risk for a high-grade squamous intraepithelial lesion (HSIL).

Apgar BS, Zoschnick L, Wright TC Jr. The 2001 Bethesda System terminology. American Family Physician. 2003 Nov 15;68(10):1992-8.

2. **D** NIL; negative for intraepithelial lesion or malignancy

Pap slides that have no epithelial abnormalities are listed under the category negative for intraepithelial lesion or malignancy (NIL)—replacing the previous 1991 categories of "within normal limits" and "benign cellular changes." If present, organisms may be included as a comment in the NIL category. The presence of atrophy, radiation, and inflammation may also be optionally included.

Apgar BS, Zoschnick L, Wright TC Jr. The 2001 Bethesda System terminology. American Family Physician. 2003 Nov 15;68(10):1992-8.

3. **C** "other" category to include endometrial cells in women at least 40 years of age

The 2001 Bethesda system of classification has an "other" category for reporting normal or abnormal endometrial cells in females over the age of 40. This is paramount because the presence of endometrial cells (even normal by morphology) seen from women 45 years or older may be associated with endometrial hyperplasia or even adenocarcinoma as opposed to a benign endometrium.

Apgar BS, Zoschnick L, Wright TC Jr. The 2001 Bethesda System terminology. American Family Physician. 2003 Nov 15;68(10):1992-8.

4. **B** endocervical adenocarcinoma in situ

Atypical glandular cells (AGC) "favor reactive" was eliminated due to confusing clinical implications and AGC is simply modified as either endocervical, endometrial, or unqualified using Bethesda 2001. Since the previous classification system was written, the diagnostic criteria of adenocarcinoma in situ has been well established and is now included as a descriptive diagnosis as well as the diagnosis of "AGC, favor neoplastic," indicating those cells that have clear morphologic features (overlapping cells, hyperchromasia) but lack full spectrum of diagnostic criteria for AIS (stratification of the cells, or a feathering and splattering effect with abnormal nuclear features).

Apgar BS, Zoschnick L, Wright TC Jr. The 2001 Bethesda System terminology. American Family Physician. 2003 Nov 15;68(10):1992-8.

5. **B** ancillary testing

Should HPV DNA co-testing be performed (concurrent with the Pap slide from a liquid-based specimen) this should be reported in parallel with the cytology results. In addition, if the laboratory utilizes an automated (computer-assisted) screening system, the specific type of system used and the result should be provided on the final report.

Apgar BS, Zoschnick L, Wright TC Jr. The 2001 Bethesda System terminology. American Family Physician. 2003 Nov 15;68(10):1992-8.

6. **A** true

The 2001 Bethesda system of classification has an "other" category for reporting normal or abnormal endometrial cells in females over the age of 40. This is paramount because the presence of endometrial cells (even normal by morphology) seen from women 45 years or older may be associated with endometrial hyperplasia or even adenocarcinoma as opposed to a benign endometrium.

Apgar BS, Zoschnick L, Wright TC Jr. The 2001 Bethesda System terminology. American Family Physician. 2003 Nov 15;68(10):1992-8.

7. **B** false

Pap tests are considered primarily a screening test for squamous epithelial lesions and cancer but should not be used for the detection of endometrial adenocarcinoma. A NIL Pap does not imply absence of an endometrial lesion due to the fact that the endometrium is not sampled by the clinician during the Pap test and the fact that many endometrial lesions to do not shed.

Apgar BS, Zoschnick L, Wright TC Jr. The 2001 Bethesda System terminology. American Family Physician. 2003 Nov 15;68(10):1992-8.

8. **A** true

If the laboratory utilizes an automated (computer-assisted) screening system, the specific type of system used and the result should be provided on the final report.

Apgar BS, Zoschnick L, Wright TC Jr. The 2001 Bethesda System terminology. American Family Physician. 2003 Nov 15;68(10):1992-8.

9. **C** 5,000

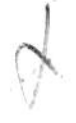

A minimum of 5,000 cells are required to render a liquid-based Pap specimen adequate for evaluation, whereas 8,000-12,000 cells are considered optimal for analyzing conventional Pap smears.

Solomon D, et al, JAMA. 2002;287(16), pp. 2114–2119.

10. **B** 10

The presence or absence of a transformational zone component should be reported in the specimen adequacy section of the cytology report, as should presence of a minimum of 10 well-preserved transformation zone cells (endocervical and/or squamous metaplastic cells) as individuals and/or groups. Mucus or parabasal cells do not count in this computation.

Solomon D, et al, JAMA. 2002;287(16), pp. 2114–2119.

11. **B** air drying that obscures evaluation of at least 75% of the epithelial cells

If air drying, or any other factor, obscure 75% or more of the epithelial cells on the surface of the slide, the case is rendered unsatisfactory.

DeMay RM, The Art & Science of Cytopathology.
Specimen adequacy, p. 148.

12. **A** ASCCP

In 2005, the American Society for Colposcopy and Cervical Pathology (ASCCP), along with its partner societies (as well as federal and international organizations) developed the new guidelines at an NIH conference in September 2006; subsequently, "The 2006 Consensus Guidelines for the Management of Women with Abnormal Cervical Cancer Screening Tests" were published.

Obstet Gynecol 2007 Oct;197(4): 346-355.

13. **B** high-risk HPV test (-) repeat cytology in 12 months

HPV cotesting with cytology eliminates the need for women to return to the office for an additional DNA test. Moreover, women with HPV negative Paps diagnosed as ASCUS are allowed to be re-evaluated by the clinician in 12 months as opposed to undergoing unnecessary colposcopy (which would otherwise affect 40-60% of women).

Wright TC Jr, Massad LS, Dunton CJ, Spitzer M, Wilkinson EJ, Solomon D; 2006 American Society for Colposcopy and Cervical Pathology-sponsored Consensus Conference. 2006 consensus guidelines for the management of women with abnormal cervical cancer screening tests. Am J Obstet Gynecol. 2007 Oct;197(4):346-55.

14. **B** high-risk HPV test(+); requires colposcopy

HPV cotesting with cytology eliminates the need for women to return to the office for an additional DNA test. Moreover, women with HPV-positive Paps diagnosed as ASCUS are forwarded to the clinician for immediate colposcopy.

Wright TC Jr, Massad LS, Dunton CJ, Spitzer M, Wilkinson EJ, Solomon D; 2006 American Society for Colposcopy and Cervical Pathology-sponsored Consensus Conference. 2006 consensus guidelines for the management of women with abnormal cervical cancer screening tests. Am J Obstet Gynecol. 2007 Oct;197(4):346-55.

15. **A** repeat cytology at 6 and 12 months or HPV test in 12 months

HPV testing performed 12 months after the initial colposcopy or two repeat cytology examinations performed at 6 month intervals are both equally effective means for following a patient with a HPV positive ASCUS Pap for which colposcopy reveals no lesion.

Wright TC Jr, Massad LS, Dunton CJ, Spitzer M, Wilkinson EJ, Solomon D; 2006 American Society for Colposcopy and Cervical Pathology-sponsored Consensus Conference. 2006 consensus guidelines for the management of women with abnormal cervical cancer screening tests. Am J Obstet Gynecol. 2007 Oct;197(4):346-55.

16. **B** repeat cytology at 6 and 12 months or HPV test in 12 months

HPV testing performed 12 months after the initial colposcopy or two repeat cytology examinations performed at 6 month intervals are both equally effective means for following a patient with a HPV positive ASCUS Pap for which colposcopy reveals LSIL due to the fact that LSIL is likely to regress and may involve non-oncogenic HPV virotypes.

Wright TC Jr, Massad LS, Dunton CJ, Spitzer M, Wilkinson EJ, Solomon D; 2006 American Society for Colposcopy and Cervical Pathology-sponsored Consensus Conference. 2006 consensus guidelines for the management of women with abnormal cervical cancer screening tests. Am J Obstet Gynecol. 2007 Oct;197(4):346-55.

17. **A** **immediate colposcopy**

Among women with LSIL, the prevalence of CIN 2,3 identified at colposcopy is 12-16%—the same as women with ASC-US and HPV positivity; ergo, managing both groups of women in similar fashion is recommended (except in postmenopausal women).

Wright TC Jr, Massad LS, Dunton CJ, Spitzer M, Wilkinson EJ, Solomon D; 2006 American Society for Colposcopy and Cervical Pathology-sponsored Consensus Conference. 2006 consensus guidelines for the management of women with abnormal cervical cancer screening tests. Am J Obstet Gynecol. 2007 Oct;197(4):346-55.

18. **A** **repeat cytology at 6 and 12 months or HPV test in 12 months**

HPV testing performed 12 months after the initial colposcopy or two repeat cytology examinations performed at 6-month intervals are both equally effective means for following a patient with a LSIL Pap for which colposcopy was negative.

Wright TC Jr, Massad LS, Dunton CJ, Spitzer M, Wilkinson EJ, Solomon D; 2006 American Society for Colposcopy and Cervical Pathology-sponsored Consensus Conference. 2006 consensus guidelines for the management of women with abnormal cervical cancer screening tests. Am J Obstet Gynecol. 2007 Oct;197(4):346-55.

19. **C** **repeat cytology at 6 and 12 months or HPV test in 12 months**

HPV testing performed 12 months after the initial colposcopy or 2 repeat cytology examinations performed at 6-month intervals are both equally effective means for following a patient with a LSIL Pap for which colposcopy was CIN I.

Wright TC Jr, Massad LS, Dunton CJ, Spitzer M, Wilkinson EJ, Solomon D; 2006 American Society for Colposcopy and Cervical Pathology-sponsored Consensus Conference. 2006 consensus guidelines for the management of women with abnormal cervical cancer screening tests. Am J Obstet Gynecol. 2007 Oct;197(4):346-55.

20. **D** **LEEP with ECC**

A loop electrosurgical excision (LEEP) or and endocervical curettage should be immediately implemented for women with colposcopically confirmed CIN 2 or 3 (except when pregnant).

Wright TC Jr, Massad LS, Dunton CJ, Spitzer M, Wilkinson EJ, Solomon D; 2006 American Society for Colposcopy and Cervical Pathology-sponsored Consensus Conference. 2006 consensus guidelines for the management of women with abnormal cervical cancer screening tests. Am J Obstet Gynecol. 2007 Oct;197(4):346-55.

21. **B** **repeat Pap in 12 months**

Follow-up with annual cytologic testing is recommended. Upon follow up, only those adolescents with a cytologic diagnosis of HSIL or greater should be referred to colposcopy.

Wright TC Jr, Massad LS, Dunton CJ, Spitzer M, Wilkinson EJ, Solomon D; 2006 American Society for Colposcopy and Cervical Pathology-sponsored Consensus Conference. 2006 consensus guidelines for the management of women with abnormal cervical cancer screening tests. Am J Obstet Gynecol. 2007 Oct;197(4):346-55.

22. **B** **repeat Pap in 12 months**

Adolescents (women under 20) with a cytologic diagnosis of LSIL have a high rate of regression; however, immunologic clearance, followed by regression, may take several years. Because of the regressive feature of LSIL in adolescents, follow-up with annual cytologic testing is only recommended. Upon annual follow up, only those adolescents with a cytologic diagnosis of HSIL or greater should be referred to colposcopy.

Wright TC Jr, Massad LS, Dunton CJ, Spitzer M, Wilkinson EJ, Solomon D; 2006 American Society for Colposcopy and Cervical Pathology-sponsored Consensus Conference. 2006 consensus guidelines for the management of women with abnormal cervical cancer screening tests. Am J Obstet Gynecol. 2007 Oct;197(4):346-55.

23. **D** **inadvertent HPV test should be ignored regardless of positivity; colposcopy is not warranted; repeat Pap in 12 months**

HPV DNA testing and colposcopy is not warranted for adolescents with ASC-US or LSIL. Inadvertent HPV testing should be ignored and not considered when managing the patient.

Wright TC Jr, Massad LS, Dunton CJ, Spitzer M, Wilkinson EJ, Solomon D; 2006 American Society for Colposcopy and Cervical Pathology-sponsored Consensus Conference. 2006 consensus guidelines for the management of women with abnormal cervical cancer screening tests. Am J Obstet Gynecol. 2007 Oct;197(4):346-55.

24. **B** **colposcopy**

Colposcopy is warranted if the patient has a cytologic diagnosis of HSIL. If confirmed by colposcopy as CIN 2 or 3, a loop electrosurgical excision (LEEP) with endocervical curettage should be immediately implemented (except when pregnant).

Wright TC Jr, Massad LS, Dunton CJ, Spitzer M, Wilkinson EJ, Solomon D; 2006 American Society for Colposcopy and Cervical Pathology-sponsored Consensus Conference. 2006 consensus guidelines for the management of women with abnormal cervical cancer screening tests. Am J Obstet Gynecol. 2007 Oct;197(4):346-55.

25. **C** **HPV testing in 12 months.**

HPV testing performed 12 months after the initial colposcopy or two repeat cytology examinations performed at 6-month intervals are both equally effective means for following a patient with a ASC-H Pap for which colposcopy was negative.

Wright TC Jr, Massad LS, Dunton CJ, Spitzer M, Wilkinson EJ, Solomon D; 2006 American Society for Colposcopy and Cervical Pathology-sponsored Consensus Conference. 2006 consensus guidelines for the management of women with abnormal cervical cancer screening tests. Am J Obstet Gynecol. 2007 Oct;197(4):346-55.

26. **B** **HPV testing in 12 months**

HPV testing performed 12 months after the initial colposcopy or two repeat cytology examinations performed at 6 month intervals are both equally effective means for following a patient with a ASC-H Pap for which colposcopy was LSIL.

Wright TC Jr, Massad LS, Dunton CJ, Spitzer M, Wilkinson EJ, Solomon D; 2006 American Society for Colposcopy and Cervical Pathology-sponsored Consensus Conference. 2006 consensus guidelines for the management of women with abnormal cervical cancer screening tests. Am J Obstet Gynecol. 2007 Oct;197(4):346-55.

27. **A** **colposcopy**

For pregnant (non-adolescent) patients with a cytologic diagnosis of LSIL, colposcopy is recommended, but an endocervical curettage (ECC) is not recommended. If the patient or the clinician chooses, postponing the follow up colposcopy until 6 weeks postpartum is considered an acceptable management paradigm for patients with this diagnosis.

Wright TC Jr, Massad LS, Dunton CJ, Spitzer M, Wilkinson EJ, Solomon D; 2006 American Society for Colposcopy and Cervical Pathology-sponsored Consensus Conference. 2006 consensus guidelines for the management of women with abnormal cervical cancer screening tests. Am J Obstet Gynecol. 2007 Oct;197(4):346-55.

28. **D** **repeat colposcopy and cytology in 6-month intervals for up to 2 years**

Should a patient have a negative colposcopy and endocervical curetting after a cytologic diagnosis of HSIL, the recommended management is for clinical observation with colposcopy and repeat cytology at 6-month intervals for up to 2 years .

Wright TC Jr, Massad LS, Dunton CJ, Spitzer M, Wilkinson EJ, Solomon D; 2006 American Society for Colposcopy and Cervical Pathology-sponsored Consensus Conference. 2006 consensus guidelines for the management of women with abnormal cervical cancer screening tests. Am J Obstet Gynecol. 2007 Oct;197(4):346-55.

29. **D** **biopsy**

A biopsy should be performed on adolescent patients with persistent HSIL after repeated negative colposcopies. If the biopsy is subsequently positive, the management should follow ASCCP guidelines as related to the severity of disease.

Wright TC Jr, Massad LS, Dunton CJ, Spitzer M, Wilkinson EJ, Solomon D; 2006 American Society for Colposcopy and Cervical Pathology-sponsored Consensus Conference. 2006 consensus guidelines for the management of women with abnormal cervical cancer screening tests. Am J Obstet Gynecol. 2007 Oct;197(4):346-55.

30. **B** **colposcopy with ECC, HPV testing**

HPV testing and/or a repeat Pap test have poor sensitivity in the initial triage for AGC; therefore, multiple clinical modalities are recommended, including colposcopy, endocervical curetting, HPV testing, and endometrial evaluation (if the patient is over the age of 35).

Wright TC Jr, Massad LS, Dunton CJ, Spitzer M, Wilkinson EJ, Solomon D; 2006 American Society for Colposcopy and Cervical Pathology-sponsored Consensus Conference. 2006 consensus guidelines for the management of women with abnormal cervical cancer screening tests. Am J Obstet Gynecol. 2007 Oct;197(4):346-55.

31. **B** **endometrial and endocervical sampling**

Both of these clinical modalities are recommended for patients with cytologic diagnoses of AGC specifying endometrial morphology. Colposcopy may be concominently performed or deferred until determination of its relevance is established after the histologic results have been analyzed from the endometrial and endocervical sampling.

Wright TC Jr, Massad LS, Dunton CJ, Spitzer M, Wilkinson EJ, Solomon D; 2006 American Society for Colposcopy and Cervical Pathology-sponsored Consensus Conference. 2006 consensus guidelines for the management of women with abnormal cervical cancer screening tests. Am J Obstet Gynecol. 2007 Oct;197(4):346-55.

32. **C** **colposcopy with ECC, HPV testing, endometrial sampling.**

HPV testing and/or a repeat Pap test have poor sensitivity in the initial triage for AGC; therefore, multiple clinical modalities are recommended, including colposcopy, endocervical curetting, HPV testing, and in this case of a 37-year-old female, endometrial evaluation (included in the work up for patients over the age of 35).

Wright TC Jr, Massad LS, Dunton CJ, Spitzer M, Wilkinson EJ, Solomon D; 2006 American Society for Colposcopy and Cervical Pathology-sponsored Consensus Conference. 2006 consensus guidelines for the management of women with abnormal cervical cancer screening tests. Am J Obstet Gynecol. 2007 Oct;197(4):346-55.

33. **D** diagnostic excisional procedure

Confirmation that there is no invasive disease is followed by an immediate excisional procedure for these adenocarcinomas in situ glandular lesions, based on cytology alone.

Wright TC Jr, Massad LS, Dunton CJ, Spitzer M, Wilkinson EJ, Solomon D; 2006 American Society for Colposcopy and Cervical Pathology-sponsored Consensus Conference. 2006 consensus guidelines for the management of women with abnormal cervical cancer screening tests. Am J Obstet Gynecol. 2007 Oct;197(4):346-55

34. **D** repeat HPV and Pap test at 12 months

Conservative follow-up with repeat cytology and HPV testing at 12 months is the best management paradigm due to the fact that these may be subclinical lesions that are not clinically detectable. Should repeat testing be persistently as HPV-positive and cytology negative, colposcopy is warranted.

Wright TC Jr, Massad LS, Dunton CJ, Spitzer M, Wilkinson EJ, Solomon D; 2006 American Society for Colposcopy and Cervical Pathology-sponsored Consensus Conference. 2006 consensus guidelines for the management of women with abnormal cervical cancer screening tests. Am J Obstet Gynecol. 2007 Oct;197(4):346-55

35. **A** repeat cytology at 12 months

Considering the HPV test is now negative, the patient should be managed per ASCCP protocol. In that case, management recommendations would be to repeat cytology in 12 months with or without an HPV test.

Wright TC Jr, Massad LS, Dunton CJ, Spitzer M, Wilkinson EJ, Solomon D; 2006 American Society for Colposcopy and Cervical Pathology-sponsored Consensus Conference. 2006 consensus guidelines for the management of women with abnormal cervical cancer screening tests. Am J Obstet Gynecol. 2007 Oct;197(4):346-55

Selected Bibliography

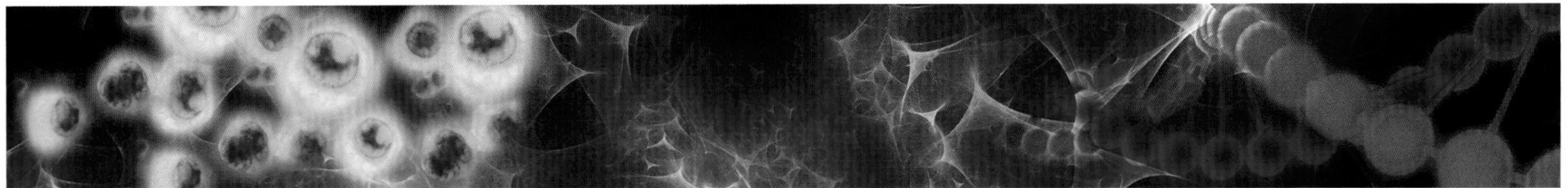

al-Saleh W, Delvenne P, Greimers R, et al. Assessment of Ki-67 antigen immunostaining in squamous intraepithelial lesions of the uterine cervix. Correlation with the histologic grade and human papillomavirus type. *Am J Clin Pathol.* 1995;104:154–160.

American Cancer Society Facts and Figures; 2002: http://cancer.org.

Aponte-Cipriani SL, Teplitz C, Rorat E, et al. Cervical smears prepared by an automated device versus the conventional method of comparative analysis. *Acta Cytologica.* 1995;39:623–630.

Ashfaq R, Birdsong G, Salinger F, et al. Diagnostic comparison of ThinPrep slides in Papanicolaou smears with and without infections. *Acta Cytol.* 1996;40:1047.

Ashfaq R, Gibbons D, Vela C, et al. ThinPrep Pap Test accuracy for glandular disease. *Acta Cytol.* 1999;43:81–85.

Atkinson BF. *Atlas of Diagnostic Cytopathology.* Philadelphia: Saunders; 1992.

Ayre JE. *Cancer Cytology of the Uterus.* New York: Grune & Stratton; 1951.

Bancroft JD, Stevens A, eds. *Theory and Practice of Histological Techniques,* 3rd ed. New York: Churchill Livingstone; 1990.

Bibbo M, ed. *Comprehensive Cytopathology.* Philadelphia: Saunders; 1991.

Bigner SH, Johnson WW. *Cytopathology of the Central Nervous System.* Chicago: ASCP Press; 1994.

Buckingham L and Flaws M. *Molecular diagnostics: fundamentals, methods & clinical applications.* FA Davis; 2007.

Clinical Laboratory Improvement Amendments of 1988. *Federal Register.* 1990;55:9538–9610.

Clinical Laboratory Improvement Amendments of 1988. *Federal Register.* 1992;57:7218–7243.

Corkill M, Knapp D, Martin J, et al. Specimen adequacy of ThinPrep sample preparations in a direct-to-vial study. *Acta Cytol.* 1997;41:39–44.

Daniely M, Rona R, Kaplan T, et al. Combined morphologic and fluorescence in situ hybridization analysis of voided urine samples for the detection and follow-up of bladder cancer inpatients with benigh urine cytology. *Urol Oncol.* 2008;26(3):332.

Davey DD, Zaleski S, Sattich M, et al. Prognostic significance of DNA cytometry of postirradiation cervi-covaginal smears. *Cancer.* 1998;84:11–16.

Dehn D, Torko KC, Shroyer KR. Human papillomavirus testing and molecular markers of cervical dysplasia and carcinoma. *Cancer.* 2007; 111(1):1-14.

DeMay RM. *The Art & Science of Cytopathology.* Chicago: ASCP Press; 1996.

DeMay RM. *Practical Principles of Cytopathology Revised edition.* Chicago: ASCP Press; 2007.

DeMay RM. *The Pap Test.* Chicago, IL: ASCP Press; 2005.

Department of Labor, Occupational Safety and Health Administration. Occupational exposure to blood-borne pathogens: final rule (29 CFR 1910.1030). *Federal Register.* 1991;56:64004–64182.

Douglass K. *ThinPrep Pap Test: Morphology Reference Manual.* Boxborough, MA: Cytyc; 1996.

Evans SK, Wilbur DC. Identification of endocervical cells and microorganisms on cervical thin-layer cytology specimens: Comparison to paired conventional smears. *Acta Cytol.* 1993;37:776.

Feldman P, Covell J, Karkos T. *Fine Needle Aspiration Cytology: Lymph Node, Thyroid, and Salivary Gland.* Chicago: ASCP Press; 1989.

Feldman PS, Covell JL. *Fine Needle Aspiration Cytology and Its Clinical Applications: Breast and Lung.* Chicago: ASCP Press; 1985.

Ferenczy A. Viral testing for genital human papillomavirus infections: recent progress and clinical potentials. *Int J Gynecol Cancer.* 1995;5:321–328.

Frable W J, Bennington JL, eds. *Thin-Needle Aspiration Biopsy.* Philadelphia: Saunders; 1983.

Frost JK. *The Cell in Health and Disease.* Monographs in Clinical Cytology. Basel, Switzerland: S. Karger; 1969.

Geisinger K, Silverman J, Wakely P. *Pediatric Cytopathology.* Chicago: ASCP Press, 1995.

Gill GW, Miller KA. *Laboratory Techniques for Specimen Preparation,* 5th ed. Baltimore: The Johns Hopkins School of Medicine; 1973.

Gitman LJ. *Principles of Managerial Finance,* 5th ed. New York, NY: Harper & Row; 1988.

Goodman A, Hutchinson ML. Cell surplus on sampling devices after routine cervical cytologic smears. *J Reprod Med.* 1996;41:239–241.

Guo M, Patel SJ, Chovanec M, et al. A human papillomavirus testing system in women with abnormal Pap resuls. A comparison study with follow-up biopsies. *Acta Cytol.* 2007; 51(5):749-754.

Holladay EB, Logan S, Arnold J, et al. A comparison of the clinical utility of p16^{ink4a} immunolocalization to the presence of HPV by Digene Hybrid Capture 2 for the detection of cervical dysplasia/ neoplasia. *Cancer Cytopathol.* 2006: 108(6).

Johnson WW. Histologic and cytologic patterns of lung cancer in 2580 men and women over a 15-year period. *Acta Cytol.* 1998;32:163–168.

Keebler CM, Somrak TM. *The Manual of Cytotechnology,* 7th ed. Chicago, IL: ASCP Press; 1993. Kline RS. Handbook of Fine Needle Aspiration Biopsy Cytology, 2nd ed. New York: Igaku-Shoin; 1992.

Kline TS, Kline IK. Guides to Clinical Aspiration Biopsy: Breast. New York: Igaku-Shoin; 1989.

Koss LG. *Diagnostic Cytology,* 4th ed. Philadelphia: J. B. Lippincott; 1992.

Koss LG. *The Papanicolaou test for cervical cancer detection: A triumph and a tragedy. JAMA* 1989;261:737–743.

Koss LG, Woyke W, Olszewski W. *Aspiration Biopsy: Cytologic Interpretation and Its Histologic Basis,* 2nd ed. New York: Igaku-Shoin; 1992.

Kurman RJ, ed. *Blaustein's Pathology of the Female Genital Tract,* 3rd ed. New York: Springer-Verlag; 1987.

Laboratory Accreditation Committee. *Criteria for Cytopathology Laboratory Accreditation.* Philadelphia: American Society of Cytopathology; 1988.

Layfield L, Glasgow B, Cramer H. *Cytopathology of the Head and Neck.* Chicago: ASCP Press; 1997.

Lee KR, Ashfaq R, Birdsong GG, et al. Comparison of conventional Papanicolaou smears and a fluid-based, thin-layer system for cervical cancer screening. *Obstet Gynecol.* 1997;90:278–284.

Lee KR, Manna EA, St John T. Atypical endocervical glandular cells: Accuracy of cytologic diagnosis. *Diagn Cytopathol.* 1995;13:202–208.

Liang XM, Wieczorek RL, Koss LG. In situ hybridization with human papillomavirus using biotinylated DNA probes on archival cervical smears. *J Histochem Cytochem.* 1991;39:771–775.

Linder J, Zahniser D. ThinPrep Papanicolaou testing to reduce false-negative cervical cytology. *Arch Pathol Lab Med.* 1998;122:139–144.

Linsk JA, Franzen S. *Clinical Aspiration Cytology,* 2nd ed. Philadelphia: J. B. Lippincott; 1989.

Manos MM, Kinney WK, Hurley LB, et al. Identifying women with cervical neoplasia: using human papillomavirus DNA testing for equivocal Papanicolaou results. *JAMA.* 1999;281:1605–1610.

Masood S. *Cytopathology of the Breast.* Chicago: ASCP Press; 1996.

Meisels A, Morin C. *Cytopathology of the Uterus.* Chicago: ASCP Press; 1997.

Murphy W. *Urological pathology.* Philadelphia: Saunders; 1989.

Naib ZM. *Exfoliative Cytopathology,* 3rd ed. Boston: Little, Brown; 1985.

O'Shaughnessy JA, Ljung BM, Dooley WC, et al. Ductal lavage and the clinical management of women at high risk for breast carcinoma: a commentary. *Cancer.* 2002;94:292–298.

Oertel YC. *Fine Needle Aspiration of the Breast.* Stoneham, MA: Butterworth; 1987.

Orell SR, Sterrett GF, Walters MN-I, et al. *Manual and Atlas of Fine Needle Aspiration Cytology,* 2nd ed. New York, NY: Churchill Livingstone; 1992.

Papanicolaou GN, Traut HF. *Diagnosis of Uterine Cervix by the Vaginal Smear.* Cambridge: Harvard University; 1943.

Papanicolaou GN. *Atlas of Exfoliative Cytology.* Cambridge: Harvard University; 1954.

Patten SF Jr. *Diagnostic Cytopathology of the Uterine Cervix,* 2nd ed. Monographs in Clinical Cytology. Basel: S Karger; 1978.

Qui W, Carson-Walter E, Liu H. PUMA regulates intestinal progenitor cell radiosensitivity and gastrointestinal syndrome. *Cell Stem Cell.* 2;576-583.

Raab SS, Snider TE, Potts SA, et al. Atypical glandular cells of undetermined significance: Diagnostic accuracy and interobserver variability using select cytologic criteria. *Am J Clin Pathol.* 107:299–307, 1997.

Reagan JW, Ng ABP. *The Cells of Uterine Adenocarcinoma,* 2nd ed. In: Weid GL, ed. Monographs in Clinical Cytology. Basel, Switzerland: S. Karger; 1973.

Roberts JM, Thurloe JK, Bowditch RC, et al. Comparison of ThinPrep and Pap smear in relation to prediction of adenocarcinoma in situ. *Acta Cytol.* 1999;43:74–90.

Rosenthal DL. *Cytopathology: Pulmonary Disease.* In: Weid GL, ed. Monographs in Clinical Cytology. Basel, Switzerland: S. Karger; 1988.

Schmitt FC, Longa Ho-Filho A, Valent A, et al. Molecular techniques in cytopathology practice. *J Clin Pathol.* 2008; 61(3):258-267.

Silverman JF, ed. *Guides to Clinical Aspiration Biopsy: Infectious and Inflammatory Diseases and Other Nonneoplastic Disorders.* New York: Igaku-Shoin; 1991.

Siñczak-Kuta A, Tomaszewska R, Rudnicka-Sosin L, et al. Evaluation of HER2/neu gene amplification in patients with invasive breast carcinoma; Comparison of in situ hybridization methods. Polish Journal of Pathology. 2007;58(1): 41-50.

Snyder JR, Wilkinson DS, eds. *Management in Laboratory Medicine.* Philadelphia: Lippincott-Raven; 1998.

Solomon D, Davey D, Kurman R, et al. The 2001 Bethesda System: terminology for reporting results of cervical cytology. *JAMA.* 2002;287:2114–2119.

Spriggs AI, Boddington MM. *Atlas of Serous Fluid Cytopathology: A Guide to the Cells of Pleural, Pericardial, Peritoneal and Hydrocele Fluids.* In: Gresham GA, ed. *Current Histopathology Series,* vol 14. Dordrecht, the Netherlands: Kluwer; 1989.

Spasenija S, Glatz K, Schoenegg R, et al. Multitarget fluorescence in situ hybridization elucidates equivocal lung cytology. Chest. 2006; 129; 1629-1635.

Takeda M. *Atlas of Diagnostic Gastrointestinal Cytology.* New York: Igaku-Shoin; 1983.

Tao L. *Cytopathology of the Endometrium.* Chicago: ASCP Press; 1993.

Tao L. *Cytopathology of Malignant Effusions.* Chicago: ASCP Press; 1996.

Triol JH, ed. *ASCT Cytopathology Quality Assurance Guide I.* Raleigh, NC: American Society for Cytotechnology; 1992, 1994.

Walensky G. Medicare, Medicaid and CLIA programs: regulations implementing the Clinical Laboratory Improvement Amendments of 1988 (CLIA '88). *Federal Register.* 57:7002–7243, February 28, 1992.

Wilbur DC, Dubeshter B, Angel C, et al. Use of thin-layer preparations for gynecologic smears with emphasis on the cytomorpholoty of high-grade intraepithelial lesions and carcinomas. *Diagn Cytopathol.* 14:201–211.

Wied GL, Keebler CM, Koss LG, et al., eds. *Compendium on Diagnostic Cytology,* 6th ed. Chicago: Tutorials of Cytology; 1990.

Wong AK, Chan RC, Nicholas WS, et al. Human papillomavirus (HPV) in atypical squamous cervical cytology: the Invader HPV test as a new screening assay. J Clin Microbiol. 2008; 46(3):869-875

Wright TC, Kurman RJ, Ferenczy A, eds. *Blaustein's Pathology of the Female Genital Tract,* 4th ed. New York: Springer-Verlag; 1994.

Wright TC Jr, Massad LS, Dunton CJ, et al. 2006 American society for colposcopy and cervical pathology-sponsored consensus conference. 2006 consensus guidelines for the managament of women with abnormal cervical cancer screening tests. *Am J Obstet Gynecol.* 2007 Oct; 197(4):346-355.

Index

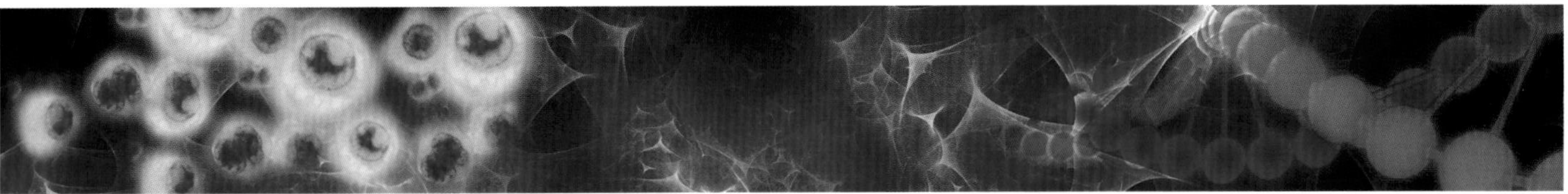

A

B

C

D

E

F

G

H

I

J

K

L

M

N

O

P

R

S